Brain Damage in the Newborn and its Neurologic Sequels

Pathologic and Clinical Correlation

Abraham Towbin, M.D.

Medical Director
Mental Retardation Research Institute
Danvers, Massachusetts

PRM Publishing Company, Inc., Danvers, Massachusetts

Library of Congress Catalog Card Number: 98-66285

ISBN# 0-9660551-0-1

Published by PRM Publishing Company, Inc., 130 Centre Street, Danvers, MA 01923.

Printed in the United States of America by World Color Book Services, Inc.

Dedicated to my associate
GERTRUDE L. TURNER
for her help, her commitment to this work through the years

Acknowledgments

The author wishes to express his appreciation—

To Susan Hayes Enterprises, to Susan M. Hayes, for consultation in planning the publication of this book.

To Julie Hagen, copyeditor, for reviewing the manuscript of this book.

To Primary Design, Inc., to Jules Epstein, for the design and composition of the book.

To Eastern Rainbow, Inc., to Rick Cordeau, Color Manager, for his efforts in the preparation of the illustrations.

To World Color Book Services, Inc., for its assistance in printing this book.

Foreword by

HARRY M. ZIMMERMAN, M.D.
Emeritus Professor of Pathology, Albert Einstein College of Medicine,
  New York, New York
Emeritus Director of Laboratories, Montefiore Hospital and Medical Center,
  Bronx, New York
Past President of the American Association of Neuropathologists

LAWRENCE T. TAFT, M.D.
Professor of Pediatrics, UMDNJ, New Jersey's University of Health Sciences,
  and Robert Wood Johnson Medical School, New Brunswick, New Jersey

PHILIP P. McGOVERN, Jr., M.D.
Clinical Professor of Obstetrics and Gynecology,
  Tufts New England Medical Center, Boston, Massachusetts

NORMAN FRANKEL, Ph. D.
Psychologist,
  Lake Forest, Illinois

Foreword

The author of this book, Abraham Towbin, has devoted more than 40 years to the study of this subject. Publication of the work, much of it innovative, presents the last word on the pathogenesis of the anatomic lesions in the fetus and newborn that account for the clinical syndromes of cerebral palsy, mental retardation, some epileptiform attacks, and certain obscure cerebral dysfunctions.

The greatest strength of this publication lies in the meticulous and extensive detailing of the anatomic lesions in over 200 cases. There is no greater student of this field than Dr. Towbin. For many years he has dominated the area of neonatal neuropathology. His many original publications through the years have emphasized the pathogenesis of cerebral lesions in the neonate. Now we have a compendium of his many original contributions. But this author has not written for the neuropathologist alone. He has in mind the neurologist, the neonatologist, the pediatrician, and even the obstetrician. There are also many suggestions for the practicing clinician faced with litigation.

An unusual feature of this work is the arrangement of the subject matter in the two parts. In the first, the predominating emphasis is on the anatomic changes and their pathogenesis, with frequent reference to the clinical features illustrated by the Case Studies in the second part of the book. In the latter, the histories of the 238 cases are explained with references to the pertinent considerations of pathogenetic factors described in detail in the text. The casual reader is apt to feel a certain repetitiousness if he attempts to read this work as an ordinary text. The clear intent is for it to serve as a book of reference, with the reader referring to specific subjects in the text and in the case studies. As a book of reference, this volume will be found invaluable.

HARRY M. ZIMMERMAN, M.D.

Dr. Zimmerman reviewed the manuscript of this book before his death.
For this forward and for his interest in this work, the author is grateful.

This book is a monumental accomplishment by an ageless neuropathologist whose career has been devoted to assessing the development of the fetal, natal, and early postnatal brain and how genetic factors, intrauterine environment, the birth process, and neonatal experiences affect brain structure. This book offers a wealth of information to geneticists, neuropathologists, developmental pediatricians, neurologists, perinatologists, and developmental neuroscientists.

LAWRENCE T. TAFT, M.D.

In the history of obstetrics we physicians primarily focused our attention on the mother. In the last quarter of a century the studies of Dr. Abraham Towbin brought to the attention of clinicians the importance of the processes of pregnancy as they affect the fetus. This book, encompassing the teaching and the pathology research of Dr. Towbin, has important application in the management of pregnancy.

This book should be read by all obstetricians.

PHILIP P. McGOVERN, Jr., M.D.

The new concepts in the fields of pathology and especially neonatal neuropathology could not have developed during the past 40 years without the intellectual devotion and the excited and driven detail provided in the works of Dr. Abraham Towbin. This reference book and outstanding case study approach by Dr. Towbin provides the reader with the opportunity to view neuropathology as a true plot in a continuous story line that leads to rational answers as to the cause of fetal-neonatal brain damage and its sequels.

For years Dr. Towbin created novel methods and experimental designs and traveled into unknown territory seeking reasons for neurological disabilities, for mental retardation, cerebral palsy, epilepsy, and other cerebral disorders.

The developing theme — the sequence of hypoxia in the immature premature fetus causing fetal cardiac failure leading to venous infarction, especially in the germinal matrix tissue — accurately establishes the chronology of the pathogenesis of fetal-neonatal hypoxic cerebral damage and sequelant neurologic disabilities.

The unique textual and photographic examples create the true "reference library" in neonatal neuropathology. The reader feels that an important message has been dedicated to the history and future knowledge of neonatal problems and their sequels.

NORMAN FRANKEL, Ph.D.

Preface

Clinicians—obstetricians, neonatologists, pediatricians, and neurologists — increasingly recognize the need for more information about the pathology of fetal-neonatal brain damage, damage that leads to cerebral palsy and other developmental disabilities. In medicine, it is a given that in order to prevent a disease, in order to effectively treat a disease, there must be a good understanding of the cause, the pathogenesis. In practice, clinicians often are called upon to provide an interpretation of the cause, the pathogenesis, of brain damage present in an infant, as required in documenting the patient's chart, in teaching, or in giving court testimony. Interpretations given are based on concepts acquired in training or obtained in the clinical literature — concepts that often are not current, not comprehensive.

Obstetricians, traditionally preoccupied with the well-being of the mother, in current times have increasingly faced the need to know more about what goes on with the fetus, the fetal brain, when the mother is sick. In the past obstetricians readily conceded that pathology of the brain was not their province. Today the obstetrician, in practice, in litigation — held directly responsible for what happens to the fetus, to the fetal brain — needs to be knowledgeable about fetal-neonatal brain damage.

Pediatricians and neonatologists, in the management of neurologically depressed newborn infants, are concerned about the cause of fetal-neonatal brain damage. It is increasingly evident pathologically that neurologic manifestations in the newborn, in the past generally assumed to be due to acute brain damage incurred during labor and delivery, are at times due to the effects on the fetus of antecedent pregnancy complications, intrauterine pathologic processes ongoing long before birth, with the fetus surviving and born with accumulated old brain damage.

Neurologists, particularly pediatric neurologists, are often called as consultants when newborn infants present with neurologic depression, with seizures, and they later undertake the follow-up management of brain-damaged infants that develop cerebral palsy or other cerebral disability. Although obstetrics is at the other end of the spectrum of medical specialties, it is requisite that the neurologist in such cases, seeking to understand causation, be well informed about the sequence of pathologic processes that affect the maternal-placental-fetal complex, processes that cause fetal-neonatal brain damage.

The pathology of fetal-neonatal brain damage, long the subject of speculation and misinformation, gradually became elucidated in recent decades, mainly through pathology research in the 1960s and 1970s. However, this information, lodged mainly in the pathology literature, has not become common knowledge in the medical world. Publications dealing with newborn brain damage available to doctors in recent times still present anachronistic pathology information, concepts of a time past. The National Institutes of Health (NIH) book *Prenatal and Perinatal Factors Associated with Brain Disorders,* published in 1985, while commonly cited and presenting valuable clinical perspectives, fails to incorporate comprehensive pathology research information that has become available in recent decades.

The interpretation of pathogenesis is primarily the province of the pathologist —to present valid information concerned with intrinsic organic causal mechanisms, the interpretation of visceral disease that takes place within the body. Through his experience in correlating clinical information with autopsy studies, the pathologist is able to provide basic information about causal factors that initiate structural damage in the body, and to define the subsequent organ changes. Clinicians do not have the opportunity to gain this experience, this knowledge.

The discipline of pathology, the practice of interrelating clinical information with visceral changes observed at autopsy, provides the capability of interpreting disease in the living. The pathologist uses this discipline to define the pathogenesis of brain damage in newborn infants and in the interpretation of causal processes in cases of cerebral palsy and related chronic cerebral disabilities.

The sphere of pathology dealt with here is multifaceted. In interpreting the pathogenesis of newborn brain damage, of cerebral palsy, there must be a comprehensive knowledge of (1) **obstetric pathology** — disease processes in the mother that adversely affect the fetus, placental and umbilical cord disorders, meconium contamination of the amniotic fluid, and other intrauterine complications that may compromise the fetus; (2) **the general visceral pathology of the fetus and newborn,** especially with regard to circulatory disturbances and neonatal pulmonary disease; (3) **pathology of the brain, fetus and newborn;** and (4) **the neuropathology of cerebral palsy and other related chronic cerebral disabilities.**

Plainly, assessment of the pathogenesis of fetal-neonatal brain damage requires more than a study of brain specimens, more than CT scan studies. Neuroradiologists and neuropathologists, focusing their attention on changes in the brain, have in recent times written extensively about patterns of damage in the newborn infant; however, most have not been able to deal comprehensively with causative mechanisms, with pathogenesis, because they do not have the background, the grasp of pathologic obstetrical processes and fetal-neonatal processes that antecede the development of the brain damage. Many current texts dealing with newborn brain damage and cerebral palsy convey anachronisms, the interpretations of a time past that fail to reflect current information available in research studies in the pathology literature. Much of the present literature portraying the pathology of fetal-neonatal brain damage continues to be written, not by pathologists, but by pediatricians and neurologists, by authors who lack direct personal experience in pathology, by doctors who have not themselves researched cases correlating the clinical data with their examination of the placenta and their autopsy findings in the cases.

Doctors dealing with cases of newborn brain damage and cerebral palsy, concerned with causation, with pathogenesis, have not had available a comprehensive sourcebook based on established valid pathology principles — bringing together the interrelated facets, the spectrum of obstetrical pathology, placental pathology, fetal-neonatal systemic pathology and brain pathology — central to these cases. It is the purpose of this volume to make available, to interrelate, these basic components of pathogenesis.

Experience in the field

My research work in the field of cerebral palsy pathology began in 1952 in the Department of Pathology at Ohio State University. There, as pathologist at Columbus State School, a large custodial institution where autopsies had never been done previously, I had the opportunity to investigate a large series of cases of cerebral palsy, to study the clinical data, and to analyze the brain specimens. There was little in the American literature about the pathology of cerebral palsy. After publishing my studies of these cases (*Archives of Pathology,* 1955) (see bibliography, page xii), I was invited, as a Fulbright Research Scholar, in 1957, to study this kind of case material at the Neuropathology Institute (Max-Planck) in Munich. Combining my experience at Ohio State University with that at the Max-Planck, I published the monographic study, *The Pathology of Cerebral Palsy* (1960) (see bibliography, page xii), reflecting the state of knowledge at the time, but I realized that the level of knowledge at that time permitted mainly only a presentation of the end pattern of the damage in the cerebrum in cerebral palsy, and offered little information about pathogenesis.

Clearly, a resolution of the question of pathogenesis lay in studying the origin of the pathologic process, studying the fresh acute processes of damage in the fetus and newborn. I undertook this pursuit in 1958, as a hospital pathologist at LaGrange Memorial General Hospital, in LaGrange, Illinois, a hospital with a large obstetrical census (it was the "baby-boom" era). My progress was limited because of technical problems, difficulties in making detailed pathologic studies of the very soft gelatinous texture of the fetal and newborn brain.

In 1962 I was invited by Dr. Paul Yakovlev to participate as pathologist in research in the NIH Collaborative Perinatal Project, in the Neuropathology Department at Harvard Medical School. Applying Yakovlev's technique, embedding the entire brain specimen in plastic and preparing whole-brain sections for microscopic study, I was able to define the basic pathologic nature of hypoxic cerebral damage in the fetus and newborn, correlating antecedent gestational causal complications with sequelant cerebral damage.

Clinical experience. For a period of 3 years beginning in 1977, as a staff physician at Fernald State School, Waltham, Massachusetts, I had the opportunity to gain clinical knowledge to complement my years of pathology studies. Under the seasoned guidance in pediatric neurology and psychiatry of Dr. Benjamin Matzilevich and Dr. David T. Gavin, I had firsthand experience caring for people with cerebral palsy, epilepsy and other neurologic disabilities.

Subsequently, returning to the laboratory, working with my associate, Gertrude L. Turner, I pursued further the link between gestational complications and sequelant brain damage in the newborn. This research program was conducted in suburban Boston hospital pathology departments. In later neuropathology research, the relationship between fetal-neonatal brain damage and cerebral palsy was investigated in transitional studies linking patterns of cerebral damage in the newborn with damage in infants who survived for short periods, with patterns of damage in cases of long survival, cases of cerebral palsy. These studies continue in the pathology laboratory at the Mental Retardation Research Institute in Danvers, Massachusetts.

Bibliography

Towbin A. (1955). The pathology of cerebral palsy: I. Developmental defects of the brain as a cause of cerebral palsy. *Arch Path* 59: 397–411.

Towbin A. (1955). Cerebral palsy due to encephaloclastic processes. *Arch Path* 59: 529–552.

Towbin A. (1960). *The Pathology of Cerebral Palsy*. Springfield, Illinois: Charles C Thomas.

Towbin A. (1964). Spinal cord and brain stem injury at birth. *Arch Path* 77: 620–632.

Towbin A. (1966). Massive cerebral hypoxic damage in the fetus near term. *Proc Fifth Internat Congr Neuropathology*. Pp. 724–729.

Manterola A., Towbin A., and Yakovlev P. (1966). Cerebral infarction in the human fetus near term. *J Neuropath & Exper Neurol* 25: 479–488.

Towbin A. (1968). Cerebral intraventricular hemorrhage and subependymal matrix infarction in the fetus and premature newborn. *Am J Pathol* 52: 121–140.

Towbin A. (1969). Latent spinal cord and brain stem injury in newborn infants. *Dev Med Child Neurol* 11: 54–68.

Towbin A. (1969). Mental retardation due to germinal matrix infarction. *Science* 164: 156–161.

Towbin A. (1969). Cerebral hypoxic damage in the fetus and newborn. *Arch Neurol* 20: 35–43.

Towbin A. (1969). Cerebral hypoxic damage in the fetus and newborn. *Obstet & Gynec Survey* 24: 628–632.

Towbin A. (1969). Nervous system damage related to hyaline membrane disease. *Lancet* i: 890.

Towbin A. (1970). Neonatal neuropathologic examination. Chapter 5 in: Tedeschi C. G, ed., *Neuropathology: Methods and Diagnosis*. Boston: Little, Brown & Co. Pp. 215–224.

Towbin A. (1970). Neonatal damage to the central nervous system. Chapter 23 in: Tedeschi C. G., ed., *Neuropathology: Methods and Diagnosis*. Boston: Little, Brown & Co. Pp. 609–653.

Towbin A. (1970). Central nervous system damage in the human fetus and newborn. *Am J Dis Child* 119: 529–542.

Towbin A. (1970). Central nervous system damage in the premature related to the occurrence of mental retardation. In: Angle C. R., Bering E. A., eds., *Physical Trauma as an Etiological Agent in Mental Retardation*. Proceedings of a Conference on the Etiology of Mental Retardation. Bethesda, MD.: National Institute of Neurological Diseases and Stroke. Pp. 213–239.

Towbin A. (1971). Cerebral palsy. Chapter 138 in: Minckler J., ed., *Pathology of the Nervous System.* New York: McGraw-Hill. Pp. 1832–1850.

Towbin A. (1971). Organic causes of minimal brain dysfunction. *JAMA* 217: 1207–1214.

Towbin A. (1972). Organic causes of minimal brain dysfunctions: Perinatal origin of minimal cerebral lesions. *Obstet & Gynec Survey* 27: 362–367.

Towbin A. (1972). Mental retardation. Chapter 186 in: Minckler J., ed., *Pathology of the Nervous System.* New York: McGraw-Hill. Pp. 2612–2626.

Towbin A., and Turner G. L. (1972). Norwood Project: Placental studies (unpublished manuscript).

Towbin A. (1977). Trauma in pregnancy: Injury to the fetus and newborn. Chapter 7 in: Tedeschi C. G., ed., *Forensic Medicine.* Philadelphia: W. B. Saunders. Pp. 436–486.

Towbin A., and Turner G. L. (1978). Obstetric factors in fetal-neonatal visceral injury. *Obstet Gynecol* 52: 113–124.

Towbin A. (1978). Cerebral dysfunctions related to perinatal organic damage: Clinical-neuropathologic correlations. *J Abnorm Psychol* 87: 617–635.

Towbin A. (1980). Neuropathologic factors in minimal brain dysfunctions. Chapter 8 in: Rie H. E., Rie E. D., eds., *Handbook of Minimal Brain Dysfunctions.* New York: John Wiley & Sons. Pp. 185–209.

Towbin A. (1981). Perinatal brain damage and its sequels. Chapter 4 in: Black P., ed., *Brain Dysfunctions in Children.* New York: Raven Press. Pp. 47–77.

Towbin A. (1981). The brain damaged newborn. *MRRI Journal* 1: 2–3.

Towbin A. (1982). The minimal brain dysfunctions. *MRRI Journal* 2: 2–3.

Towbin A. (1982). Brain damage and mental retardation. *MRRI Journal* 2: 6–7.

Towbin A. (1984). Epilepsy — What causes it? *MRRI Journal* 4: 2–3.

Towbin A. (1986). Obstetric malpractice litigation: The pathologist's view. *Am J Obstet Gynecol* 155: 927–935.

Towbin A. (1987). The depressed newborn; pathogenesis and neurologic sequels. *Perinatology Neonatology* 11: 16–18.

Towbin A. (1987). Neuropathologic correlates. Chapter 7 in: Tupper D. E., ed., *Soft Neurological Signs.* New York: Grune & Stratton. Pp. 157–178.

Towbin A. Pathogenesis of fetal-neonatal hypoxic visceral damage. Presentation at the American Society of Clinical Pathology/College of American Pathologists, Scientific Assembly, San Francisco: March 31, 1987.

Towbin A. (1989). Behavior disorders of mentally retarded persons, the dually diagnosed: Factors of pathogenesis. *J Clin Psychol* 45: 910–918.

Format of the book

This book comprises an expository text and case studies.

The **text** deals with brain damage in the fetus and newborn, its underlying causes, and the pathologic processes that ensue in infants surviving. Concerned here are a broad range of clinical and pathologic disciplines: (1) Obstetrical factors — taken into account are complications of pregnancy that adversely affect the fetus; placental and umbilical cord disorders and other intrauterine pathologic processes that compromise the fetus. (2) Pathology of the fetus and newborn — the effects of gestational complications in producing pathologic visceral changes in the fetus and newborn. (3) Fetal-neonatal neuropathology — pathologic changes in the brain incurred during gestation and birth. (4) Neuropathology of cerebral palsy and other disabilities sequelant to fetal-neonatal brain damage.

The first chapter of the book deals with the pathogenesis of cerebral damage in the fetus and newborn. The second chapter is a clinical-pathologic correlation of the neurologic status of the depressed newborn. The last chapters are a consideration of the sequels of fetal-neonatal brain damage, the pathogenesis of cerebral palsy and related cerebral disabilities.

The text presentation is followed by case studies amplifying factors of pathogenesis newborn brain damage and sequelant cerebral disabilities. The use of case studies is a time-honored method of teaching.

The **case studies** presented here — 238 relevant case examples — are of two types: pathology studies and clinical case studies.

The pathology studies, cases of newborn infants with brain damage, illustrate basic processes of pathogenesis linking gestational complications with consequent newborn brain damage. Most of the cases deal with hypoxia-producing pathologic processes that lead to fetal-neonatal brain damage. Also presented are cases of brain damage due to infectious disease and physical injury and abnormalities due to malformation.

The clinical case studies presented here deal with pathogenesis of cerebral palsy and related organic neurologic disabilities. These cases illustrate the adverse effects of gestational complications on the fetus and newborn that lead to brain damage, and ultimately to cerebral palsy, mental retardation, and other cerebral disabilities. The clinical cases for the most part were collected in the course of years, in participating as a consultant in the litigation of cases of newborn brain damage and related cerebral disabilities.

The text material is closely geared to the case studies; in the text, in dealing with specific clinical and pathologic processes, relevant cases are cited. The case examples, likewise, are cross-referenced to relevant discussions in the text.

Contents

1 Brain Damage in the Fetus and Newborn: Pathogenesis

Hypoxic cerebral damage

Infectious diseases of the fetus and newborn

Physical injury of the nervous system

Malformations of the nervous system

Other visceral damage associated with neonatal brain damage

Hypoxic cerebral damage is the most important form of brain damage in the fetus and newborn. Three other basic pathologic processes exercise their effects on the brain: infectious disease, physical injury, and malformations.

During gestation and birth, during intrauterine life and in the descent through the birth canal, the exposure of the fetus to hypoxic damage, to other adverse processes, particularly the risk of damage to the central nervous system, makes the period of gestation and birth the most endangering experience to which most individuals are ever subjected. The perinatal period has a death rate greater than that of any other time of life. Neonatal death occurs in over 3 percent of births. The high mortality is in large measure due to the broad incidence of central nervous system damage.

In the neonate, in autopsy studies in cases with central nervous system damage, often there is associated damage in other viscera. However, it is the damage to the central nervous system that is the most frequent process contributing to death.

In addition to the high mortality, of critical significance is the high morbidity associated with central nervous system damage at birth. The damage may be slight, unrecognized—or it may be extensive, but sublethal. In the population of this country there are estimated to be 2 to 4 million persons with cerebral palsy, epilepsy, and mental retardation of a form attributable to organic cerebral damage incurred during fetal-neonatal life.

The causal factors involved in neonatal central nervous system damage are concerned with complications—at times in the mother, at times in the neonate, or in the delivery process, or postnatally in the newborn.

Hypoxic Cerebral Damage in the Fetus and Newborn

Anatomic factors
Pathogenesis of fetal-neonatal hypoxic cerebral damage
Imaging studies of hypoxic cerebral damage
Complications of pregnancy contributing to fetal-neonatal hypoxic brain damage

The pathology of hypoxic brain damage is presented as follows:

Anatomic factors concerned with hypoxic cerebral damage will be defined.

Pathogenesis of fetal-neonatal hypoxic damage will be detailed. When the fetus or the newborn infant is subjected to oxygen deprivation, the body of the fetus, of the newborn, undergoes a step-by-step sequence of pathologic changes. These bodily processes that occur with hypoxia ultimately target the brain, resulting in hypoxic cerebral damage.

Imaging studies of the brain, CT and MRI studies, are correlated with the pathologic changes that occur consequent to fetal-neonatal hypoxia.

Complications of pregnancy that cause hypoxia in the fetus and newborn are analyzed: complications in the mother, in the placenta, in the fetus, and complications that affect the newborn infant postnatally, causing hypoxic cerebral damage.

The interpretation of the pathogenesis of fetal-neonatal cerebral damage, the interpretation of the pathogenesis of cerebral palsy and other sequelant cerebral disabilities presented here, is based on facets of basic pathology established by research workers in the past, by research workers in recent decades. These basic principles of pathology form the foundation for interpreting the pathogenesis of fetal-neonatal brain damage and sequelant cerebral palsy and other neurologic disabilities:

- In the fetus and newborn two basic patterns of acute hypoxic cerebral damage occur, related to gestational age. In the premature immature fetus and newborn, hypoxic damage consistently affects the deep cerebral strata, involving germinal matrix and neighboring basal ganglia and periventricular white matter. At term, hypoxia causes damage to the surface strata, the cerebral cortex.
- Hypoxic cerebral damage in the fetus and newborn, in its pathogenesis, is due to venous stasis-thrombosis with consequent hemorrhagic infarction.
- Subacute old cerebral hypoxic damage is present at times in newborn infants.

In times past, pathology studies of brain damage in the fetus and newborn were limited because of laboratory technical difficulties. Brain tissue of the fetus and newborn is by nature soft and friable, gelatinous, sometimes diffluent. Pathologists in the past, using small histologic sections, were confronted with insurmountable difficulties in attempting to demonstrate focal small lesions in the newborn brain.

In current research studies in the pathology laboratory, special investigation methods were introduced, techniques that permitted the consistent preservation and identification of focal cerebral lesions, especially small lesions.

The technical breakthrough, the development of an adequate methodology for studying the soft gelatinous brain tissue, was accomplished by Yakovlev (1970) working in the Collaborative Perinatal Project (1965). With the Yakovlev technique, the whole brain specimen is embedded in a plastic material (celloidin), then whole-brain histologic sections, cut serially, are produced, making it possible to identify with consistency focal lesions, large and small, and to establish their geographic relationship in the brain specimen.

Anatomic Factors: *Structures Involved in Fetal~Neonatal Hypoxic Cerebral Damage*

Cortex
Basal ganglia
Germinal matrix

In interpreting fetal-neonatal cerebral damage, the structures that are mainly involved are the cortex, the basal ganglia, the germinal matrix tissue (present in the immature cerebrum), and the periventricular white matter. These structures are indicated in Figures 1 through 3.

Figure 1 notes essential structures in the cerebrum. Correspondingly, Figure 2 indicates changes that take place in these structures consequent to hypoxic damage to the immature cerebrum — damage that leads to cerebral palsy; relevant to this example, an elaboration of underlying pathologic and clinical processes is the basic direction of this text.

Figure 1. Cerebrum: essential anatomic structures dealt with in this text.

Figure 2. Cerebrum showing residual pathologic changes consequent to damage originating during early fetal life (basal ganglia scarring, loss of cerebral white matter with enlargement of ventricles); pattern of changes characteristic of cerebral palsy and related neurologic disability.

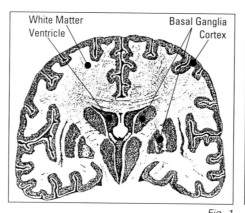

Fig. 1

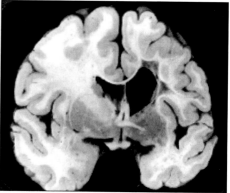

Fig. 2

The **cortex** covering the surface of the cerebrum is a layer of gray matter made up of nerve cells and supporting glial elements. The cortex in the frontal region is concerned with the function of intellect; damage to the frontal cortex leads to a reduction of mental function, mental retardation, or leads to a distortion of mental function, to psychopathy. Damage to the temporal portion of the cortex at times leads to epilepsy.

Basal ganglia, thick deposits of nerve cells in the deep portion of the cerebrum, near the ventricles, are commonly referred to as the extrapyramidal system. The basal ganglia are concerned with the control of muscle tone, with fine motor function. It is damage to the deep portions of the cerebrum, damage to the basal ganglia, occurring in the premature, that leads to manifestations of cerebral palsy.

Germinal matrix deposits (Figure 3) are present in the premature immature cerebrum, appearing as masses of tissue bulging from the lining of the ventricles into the ventricle spaces. Matrix deposits are located immediately adjoining basal ganglia. Matrix is composed of primitive immature cells, depots of source material that contribute to the formation of the basal ganglia and other neuronal structures in the cerebrum.

Figure 3. Germinal matrix tissue present in the immature cerebrum. Matrix deposits projecting into the cerebral ventricles appear as polypoid deep staining tissue (black in the illustration). Premature cerebrum; 19 weeks' gestation.

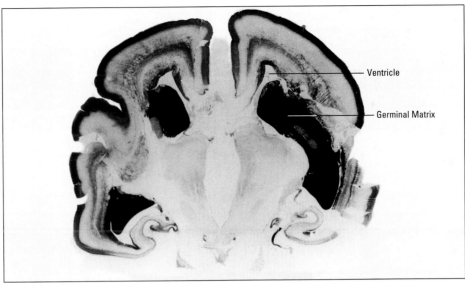

Fig. 3

The germinal matrix, highly vulnerable tissue, is the primary site of hypoxic damage in the immature premature cerebrum. The damage at times extends outward into the periventricular strata, into the basal ganglia and white matter.

As the premature fetus advances in gestational age, the germinal matrix is gradually used up and matrix deposits are not evident after 35 weeks of gestation, not present in the mature cerebrum.

In the mature cerebrum, with the germinal matrix gone, the cortex becomes the primary target of hypoxic damage.

Pathogenesis; Transition of Hypoxic Cerebral Damage: *Acute to Subacute to Chronic*

Acute hypoxic cerebral damage
      Hypoxic onset
      Cardiac failure, congestive heart failure
      Venous infarctional damage
     Patterns of acute cerebral damage
        Premature cerebrum — deep damage
        Mature cerebrum — cortical acute hypoxic damage
    Arterial versus venous pathogenesis of hypoxic cerebral damage
    "Hypoxic ischemic encephalopathy"
    Quantitative relationship between hypoxia and brain damage
Subacute cerebral damage present in the newborn
Chronic (late) sequels of fetal-neonatal cerebral damage
      Porencephaly (encephaloclastic)
      Hydrocephalus ex vacuo
      Hydranencephaly
      Status marmoratus
      Microcephaly

Acute fresh hypoxic cerebral damage undergoes a transitional pattern of changes to the **subacute** stage, and subsequently the tissue — months and years later — undergoes **chronic** changes, with the end picture of scarring and cavitation.

Acute Hypoxic Cerebral Damage

How does exposure to hypoxia end up making lesions of acute brain damage? What is the sequence of pathologic processes that begins with exposure to hypoxia, that leads to pathologic changes in the body of the fetus, and ends with damage to the brain, damage present in the newborn?

The causal mechanisms involved in the pathogenesis of fetal-neonatal hypoxic damage, the sequence of the step-by-step bodily changes that occur in the interval between hypoxic exposure and the appearance of cerebral damage, long remained obscure. All that was known for certain was that fetal-neonatal hypoxia led to cerebral damage; the intermediate pathologic processes were a matter of speculation.

In the 1960s, studies in the NIH Collaborative Perinatal Project provided basic information about the pathogenesis of fetal-neonatal hypoxic cerebral damage (Towbin, 1968). These studies confirmed that the hemorrhagic cerebral lesions were **venous infarctions.** The studies showed that the acute infarctional damage that occurs in the brain and other organs with fetal-neonatal hypoxia is not a limited local phenomenon. The hemorrhagic infarcts represent the final segment in a series of pathologic systemic body processes that involve antecedent fetal-neonatal factors, processes that may have their origin before, during, or after birth. The development of the underlying processes leading to cerebral infarctional damage evolves through three stages, each precipitating the next:

(1) The **hypoxic onset**, fetal-neonatal hypoxia-producing complications, leads to (2) **cardiac failure**, to myocardial oxygen deprivation, and results in (3) **venous thrombosis** and **infarction** (Table 1).

Hypoxic onset

The hypoxia-producing complication, prenatally, intranatally, or postnatally, may have its origin in any of the components of the maternal-placental-fetal organization. During gestation, fetal malnutrition and oxygen deprivation may be due to maternal illness (page 35) (Case 109, page 500; Case 179, page 618; Case 185, page 630; Case 200, page 661; Case 215, page 702). The placenta is often faulty; its function, to transfer oxygen and nutriment from the maternal blood to the fetal blood, may be inadequate due to pathologic changes present, such as placental infarction (page 71) or premature detachment of the placenta (page 66). At times the umbilical cord, the supply conduit between the placenta and the fetus, becomes compressed or knotted (page 84). These same complications may appear, often catastrophically, intranatally — during labor and delivery. Frequently the hypoxic state initiated prior to birth is extended postnatally, especially with prematures, with the postnatal development of hyaline membrane disease, pneumonia, or other pulmonary complication (page 105).

Table 1.

Pathogenesis of Fetal-Neonatal Hypoxic Cerebral Damage

(1) THE HYPOXIC ONSET

In the fetus:
Hypoxia-producing gestational complications; maternal illness, placental disorders, umbilical cord compression, and other conditions that compromise the maternal-placental-fetal organization

In the newborn:
Hypoxia-producing postnatal complications: apnea, hyaline membrane disease, pneumothorax, and other respiratory disturbances; anemia; heart defects

(2) CARDIAC FAILURE; CIRCULATORY STASIS

Generalized Bodily Venous Congestion

Oxygen deprivation causes the heart muscle to weaken; leads to "backward" circulatory failure, to stasis-thrombosis of veins of the body

In the premature (immature) fetus or newborn

(3) Stasis-thrombosis of deep cerebral veins

Infarction (hemorrhagic) of subependymal germinal matrix

Extension into periventricular white matter, to basal ganglia and other deep structures

Penetration of hemorrhagic infarction through the ependyma, leading to cerebral intraventricular hemorrhage

Extension of hemorrhage into the third and fourth ventricles and out into subarachnoid space about the brain stem, into the posterior fossa

In the mature, term, fetus or newborn

(3) Stasis-thrombosis of surface cerebral veins

Infarction (hemorrhagic) of the cerebral surface, cortex

Subarachnoid hemorrhage

Cardiac failure; circulatory stasis: congestive heart failure

Prolonged hypoxia imposed on the body, whether fetus, newborn, or adult, leads to weakening of the heart, to myocardial exhaustion, to cardiac slowing, to cardiac decompensation, to cardiac failure.

The heart functions as a double-action pump, drawing out blood from the venous side of the circulation and propelling it forward into the arteries. In the fetus and newborn, as in the adult, when the oxygen available to the body is inadequate, manifestly the tissue that suffers first is the constantly working, contracting heart muscle. The pump falters. Failure of the heart to adequately pump out the blood from the venous side of the circulatory system leads to backward failure, to venous engorgement, a stagnant backlog of blood in the veins of the body — congestive circulatory failure. The venous engorgement is most extensive in the peripheries of the body — locally, in the legs, and intracranially, in the brain (Figure 4).

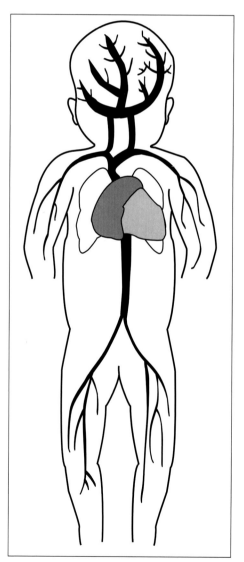

Figure 4. Congestive heart failure. Diagram demonstrates engorgement of veins, especially in the cranial circulation and lower extremities. With congestive heart failure, the heart fails to adequately pump out the blood from the venous side of the circulatory system, leading to "backward failure," to venous stasis-thrombosis.

Fig. 4

With mounting congestive heart failure, the heart becomes enlarged, dilated, distended with blood. Edema of the soft tissues develops. Subcutaneous tissues become waterlogged; extremities become swollen, turgid, suffused with edema fluid (hydrops fetalis) (Figure 5). Body cavities accumulate edema fluid, hydrothorax, hydropericardium. The abdomen becomes enlarged, distended with ascites fluid. Cerebral congestion, cerebral edema, results. The liver and spleen become congested, enlarged, congestive hepatosplenamegaly.

Figure 5. Congestive heart failure causing hydrops fetalis, characterized by severe edema of the subcutaneous tissue, most pronounced about the face and the extremities.

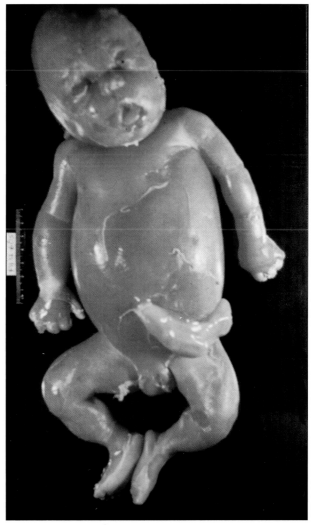

Fig. 5

The illustrations in Figure 6 demonstrate the pathologic sequence of an hypoxia-producing complication leading to congestive heart failure: Premature detachment of the placenta with retroplacental hemorrhage resulted in intrauterine hypoxia, with the stillborn infant consequently showing classical manifestations of congestive heart failure — severe cyanosis, cardiac dilatation, venous engorgement, hydrothorax, venous congestion of the brain.

Figure 6(a). Placenta, premature detachment with retroplacental hemorrhage. Stillborn infant cyanotic due to intrauterine hypoxia with congestive heart failure.

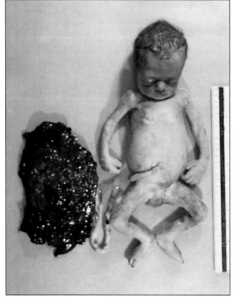

Fig. 6(a)

Figure 6(b). Congestive heart failure due to intrauterine hypoxia; cardiac failure, with heart enlarged, dilated; large veins engorged; hydrothorax. View of thoracic viscera at autopsy.

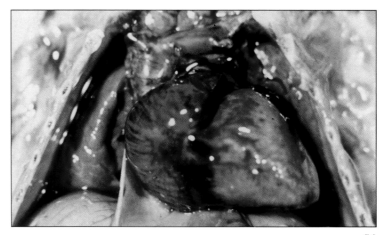

(b)

Figure 6(c). Cerebral congestion and edema, with flattening of the convolutions, consequent to congestive heart failure in this case.

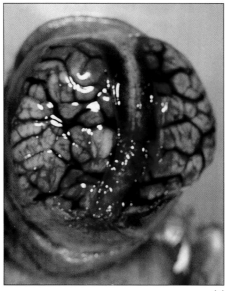

(c)

Venous thrombosis; infarction (cerebral)

The slowing and stasis of venous flow leads to in vivo intravascular blood clotting, venous thrombosis. This interference with local circulation, stasis-thrombosis of veins, leads to local infarction, infarction of the portion of the organ drained by the occluded vein.

Figure 7 demonstrates the mechanism of venous infarction in the deep cerebral tissues in the premature brain. Occlusion of the deep cerebral vein causes interference with circulation, blocking of the outflow of the blood from the region with consequent devitalization and suffusion of blood in the affected tissues, hemorrhagic infarction.

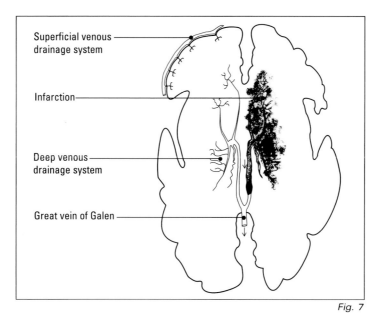

Figure 7. Mechanism of hypoxic deep cerebral venous infarction in premature brain. At right, deep venous tributaries show dilatation and stasis-thrombosis, with corresponding hemorrhagic infarction of the deep cerebral structures. Deep venous structures prominently developed in contrast to rudimentary cortical veins.

Fig. 7

The link between cerebral venous thrombosis and cerebral infarction is demonstrated in Figure 8. The germinal matrix on the lateral aspect of the ventricle walls shows patches of infarction due to thromboses of the germinal matrix veins.

Figure 8. Thromboses of germinal matrix veins with associated matrix infarction. **(a).** Deposits of germinal matrix appear as dark pads of periventricular tissue on the lateral aspect of the ventricles. Premature brain; whole brain serial section. **(b).** Midline periventricular cerebral structures with germinal matrix, as in (a). The higher magnification shows germinal matrix veins distended with thrombus material, surrounded by areas of matrix infarction.

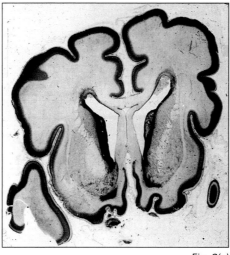
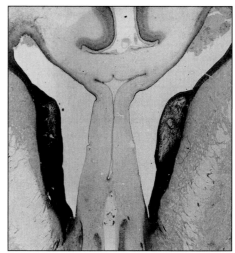

Fig. 8(a)   *(b)*

Figure 9(a) likewise shows thrombosis of a large intracranial venous sinus. Extension of the process retrograde, upward into the cerebrum, resulted in periventricular hemorrhagic infarctions, as evident in Figure 9b.

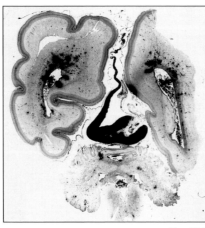 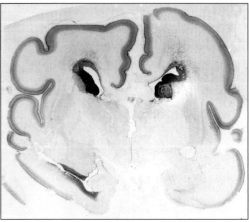

Fig. 9(a) *(b)*

Figure 9(a). Thrombosis of the Galen vein and tributaries, draining the cerebrum, resulting periventricular hemorrhagic infarction. The Galen vein (black staining) extends medially in a tortuous, expanding course. Retrograde thrust of venous engorgement evident in periventricular tributaries; dilated veins, petechiae, and confluent areas of hemorrhagic necrosis present. Premature infant of 29 weeks' gestation; lived 30 hours. Abruptio placentae, hyaline membrane disease. Frontal-horizontal section of brain. **(b).** Section taken more anteriorly in the cerebrum shows the lateral ventricles with dark staining deposits of germinal matrix overlying the caudate nuclei. On the right, the germinal matrix shows a centrally placed dilated vein with a thrombus; surrounding this is a pale marginal area: perivenous hemorrhagic infarction.

In the fetus and newborn, venous infarctional damage may occur not only in the brain but also in the kidneys, adrenal glands, and other structures (Case 27, page 301) (Towbin and Turner, 1978). However, in pathologic studies, hypoxic infarctional damage in organs other than in the brain appears infrequently. The brain proves to be the most vulnerable organ, the most common target, and in this respect, the site with the most serious consequences.

Patterns of acute hypoxic cerebral damage: premature; mature

Premature cerebrum: deep damage
Mature cerebrum: cortical damage

The location of acute hypoxic damage in the cerebrum occurs in two distinctive patterns. In the **premature immature** cerebrum, hypoxia causes damage specifically in the **deep** structures of the cerebrum. In the **mature** cerebrum, acute hypoxic damage occurs not in the deep structures, but consistently in the **surface cortical** strata (Figure 10) (Schwartz, 1961; Larroche, 1968; Towbin, 1968, 1969, 1970a, 1977; Csermely, 1972; Okazaki, 1983).

Figure 10. Two basic patterns of hypoxic cerebral damage, related to gestational age. In the premature, damage originates in the deep cerebral strata. At term, in the mature cerebrum, damage is limited to the surface, to the cortex.

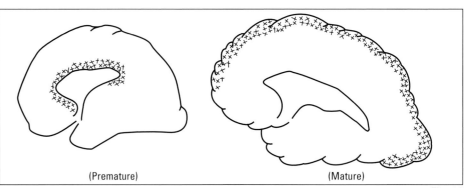

(Premature) (Mature)

Fig. 10

Premature cerebrum: deep hypoxic damage

The effects of hypoxia in the premature, deep cerebral hemorrhagic infarctional damage, are demonstrated in Figures 8, 9, 11, and 12. The damage appears as irregular areas of hemorrhagic necrotic tissue deep in the cerebrum. Massive deep cerebral infarction is present, with blood from the hemorrhagic infarcts escaping into the ventricles.

The following two illustrations present a comparison of the pattern of damage as it occurs in a very early premature cerebrum (Figure 11) with the pattern of damage that occurs in a premature cerebrum of more advanced gestational age (Figure 12).

Figure 11. Early premature brain (approximately 20 weeks gestational age) showing massive periventricular hemorrhagic infarction wiping out the germinal matrix and extending into the adjoining white matter and basal ganglia.

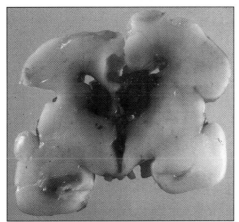

Fig. 11

Figure 12. Premature brain of more advanced gestational age, approximately 36 weeks' gestation, showing characteristic pattern of acute hypoxic damage in the premature cerebrum: deep cerebral periventricular hemorrhagic infarction extending to the white matter and basal ganglia. The ventricles contain clots of blood.

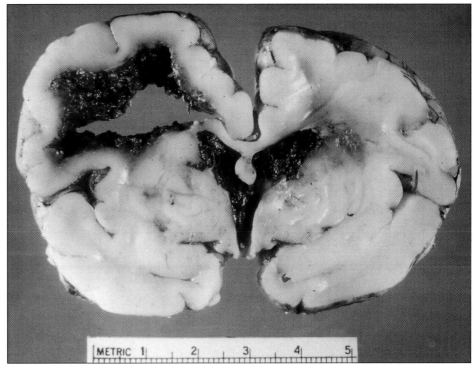

Fig. 12

Pathogenesis of hypoxic deep cerebral damage in the premature

What determines the location of acute hypoxic cerebral damage? Why deep in the premature and surface in the mature cerebrum?

The specificity in location of fetal-neonatal acute cerebral hypoxic damage, deep in the premature, cortical at term, is not a random occurrence but is influenced by three biologic factors, all related to gestational age (Towbin, 1977): the presence or absence of germinal matrix tissue, the momentum of local organogenesis, and the degree of development of local vascular elements.

The location of acute brain damage in the premature in the deep strata of the cerebrum is determined by the presence of germinal matrix, the rapid local organogenesis, and by increased vascularity of the deep structures.

Illustrative Cases:

Germinal matrix infarction

Germinal matrix tissue (Figure 3, page 5) is extremely soft and friable, is manifestly vulnerable to hypoxia, and readily undergoes hemorrhagic disintegration, infarction. Hypoxia in the premature leads to deep cerebral damage because the target tissue, the primary site of origin, the germinal matrix, is deeply located. The process of infarction in the germinal matrix, extending peripherally, leads to hemorrhagic necrosis of the basal ganglia and, extending centrally, causes bleeding into the ventricles.

Hypoxic damage to the deep cerebral structures occurs in the premature brain prior to 35 weeks of gestation. With the germinal tissue becoming attenuated near term, with this target tissue no longer present in the deep cerebrum, the primary site of hypoxic damage at term (as in the adult) shifts to the cortex.

Organogenesis

This process, pertaining to the time during which the structures of an organ are undergoing active elaboration, is a period of manifestly increased vulnerability to injury. During early fetal life, local organogenesis in the cerebrum is most prominent in the deep strata, where elaboration of cerebral structures from the deposits of germinal matrix is highly visible. The deep structures, undergoing rapid maturation, are immediately susceptible to hypoxic infarctional injury. Later, as the fetus becomes mature, with the basal ganglia and other deep structures now well formed, and with the germinal matrix depleted, structural activity shifts to the surface, where the cortex, previously biologically inert, now undergoes accelerated organogenesis—and, at term, becomes the main target of hypoxic injury.

Vascularization

Vascular development, particularly the elaboration of venous elements, directly influences the occurrence of hypoxic damage in the fetal-neonatal brain. In the premature, coincident with active organogenesis, vascularization of the deep cerebral structures proceeds early, providing a broad venous network. Hypoxia leads to thrombotic occlusion of the deep veins, with consequent infarctional damage in the deep structures of the premature cerebrum. At term, the cortex, previously an avascular layer of tissue, rapidly undergoes development and acquires a prominent vascular system. With hypoxia, thrombosis of the newly formed surface veins results in infarctional damage.

Periventricular hemorrhagic infarction, intraventricular hemorrhage, subarachnoid hemorrhage

At times, hemorrhagic infarction in the periventricular germinal matrix breaks through into the lateral ventricles, causing intraventricular hemorrhage (Figure 13).

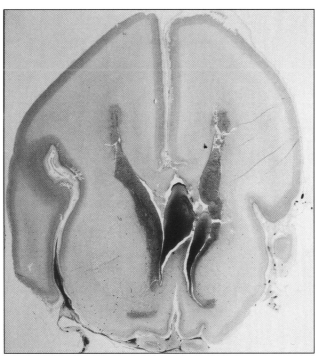

Fig. 13

Figure 13. Germinal matrix hemorrhagic infarction with intraventricular hemorrhage. Histologic section of cerebrum. Germinal matrix appearing as purple-staining periventricular deposits of tissue. On the right, the germinal matrix with hemorrhagic infarction, with extension of hemorrhage into the lateral ventricle.

The blood, extending into the third ventricle, through the aqueduct, and into the fourth ventricle, reaches the subarachnoid space, with subarachnoid hemorrhage appearing over the ventral surface of the brain (Figures 14 and 15).

Figure 14. Midsagittal section through the brain. Extension of intraventricular hemorrhage into the subarachnoid space. Blood from hemorrhagic infarction of the cerebral subependymal matrix tissue. Blood traversed through the aqueduct, through the fourth ventricle, through the foramen of Luschka, and out into the subarachnoid space. Premature infant. At autopsy, the ventral surface of the brain presented a layer of blood, up to 3 mm thick, in the subarachnoid space of the interpeduncular fossa and around the pons and medulla.

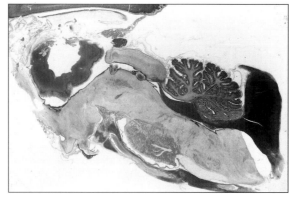

Fig. 14

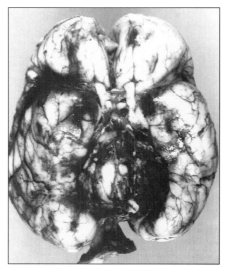

Fig. 15(a)

Figure 15. Subarachnoid hemorrhage due to extension of the intraventricular hemorrhage through the ventricles and out into the subarachnoid space. Newborn, 29 weeks' gestation. **(a).** Brain, ventral surface, with subarachnoid blood at the base of the brain, surrounding the brain stem and cerebellum. Subarachnoid blood originating from intraventricular hemorrhage. **(b).** Intraventricular hemorrhage. Brain section at the level of the lateral ventricles. **(c).** Extension of intraventricular hemorrhage through the ventricular system into the third ventricles. Brain section at the level of the thalami. **(d).** Extension of hemorrhage out into the subarachnoid space around the brain stem and cerebellum; compare with (a).

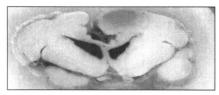

(b)

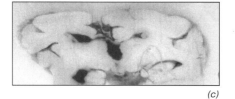

(c)

(d)

Clot formation in the intraventricular drainage system may lead to obstruction of cerebrospinal fluid outflow, with consequent development of obstructive hydrocephalus (page 157).

As previously described, damage to the germinal matrix extending outward into the periventricular strata, into basal ganglia and periventricular white matter, leads to cerebral palsy in surviving infants (Chapter 3). At times, with severe hypoxic exposure in the premature, the damage beginning in the germinal matrix extends outward beyond the basal ganglia, through the cerebrum to the cortex (Figures 16 and 17).

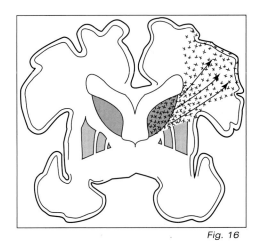

Fig. 16

Figure 16. Pattern of hypoxic cerebral damage in the premature newborn. In the premature, deep cerebral damage beginning in the periventricular germinal matrix extends to the basal ganglia and at times through the cerebrum to the cortex.

Infants surviving with this pattern of damage, in addition to cerebral palsy, also develop cortical disabilities of mental retardation, epilepsy, and psychopathy.

The distribution of hypoxic cerebral damage present at birth in most cases is bilateral, but often is more extensive in one cerebral hemisphere than in the other (Figure 17). Reflecting this, clinically in infants that survive, the neurologic signs — spasticity, abnormal reflexes — are more pronounced on one side of the body than on the other. These children may be diagnosed as having hemiplegic cerebral palsy.

Figure 17. Massive deep cerebral hypoxic damage, asymmetric hemorrhagic infarction extending from the germinal matrix through the cerebrum to the cortex on the right. On the left, the germinal matrix with a large distended thrombosed vein. Delivery at 27 weeks of gestation; premature detachment of the placenta and prolapse of the umbilical cord.

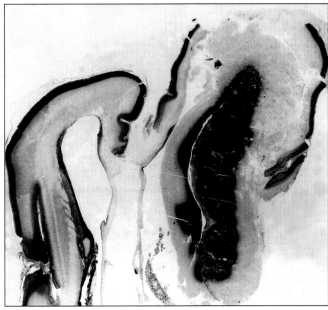

Fig. 17

Minimal deep cerebral hypoxic damage

The severity of hypoxic deep cerebral damage in the premature brain varies, at times massive (Figures 11, 12), at times of minimal nature (page 220; Case 2, page 230), appearing as focal infarcts in the germinal matrix or in the deep cerebral white matter, as small islands of periventricular leucomalacia.

Periventricular leucomalacia (PVL)

Illustrative Case:
Case 40   *p. 328*

Periventricular leucomalacia (*leuco-*, white; *-malacia*, softness) is another form of deep damage that appears specifically in the deep periventricular white matter in the premature brain following hypoxia. This pattern of damage is commonly associated with germinal matrix infarction. PVL consists of small islands of necrosis, small venous infarcts, in the deep white matter (Figure 18).

Figure 18. Periventricular leucomalacia (PVL), small foci of venous infarction in periventricular white matter appearing as confluent "smudged" islands surrounding dilated engorged small capillaries and thrombosed veins.

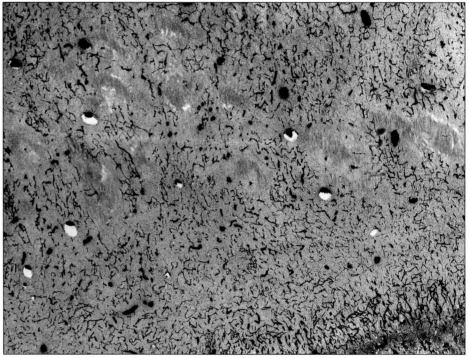

Fig. 18

Incidence of premature hypoxic cerebral damage

Some degree of deep hypoxic cerebral damage is evident at autopsy in prematures, almost universally (Collaborative Perinatal Project, 1965; Yakovlev and Rosales, 1970). In pathology studies, in postmortem examination of 140 premature newborn infants of 22 to 35 weeks' gestation, deep cerebral infarctional damage of severe to moderate degree was present in 48 percent of cases. In the other 52 percent of cases, damage of minimal form was present, often with lesions scattered diffusely through the germinal matrix and adjoining tissue (Towbin, 1970a).

Mature cerebrum: cortical hypoxic damage

Illustrative Cases:
Case 31   *p. 312*
Case 34   *p. 316*

As previously noted, acute hypoxic brain damage occurs in the newborn in two different patterns: in the premature, damage in the cerebrum is deep; hypoxic cerebral damage in the mature brain affects the cerebral surface, the cortex (Figure 10). In the mature fetus and newborn (with germinal matrix attenuated, no longer present), the primary target of hypoxia is the cerebral surface, the cortex. The damage to the cortex varies, from severe to intermediate to minimal.

Severe hypoxic cortical damage in a term newborn is shown in Figure 19; the surface tissue, the cortex and subcortical white matter, have become hemorrhagic and necrotic, through the process of venous infarction.

Figure 19. Cortical cerebral hypoxic damage, hemorrhagic infarction in the mature fetus. Term delivery; heart malformation; progressive circulatory failure; survival of three weeks.

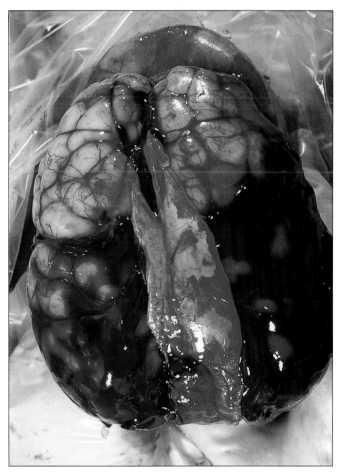

Fig. 19

Intermediate hypoxic damage in the form of cortical necrosis is shown in Figure 20. This pattern of damage at times is focal, at times diffuse over the cerebrum (Case 31, page 312).

Figure 20. Cortical necrosis. Hypoxic damage in the cerebral cortex in a mature fetus. Intrauterine death prior to labor, due to premature detachment of the placenta. **(a).** Whole brain histologic section. In the posterior areas, the parieto-occipital region, appearing in the lower portion of the illustration, the cortex shows a patchy distribution of pale "moth-eaten" areas, characteristic of hypoxic cortical necrosis.

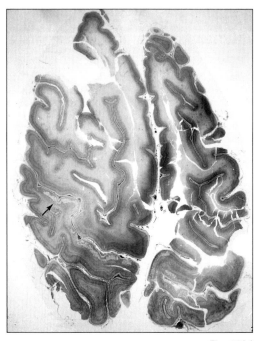

Fig. 20(a)

Figure 20(b). Cortex showing irregular hypoxic devastation. Higher magnification of an area in the mid-portion of the left cerebral hemisphere as shown in (a). The damaged cortex, in the mid-lower portion of the illustration, shows pale confluent patches with cellular elements wiped out; this is in contrast to the preserved cortex, in the mid-upper portion of the illustration. The intact cortex shows the normal laminar pattern, with six stratified layers of cells. The surface of the damaged cortex is indented by a dilated vein occluded by a thrombus, responsible for the underlying hypoxic necrosis of the cortex.

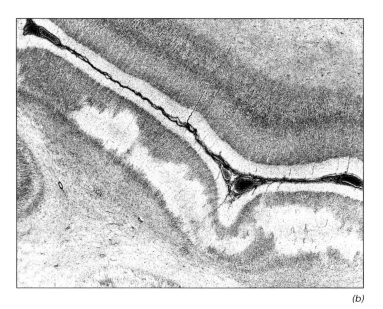

(b)

The mature cerebral cortex microscopically is composed of six lamina (layers) of neurones. Laminar necrosis is the pattern of damage that is commonly observed in adults who have suffered severe hypoxia, asphyxial accidents, and survived for a period of days. With hypoxic laminar necrosis, the third and fifth laminae of neurones are wiped out, leaving the cortex with patchy necrotic pale areas depleted of nerve cells.

Minimal hypoxic cortical neuronal damage (Chapter 7) is of cellular order, with varying numbers of nerve cells injured, eliminated. Distinctive changes are evident histologically; the cortex becomes punctuated with shrunken, deeply staining neurones, which appear singly or in clusters, as demonstrated in Figure 21 (a section of cortex from a term infant with respiratory depression at birth who lived one day). Some of the affected neuronal elements that are more labile become shriveled and necrotic, and are quickly wiped out by the oxygen deprivation; neighboring cells, of similar caste and form, having a higher threshold and proving more durable, appear unchanged and survive.

In the newborn infant, as in the adult after hypoxic exposure, such damage may affect broad areas of the cerebrum. The ultimate decrease in neuronal population, although sufficient to contravene function, may be so lightly distributed as to escape detection when the tissue is later examined microscopically. A depletion of cells up to 30% may go unrecognized even by experienced neuropathologists.

Figure 21. Minimal cortical neuronal hypoxic cerebral damage. Section of precentral (motor) cortex. In the upper part of the illustration large pyramidal-shaped neurones (Betz cells) show acute hypoxic damage, appearing shrunken, deeply stained, with loss of fine architectural markings. In contrast, nerve cells in the lower portion of the illustration are anatomically more preserved with nuclei and nucleoli well defined. Term infant with respiratory depression; lived one day.

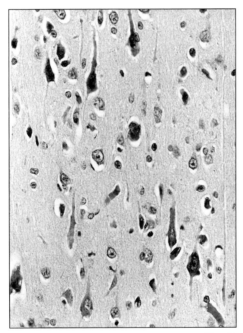

Fig. 21

Pathogenesis of cortical hypoxic damage in the mature cerebrum

The effect of hypoxia in the mature cerebrum, surface cerebral damage, results from stasis-thrombosis of the superficial cerebral veins over the surface of the cerebrum. Blood oozing from the infarcted cerebral surface gives rise to subarachnoid hemorrhage.

Pertinently, the surface cerebral damage that occurs with hypoxia at term, affecting the cortex, does not penetrate downward to the deep cerebral structures (Figure 22). Hypoxia at term does not cause cerebral palsy.

For the mature newborn, the sequels of hypoxic exposure are the same as occur in the adult subject; adults who survive after asphyxial exposure often show cortical manifestations, with a reduction in mental facilities, at times with psychopathy, at times with epilepsy. Affected adults do not have basal ganglia manifestations, do not develop cerebral palsy. The same applies to the mature newborn consequent to hypoxia.

Figure 22. In the mature (term) newborn, cortical damage extends to the superficial strata; damage does not penetrate deeply to the basal ganglia.

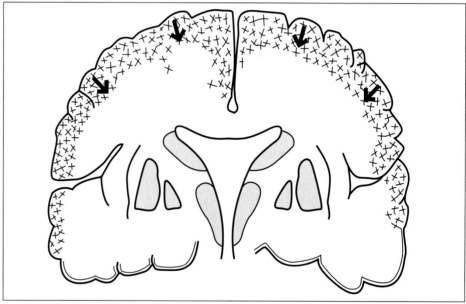

Fig. 22

Arterial versus venous pathogenesis of hypoxic cerebral damage

Pathology studies in the Collaborative Perinatal Project (Towbin, 1968) and in other investigations (Macgregor, 1946; Young and Courville, 1962; Kalbag and Woolf, 1967; Okazaki, 1983) show conclusively that fetal-neonatal acute hypoxic cerebral damage is of venous origin, due to venous stasis-thrombosis leading to hemorrhagic infarction. Although it has been thought by some writers that the acute hypoxic lesions in the fetus and newborn were due to arterial infarction, it is clear that the pathologic processes, as evident in Figures 8, 9, 17, and 218, are of venous origin, venous stasis-thrombosis, venous infarction.

"Hypoxic ischemic encephalopathy" (HIE)

The misinterpretation that the cerebral damage is of arterial origin gave rise to the clinical concept of "hypoxic ischemic encephalopathy," a concept pathologically invalid.

"Hypoxic ischemic encephalopathy" —conceived by clinicians, based on the idea that acute hypoxic cerebral damage is due to an arterial mechanism — although widely used, is contradictory, misleading. The term is usually applied by clinicians in reference to clinical manifestations of newborn brain damage, to newborn neurologic depression. The implication conveyed is that hypoxic brain damage has occurred due to "ischemia," due to lack of arterial blood supply to the brain. Ischemia means lack of blood (*isch-*, lack; *-emia*, blood).

Of the three words in the term "hypoxic ischemic encephalopathy," the first word, "hypoxic," and the last word, "encephalopathy," brain damage, are appropriate. The middle word, "ischemic," meaning lack of arterial perfusion, defines the pathologic process incorrectly. Hypoxia-produced lesions present at birth, whether acute or subacute, are infarcts —hemorrhagic venous infarcts. They are bloody lesions, stuffed with blood, causing bleeding, often intraventricular hemorrhage. The lesions visibly are not "ischemic."

Hypoxia causes brain damage, encephalopathy. There is no argument about that. The issue is the use of the word "ischemic," applying this term, meaning lack of blood, to the hemorrhagic infarcts in the newborn brain. Although the matter is academic, with little bearing on clinical outcome, use of this contradictory term, "hypoxic ischemic encephalopathy," should be avoided.

The clinical literature dealing with the pathogenesis and diagnosis of fetal-neonatal brain damage has become confused, vacillatory. To illustrate, one article appears indicating that the writer believes that the damaging process is of venous origin (Volpe, 1979), while in another publication the same writer, a clinician, opines that the cause is arterial, applying the concept of hypoxic ischemic encephalopathy (Volpe, 1987).

Clinicians are gradually becoming informed about the pathology of fetal-neonatal brain damage. However, the use of HIE is a sort of clinical reflex, a mindset, and the use of this term may go on and on —but it will not be used by knowledgeable pathologists.

Hypoxia duration: degree of cerebral damage

How long can a human fetus be exposed to hypoxia before acute hypoxic damage occurs? There is no pat answer to this question. This issue is often posed during obstetrical malpractice suits, often with reference to a period of abnormal monitor tracing or in cases of umbilical cord prolapse, when the umbilical cord protrudes into the vagina ahead of the fetus and becomes compressed. The assertion that a certain number of minutes of cord compression, of hypoxia, causes brain damage —is not valid. The development of hypoxic damage is not governed solely by the duration of the hypoxic complication. A fetus may tolerate for prolonged periods hypoxia of a mild degree without manifest effects. The development of cerebral acute hypoxic damage in the fetus depends to a major degree on the intensity of the hypoxia and on the individual constitutional susceptibility of the fetus to oxygen deprivation. The intensity, the degree to which the oxygen supply is cut off, cannot be precisely judged; in cases of cord compression, the tightness of the compression, the compromise of circulation through the cord, cannot be measured. Monitor record abnormalities do not specifically indicate, measure, hypoxia. Constitutionally, fetuses, like adults, have a broad range of difference in their susceptibility to hypoxia. Experimentally, in animals, in fetuses and mature animals subjected to a set amount of hypoxia, the severity of resulting cerebral damage varies broadly among the members of the experimental group.

Subacute cerebral damage present in the newborn

What happens to an area of acute hypoxic brain damage if the damage is sublethal and the fetus, the newborn, survives?

The damaged tissue gradually undergoes changes characterized pathologically as **subacute**. The area of acute hemorrhagic infarction gradually undergoes disintegration (Figure 23). Deposits of blood become circumscribed, inspissated, and, with breakdown of the hemoglobin, the deposits lose their red coloration and become tan.

In the surviving fetus, newborn, the necrotic tissue becomes softened and may ultimately be absorbed or converted to scar tissue (Figure 24).

Most people, many doctors, still have the idea that in newborn infants with brain damage, the damage is attributable to something that went wrong during labor and delivery. This idea is erroneous. Newborn infants at times harbor old subacute cerebral hypoxic damage. The occurrence of subacute cerebral damage in the newborn is well documented in the pathology literature.

In autopsy studies of hypoxic brain damage in the newborn, while in most cases the damage is acute, fresh, in some cases the damage, as determined by pathologic analysis, is subacute, old, recognized to have originated weeks, months prior to birth.

Figure 23. Subacute (old) cerebral hypoxic damage in a term newborn. The devitalized areas, old infarcts pathologically, appear as confluent pale patches deep in the cerebrum, adjoining the ventricles. History of complicated pregnancy with maternal viral infection, excessive weight gain, and polyhydramnios.

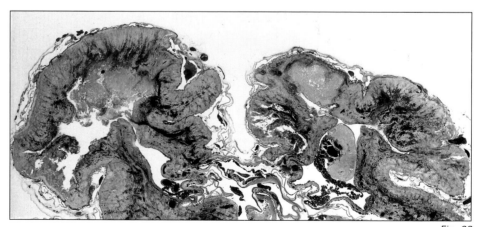

Fig. 23

Figure 24. Subacute cerebral damage present at birth in a term infant. The surface of the right frontoparietal region is smooth and leathery, with loss of convolutional structure. (Refer to Case 39, page 326.)

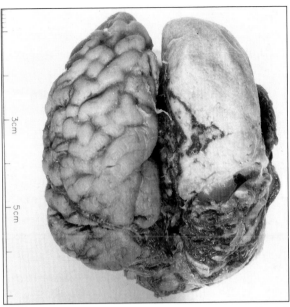

Fig. 24

Subacute cerebral damage in newborn infants was first observed by Neuburger (1934) and Hallervorden (1949). These pioneer case studies present key evidence relating hypoxic exposure of the fetus during premature intrauterine life to the occurrence of deep subacute cerebral damage in the infants born at term. In these cases the mothers had attempted suicide by asphyxia during pregnancy, months before delivery, with the infants surviving to term, dying after birth. The brain specimens of the infants showed extensive scarring and cyst formation in the cerebral white matter and in the basal ganglia. Gossey and Golaire et al. (1982) presented a similar case of a mother who attempted suicide at 30 weeks of pregnancy and delivered at 36 weeks; the newborn died. At autopsy, the cerebrum showed cystic areas and calcification in the basal ganglia, together with widespread necrosis in the white matter. Ellis and Goetzman et al. (1988) reported neuropathology studies of 15 newborn cases that showed lesions in the brain prior to the time of birth. Other cases of subacute hypoxic cerebral damage in the newborn have been reported by Manterola, Towbin and Yakovlev (1966), Towbin (1968, 1977), Towbin and Turner (1978), Csermely (1972), Cohen and Roessmann (1994), and others.

In imaging studies, subacute cerebral damage is at times evident in the brain in newborn infants. In such cases, CT and MRI studies, done directly after birth, show areas of rarefaction indicating a far-advanced loss of tissue substance, old subacute cerebral damage, destruction originating long before birth (page 33). In such cases, the cerebrum (previously edematous during the acute stage) shows no signs of edema in the CT scans; the brain is not swollen, the ventricles are patent. Correspondingly, clinically, the fontanelles are flat, not bulging.

Subacute lesions are usually surrounded by a margin of hemorrhagic tissue; at times blood oozes from the still bloody subacute lesion into the ventricles. The presence of intraventricular blood in a CT scan does not prove the presence of acute brain damage.

Correlating clinical and pathologic factors—when hypoxia-producing pregnancy complications, such as maternal illness or placental disorders, occur during early fetal life, weeks or months before term, the premature fetus may succumb soon after the hypoxia, be stillborn, and show acute deep cerebral damage at autopsy. Or the fetus may survive the episode of transient intrauterine hypoxia, with the gestation going on to term, with the deep cerebral damage becoming subacute, old; in such cases, at times the compromised fetus dies during the stress of labor, or the neonate dies soon after birth; postmortem studies of the brain reveal deep cerebral lesions that pathologically are of subacute pattern, old (Figures 23 and 24).

If the fetus with hypoxic cerebral damage incurred in early fetal life survives to term, with the deep cerebral damage becoming subacute, with the damage extending to the basal ganglia, the affected infant subsequently will develop cerebral palsy (Chapter 3).

Thus, although cerebral palsy is known as "the disease of prematurity," it often develops in children born at term. *The occurrence of deep cerebral damage, incurred during premature fetal life, with the fetus surviving to term bearing subacute cerebral damage, explains the common occurrence of cerebral palsy in children born at term.*

When hypoxia-producing complications occur late in gestation, near term, cerebral damage that occurs is limited to the surface strata, to the cortex. In such circumstances, with the infant born weeks after the gestational insult occurred, the cerebrum in the newborn infant shows a pattern of surface damage that, pathologically, is subacute, old, as illustrated in Figure 23. Infants that survive develop cortical manifestations of mental retardation, epilepsy, and other cortical disabilities, but do not develop cerebral palsy (Chapters 4–6).

Infants previously compromised, damaged during early intrauterine life, surviving to term with old subacute brain damage, often do not tolerate the ordinary stress of labor, with consequent fetal monitor abnormalities appearing — not because of excessive hypoxic exposure — but because the compromised, enfeebled fetus is unable to cope with the intranatal stress. These babies are born depressed.

The postnatal performance of infants with subacute cerebral damage is distinctive, different from the clinical course of the newborn with acute cerebral damage: Infants born with acute hypoxic cerebral damage show a persisting pattern of depression of vital function, with coma and congestive heart failure extending over a period of many days. In contrast, infants with subacute cerebral damage, being previously compromised during fetal life, are depressed at birth but usually respond to resuscitation in the delivery room and are active and alert after a short period. The difference in the postnatal clinical pattern is of direct importance in determining the time of incurrence of brain damage in infants who later develop neurologic disability (Chapter 2).

Recognition of the phenomenon of subacute cerebral damage in the newborn is of major importance in obstetrical malpractice litigation. Although well known to pathologists, the occurrence and significance of subacute cerebral damage, the result of prior gestational hypoxic exposure, is not generally realized by clinicians. Consequently, in infants born at term who develop cerebral palsy, clinicians often fail to recognize the effects of adverse gestational processes in causing fetal subacute cerebral damage and are prone to attribute the cause of cerebral palsy to events of labor and delivery.

Chronic (late) sequels of fetal-neonatal hypoxic cerebral damage

What is the end stage, the pathologic pattern of brain damage, in infants who survive and develop manifestations of cerebral palsy and other neurologic disabilities?

The late chronic pattern reflects the pathologic process of atrophy, with scarring and contraction of tissue, often with cavitations and focal calcification. When damage to a portion of the cerebrum is severe, extreme, the disintegrated tissue is absorbed, later creating a cavity (Figures 25, 26, 27).

Figure 25. Periventricular cysts at the caudo-thalamic angle, in the region previously occupied by germinal matrix during early fetal life. Each side shows a loculated cystic structure. It is apparent that large matrix deposits present during early fetal life became infarcted; with the fetus surviving, the infarctional process became chronic, with the damaged tissue absorbed, leaving large cysts.

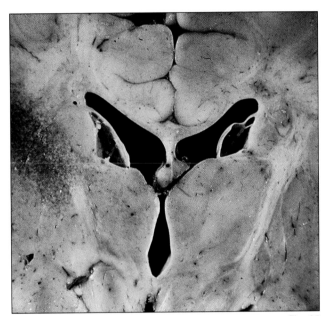

Fig. 25

Figure 26. Chronic deep cerebral lesions; cerebral palsy clinically in a 9-year-old child with history of premature birth. Section of brain shows residues of hypoxic perinatal deep cerebral infarctional damage, with cystic scarring, destruction of basal ganglia and adjoining periventricular structures. Ventricles much enlarged due to loss of cerebral white matter, ex vacuo hydrocephalus.

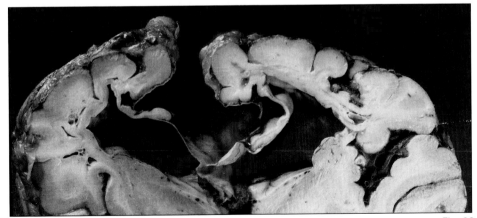

Fig. 26

In the late chronic stage of cerebral hypoxic damage, overall wasting of the cerebral structures is present. Scarring of the cerebral tissue affects the gray matter of the cortex and deep structures, the basal ganglia, with decimation of nerve cell population. White matter is also decreased and replaced in varying degree by scar tissue. Cavitations appear in the white matter and basal ganglia (Figure 27). With the underlying white matter decimated, the cerebral surface shows shrunken, narrowed convolutions, with increased space between convolutions.

Porencephaly (encephaloclastic)

Figure 27. Porencephaly (encephaloclastic). Cerebral white matter replaced by porencephalic cysts. Frontal section through the anterior of the cerebrum. Cerebral palsy in an infant, age 2 months; severe seizures and profound developmental delay.

Large cavitations in the cerebral wall, the result of remote hypoxic breakdown of cerebral tissue, are referred to as encephaloclastic porencephaly (Figure 27). The cavities are lined with scar tissue and contain watery clear fluid. Encephaloclastic porencephaly is distinguished from malformation porencephaly, the result of faulty formation of the cerebrum (page 150).

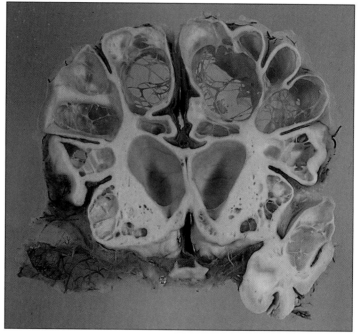

Fig. 27

Basal ganglia damage

Pathologically, the end stage of hypoxic deep cerebral damage, in many cases, presents basal ganglia scars, cavitations, and focal calcification. This is the characteristic pattern of damage in cases of cerebral palsy (page 188).

Damage to the basal ganglia leads to forms of cerebral palsy: **hypertonic**, spastic cerebral palsy with increased muscle tone; **hypotonic** cerebral palsy, with decreased muscle tone; **athetosis**, a disturbance in motor control, with recurring, squirming, purposeless motions and grimacing.

Hydrocephalus ex vacuo

The diffuse loss of cerebral white matter results in a secondary enlargement of the ventricles, **ex vacuo hydrocephalus**. (Figures 35, 36). With the overall compromise of the cerebrum, the brain fails to grow appropriately, resulting in microcephaly.

Ex vacuo hydrocephalus is the condition that develops over the course of months and years, leading to enlargement of cerebral ventricles, characteristic of cases of cerebral palsy. The enlargement of the ventricles is the result of hypoxic damage to the cerebral periventricular strata in the premature immature brain. The damaged tissue later becomes absorbed, contracted, and scarred. In the late stages there is visible loss of periventricular white matter, leaving the ventricles enlarged. Ex vacuo hydrocephalus is usually evident by CT scans in cases of cerebral palsy.

Hydranencephaly

Hydranencephaly appears as an extreme form of hydrocephaly. The picture here is of the cerebral walls almost wiped out, leaving a thin walled bag filled with cerebrospinal fluid (Figures 28a and b).

With hydranencephaly, as with hydrocephalus, the pathogenesis in a given case is often problematic as to whether the defect stems from embryonic life, as a developmental malformation, or is due to total loss of structural substance resulting from encephaloclastic processes during fetal life (Case 39, page 326).

Hydranencephaly is associated with loss of basic cerebral function, leaving brain stem control of vital function more or less intact.

Figure 28(a). Hydranencephaly demonstrated by air ventriculography. (Also see 28(b) next page.)

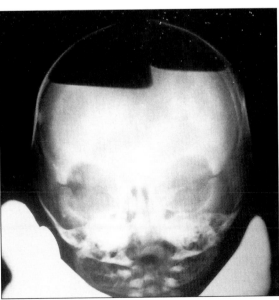

Fig. 28(a)

Figure 28(b). Hydranencephaly. The newborn infant was microcephalic, lived briefly. At autopsy, the cerebrum appeared as a ballooned, thin-walled bag distended with cerebrospinal fluid.

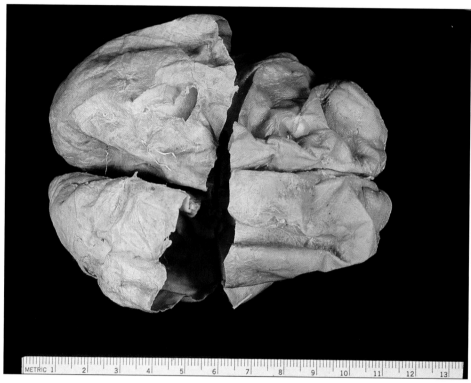

Fig. 28(b)

Status marmoratus

The Vogts (1920) described the condition of status marmoratus, in which the basal ganglia are damaged, scarred, and grossly show confluent mottled white areas resembling the appearance of marble, giving the condition its name (Figure 29). Clinically, the condition, thought to be due to early hypoxic damage, is associated with cerebral palsy. The "marbling" appearance is due to an excessive production of myelin, the fatty material that surrounds nerve fibers.

Figure 29(a). A section through the cerebral basal ganglia showing changes of status marmoratus, small confluent puffy white areas distributed through the gray. From a 19-year-old woman with cerebral palsy, epilepsy, and mental retardation. **(b).** For comparison, basal ganglia with normal structure.

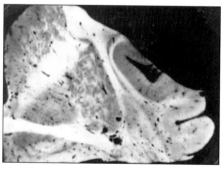

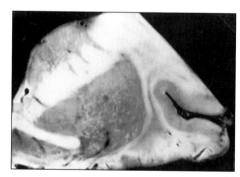

Fig. 29(a)   *(b)*

Microcephaly (encephaloclastic)

Microcephaly, smallness of the cerebrum, with corresponding small size of the head, develops in cases of cerebral palsy as a consequence of deep cerebral damage incurred in the early premature immature fetal life.

The brain normally enlarges due mainly to elaboration, growth, of the deep strata of the cerebrum (not from the cortex). When the deep structures of the cerebrum are damaged during fetal life, the development, growth, of the brain eventually is attenuated, ultimately becoming noticeable as microcephaly during infancy.

Newborn infants at times are microcephalic, with head circumference less than average, the consequence of encephaloclastic deep cerebral damage originating during early fetal life.

The brain in cases of cerebral palsy commonly shows enlarged ventricles of ex vacuo hydrocephalus and overall is small, microcephalic. This is the paradox of microcephaly and hydrocephaly that characterizes the brain in cerebral palsy.

Encephaloclastic microcephaly is to be distinguished from genetic micro-cephaly (page 198).

Imaging studies of hypoxic cerebral damage

Acute hypoxic cerebral damage, fetus and newborn
Subacute hypoxic cerebral damage, fetus and newborn
Chronic (late) hypoxic cerebral damage (in cerebral palsy)

CT studies, as well as ultrasound and MRI studies, in cases of brain damage, reveal evidence, to a greater or lesser degree, of structural changes present.

CT scans show shadows, blacks, grays, and pale translucent areas. Scans can accurately diagnose the size of ventricles, the presence of blood and calcifications, and cavitations, if present. The radiologist, on the basis of scans, cannot validly make pathologic tissue diagnoses, except for speculative interpretation.

Cerebral tissue that has severe damage with diffuse loss of nerve cells (evident on microscopic examination) often is not grossly evident, not evident to the naked eye. Accordingly, it cannot be expected that radiologic studies, ultrasound, CT scans, would validly diagnose the presence or absence of such tissue damage. A CT scan interpretation that says no changes are evident in the cerebral structure does not mean there is no damage to the tissue.

Accordingly, in cases in which the brain scans reveal no change in the basal ganglia, or in the cortex, there may be in fact far-advanced damage, scarring, and nerve cell depletion. In cases of cerebral palsy, the basal ganglia, grossly and on CT and MRI scan, may appear unchanged, but on microscopic exam show devitalized tissue.

In the healthy newborn in the CT scan of the cerebrum, the lateral ventricles are patent (Figures 30 and 31).

Figure 30. Diagram of brain section indicating patent lateral ventricles as in a normal term newborn brain.

Figure 31. CT scan of brain of 1-day-old term newborn; normal ventricles are patent and appear on each side of the mid-upper portion of the cerebrum as semilunar areas of low density. The third ventricle appears as an elongated density in the center of the brain. (Patchy densities posteriorly, subarachnoid hemorrhage in the posterior fossa.)

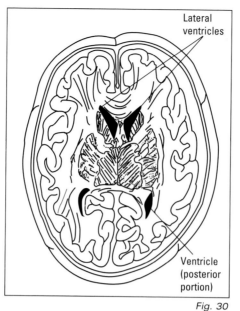

Fig. 30

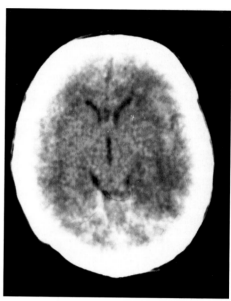

Fig. 31

Imaging studies of acute hypoxic cerebral damage

Illustrative Case:
Case 140   p. 554

In cases of acute hypoxic brain damage, damage of varying severity, the ventricles in the cerebrum become compressed by the edematous swelling of the cerebrum. As seen in the CT scan, the ventricles are obliterated (Figures 32 and 33).

The pattern of acute hypoxic cerebral damage, as evidenced in CT scans and other imaging studies, varies. When the damage is present as a fresh acute hemorrhagic infarct, it is usually readily evident in the CT scan, appearing as areas of increased density.

Figure 32. Diagram of brain illustrating compression of ventricles due to cerebral swelling.

Figure 33. CT scan of the cerebrum; newborn; obliteration of the lateral ventricles due to hypoxic cerebral edema.

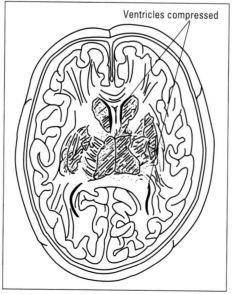

Fig. 32

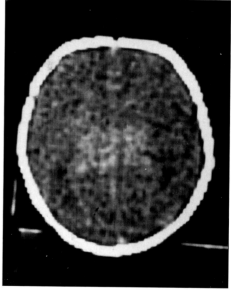

Fig. 33

However, at the other extreme, early acute brain damage, when present extensively, may not show up in the CT scan. In cases studied at autopsy, with CT scans taken prior to death, microscopic studies of the brain at times show areas of acute brain damage, while the CT scan shows no evidence of structural changes.

The presence or absence of obliteration of the ventricles, evident in CT studies of the newborn brain, is of direct major importance in litigation: If there is evidence of cerebral damage in the CT scan, and if the ventricles are clearly patent, it means there is no cerebral edema, no acute pathologic process in the brain; it means the cerebral damage is old, subacute.

Imaging studies of subacute hypoxic cerebral damage

In newborn infants the CT scan at times shows (1) patent cerebral ventricles and (2) focal areas of damage, areas of increased translucency, reflecting damage faradvanced, having origin weeks, months, prior to birth (Figure 34).

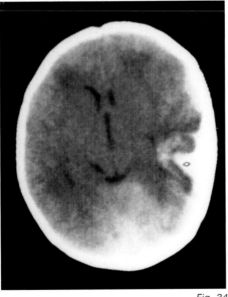

Fig. 34

Figure 34. Newborn CT scan showing large focal lesion in the left temporal parietal region appearing on the right in this image. The lateral ventricles are widely patent. These findings, a large cerebral lesion with patent ventricles, are consistent with subacute cerebral damage incurred some period of time prior to birth.

It is important to emphasize, with regard to cases in litigation, that in such neonatal CT scans, if there is evidence of cerebral damage, and if the cerebral ventricles are visible, patent, it means there is no acute cerebral swelling; it means the damage is old, subacute, not recent, not incurred intranatally during labor and delivery.

Imaging studies of the chronic (late) stage of hypoxic cerebral damage

The (late) chronic cerebral changes that appear in CT scan studies following hypoxic damage incurred in early premature fetal life, in cases of cerebral palsy, show a characteristic pattern; in the CT scans the cerebral ventricles are enlarged (ex vacuo hydrocephalus) due to loss of periventricular white matter; cavitations at times are evident in the cerebral walls, in the basal ganglia (Figure 35). These structural changes correspond to changes observed in pathology studies of brain specimens in cases of cerebral palsy (Figure 36).

Figure 35. CT scan of brain in a case of cerebral palsy. Arrows indicate cavitations in the basal ganglia; ventricles dilated. Compare to Figure 36.

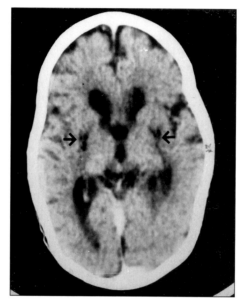

Fig. 35

Figure 36. Cerebral palsy lesions; 8-year-old. Residue of deep cerebral damage incurred during premature fetal life affecting basal ganglia; loss of periventricular white matter and enlargement of ventricles.

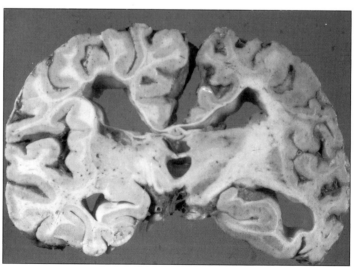

Fig. 36

In cases of severe hypoxic damage in early premature life, with infants surviving, tissue in the cerebral wall disintegrates leaving little or no substance, with the cerebral wall converted to confluent cysts. Infants surviving show severe cerebral palsy and other severe cerebral disability (Figure 37).

Figure 37. CT scan of brain showing chronic pattern of changes with extreme loss of cerebral substance; the cerebral wall is destroyed, replaced by confluent cystic structures. A case of severe cerebral palsy.

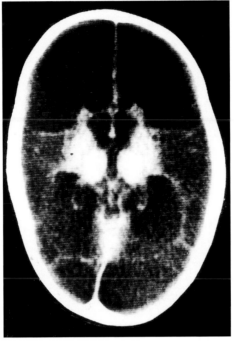

Fig. 37

Hypoxia-producing complications of gestation leading to fetal-neonatal cerebral damage

Maternal complications
Placental defects
Umbilical cord complications
Amniotic sac abnormalities
Amniotic fluid abnormalities
Fetal complications causing hypoxia
Postnatal hypoxia-producing conditions

Biologically, the maternal-placental-fetal complex is delicately balanced, with a narrow margin of safety for the fetus, for the newborn. Considered pathologically, there are, accordingly, four gestational components — maternal, placental, fetal, neonatal — that are subject to complicating pathologic processes that lead to hypoxia, to hypoxic cerebral damage in the fetus and newborn.

Maternal factors — it is a given, clinically and pathologically, that the well-being of the fetus is dependent on the good health of the mother. Illness in the mother exercises its effect directly on the fetus, leading to deprivation of nutrition and oxygenation.

The placenta is the supply organ for the fetus, transferring oxygen from the mother's blood to the fetus' blood in the placenta, with the oxygenated blood then conducted through the umbilical cord circulation to the fetus. Compromise of the structures of the placenta or the cord leads to fetal hypoxia.

The fetus is subject to most all the diseases that affect the adult. The fetus, rendered anemic due to infection or other pathologic processes, becomes chronically hypoxic.

Maternal complications: fetal-neonatal hypoxic cerebral damage

Premature (preterm) labor
    Cervical incompetence
    Tocolytic agents
    Cesarean section with premature labor
Postmature (postterm) labor
Dystocia
Duration of delivery: prolonged, precipitous
Poor reproductive background
Teenage pregnancy
Advanced maternal age
Multiparity
Trauma, maternal
Infectious disease in the mother
    Influenza
    Cytomegalic viral infection
    Herpes simplex
    Rubella
    HIV
    Syphilis
    Gonorrhea
    Chlamydia
Vaginal bleeding
    Postconception vaginal bleeding (vicarious bleeding)
Hyperemesis gravidarum
Maternal anemia
Metabolic disorders
    Low maternal weight gain
    Maternal obesity
    Diabetes mellitus
    Thyroid disease
Heart disease in the mother
Pulmonary disease in the mother
Toxemia: preeclampsia; eclampsia; gestational hypertension
Hypertension
Psychiatric stress
Toxic agents affecting gestation

In many cases, brain damage present at birth is attributable to maternal illness during gestation. Any kind of maternal illness during pregnancy, physical or emotional stress, directly affects the maternal-placental-fetal organization, potentially causing fetal deprivation, debility.

Most forms of maternal illness, acute or chronic, exercise their damaging effect on the fetus through the common denominator of oxygen deprivation, hypoxia. Although all the structures of the body are vulnerable to hypoxic injury during gestation and delivery, the most sensitive target proves to be the brain. Pathologically, hypoxic brain damage at birth is not primarily a brain disorder, is not primarily a local intracranial process; rather, the brain, as a target organ, incurs damage that in effect is the end stage of a syndromic sequence of pathologic processes, processes often originating due to maternal illness (page 6).

The severity of the maternal illness does not necessarily correspond to the degree of fetal damage. A mild maternal illness may prove disastrous for the fetus; at other times the fetus seems to escape manifest damage. The observation that maternal illness is common during pregnancy, with the fetus, the offspring, usually appearing to escape damage — does not alter the fact that in some cases even minor illness in the mother may have devastating effects on the fetus, may lead to miscarriage. Nevertheless, the occurrence and significance of maternal illness during pregnancy often is minimized by clinicians, and often is overlooked, unrecorded.

The clinical record in a case under review often does not supply medical information about the first months of the pregnancy, the first prenatal visit usually coming a month or two after a missed menstrual period. The delivery record commonly notes, perfunctorily, that the course of the pregnancy was "uncomplicated." Often overlooked are details such as an episode of midpregnancy vaginal bleeding. The citation "uncomplicated" would lead one to think that the mother went through the nine months of pregnancy — through a winter — without so much as a cold or URI (upper respiratory infection). This is unlikely. Pregnant women are highly susceptible to colds, to viral infections. Often mothers hesitate to report colds and other illnesses, or they forget. Certainly, in cases under litigation being pursued years after the pregnancy, the mother would not likely recall the occurrence of all her acute illnesses during pregnancy, illnesses adversive to the well-being of the fetus.

Adverse maternal pregnancy factors affecting the fetus are of a wide range. Some factors, such as teenage pregnancy, obesity, psychiatric stress, are of indirect causal nature, unfavorable to the gestation, contributing to increased fetal-neonatal morbidity and mortality. Other maternal factors, complications such as acute maternal infectious disease, especially illnesses with fever, lead directly to fetal damage, to hypoxic cerebral damage.

Premature (preterm) labor

Premature labor is a problem often encountered in obstetric malpractice litigation. Questions arise concerning the effect on the fetus of the treatment of premature labor, the use of tocolytic agents (medication to halt labor), surgical procedures on the uterine cervix to prevent abortion and, with these problems, the early resort to cesarean section.

What are the **pregnancy complications**, the elementary pathologic processes, that develop in the uterus that ultimately lead to the onset of premature labor contractions? Do these antecedent pathologic processes affect the fetus adversely?

The very nature of premature labor implies that something is going wrong in the maternal-placental-fetal complex. At times this "something" is a preexisting pathologic process ongoing over a prolonged period, or is recurrent; many times these intrauterine complications in their beginning are clinically silent, without maternal symptoms. Etiologically, these pathologic processes at times are of maternal origin (maternal anemia, endocrine and metabolic disorders, viral infectious disease, etc.), but more often are of placental origin (placental infarction, placenta previa, premature detachment of the placenta).

The most common cause of premature labor with excessive bleeding at the onset is placental defect, either (1) placenta previa, or (2) premature detachment of the placenta.

Pathologically the effects on the fetus due to premature labor occur in two time periods: the period that antecedes the onset of active uterine contractions, and the period related to the intranatal processes of active labor (page 92).

In the first part of the complication, prior to the onset of active labor, there is a period of varying duration during which the mother is sick, as with an episode of the flu, or a placental detachment or other disorder is beginning — a period during which the fetus is being subjected to varying severity of hypoxia and other deprivation. The damage to the fetus may be far advanced before the onset of labor. Stillborn premature infants may show the effects of prolonged deprivation, subacute and acute hypoxic cerebral damage. It is a mistake to conclude that the brain damage incurred by a prematurely born infant is incurred altogether during the time of the premature labor.

In the second part of the complication, beginning with the onset of active labor, the risk of injury to the premature, immature fetus rises to a climax. The fragile immature fetus is subjected to both mechanical injury and hypoxic damage as it is forced through the rigid, physically unprepared birth canal. It is a misconception to think that the premature fetus, being small, will easily slip through the birth canal.

This sequence of prenatal and intranatal brain damage that affects premature infants obviously varies from case to case, with many infants appearing to escape damage. Obviously too, some premature infants do not escape damage, show acute postnatal and later neurologic disabilities.

Maternal illness, acute viral disease, toxemia, are processes that are associated with a high incidence of premature labor with miscarriage. Uterine disease, cervical incompetence, placental disorders are common causes of premature labor. It is not the province of this volume to detail all the causes of premature labor; this subject is dealt with appropriately in obstetric texts. However, certain aspects of the problem of premature labor do commonly appear in malpractice litigation.

Cervical incompetence: Premature labor

Cervical incompetence refers to the painless dilatation of the uterine cervix during the second or early third trimester, with the consequent onset of premature labor and miscarriage. The application of surgical treatment is a matter of debate. The surgical treatment — the Shirodkar operation cerclage — consists of reinforcing the cervix with an encircling, purse-string, suture during midpregnancy. This treatment often leads to bacterial infection of the cervix, with extension to the intrauterine strata, with chorioamnionitis and placentitis.

Tocolytic agents

The use of tocolytic agents, of medication to halt premature labor, is at times a matter brought up during litigation. The pathologic effects on the fetus are at times questioned. Ethyl alcohol had wide usage in the past to halt labor; its efficacy is doubtful, and it certainly rendered the mother and the fetus and newborn drunk. The adversive effect of other tocolytic agents, isoxsuprine, ritodrine, terbutaline — because of multiple factors involved in assessing fetal-neonatal morbidity and mortality in premature births — remains open to question (page 56).

Cesarean section, with premature labor

Cesarean section is increasingly practiced to terminate premature labor, when labor cannot be halted and birth is inevitable. In such circumstances it is considered better to deliver a relatively intact premature infant by cesarean section early on, before far-advanced brain damage has accrued, and not to subject the fragile fetus to injury by vaginal delivery. The neonatal mortality is two to three times greater in premature infants delivered vaginally than in premature infants born by cesarean section.

Postmature (postterm) labor

Illustrative Cases:
Case 69 *p. 406*
Case 117 *p. 513*
Case 211 *p. 692*

There is an important difference clinically and biologically between postterm gestation and postmature gestation. Prolongation of pregnancy beyond 42 weeks, postterm gestation, is an abnormality of the maternal reproductive function, the cause of which is not clearly known (page 93). In some cases of postterm gestation, the newborn infant, physically and neurologically, is like a baby two or three weeks old — is truly postmature.

Postmaturity per se does not cause hypoxic brain damage. In infants who are postmature, cerebral damage, if present, is attributable to concomitant pathologic processes, at times to placental disorders.

Often postterm babies are not biologically *postmature*. In such cases of postterm gestation, gestation extending beyond 42 weeks, the newborn infants plainly have the physical appearance and neurologic development of an ordinary 40-week gestation. They are simply mature newborn.

Dystocia

Illustrative Cases:
Case 38 *p. 325*
Case 203 *p. 669*

Dystocia (*dys-*, abnormal; *-tocia*, birth) usually refers to a disproportion between the size of the fetus and the size of the birth canal, cephalopelvic disproportion. Accordingly, dystocia may be due to maternal factors or fetal causes. Regarding maternal causes, this condition may be due to a malformed small maternal pelvis. Small women usually have a small pelvis. Or, the bony pelvis may have been deformed by trauma or disease.

Fetal disproportion occurs in cases of maternal diabetes, with the fetus being oversize, macrosomic. It occurs in cases of excessive enlargement of the fetal head.

Dystocia occurs with abnormal fetal presentation, conditions in which the presenting part cannot traverse the birth canal, as with face presentation, with shoulder presentation, with transverse presentation, in which the body of the fetus blocks the birth canal, and with compound presentation as when a limb prolapses alongside the head in traversing the birth canal.

Dystocia per se does not cause hypoxia directly, but if unrelieved, if descent of the fetus is blocked, with labor prolonged for days, the condition becomes ominous for the mother and the fetus. When unrelieved, dystocia may cause rupture of the uterus. More directly, fetal injury—cranial trauma, intracerebral damage, and at times spinal injury — occurs as the head is forced through the birth canal (pages 134, 138). The newborn infant, surviving, harboring intracranial injury, spinal injury, with depression of vital function, depression of respiration, may develop superimposed hypoxic cerebral damage.

Duration of labor

In the clinical-pathologic correlation of neonatal central nervous system damage, it is manifestly evident that the *duration* of labor is a most significant factor. The extremes — prolonged labor and precipitous labor — both are associated with a high incidence of neonatal morbidity and mortality.

Prolonged labor

Prolonged labor connotes the existence of obstetric complications — the presence of factors offering resistance to parturition, impediments producing fetal trauma and hypoxia.

Precipitous labor

Precipitous delivery, with the unmolded head traversing the inadequately relaxed birth canal, fosters intracranial injury and predisposes to spinal injury. It is evident that the safest parturition is that of moderate length.

Poor reproductive background of the mother

Pregnancy outcome is at risk in cases of mothers with poor reproductive history, past pregnancies with vaginal bleeding, premature labor, miscarriages. Often mothers with this history produce compromised infants, with low birth weight, with manifest hypoxic damage.

With a clinical history of poor reproductive performance of the mother in past pregnancies, there is an increased incidence of cerebral palsy in the offspring (Stanley and Alberman, 1984).

Induced abortions are said to be essentially innocuous. Perhaps so. On the other hand, in the clinical prenatal assessment of a pregnancy, a history of multiple (induced) abortions is commonly considered a risk hazard. Pathologically, with multiple abortions — with the endometrial cavity repeatedly invaded, exposed to infection — there often results a smoldering low-grade chronic endometritis, which becomes manifest during gestation as chorioamnionitis.

Teenage pregnancy

Teenage pregnancies have a common scenario: The mother, a high school student, about 16 years old, unwed, unemployed, a primipara, often with problems at home, problems about religion.

Implicit in this circumstance is a substantial element of psychiatric stress added to the pragmatic problems of being pregnant, stress adversive to the mother and to the fetus. Often prenatal care is delayed, with the mother at first trying to hide the pregnancy, coming for prenatal care in midpregnancy. The young mother, not knowledgeable about pregnancy, how to take care of herself, often becomes malnourished, anemic.

There is an increased incidence of fetal and neonatal morbidity and mortality with young primiparous mothers. There is an increased incidence of cerebral palsy in the offspring of young primiparous mothers (Stanley and Alberman, 1984).

Advanced maternal age

Advanced maternal age, over 35 years at the time of pregnancy, is associated with increased fetal morbidity and mortality and low birth weight of the newborn. Advanced maternal age is associated with increased incidence of cerebral palsy.

Multiparity

The number of previous pregnancies influences the outcome of pregnancy. With parity over three, there appears an increase in neonatal morbidity and mortality. The incidence of cerebral palsy is increased in mothers with parity over three.

Trauma, maternal

Trauma is common in late pregnancy, said to occur in varying degree in over 50 percent of pregnancies. Severe trauma of the mother associated with direct trauma to the fetus is rare, the fetus being cushioned, floating in amniotic fluid.

Complications resulting from blunt trauma to the abdomen in pregnant women are rare. When complications occur, they are usually related to premature detachment of the placenta, with the resulting fetal hypoxia (page 68). Blunt trauma to the abdomen with injury to the placenta, at times leads to massive fetal-maternal transfusion (page 97), at times lethal to the fetus.

Severe bodily injury to the mother during pregnancy, as in highway accidents, causing a prolonged state of shock in the mother, leads to cardiac failure, with compromise of circulation to the placenta, rendering the fetus hypoxic.

Infectious disease in the mother during pregnancy

With most forms of acute maternal infectious disease, the damaging effects on the fetus that occur are brought about, not by the fetus becoming infected, but are due secondarily to the factor of maternal sepsis with fever, fever causing fetal hypoxia. Fever in the mother results in increased metabolic oxygen demands by the mother's body. This results in fetal oxygen deprivation, as much as 50 percent decrease with fever of 104 degrees.

Some infectious agents, transmitted to the fetus from the mother, cause damage directly to the brain of the fetus, the most important clinically being rubella (German measles), cytomegalic viral infection (CMV), syphilis, and HIV infection.

Influenza, maternal

Influenza, the flu, in the form of episodes of upper respiratory infection, colds, viral sore throat — when prolonged, with fever, prostration, and weight loss — is a hazard to the mother and fetus (page 118).

Cytomegalic viral infection

CMV in the mother is now recognized as causing serious brain damage in the fetus (page 118).

Herpes simplex

This genital infection, present during pregnancy, is of broad occurrence, with the fetus becoming infected during delivery (page 119).

Rubella

This acute infection, German measles, in the mother during the early months of pregnancy, is well known to cause severe inflammatory damage in the fetal brain (page 120).

HIV infection (AIDS)

HIV infection in the mother, and the effects on the fetus, are of mounting concern clinically. With seropositive mothers, premature labor and low birth weight babies appear frequently. However, the interpretation of the effects of the HIV virus on the fetus in cases of seropositive mothers is complicated by multifactorial fetus-damaging gestational processes, such as maternal malnutrition and drug abuse, processes that are often also present in AIDS mothers (page 121).

Syphilis

Congenital syphilis historically has been noted as a menace to the fetus (page 122).

Gonorrhea

Gonorrhea infection usually remains latent during pregnancy. In some cases, during the first trimester, the infection may reach the fallopian tubes with resulting acute salpingitis and local peritonitis, referred to as PID, or pelvic inflammatory disease. Clinically, fever and sepsis, with abdominal pain, develop.

Chlamydia

Chlamydia infection is a sexually transmitted disease due to the tiny bacterium *Chlamydia trachomatis*. Chlamydia infection is known to be injurious to the newborn.

Vaginal bleeding

Vaginal bleeding is a common and often serious pregnancy condition. It is not a pathologic entity in itself but is symptomatic of an underlying pathologic process, most often a placental disorder. Accordingly, the subject of vaginal bleeding will be dealt with in the section on placental pathology (page 68). The most important pathologic processes of the placenta giving rise to hemorrhage are (1) premature detachment, referred to as placental abruption, and (2) placenta previa, the placenta located abnormally, over the entrance to the cervix (pages 66, 69).

Postconception vaginal bleeding (vicarious bleeding)

A third common form of vaginal bleeding, postconception bleeding, although benign, is of much importance clinically, its occurrence often leading to confusion about gestational age.

Anatomically, the pregravid uterine cavity is lined with a thick mucosa, the endometrium. With menstruation, hemorrhagic desquamation of the endometrial lining takes place.

With pregnancy, bleeding at times occurs near the end of the first month after conception. At this time in the gestation, the endometrial cavity is still partly open, with the enlarging fetus and amniotic sac occupying only part of the uterine cavity. With the endometrial cavity decreased but still patent, oozing hemorrhage from the endometrial lining into the still patent endometrial cavity results in an episode of vaginal bleeding, like a light menstrual period. This process per se does not compromise the gestation; the pregnancy remains intact.

This pattern of vicarious vaginal bleeding is of importance, clinically, commonly leading to errors in calculating the duration of pregnancy. For example, in a case with reported normal menstrual bleeding early, in January, with conception occurring later that month, and with vaginal bleeding, less than usual, in February (vicarious postconception bleeding), if the mother counts her last menstrual period (LMP) as being in February, the calculation of the pregnancy duration, by dates, will be flawed. The gestational age will in fact be older than indicated by the mother's reported LMP.

Although vicarious postconception type bleeding does not compromise the gestation, other causes of bleeding, especially placental abruption and placenta previa, are a hazard to both the mother and the fetus, with the mother becoming anemic, systemically hypoxic, and consequently the fetus is rendered hypoxic.

The importance of vaginal bleeding is sometimes minimized clinically, in that often there appears to be no impact on the pregnancy outcome. However, pathologic processes, such as partial detachment of the placenta, in their origin are often latent, subtle, so that the adverse effects on the fetus are far advanced by the time clinical symptoms of maternal bleeding occur. Throughout this silent period the fetus is compromised, deprived, hypoxic. The amount of vaginal bleeding is not necessarily proportional to the degree of placental disease or to the severity of the fetal damage.

While it may be pointed out that maternal bleeding during pregnancy in some instances appears to be innocuous, and may seem to have no harmful effect on the fetus, the fact is that such episodes of bleeding are often followed by miscarriage, and the fetus at autopsy shows varying severity of acute and subacute hypoxic cerebral damage.

The intrauterine pathologic processes associated with pregnancy bleeding are not an all-or-none thing. While this complication in some instances leads to fetal death and miscarriage, in other instances, with sublethal complications, the compromised fetus survives, with pregnancy maintained to term, with the infant harboring accrued old subacute cerebral lesions, present at birth.

Hyperemesis gravidarum (pernicious vomiting)

Illustrative Cases:
Case 170 *p. 602*
Case 185 *p. 630*

Uncontrollable vomiting may occur during pregnancy, beginning in the second or third month and lasting for months. Emotional problems contribute to the condition. If the pregnancy is undesired the mother may protest, consciously or subconsciously, by vomiting.

Vomiting may lead to serious adverse effects on the mother, compromising the fetus. Anorexia, anemia, and, at times, weight loss occur. Fluid loss, dehydration, electrolyte imbalance develop. The condition usually subsides spontaneously, or with treatment, and the pregnancy is maintained.

Maternal anemia as a cause of fetal hypoxia

Illustrative Cases:
Case 170 *p. 602*
Case 198 *p. 655*
Case 210 *p. 689*

The anemia that occurs in mothers during pregnancy is usually regarded as a deficiency anemia, due to an inadequate diet or, more specifically, due to deficient iron intake. At times maternal anemia is due to recurrent vaginal bleeding.

Anemia in pregnancy is usually of the type characterized as "microcytic, hypochromic," meaning the red blood cells are smaller than normal and under-colored due to deficient hemoglobin in the red cells.

The determination of anemia in the mother is concerned mainly with the hematocrit and hemoglobin levels.

The **hematocrit** reflects the bulk amount of red cells in the blood. This is determined by centrifuging a tube of blood and measuring the height of the blood cell level in the tube, then comparing this to the height of the entire blood column; this is expressed as a percentage. Ordinarily the average hematocrit for women is 38 to 47 percent.

The **hemoglobin** determination is a measure of the amount of hemoglobin, the number of grams per 100 milliliters of blood. The average for women is 12 to 16 grams.

Hematocrit of less than 37 percent, or hemoglobin of less than 11 grams, in pregnant women is a significant abnormality.

Anemia involves a decrease in the red cells in the blood, a decrease in hemoglobin. Hemoglobin is the oxygen-carrying vehicle in the blood. Accordingly, anemia compromises oxygenation of the mother, with resulting decreased oxygen supply to the placenta and to the fetus. While this kind of pregnancy complication may be tolerated by the fetus in many cases, in other instances such oxygen deprivation may lead to intrauterine fetal death or may be sublethal and cause fetal damage, lasting cerebral damage.

Maternal anemia is associated with fetal deprivation that leads to intrauterine growth retardation (Taylor, 1976).

Metabolic disorders

Metabolic disorders in pregnant mothers may substantially compromise the fetus, causing chronic fetal malnutrition and hypoxia. The problems commonly encountered are maternal malnutrition with low pregnancy weight gain, maternal obesity, diabetic conditions, and thyroid disease.

Pregnancy exerts stress on the mother's metabolic equilibrium. In mothers functioning in marginal metabolic balance, the added stress of providing adequate nutrition and oxygenation for a fetus commonly causes latent metabolic disorders to become clinically manifest.

Low pregnancy weight gain

Illustrative Cases:
Case 97   *p. 473*
Case 164   *p. 593*
Case 187   *p. 634*
Case 192   *p. 644*
Case 195   *p. 649*
Case 207   *p. 682*

Low maternal weight gain during pregnancy in many instances is the consequence of an inadequate diet, malnutrition. In other cases, concomitant illness, prolonged nausea and vomiting during pregnancy, or emotional stress are contributory. Other cases are due to subtle, obscure, metabolic factors, difficult to diagnose precisely.

Low maternal weight gain is an ominous sign. Low weight gain compromises fetal well-being and is associated with impaired neonatal outcome, at times accompanied by intrauterine growth retardation of the fetus (Bolognese, Schwartz, and Schneider, 1982).

Maternal obesity

The term "morbid obesity" is applied to women who are extremely overweight, weighing 200 to 300 pounds. Marked obesity is a hazard to the pregnant mother and her fetus (Pritchard, MacDonald, and Gant, 1985). Morbid obesity is reflective of a metabolic endocrine disorder. Obesity per se predisposes to hypertension and to diabetes.

Excessive pregnancy weight gain

Excessive weight gain during pregnancy at times occurs in obese mothers, and also in mothers of average weight. The average optimal weight gain during pregnancy is 20 to 30 pounds. In some instances, in cases of disordered metabolism, the gain may reach 60 to 80 pounds. Excessive weight gain occurs at times in mothers with diabetic conditions.

Diabetes mellitus

Overt diabetes
Prediabetes
"Gestational diabetes"

In pregnancy, diabetes is a hazard to the mother and to the well-being of the fetus and the newborn. The placenta is affected; placental function is compromised. Excessive production of amniotic fluid, hydramnios, is common. The diabetic mother is predisposed to toxemia, eclampsia, and infection; delivery may be complicated by dystocia due to fetal overgrowth, macrosomia.

The severity of fetal hazard is generally related to the severity of the mother's diabetes. Even with diligent control, fetal morbidity is high, with fetal mortality up to 15 percent. There is an increased incidence of miscarriage, with examination of the stillborn fetus showing pathologic changes of hypoxic cerebral damage.

Diabetic conditions are encountered in pregnant women in varied patterns, reflecting the severity of the manifestations.

Overt diabetes

Overt diabetes refers to mothers with known diabetes, insulin-dependent cases (class A diabetes). These women have abnormal carbohydrate metabolism, and when untreated, they have excessive urinary glucose (glucosuria), elevated blood levels of glucose (hyperglycemia), ketoacidosis (acidosis due to high levels of ketones in the blood and urine). Characteristically these women are obese and hypertensive and often present a family history of diabetes.

In the clinical diagnosis of diabetes, the absence of a precise marker continues to be a problem. Clinically, the diagnosis of diabetes is suspected with the finding of an elevated fasting blood glucose over 105.

The **glucose tolerance test** is the common clinical test for diabetes mellitus. The subject ingests a measured amount of a carbohydrate test meal; the level of blood glucose is measured during the subsequent three hours. A rapid and persisting elevation of the blood glucose level is indicative of diabetes. A failure of the blood glucose to return to a normal level at three hours is diagnostic of diabetes.

Hypoglycemia, in mothers treated with insulin medication, at times occurs following exercise or other transient episodes of stress. These brief periods of maternal hypoglycemia do not appear to injure the fetus; the fetus during intrauterine life is known to have physiologically, normally, a relatively low blood glucose level. However, in mothers with poorly controlled diabetes, with recurrent periods of hypoglycemia and keto-acidosis leading to diabetic coma, often the pregnancy ends in miscarriage.

Hypoglycemia in the newborn occurs in some cases of maternal diabetes. The fetus tends to overproduce insulin, to compensate for the mother's deficient production of insulin. This leaves the infant, after birth, with an overproduction of insulin, with consequent hypoglycemia. These cases are often complicated by hypoxia-producing complications. However, hypoglycemia per se does not cause cerebral damage.

The **placenta** in diabetes shows pathologic changes, evident in microscopic examination. At times the function of the placenta is compromised, leading to a state of placental insufficiency, with fetal nutrition and oxygenation becoming defective. In such circumstances, the fetus fails to grow and, paradoxically, the fetus instead of being oversize is small, dysmature.

The fetus and newborn, in cases of maternal diabetes, are often adversely affected. This occurs even in mothers given optimal care, in mothers with good diabetic control. The pathologic mechanisms causing the injurious effects on the fetus are not precisely known.

Macrosomia

At birth, the most characteristic feature in affected infants, in offspring of diabetic mothers, is gigantism, macrosomia (*macro-,* large; *-somia,* body), a newborn weighing 9 or 10 pounds or more (Figure 38). The large newborn infants, despite their hefty appearance, for reasons not well understood, do not do well postnatally, do not thrive. The infants commonly develop respiratory distress syndrome, hyaline membrane disease.

At times, however, offspring of diabetic mothers are small, reflective of intrauterine growth retardation (IUGR).

Malformations in offspring of diabetic mothers

Malformations, especially cardiac and spinal defects, are of high incidence in offspring of diabetic mothers. These defects are apparently of *induced* nature, originating in damage to the embryo or early fetus due to the unfavorable diabetic intrauterine environment (page 141).

Clinical and pathology studies indicate that during early intrauterine life at times the fetus incurs hypoxic cerebral damage and, with the fetus surviving to term, is born harboring old, subacute, cerebral damage of hypoxic origin. In

Illustrative Cases:

Case 5	p. 238
Case 15	p. 269
Case 130	p. 536
Case 149	p. 571
Case 157	p. 583
Case 167	p. 598
Case 177	p. 614
Case 183	p. 626
Case 191	p. 642
Case 203	p. 669
Case 208	p. 684

Illustrative Cases:

Case 167	p. 598
Case 191	p. 642
Case 199	p. 658
Case 203	p. 669
Case 226	p. 724

Figure 38. Macrosomic baby compared to an average-size baby. **(a).** Macrosomic term stillborn infant, early maceration; weight 10 pounds, 6 ounces. Mother had delivered 4 term babies previously, all with birth weight less than 7 1/2 pounds. With this macrosomic newborn, mother suspected of having latent diabetes. **(b).** Term newborn, weight 7 pounds, 13 ounces.

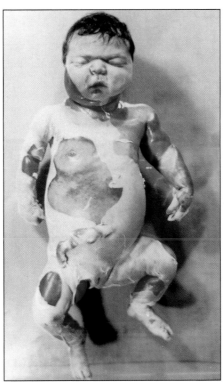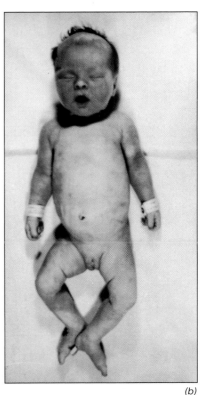

Fig. 38(a)   *(b)*

offspring of mothers with diabetic conditions, there is an increased incidence of cerebral palsy and other cerebral disabilities.

The current standard obstetric practice is to terminate pregnancy in diabetic mothers at 36 to 40 weeks, usually by elective cesarean section. Delivery is accomplished to avoid physical injury and metabolic complications of delivery of an oversize fetus at term.

Prior to delivery the pregnancy is monitored to determine the stage of maturity of the fetus; amniotic fluid is obtained by amniocentesis to test the L-S ratio (lecithin-sphingomyelin ratio; normal at term is 2.0). However, at times the information provided in the L-S monitoring proves misleading, with the infant delivered apparently prematurely, developing treatment-caused, iatrogenic, complications, with subsequent brain damage and later development of neurologic disability—and this forming the basis of a malpractice suit.

Prediabetes

Prediabetes, latent diabetes, refers to cases with a high potential for future development of symptomatic diabetes. Prediabetes is a subclinical disorder of carbohydrate metabolism that may exist for fifteen to twenty years prior to the development of overt diabetes. These women are usually obese, mildly hypertensive, and usually have a family history of diabetes. The glucose tolerance test usually is equivocal or negative; there may be occasional glucosuria.

The first suspicion of prediabetes is the delivery by a primipara of an oversize macrosomic baby weighing nine or ten pounds or more. The hallmark of prediabetes is a succession of oversize babies.

During the latent period of prediabetes, during the nascent period of this disorder, subclinical maternal metabolic, renal, and circulatory changes evolve. These pathologic maternal processes exercise an adversive effect on the fetus. Although the mother shows no outward manifestations, no positive laboratory tests, prediabetes (or diabetes) effects an unfavorable intrauterine environment. The fetus is exposed to adverse intrauterine processes analogous to the damaging processes of untreated overt diabetes. As with maternal overt diabetes, there is an increased incidence of fetal-neonatal morbidity and mortality. Surviving infants at times develop manifestations of cerebral palsy and other developmental disability.

Although the syndrome of prediabetes is well established in medical literature, in obstetric malpractice litigation the occurrence and significance of prediabetes, even when the manifestations are present in the mother, are often overlooked by clinicians, not taken into consideration. In a given case, the link between maternal prediabetes and the development of cerebral disability in the offspring may become substantiated years after the delivery, when the latent prediabetes of the mother emerges as overt diabetes. In cases in which prediabetes is a consideration, cases that come to trial five or ten years after delivery, it is relevant to obtain information about a recent glucose tolerance test and other current information regarding diabetes in the mother.

Gestational diabetes

Gestational diabetes is a clinical diagnosis applied to mothers who initially present with a clinical background pattern characteristic of prediabetes, who during pregnancy develop elevated blood glucose levels and urine positive for glucose; these manifestations of diabetes may persist or disappear after delivery.

Follow-up studies in cases with prediabetes, with gestational diabetes, indicate that overt diabetes develops in 10 to 30 percent of these women in the course of years.

In times past, before the discovery of insulin for the treatment of diabetes, most diabetic women were too ill to conceive. When pregnancy did occur, it was considered a serious complication, often with rapid deterioration of the diabetes, with consequent high rate of maternal and fetal-neonatal mortality.

The advent of insulin treatment dramatically improved the prognosis for pregnancy in diabetic women; with appropriate treatment, today gestation in most cases is maintained, and most offspring develop without manifest disability.

However, despite the present-day improvement in outcome, the pregnant diabetic and her newborn can both be classified as high risk patients.

Despite the well established clinical and pathology evidence showing the damaging effects on the fetus caused by maternal diabetic conditions, in litigation the significance of maternal diabetes in a given case commonly is sublimated, given little consideration with regard to pathogenesis of fetal-neonatal cerebral damage. The fact that the prenatal record indicates a fairly well controlled diabetic status or "gestational diabetes" that reverts after delivery, should not be interpreted clinically or legally as meaning that the gestational diabetic process had no pathologic effect on the fetus, on the newborn.

Thyroid disease in the mother

The thyroid exercises a major role in maintaining a normal gestation. The hazards to the fetus of maternal hypothyroidism or hyperthyroidism are well known.

Both hyperthyroidism and hypothyroidism are adversive to the well-being of the fetus, resulting in an increased occurrence of fetal and neonatal death. Hyperthyroidism, with its associated increased bodily oxygen demand, when present during pregnancy, leads to a relative oxygen deprivation of the fetus.

Heart disease in the mother

Chronic cardiac insufficiency during the child-bearing age is commonly due to old rheumatic heart disease with sequelant heart valve defects. The scarring of the heart valves, particularly the mitral valve, causes heart murmur, "leakage" of the valve, chronically compromising the pump function of the heart. Rheumatic fever also creates scarring of the myocardium; there is no way to reverse this damage. The total effect of old rheumatic heart disease is a chronic compromise of cardiac performance.

With conditions of stress, with the stress of pregnancy, varying severity of cardiac failure, congestive circulatory failure, may appear, rendering the mother hypoxic and, consequently, rendering the fetus hypoxic.

Pulmonary disease in the mother

Obvious pulmonary disease in the mother is an hypoxia-producing hazard for both the mother and the fetus. During pregnancy the body's metabolism, its oxygen requirement, is increased up to 25 percent.

Asthma, pulmonary allergy, often encountered in mothers during pregnancy, is associated with episodes of respiratory insufficiency, especially when complicated by acute respiratory infection. Asthma at times is exacerbated during pregnancy, with the occurrence of severe attacks of respiratory distress exposing the mother and fetus to serious episodic hypoxia.

Toxemia: preeclampsia, eclampsia, gestational hypertension

Toxemia of pregnancy, in the present-day concept, includes clinical patterns of preeclampsia, eclampsia, and gestational hypertension.

(The term "toxemia," implying that the process is due to a toxic agent, is not well chosen; the cause of toxemia remains unclear.)

During pregnancy, affected women develop increasing albuminuria, peripheral edema, retention of fluids, leading to rapid weight gain and increased blood pressure, above 140/90.

When, in addition to these manifestations, there appear neurologic symptoms of headache, dizziness, blurring of vision, and other visceral abnormalities, and when hyperactive reflexes appear, the diagnosis of preeclampsia is made. With the oncoming of lethargy, seizures, and coma, the condition is diagnosed as overt eclampsia.

Toxemia of pregnancy broadly affects the maternal-placental-fetal complex. The visceral changes in this disease — compromise of maternal kidney, liver, cardiovascular, and other visceral functions — begin in a prelusive period, at a time before signs and symptoms appear in the mother. The adversive effects on the mother and fetus begin before albuminuria and hypertension appear. With toxemia, the maternal renal, hepatic, and other metabolic disturbances that occur affect not only the mother, but also the well-being of the fetus.

In the mother, in toxemia, in eclampsia, pathologically the underlying process appears primarily to affect small arteries and arterioles, an arteritis that is associated with thrombotic occlusion of the vessels. These vascular changes appear in the kidney, liver, brain, and other viscera, and in the placenta.

The arterial changes are associated with spasm, causing hypertension and causing decreased blood supply to the uterus, to the placenta, and to the other organs of the body.

In the mother, the pathologic process in the liver, liver necrosis, is analogous to changes in viral hepatitis, with consequent elevation of liver enzymes and bilirubinemia, jaundice. Liver dysfunction affects carbohydrate metabolism, causing hypoglycemia.

The placenta commonly shows gross and microscopic abnormalities. Infarcts at times occur. Microscopically, vascular changes and varied cellular changes are observed. The overall pathologic significance of the placental abnormalities in toxemia, in eclampsia, is a compromise of fetal circulation, a decrease in placental function in supplying the fetus.

There is a high incidence of fetal and neonatal mortality, from 3 to 10 percent, reported in cases of toxemia and eclampsia. In cases of fetal and neonatal death, pathology studies of the brain at times reveal far-advanced hypoxic cerebral damage.

Hypertension (chronic) in the mother

Illustrative Cases:
Case 173   *p. 608*
Case 202   *p. 666*

Hypertension makes its appearance consistently in cases of toxemia. In other cases, chronic hypertension, present previously, becomes increased during pregnancy. Hypertension is commonly found in mothers excessively obese, and in mothers with diabetic conditions.

Regarding the physiology of arterial blood pressure, two pressures are recorded: the "numerator" is the systolic pressure; the "denominator" is the diastolic. The more important, with reference to blood flow and oxygenation of the body, is the diastolic; it represents the baseline measure of arterial circulation. Systolic pressure is volatile, varying upward with physical and emotional stress.

Diastolic pressure, too high, is the fundamental of hypertension.

Ordinarily, "normal" blood pressure is around 120/80, i.e., with systolic below 140 and diastolic below 90.

Most investigators concur that hypertension jeopardizes the fetus by compromising the uteroplacental blood flow (Bolognese, Schwartz, and Schneider, 1982). Compromise of placental blood supply leads to fetal hypoxia.

Hypotension during pregnancy

Illustrative Cases:
Case 141   *p. 556*
Case 200   *p. 661*
Case 206   *p. 679*

Diastolic blood pressure, if chronically low, results in inadequate perfusion, inadequate supply of blood to the brain, and inadequate blood supply to the other organs. Translating this to the effect on the uterus, hypotension during pregnancy results in inadequate arterial perfusion of the uterus, to the placenta, and to the fetus.

This hypotensive lack of perfusion is increased in the mother during the hours of sleep; the "supine hypotensive syndrome" is well known obstetrically.

Psychiatric stress during pregnancy

Illustrative Cases:
Case 128   *p. 532*
Case 183   *p. 626*
Case 209   *p. 686*
Case 214   *p. 700*
Case 215   *p. 702*
Case 216   *p. 704*

There is increasing evidence clinically and experimentally that maternal emotional stress, in the same way as physical illness, has adverse effects on the fetus. Emotional stress disturbs the hormonal and metabolic balance of the mother, impairing her appetite and nutrition. Emotional stress commonly manifests itself in teenage pregnancies, with the mother unwed, indigent, often receiving little prenatal care.

In assessing the importance of maternal stress — in response to the question of what factors in prenatal life can lead to asphyxial neurologic damage—Niswander (1983) emphasizes that not only maternal physical illness but also psychologic disorders exercise an important role in causing fetal cerebral damage: "Quite obviously, maternal stress can and does affect the condition of the fetus." A number of clinical studies on humans and experimental studies on rhesus monkeys confirm the fact that maternal anxiety affects the fetus. It has been explained that the fetal reaction to maternal anxiety is the result of catecholamines from the mother affecting the fetus.

Niswander (1983) points out that, although it is difficult to determine directly the role of maternal emotional stress in causing prenatal fetal brain damage, "there is no reason to think it is a minor one."

Toxic agents affecting the mother during pregnancy

Medications
Anesthetics, analgesics
Pitocin
Tocolytic agents
Industrial pollutants
Addictive substances

Exposure to toxic agents, if the exposure is of a substantial degree, poses a hazard to the mother and the fetus. A great number of substances, from addictive drugs to some ordinary prescription medicines, are known to be hazardous to the fetus.

In assessing the link between toxic substances and fetal damage, it is essential to recognize the multifactorial nature of the problem. Thus, in assessing the effects of excessive smoking during pregnancy, for example, the conclusion reached will be flawed if the focus is on the factor of smoking and does not adequately take into account other adverse gestational conditions common to excessive smoking, factors of emotional stress, inadequate diet, low pregnancy weight gain.

Medications, prescribed drugs

While common sense dictates that certain drugs might harm the developing embryo and fetus, it took the thalidomide disaster, 1960-1962, to focus attention on the potential hazard of medications. Thalidomide taken during early pregnancy resulted in hundreds of deformed babies. With present-day awareness, the list of medicines incriminated as being harmful to the fetus is increasingly long and controversial.

The toxic effect of drugs is difficult to establish. Experimental studies using laboratory animals are not necessarily applicable to man. In experimental studies the high dosages that prove toxic are usually vastly greater than the dosage prescribed clinically in man.

The list of medications that are toxic to the embryo and fetus includes certain antibiotics, diuretics, psychopharmacologic drugs. Essentially, these agents exercise their harmful effects systemically, compromising metabolism and growth during intrauterine life.

Of the antibiotics, tetracycline causes decreased skeletal growth of the fetus. Of the diuretics, the thiazides cross the placenta, causing electrolyte imbalance in the fetus. Of the anticoagulants, coumarin taken during pregnancy is known to cause fetal hemorrhage and stillbirth. Barbiturates, chronically administered to the mother, can produce a withdrawal syndrome in the newborn similar to that of infants of heroin addicted mothers. Of the psychopharmacologic medications given during pregnancy, the phenothiazines may cause seizure-like manifestations in the newborn.

Anesthetics and analgesic agents

At times depression of the newborn is blamed on analgesics such as Demerol and on the anesthesia given during labor. The acute effects on the fetus of analgesics and anesthetic agents administered during labor at times occupy considerable attention with regard to depression in the newborn. This cause-and-effect relationship is open to question, with the depression in the newborn in such circumstances being attributable to factors in the case other than medication.

Experience demonstrates, as evidenced by the routine use of these agents over the years, that anesthetic agents and analgesic agents, per se, do not cause depression, do not cause acute damage in the fetus and newborn.

Pitocin

Pitocin is a synthetically produced agent that has the same pharmacologic properties as oxytocin, the naturally occurring hormone of the pituitary gland. When given during labor, small amounts of the drug probably reach the fetal circulation. There is no substantial evidence that Pitocin when used appropriately has any direct pharmacologic effect on the fetus.

Pitocin increases the contractility of the uterine musculature. Contraction of the uterus, normally and with Pitocin, causes compression of the uterine vasculature with transient decrease in blood supply to the fetus; experience indicates that this transient effect is tolerated by the fetus without damage.

The use of Pitocin requires careful supervision, continuous fetal monitoring. It is contraindicated in the presence of manifest fetal distress, fetal malposition, cephalopelvic disproportion, and with other obstetrically obvious parturitional complications. Pitocin at times is associated with uterine overstimulation, tetanic contractions.

Pitocin is appropriately used to augment uterine contractions when labor is desultory. Pitocin has been used to induce labor when delivery is considered to be in the best interests of the mother and the fetus, as in cases of maternal diabetes. However, in the present day, in such cases, cesarean section is usually done, rather than Pitocin induction.

Tocolytic agents

Medications used to suppress labor are termed tocolytic agents (*toco-*, labor; *-lytic*, dissolve). Ethyl alcohol intravenously has been used, but except in making the mother drunk, and perhaps also the fetus, it has not proven effective in preventing premature birth. No significant depression has been found in the newborn attributable to alcohol.

In present times drugs such as ritodrine have been used as tocolytic agents. Ritodrine and similar drugs sometimes have serious side effects of tachycardia and hypotension. Although these agents have been termed successful by proponents, recent studies cast doubt on their effectiveness.

Industrial pollutants

Pollution of the environment with industrial waste, with contamination of water supply and food, has been suspected as a cause of poisoning during pregnancy. Of particular concern has been pollution with lead and mercury. Ingestion of mercury-contaminated fish is thought to cause fetal death or neurologic disability in surviving infants.

Addictive substances

Heroin
Cocaine
Alcohol abuse
Nicotine (smoking)
Caffeine

There are millions of heroin and cocaine addicts in this country. A substantial portion of this addict population comprises women of childbearing age. Many pregnant women continue to use hard drugs during pregnancy. In some cities, in medical centers with large obstetric departments, maternal drug addiction occurs with an incidence of 10 percent or more of deliveries.

Heroin addiction during pregnancy

Illustrative Case:
Case 193   *p. 646*

Maternal heroin addiction is harmful to the fetus, to the newborn, in two ways, mainly causing low birth weight and causing the neonatal drug withdrawal syndrome.

Low birth weight occurs in over 50 percent of infants born of heroin addicts. Prematurity, stillbirth, and early neonatal death are frequent. The cause of the poor pregnancy outcome is multifactorial, due in large measure to prenatal neglect, poor diet, low pregnancy weight gain, anemia, or infections in the mother.

Withdrawal symptoms appear in over half of infants born to addicts and, without appropriate treatment, an appreciable number of these babies die. The withdrawal syndrome is characterized by central nervous system manifestations of irritability, jitteriness, tremulousness, and sleeplessness. Tachypnea and gastrointestinal manifestations of vomiting and diarrhea occur.

The long-term effects of maternal heroin addiction on surviving children is unclear. The IQ is usually normal. However, many children develop manifestations of hyperactivity and varied other emotional disturbances, and demonstrate neurologic "soft signs" reflecting organicity, latent cerebral damage. These sequelant problems, common generally in infants of low birth weight, are attributable to the gestational compromise of the fetus, rather than to the heroin.

The effect of heroin as a specific toxin directly damaging to the fetal nervous system remains uncertain.

Cocaine addiction during pregnancy

Cocaine appears to be gradually replacing heroin as the drug of choice among hard drug addicts. Over 10 percent of mothers take cocaine during pregnancy. Low birth weight, premature delivery, and a high incidence of perinatal death occur with maternal cocaine addiction.

Withdrawal syndrome, manifestations of irritability, tremor, and sleeplessness occur but are of lesser frequency and less severe than in offspring of heroin addicts.

The intrauterine growth retardation is attributable, as in cases of maternal heroin addicts, to fetal malnutrition brought on by maternal ill health, inadequate prenatal care, poor diet, infection, low pregnancy weight gain. These maternal factors, producing an unstable intrauterine milieu, are hypoxia-producing processes that affect the fetus. Cases have been reported with acute hypoxic cerebral damage in infants born to cocaine-addicted mothers. Pathologically, such damage is attributable to the intrauterine fetal deprivation, hypoxia, rather than to the effects of cocaine per se. Whether or not cocaine has a direct specific toxic effect on the nervous system is open to question.

Alcohol abuse during pregnancy

Fetal alcohol syndrome

Alcoholic mothers who continue to drink heavily during pregnancy give birth to babies born alcohol dependent, the fetal alcohol syndrome. The babies are underweight, enfeebled, and fail to thrive.

Does alcohol have a specific toxic effect on the brain during intrauterine life? Experimental studies in animals have mainly proven negative. However, in humans it is apparent that at times, with heavy alcoholic consumption early in pregnancy, the embryo is affected, with resulting brain abnormalities of varying severity, including anencephaly and other severe cerebral abnormality.

Lesser cerebral abnormality is often apparent in offspring of alcoholic mothers, as indicated in an abnormal EEG and defective intellectual development.

The question remains as to whether some or all of the manifestations of the fetal alcohol syndrome are due specifically to the toxic effect of ethyl alcohol, or whether the cerebral manifestations are the result of other adverse brain-damaging gestational factors present with alcoholic mothers. As with other addictions, with maternal substance abuse, the pregnancy is complicated by multifactorial problems, with maternal emotional stress, malnutrition, infections, anemia. These maternal gestational problems are potentially hypoxia-producing hazards for the fetus. The mother's gestational complications impact adversely on the fetus, with the infant at birth small and underweight, anemic, and enfeebled, and often harboring acute and subacute hypoxic cerebral damage.

Social drinking

What is the effect of social drinking on gestation? Will a glass of wine or a cocktail at dinner result in low birth weight babies and mentally defective children?

Warning women about *excessive* alcohol intake *is* warranted.

However, in the United States, literature that reaches the mother implies that even an occasional alcoholic drink is toxic to the fetus. Experience dictates that this is a fallacy: In Europe — in France, Italy, Spain — wine is traditionally an everyday drink, yet these countries do not breed a population of low birth weight babies and mentally defective children.

Smoking during pregnancy; nicotine addiction

At the first prenatal examination, routinely the mother is asked about smoking; the prenatal record always has an entry regarding smoking, and the amount. The implication here is that smoking during pregnancy is bad, a no-no.

The case against tobacco is strengthened by substantial statistical research reports indicating that excessive smoking during pregnancy, one and a half packs a day, increases stillbirths and low birth weight babies. Other research reports contend that some statistical reports are flawed, that often overlooked in these studies are the coincident factors of poverty, poor diet, low pregnancy weight gain, and emotional stress common to mothers that are heavy smokers.

However, it remains problematic whether or not an occasional cigarette smoked during pregnancy is harmful. Nevertheless, if problems develop in the outcome of the pregnancy, and if the mother smoked during the pregnancy, commonly the smoking is pointed to as having contributed to the pregnancy problem.

Caffeine: coffee and tea consumption during pregnancy

Many agents encountered in daily living, like caffeine, have been indicated in medical and lay literature as harmful to pregnancy. Many of these conclusions are based on rationalization, unsupported by comprehensive clinical or pathologic studies.

In early studies, caffeine consumption during pregnancy was linked to various adverse outcomes, including spontaneous abortion, birth defects, and low birth weight. In 1980, the Food and Drug Administration removed caffeine from the list of substances regarded as safe during pregnancy. Subsequent clinical studies refuted this reported link between caffeine consumption and adverse gestational outcome. In 1993 the National Institutes of Health completed a multicenter study of a cohort of 431 pregnant women, monitoring caffeine exposure, exposure to other risks, fetal growth by ultrasonography, and pregnancy outcome. The study concluded that there was no evidence that moderate caffeine use increased the risk of spontaneous abortion, intrauterine growth retardation, or microcephaly, after accounting for other risk factors (Mills et al., 1993).

Placental defects: fetal hypoxia

Pathologic processes affecting the placenta, especially premature detachment and infarction, in many cases cause fetal hypoxia, with hypoxic cerebral damage, with sequelant neurologic disabilities in surviving infants.

Placental anatomy

As viewed at delivery, the placenta is a discoid structure, at term about 15 to 20 centimeters in diameter and 2 to 3 centimeters thick, and usually weighing 450 to 500 grams, one pound. The weight of the placenta at term is about one-seventh that of the fetus; earlier in gestation the placenta is proportionately larger than the fetus.

The placenta and umbilical cord are essentially of fetal origin. The amniotic membrane over the placenta and lining the amniotic sac is intrinsically of the same origin structurally as the skin over the fetus.

The architecture of the placenta, the internal anatomic details that make up the placenta, are diagrammed in Figure 39. The relationship of the placenta to the uterus, the attachment of the placenta to the inner aspect of the uterine wall, is indicated.

The fetal surface of the placenta is covered by the glistening, translucent, skin-like **amnion**. At the margin of the placenta the amnionic membrane is continuous with the lining of the amniotic sac. Deep to the amnion is a cellular layer, the **chorion** (inflammation of the surface of the amniotic sac is called chorioamnionitis). At the attachment of the umbilical cord to the placenta, the amniotic membrane of the placenta continues uninterrupted to form a sheath around the umbilical cord; the amnionic membrane of the cord is, in turn, continuous with the skin of the fetus covering the abdomen.

Figure 39. Diagram of placental architecture: section through the placenta and attached wall of the uterus. Umbilical cord; umbilical arteries (two) from the fetus, carrying deoxygenated blood; large branches extending over the placental surface, under the amnion; small branches in the arborizing chorionic villi, in the placental cotyledon. Concomitant small venous tributaries arising in the chorionic villi, draining into large surface veins over the placenta, and then into the (single) umbilical vein, returning oxygenated blood to the fetus. Maternal uterine arteries emptying into the intervillous spaces supplying oxygenated blood; uterine veins exiting from the intervillous space discharging deoxygenated blood into the maternal circulation.

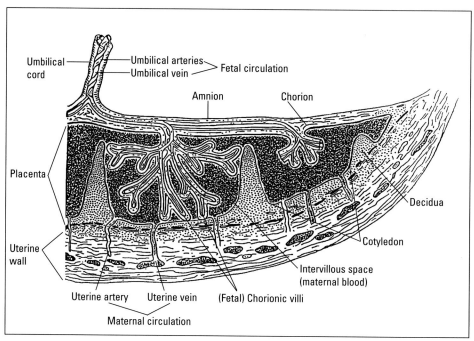

Fig. 39

The maternal surface of the placenta is composed of irregular, compact lobules, **cotyledons** (Figure 39). The tissue overall is dark red, spongy, bloody. During pregnancy the maternal surface of the placenta is tightly attached to the inner aspect of the wall of the uterus. The cotyledons are separated from the muscle layer of the uterus by a cellular tissue, the decidua, derived from elements of the endometrium that lines the nongravid uterus.

At delivery the placenta separates from the wall of the uterus along the plane indicated by the line of cleavage (broken line in Figure 39).

Histologically, the structure of the placenta as viewed on a slide under the microscope is shown in Figure 40.

In the premature placenta the chorionic villi, cut across (transected), appear as small islands, prominently vascularized. The surface of the villi in the premature placenta is covered with cuboidal epithelium (Figure 40b); the presence of cuboidal epithelium in a microscopic section of the placenta identifies the placental tissue as being of premature gestation. The chorionic villi during gestation are surrounded by (maternal) blood in the intervillous spaces (the blood usually escapes from around the chorionic villi during preparation of the pathology slide).

Figure 40(a). Histologic section of a premature placenta. Chorionic villi appear in transection as small islands; villi are relatively large, vascular, and covered with characteristic cuboidal epithelium.

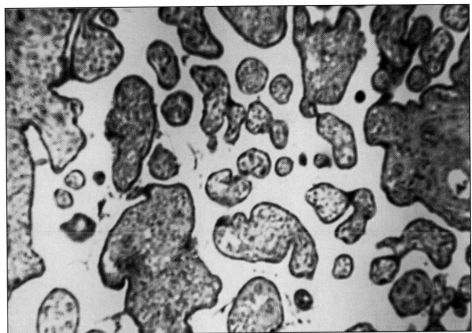

Fig. 40(a)

Figure 40(b). Chorionic villi showing cuboidal surface epithelium characteristic of the premature placenta. Higher magnification of villi appearing in center of (a).

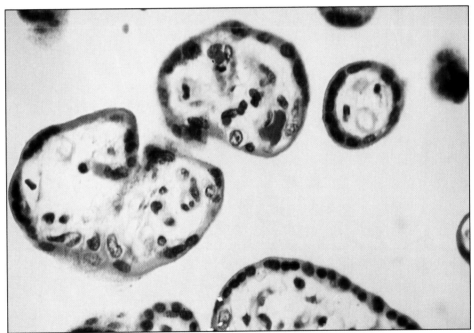

(b)

Figure 41. Histologic section; term placenta. Characteristic of the term placenta are syncytial knots, deep-staining angular concretions, on the surface of the chorionic villi.

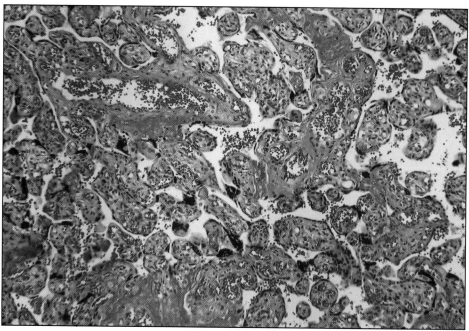

Fig. 41

At term the mature placenta microscopically (Figure 41) shows a flattening of the surface epithelium of the chorionic villi. During the last weeks of a term pregnancy, as the placenta nears maturity, the surface of the villi, here and there, acquires spotty, cellular, dark-staining accretions, "syncytial knots." The presence of syncytial knots identifies the tissue as being of mature gestation. Syncytial knots are abundant in postterm placentas. Focal calcium deposits often appear in term placentas, scattered over the maternal surface, and are usually prominent in postterm placentas.

Physiology of the placenta

In the maternal-fetal organization, the placenta functions as a physiologic interchange, a transport organ that delivers oxygen and nutriments from the mother to the fetus and, in the other direction, conveys metabolic waste products from the fetus to the maternal system.

Placental circulation

Circulation through the placenta functions through two separate vascular systems, the fetal circulation and the maternal circulation (Figure 39).

In the fetal circulation, (deoxygenated) blood from the fetus is carried through the two umbilical cord arteries to the placenta. There, the arteries branch out, ramify, in the villi as small arterioles, capillaries. In the closed vascular system of the fetus, (oxygenated) blood is returned via small tributaries in the villi to the umbilical cord vein, to the fetus.

Maternal placental circulation begins as branches of uterine arteries entering the placenta, ramifying, and opening into "lacunae" (lakes). The finger-like villi project into the maternal blood in the lacunae.

In this system, the blood of the fetus and that of the mother circulate in separate channels. The maternal blood bathes the villi in a way similar to water in the soil bathing roots of plants.

Substances that can diffuse through cellular membranes pass through from the mother's blood into the blood of the fetus — substances such as oxygen, nutritive material, antibodies. Coincidentally, substances in the blood of the fetus diffuse into the mother's blood — among them, waste products, urea, carbon dioxide, water.

Theoretically, there is no intermixture of fetal and maternal blood cells, the cells being too large to penetrate the placental filter. However, in fact, in most pregnancies, if not all, there is some breakthrough, some escape of fetal red cells into the maternal circulation.

Pathology of the placenta

The importance of systematic examination of placentas is reflected in the following study.

Laboratory examination of the placenta

Investigation of hypoxic damage incurred during fetal life, the diagnosis of underlying pathologic processes, in many cases depends on information derived from study of the placenta. The placenta should be examined in detail for pathologic changes, especially in cases with complications during pregnancy and delivery and in cases with fetal, neonatal, compromise evident at birth.

Biologically, the maternal-placental-fetus relationship is delicately balanced. The placenta has a narrow margin of safety. Maternal disease, as well as placental disorders and other intrauterine disturbances, immediately affect the fetus. The importance of the placenta pathologically, the role of this organ in the genesis of fetal disability, especially cerebral damage, is increasingly clear. Studies in the Collaborative Perinatal Project (1965) focused attention on the importance of the placenta, the role of this organ in the genesis of fetal-neonatal organic damage, especially hypoxic brain damage (Towbin, 1970b).

In our own studies, in a clinical-pathologic analysis of 1,000 consecutive deliveries, obstetric records were correlated with the routine laboratory examinations of the placentas; in this series, 23.4 percent of the placentas had significant pathologic changes (page 65) (Towbin and Turner, 1972). The occurrence of such placental defects was in general related proportionately to a decreased Apgar score. In cases with major placental defects, such as large infarctions and large retroplacental hematomas, with perinatal hypoxic death, there was consistently present moderate-to-severe infarctional damage at autopsy in the viscera, most often affecting the brain. This relationship, the frequent occurrence of cases in which disease of the placenta leads to hypoxic damage in the cerebrum, defines a consistent cause-and-effect pattern, the **placental-cerebral syndrome**.

The necessity, clinically and medicolegally, for a careful examination of placentas cannot be overemphasized. In many instances, in obstetric cases in which there is hypoxic fetal damage, basic information bearing on the etiopathogenesis can be obtained only from detailed study of the placenta. To obtain a substantial definition of the cause of a perinatal death, laboratory study of the placenta, correlated with a competently performed autopsy, is mandatory. If the placenta is not submitted to the laboratory for examination, is discarded in the delivery room as is the common practice, essential information is lost and, in many instances, the cause of the fetal-neonatal injury remains enigmatic. Consequently, with organic injury present at birth, the causal mechanism uncertain, and the underlying pathologic process overlooked, responsibility for the infant's disability or death is often misinterpreted.

The Norwood Project: Placental studies

The Norwood Project was a pathology laboratory analysis of the placentas in 1,000 consecutive deliveries, a study undertaken in 1972 at Norwood Hospital, Norwood, Massachusetts (Towbin and Turner, 1972). Table 2 details the major findings in this study.

Table 2.

Study of the Placentas in 1,000 Consecutive Deliveries:

NORWOOD PROJECT

Major Pathologic Conditions	Number
Infarct, large	55 (5.5%)
Abruption, large	76
Meconium staining, heavy	45
Postmature placenta	21

Other major lesions
    Chorioamnionitis, placenta previa, vasa previa,
    thick circumvallate, erythroblastosis fetalis, cord
    compression (tight knots), thrombosis of cord
    vessels, laceration of cord
	37

Major lesions in 1000 placentas, total	234

Major structural abnormalities were present in 234 (23.4 percent) of the placenta specimens. Of these cases, 131 placentas (13.1 percent) presented pathologic processes (large infarcts, 55; large retroplacental hematomas, 76) capable of impacting unfavorably on the gestation, on the fetus.

Minor placental abnormalities were frequent, such as small infarcts (155); small retroplacental hemorrhages (26); umbilical cord with abnormal attachment, eccentric, marginal, or membranous (190 cases); bilobed placentas (24 specimens).

The significance of the placental pathologic findings is evident in Table 3, which presents the five-minute Apgar scores in cases with major placental abnormalities. Early in the study it was evident that, paradoxically, in many cases with major pathologic placental conditions, such as large infarcts, there was no apparent immediate effect on the fetus, with the newborn in good condition, with a five-minute Apgar score of 8 to 10 (Table 3).

Table 3.

Apgar Scores (5-minute) in Cases with Major Placental Defects

Apgar score of 10, 9, 8	12% with major placenta lesions
Apgar score 7, 6	31% with major placenta lesions
Apgar score 5, 4	52% with major placenta lesions
Apgar score 3, 2, 1	72% with major placenta lesions
Apgar score 0 (stillborn)	76% with major placenta lesions

On the other hand, the majority of infants with a five-minute Apgar score of 5 or less had major placental pathologic conditions.

In the 1,000 pregnancies studied, there were 26 neonatal deaths; 20 of the deaths, 76 percent, had associated major placental abnormalities.

To further emphasize the importance of pathology laboratory examination of placentas, data in this study of 1,000 deliveries showed that in the 234 cases with major placental abnormalities that were noted in the pathology laboratory examination, in 141 of these cases, 60 percent of the deliveries, the placental abnormalities were overlooked in the delivery room, were not noted in the delivery record.

When placentas are not submitted to the laboratory for examination and are discarded in the delivery room, as is the common practice, 60 percent of placentas with major abnormalities will go undiagnosed.

The importance of this lies in the fact that often in cases with manifest newborn hypoxic brain damage, in the infants who develop cerebral palsy, lack of valid information about the placenta leads to a flawed interpretation of causation.

As noted in the Norwood Project, the two predominant placental hypoxia-producing pathologic conditions that compromise gestation are premature detachment and placental infarcts.

Abruption: premature detachment of the placenta

Premature detachment, abruption, is the most important placental complication that affects the mother and the fetus (Table 2, page 64).

Anatomically, the placenta is tightly adherent to the inner aspect of the uterine wall. At times a part of the adherent placenta becomes loosened, separated, from the uterine wall. With detachment of a part of the placenta, a pocket forms between the placenta and the uterine wall, a pocket filled with blood clot, a retroplacental hematoma (Figures 42 and 43).

The cause of premature detachment is not precisely known. Sometimes there is an underlying antecedent placental infarct at the site of the abruption (see Figure 48, page 72; Figure 382, page 448).

Figure 42. Abruption of the placenta. The illustration shows a retroplacental hematoma between the placenta and the uterine wall, with flattening of the underlying placental cotyledons. Extension of the bleeding downward, dissecting between the uterine wall and amnion through the cervix, with bleeding into the vagina.

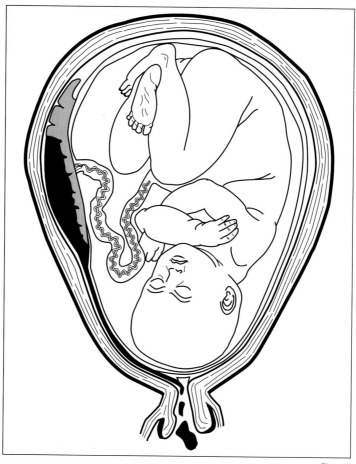

Fig. 42

Figure 43. Abruption of the placenta at 34 weeks of gestation. Placenta with adherent fresh retroplacental hematoma. The mother on admission had an upper respiratory infection and slight vaginal bleeding. Stillborn infant with cyanosis. Autopsy, fetal congestive heart failure with hydrothorax.

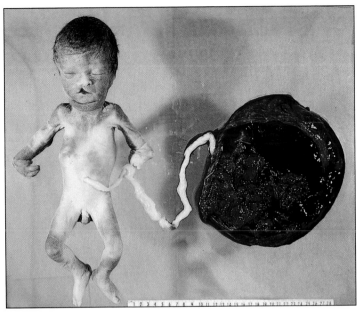

Fig. 43

Regarding the source of the blood in cases with retroplacental bleeding, the blood has its origins from the mother's circulatory system, not from the fetus. The circulatory system of the fetus is a closed system, independent of the mother's circulatory system. Anatomically, in the placenta, the vascularized fetal villi project finger-like into "lakes" of maternal blood (the intervillous spaces) that occupy the deep strata of the placenta, adjoining the uterine wall. Blood in the placental lakes comes from arteries in the adjacent uterine wall, maternal blood that empties into the "lakes." (Figure 39). With premature detachment of the placenta, the cleavage taking place between the inner aspect of the uterine wall and the adjacent deep surface of the placenta that harbors the large blood lakes, the bleeding comes from opened uterine arteries that previously supplied the blood lakes.

The size of the retroplacental hematoma varies from case to case, from a few centimeters wide to a clot that occupies half or more of the maternal surface of the placenta.

The attachment, the degree of adherence of the clot to the placenta, is important pathologically with regard to determining the age of the retroplacental clot, the duration of the abruption.

Fresh retroplacental hematomas, fresh clots of recent origin that develop just prior to delivery, are dark red, gelatinous, and, being only lightly attached, at times float away at delivery. Thus sometimes the presence of a retroplacental hematoma is missed, mistaken for a postpartum mass of clot.

Old retroplacental hematomas, clots present for weeks and months, become firm, rubbery, red-brown, indent the maternal surface of the placenta and become more or less "organized," with proliferation of cells making the clot adherent to the maternal surface. The process of organization is slow; pathologically its presence means the clot has been in place a long time.

Ultrasound studies of the mother prenatally in cases with suspected abruption may or may not reveal evidence of a retroplacental hemorrhage.

Occult retroplacental hemorrhages are clots that remain localized, walled off, organized. Small occult retroplacental hematomas are common and usually innocuous.

The effects of retroplacental hemorrhage depend on the size of the hemorrhage and, importantly, on the extension of the bleeding. There are three main dangers to the mother and to the fetus: premature labor triggered by the retroplacental hemorrhage; placental insufficiency; vaginal bleeding of various severity (bleeding into the amniotic sac).

Premature labor results at times due to the irritant effect of the blood clot on the subjacent uterine muscle.

Placental insufficiency develops in cases with large, long-present, retroplacental hematomas. That part of the placenta that is separated, walled off by the clot, is put out of function, leading to placental insufficiency, to interference with fetal oxygenation and nutrition. In this circumstance the fetus fails to thrive and is born nutritionally deprived (IUGR) and, pathologically, harboring old subacute hypoxic cerebral damage due to the chronic intrauterine hypoxia.

Vaginal bleeding is common in cases of premature retroplacental hemorrhage. Blood from the retroplacental hemorrhage dissects its way downward to the cervix and out into the vagina (Figure 42, page 66).

Of clinical importance in cases of vaginal bleeding is the problem of differentiation between placental premature detachment and placenta previa (infra). With premature separation, the onset of bleeding may occur early or at midpregnancy or near term. In contrast, placenta previa bleeding characteristically has its onset in the weeks prior to term.

In the study by Latham, Anderson, and Eastman (1954) stressing the importance of vaginal bleeding affecting pregnancy, these investigators commented, "Bleeding in pregnancy means as a rule only one thing and that is placental separation of a greater or lesser degree. In turn, placental separation, according to its degree, must necessarily mean some encroachment on the oxygen supply of the fetus and when more than one-third of the placenta is detached fetal death from anoxia usually ensues."

Vaginal bleeding may be minimal, with little apparent effect on the gestation, reported by the mother as recurrent "spotting." This spotting bleeding over a period of weeks, may ultimately render the mother anemic, cause hypoxia, adversely affecting the mother and the fetus.

Severe vaginal bleeding develops at times, catastrophically, with rapid exsanguination of the mother and, unrelieved, leads to shock and death.

At times, the retroplacental hemorrhage penetrates inward, with bleeding into the amniotic sac, with the amniotic fluid becoming "port-wine" colored. This breakthrough into the amniotic sac varies in severity, at times leading to sudden exsanguination bleeding, with the pregnant abdomen becoming even larger, rigid, of board-like hardness, as the amniotic sac fills with blood, and with the mother collapsing, in shock.

The maternal-placental-fetal complex is delicately, marginally, balanced. The intrauterine pathologic processes associated with pregnancy bleeding are not an all-or-none thing. While this complication in some instances leads to fetal death and miscarriage, in other instances, with sublethal complications, the fetus, compromised, survives.

There is a known high incidence, in my experience and that of other pathologists, of stillbirths associated with abruption, with maternal bleeding, with the fetus at autopsy showing hypoxic cerebral damage.

While it may be pointed out that maternal bleeding during pregnancy in some instances appears to be innocuous, and may seem to have no harmful effect on the fetus, the fact is that such episodes of bleeding are often followed by miscarriage, and the fetus at autopsy shows varying severity of acute and subacute hypoxic cerebral damage.

Parenthetically, in infants surviving, in cases with a history of maternal bleeding during pregnancy — there is a high incidence of cerebral palsy and related cerebral difficulties (Stanley and Alberman, 1984, p. 95; Latham, Anderson, and Eastman, 1954).

Placenta previa

Illustrative Case:
Case 123   *p. 523*

This is a cause of vaginal bleeding, much less frequent than premature placental detachment. It occurs in fewer than 1 percent of pregnancies.

The term "previa," from the Latin "ahead coming," pictures the placentation being located ahead of the fetus, with the placenta emplaced over the internal opening of the cervix (Figure 44).

Figure 44. Placenta previa. The placenta lies over the internal os of the cervix. The placental cotyledons at the cervix lie exposed, giving rise to bleeding into the cervical canal, into the vagina.

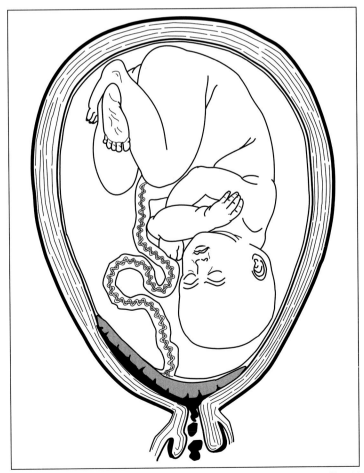

Fig. 44

The cause of placenta previa is unclear; the condition results from the ovum being implanted low in the uterus. Maternal advanced age, multiparity, and previous cesarean section appear to increase the risk of placenta previa.

Pathologic patterns of placenta previa

With the placenta located in the lower internal segment, in a part of the uterus with less nutritional power, the placenta previa tends to spread out, is large and thin.

Four forms of placenta previa occur, with reference to the relationship of the placenta to the internal opening of the cervix (internal os) (Figure 45).

Figure 45. Placenta previa. Four anatomical forms with reference to the location of the placenta to the internal os. **(a).** Total or central form, with the middle of the placenta over the internal os. **(b).** Partial, with a lateral portion of the placenta covering the internal os. **(c).** Marginal, with the edge of the placenta reaching the internal os. **(d).** Low-placed placenta, with the placenta above the internal os, in the lower uterine segment.

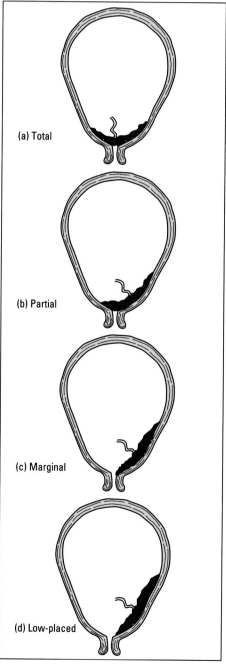

(a) Total

(b) Partial

(c) Marginal

(d) Low-placed

Fig. 45

Figure 45(a) demonstrates "total" placenta previa, sometimes called "central" placenta previa, with the center of the placenta over the internal os. Figure 45(b) shows "partial" placenta previa, in which the internal os is covered by the outer, lateral, part of the placenta. Figure 45(c) shows the "marginal" form of placenta previa, with the edge of the placenta reaching the internal os. Figure 45(d) shows the form known as "low-lying" placenta; the placenta occupies the lower segment of the uterus, the edge of the placenta not reaching the internal os.

The onset of vaginal bleeding with placenta previa, as previously noted, usually comes during the last weeks of a term pregnancy. At this time, the cervix softens, thins, and may dilate slightly, especially in the multipara. With the cervix softening and thinning, the placenta cotyledons are torn loose and bleed.

In this circumstance, with bleeding, ultrasound of the uterus usually clearly demonstrates the placental location, the placenta previa.

Clinically, in the present day, with prompt ultrasonic diagnosis and cesarean section, adversive effects in the mother and fetus have been much reduced.

Infarcts of the placenta

Clinically, placental infarcts are important, at times adversely affecting the gestation, compromising oxygenation and nutrition of the fetus, resulting in fetal intrauterine growth retardation (IUGR), at times death of the fetus. Affected fetuses accrue hypoxic cerebral damage and, surviving, the infant later develops cerebral palsy and other cerebral disabilities.

Pathology of placental infarction

An infarct, in the placenta as in other organs, is a circumscribed devitalized portion of the organ that results from local interference with circulation to the part. Infarcts of the placenta are due to obstruction of the uteroplacental circulation. The underlying cause of the circulatory obstruction is not clear. There is some evidence that the occurrence of placental infarction is increased in pregnancies complicated by maternal hypertension, toxemia, diabetes. In premature births, placental infarction occurs at times, but here cause-and-effect is unclear.

The size of infarcts in placentas varies; small infarcts of 2 to 3 centimeters are grossly recognizable, are often multiple, and are present in 10 to 20 percent of placentas.

Large placental infarcts, 4 centimeters or greater, occur in about 1 in 20 placentas (Table 2, page 64). At times the infarction occupies half or more of the placental plate (Figure 46).

Figure 46. Placental infarct.
(a). Maternal surface. The lower right half of the placental plate is infarcted; at delivery, the infarct was pale and indurated, consistent with an old infarction.
(b). Transection through the placenta with the infarcted pale portion on the right.

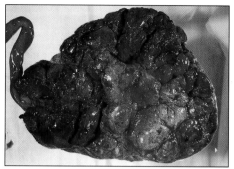 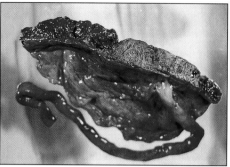

Fig. 46(a)   *(b)*

The gross and microscopic appearance of placental infarcts varies with the age of the lesion.

A fresh infarct grossly is dark red, firmer than the surrounding healthy tissue (Figure 47).

Figure 47. Fresh infarct of the placenta. The transected placenta shows a demarcated gray-red portion, tissue with fresh infarction.

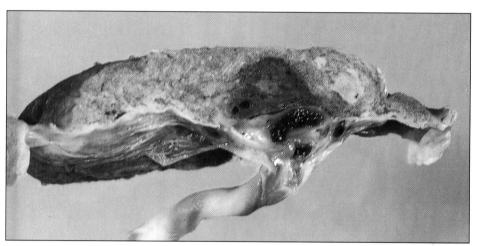

Fig. 47

As the infarct ages it becomes increasingly firm and its color changes successively from red to brown, yellow, and finally white (Figure 48).

Figure 48. Placental infarction; multiple large old infarcts. On the right, characteristic pale (indurated) infarct; on the left, a smaller infarct, appearing gray with an overlying adherent dark mass of retroplacental hematoma. Live-born infant, near term, weighing 4 pounds 15 ounces. A case of intrauterine growth retardation (IUGR) due to placental (infarction) insufficiency.

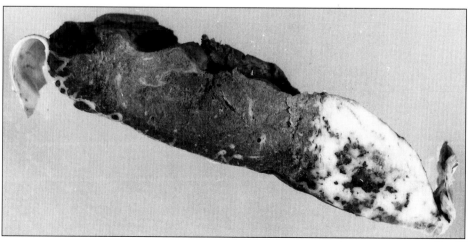

Fig. 48

At times placental infarcts give rise to retroplacental hemorrhage (Figure 48).

Microscopically, with fresh infarcts, the villi are swollen, congested, with increased syncytial knots; intervillous spaces are narrowed (Figure 49).

Figure 49. Microscopic appearance of tissue of a recent red infarct. Villi are congested, swollen, and crowded; villi with increased syncytial knots.

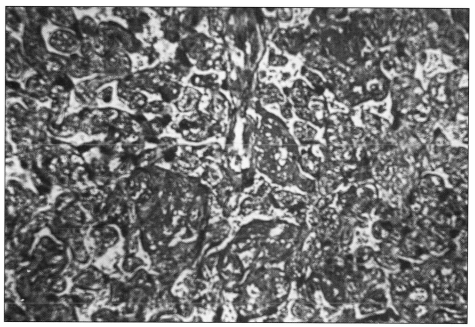

Fig. 49

Microscopically, in old infarcts, the villi become atrophied, contracted, and vessels disappear. Later the villi show obliteration of cellular detail with replacement scarring (Figure 50).

Figure 50. Microscopic section of an old infarct. On the left, scarred infarcted tissue; on the right are remnants of recognizable villi.

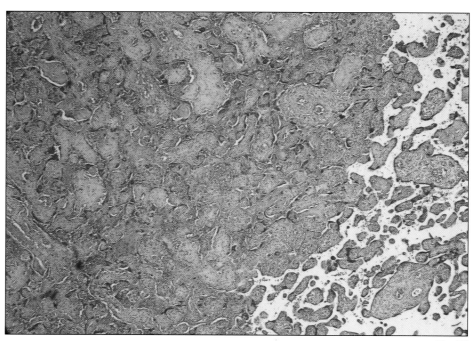

Fig. 50

Effects of placental infarction, in general, depend on the size. Small infarcts, common, appear to exercise no adversive effects. Larger infarcts, too, in many cases appear to cause no adversive effects on the fetus, on the newborn. However, large placental infarction predisposes to placental insufficiency. With large infarcts there is a high incidence of fetal death (Figure 51).

In fetuses surviving, there is a high incidence of fetal deprivation (IUGR), as in the case of the placental infarct in Figure 51. Such infants usually have a low Apgar score, often with manifestations of cerebral damage.

Figure 51. Fetal death due to massive placental infarction. Infant stillborn at 18 weeks' gestation. Placenta, maternal surface, with pale (old) infarct occupying two-thirds of the placental plate.

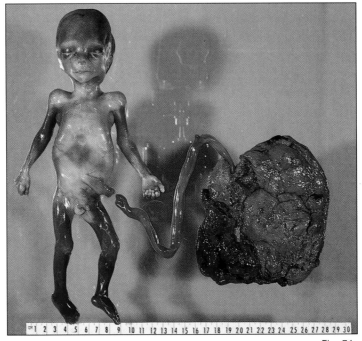

Fig. 51

Hemorrhagic endovasculitis of the placenta (HEV)

Illustrative Case:
Case 24   *p. 294*

This is a pathologic process affecting the placenta, increasingly diagnosed in recent years. Clinically in most cases the infants are either stillborn, or are born depressed, and often are small for gestational age, reflecting chronic placental insufficiency.

Hemorrhagic endovasculitis as observed microscopically affects the blood vessels, the arteries, of the placenta. The vessel walls are thickened (medial and intimal hyperplasia) with narrowing of the vascular channels. Thrombosis of vessels occurs. There is evidence of perivascular hemorrhage (Figure 52).

The cause of HEV has not been established. There is some evidence of viral infection in some cases (Sander, 1980).

Figure 52. Hemorrhagic vascular lesion of hemorrhagic endovasculitis of the placenta. The microsection of placenta shows two large arteries with necrotic hemorrhagic walls.

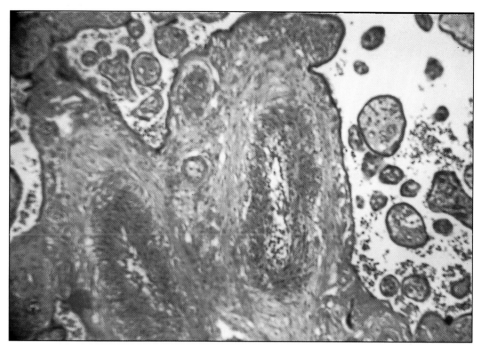

Fig. 52

Meconium staining of the placenta

Illustrative Cases:
Case 17   *p. 272*
Case 26   *p. 298*

Meconium contamination of the amniotic fluid and staining of the placenta are of common occurrence (Figure 53); attention often is focused on the presence of meconium in cases of infants born depressed. The pathology of meconium staining, its significance and effects, are dealt with on page 108 in context with the subject of meconium aspiration syndrome.

Figure 53. Meconium-stained placenta. Pronounced yellow discoloration of the fetal surface.

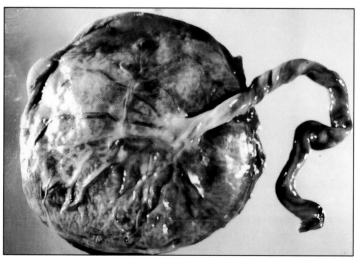

Fig. 53

Placental insufficiency; placental senescence; calcification

The placenta is the supply organ for the fetus, the intermediate transport mechanism between the mother and the fetus, providing oxygenation and nutrition for the fetus. Placental insufficiency is at times invoked clinically as a cause of fetal deprivation, intrauterine growth retardation, fetal death. Pathologically this diagnosis is warranted in cases in which the placenta is compromised by a very large infarct, or with a large old occult retroplacental hematoma. Also this applies in cases with small placentas (microplacentas).

Placental senescence is a concept applied to cases in which the placenta at term is small, atrophied, and hardened by heavy impregnation with calcium (Figure 54). This condition, with the newborn infant small, depressed at delivery, is viewed as a form of placental insufficiency.

Figure 54. Placental calcification. **(a).** Fresh placental specimen, close-up view of portion of maternal surface; surface tissue red, with sandpaper texture due to speckled white enamel-like deposits of calcium. **(b).** Microscopic appearance of placental calcification; section of deep portion of placenta; placental tissue pale pink; calcium, dark granular appearance.

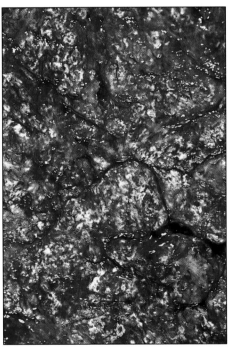
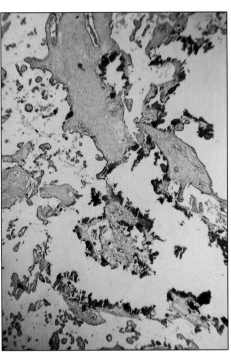

Fig. 54(a)   *(b)*

Clinically, at times, an assessment of placental insufficiency is applied in postterm birth with infants born depressed, the implication being that the fetus outgrew the capacity of the placenta to provide adequate support. This interpretation is problematic. The gross appearance of placentas from prolonged pregnancies is in no way characteristic. Studies have shown that the occurrence of focal infarcts and heavy calcification in postterm cases is no greater than in term pregnancies. Microscopically, in some cases of much prolonged gestation, chorionic villi show increased syncytial knots.

In cases of postterm gestation, with the placenta on pathologic examination showing no significant abnormality, adversive pathologic gestational processes, other than placental, must be sought in defining the cause of the fetal-neonatal compromise.

Malformations of the placenta

The two common forms of malformation, bilobe placenta and circumvallate placenta, although attracting attention at delivery, are essentially incidental findings encountered in uncomplicated births.

Bilobe placenta

The bilobe placenta usually has two equal parts (Figure 55), together having a weight about equal to that of an average placenta. Bilobe placentas occur in about 2 percent of gestations, apparently more frequently in older multiparas, with no clinical effect on the pregnancy, no effect on the well-being of the fetus.

Figure 55. Bilobe placenta, with two equal parts; weight 570 grams. Umbilical cord with marginal attachment to the two placental plates. Term pregnancy, Apgar score 10/10.

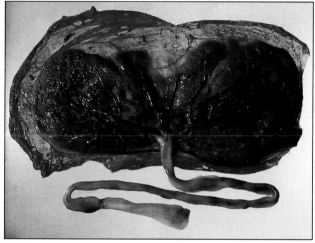

Fig. 55

Illustrative Case:
Case 58   *p. 378*

Circumvallate placenta

In this malformation, early in the development of the placenta an infolding of the membranes occurs over the fetal surface at the margin of the placental plate, resulting in an elevated, pale, callous-like ring, about 1 centimeter wide, bordering the fetal surface of the placenta (Figure 56).

Figure 56. Circumvallate placenta. **(a).** The fetal surface of the placenta shows a pale raised border characteristic of the circumvallate deformity. **(b).** The placenta, transected, showing the elevated, rolled-over circumvallate structure.

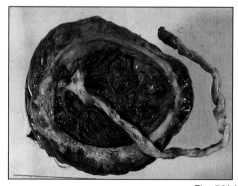 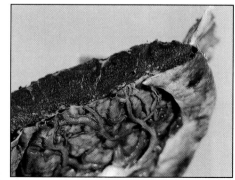

Fig. 56(a)   *(b)*

The cause of this malformation process is not known. Although manifestly innocuous clinically in most cases, its presence has at times been associated with retroplacental hemorrhage and fetal death.

Umbilical cord complications causing fetal hypoxia

Anatomy of the umbilical cord
Pathology of the umbilical cord
    Short umbilical cord
    Long umbilical cord
    Prolapse of the cord
    Nuchal cord
    Knots
    Velamentous attachment
    Vasa previa
    Umbilical cord with two vessels

Umbilical cord abnormalities, such as short cord and long cord, are potential hazards to the fetus. Likewise, mechanical compression, as with prolapse and tight knots, causes fetal hypoxia.

Anatomy of the umbilical cord

Anatomically the umbilical cord is actually a continuation of the body wall of the fetus, connecting distally with the fetal portion of the placenta and covered with skin-like amnion. The umbilical cord, the supply conduit between the placenta and the fetus, at term usually is 1.0 to 1.5 centimeters thick and about 50 centimeters, 2 feet, long. A transection of the cord shows two arteries and one vein surrounded by a gelatinous layer of cellular material, "Wharton's jelly," and a covering of amnion. The vein carries oxygenated blood from the placenta to the fetus. The two arteries, carrying deoxygenated blood, arise in the fetus as branches of the hypogastric arteries; the paired arteries coursing through the cord are spirally twisted around the vein and, often, in some segments form "varicosities," producing soft bumpy irregularities on the outer aspect of the cord (Figure 63, page 85).

Pathology of the umbilical cord

Pathologic conditions of the umbilical cord are of three main forms, all causing compression of the cord with obstruction of circulation leading to fetal hypoxia: prolapse of the cord, nuchal cord, and knots of the cord.

Clinically, compression of the cord is at times diagnosed empirically during labor, based on fetal monitor abnormalities — the concept being that the cord is transiently compressed between the descending head and the pelvic bone. This interpretation is open to question, speculative.

Malformations of the cord, in the form of abnormal attachment to the placenta, are common; of these, vasa previa, although rare, is a dangerous condition, causing maternal hemorrhage. Also of some importance are abnormalities of the cord length, short cord and long cord. Umbilical cord with two vessels is another anomaly, essentially of incidental importance.

Short umbilical cord

Illustrative Cases:
Case 58   *p. 378*
Case 62   *p. 388*

A short cord is an occult hazard that cannot be detected prenatally. The cord is considered short if it is less than 30 centimeters long. At delivery the cord must be long enough to reach from the placental site to the vulva, a length of between 30 and 35 centimeters.

Although the condition is rare, its effects can be catastrophic. If the cord is abnormally short, during descent of the fetus, tension on the cord at times leads to sudden detachment of the placenta, massive abruption. At times, stretch-tear laceration of the short cord occurs, tearing of the cord from the placenta. With tearing of the umbilical vessels, bleeding into the amniotic sac follows and blood-stained amniotic fluid appears during the delivery. With tearing of vessels in the cord, the blood that escapes is from the fetal circulation, rendering the fetus, the newborn, acutely anemic, hypoxic. Exsanguination of the fetus at times leads to intrauterine death (Figure 57).

In cases with short cord present, at times during delivery, as the fetus descends, traction on the placenta causes placental detachment with serious retroplacental hemorrhage.

Figure 57. Short umbilical cord. **(a).** At delivery, a short cord recognized; umbilical cord torn from the placenta, amniotic fluid bloody. The umbilical cord measured 24 centimeters (21 centimeters on the placenta, 3 centimeters on the fetus). Intrauterine death.

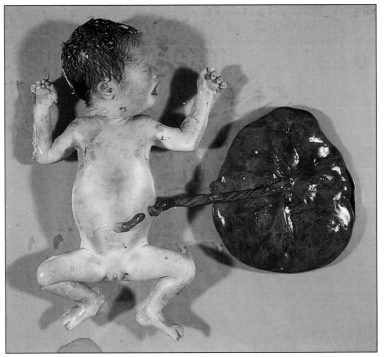

Fig. 57(a)

Figure 57(b). Stretch-tear of the cord, close-up of placental surface shown in (a). Avulsion of the placental amnion at the base of the cord.

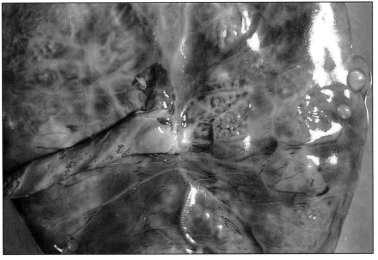

(b)

Long umbilical cord

Although the average cord length at term is about 50 centimeters (20 inches), cords that are somewhat longer, 70 to 80 centimeters, are common. Cords as long as 6 feet have been reported.

Long cords are a hazard to the fetus; with excessive length the cord is prone to prolapse at delivery. At times long cords form knots, or become entangled about the limbs of the fetus or coiled around the neck, nuchal cord (Figure 58).

Figure 58(a). Long umbilical cord with nuchal entanglement (4 coils) and premature fetal death at 22 weeks.

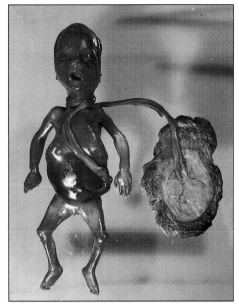

Fig. 58(a)

Figure 58(b). Same case as Figure 58(a), nuchal entanglement removed, demonstrating the excessively long umbilical cord. Note the pale ring about the neck resulting from compression by the nuchal cord.

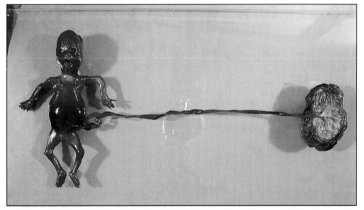

Fig. 58(b)

Prolapse of the umbilical cord

Illustrative Cases:
Case 10   *p. 256*
Case 19   *p. 276*
Case 84   *p. 450*

Prolapse of the cord is a problem of considerable concern clinically. It is the one form of cord compression that reveals itself plainly before the baby is born, creating an immediate emergency in the delivery room. Prolapse is especially prone to occur if the cord is excessively long. Prolapse usually develops when rupture of the membranes occurs before the head is engaged, with the gush of escaping amniotic fluid flushing the cord down into the vagina. After that, with contraction of the uterus, with the head descending, the loop of umbilical cord becomes compressed between the head and the pelvic bone (Figures 59 and 60).

The diagnosis of cord prolapse is usually readily evident, with the loop of cord palpable in the vagina. On vaginal examination, if pulsation of the cord is lost, this is ominous for the fetus. How long can the pulseless cord be tolerated before hypoxic cerebral damage occurs, or fetal death? Answers of six to ten minutes have been variously projected, empirically; there is no conclusive time limit, no answer based on clinical and pathologic evidence.

Figure 59. Prolapse of the umbilical cord. With premature rupture of membranes, with loss of amniotic fluid and descent of the cord, the cord becomes compressed between the head and the pelvic bones.

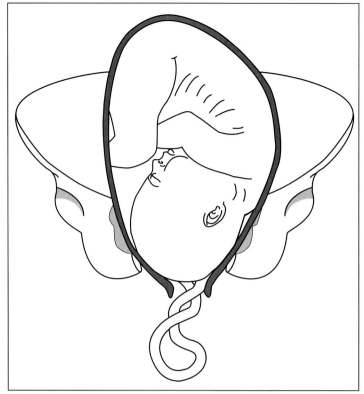

Fig. 59

Figure 60(a). Prolapse of the umbilical cord. Gestation at 22 weeks; premature rupture of membranes occurred prior to admission; on examination, pulsating umbilical cord was present in the cervical canal and vagina. Infant stillborn. Figure shows a loop of hemorrhagic cord extending down from the fetus and placenta. A white gauze tie above the prolapsed loop indicates the level of the cervical os.
(b). Segment of the prolapsed umbilical cord (enlarged); hemorrhagic, necrotic.

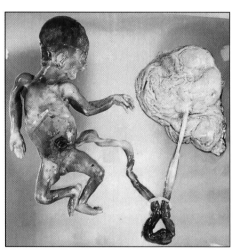

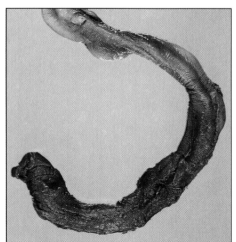

Fig. 60(a)   *(b)*

Nuchal cord

Nuchal cord, the umbilical cord coiled around the neck, is the most common form of cord entanglement (Figure 61). The presence of a long umbilical cord is a contributory factor to the occurrence of nuchal cord (Figure 58). The cord may be looped around the neck more than once, up to four times, in my experience, and up to seven times, as reported in the literature.

With the fetus moving about, changing positions, kicking, in the amniotic fluid — with the cord floating about, being tossed around by the moving parts — it is no wonder that the cord becomes fouled, entangled, wound around the neck. Entanglement of the cord around the neck and limbs is reported to occur in 10 to 20 percent of deliveries.

Pathologically, the effects of nuchal cord depend on the *tightness* and the *time factor,* the length of time the entanglement was present prior to birth.

Loose nuchal cord entanglement usually is easily reduced after delivery of the head. Most nuchal coils are loose, imposing no apparent fetal compromise.

Tight nuchal cord leads to intrauterine hypoxia, to fetal death. At autopsy, the effects of the hypoxia are evident, with cyanosis, edema, congestive heart failure, at times with acute hypoxic cerebral damage.

Figure 61. Nuchal cord. Hypoxic fetal death due to entangled umbilical cord looped around the neck. Congenital long cord. Maternal history of gradual loss of fetal activity prior to delivery. Fetus with early maceration at delivery.

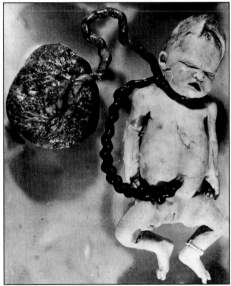

Fig. 61

A tight nuchal cord characteristically leaves a pale encircling imprint around the neck. However, the hypoxia that occurs is not due to "choking," not due to pressure on the neck; rather, the fetal hypoxia is due to the compression of the cord. Compression of the blood vessels in the cord obstructs the flow of blood to the fetus.

Regarding the degree of tightness, a nuchal cord of intermediate tightness poses a considerable problem in interpreting pathologic effects. In such cases, with the infant surviving, depressed at birth, and later developing neurologic disability, the cause-and-effect issue is problematic.

Regarding the time factor, taking into account the occult nature of this condition, a nuchal cord can be present in utero for months without clinical manifestations. In many cases, the umbilical cord becomes wound around the neck early on, months before birth. I have autopsied many cases of intrauterine death, small fetuses, with tight nuchal cord.

During intrauterine life, with the fetus floating about, with changes in position of the fetus, the pull on the nuchal cord, anchored at the neck, at times is taut, tight, at times becomes loosened. The hypoxia-producing effects of the entanglement during intrauterine life may thus be intermittent, occurring early in gestation, with the cord becoming tightened and loosened from time to time. The effects accordingly may be sublethal, with hypoxic cerebral damage being accrued.

Knots of the umbilical cord

Knots of the cord that are tight occur in about 1 percent of deliveries, causing fetal compromise, at times fetal death (Figure 62). Loose knots are common at delivery, occur in about 10 percent of cases, and manifestly do not cause hypoxia.

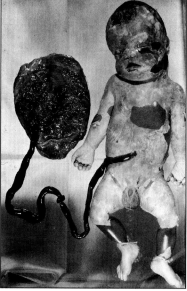 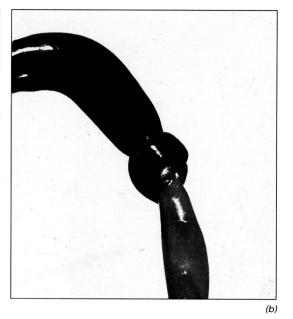

Fig. 62(a)   *(b)*

Figure 62(a). Tight umbilical cord knot; intrauterine death with maceration of the fetus. Near term pregnancy. Maternal history of decreasing fetal activity developing gradually in a period of 10 days prior to labor.
(b). Tight knot, close-up of cord knot shown in (a). At the upper right, the distal part of the cord between the placenta and the knot, swollen and congested.

During fetal life, with an umbilical cord knot present, with the fetus moving about, the knot may intermittently tighten and loosen, with the fetus correspondingly rendered hypoxic, accumulating hypoxic damage. The presence of a knot that is loose at delivery does not automatically exclude the occurrence of antecedent exposure of the fetus to hypoxia caused by the knot.

Long umbilical cord predisposes to the development of knots and prolapse of the cord.

The umbilical cord of a fetus dead in utero is prone to become knotted tightly. If the fetus is alive when an umbilical knot forms and tightens, the portion of the cord between the placenta and the knot tends to be swollen and reddened as a result of the obstruction of venous blood flow from the placenta toward the knot (Figure 62b).

Parturitional tight knots. A loose knot near the attachment of the cord to the fetus may tighten as the fetus descends; this is a serious hazard for the fetus if the cord is abnormally short, or is entangled above (Case 94, page 470).

Why is it that, paradoxically, a tight umbilical cord knot present at delivery, in some cases is manifestly innocuous, with the newborn infant lively, in good condition?

A knot may become tightened at the end of delivery when the baby is drawn away from the vagina, at a time when the cord is still anchored to the placenta. Such knots, although attracting attention, are parturitional artifacts.

False knots are bumpy irregularities that appear on the surface of the umbilical cord. The vessels of the cord are longer than the cord itself and in order to accommodate to this they twist around one another; at times arteries spiral around the vein and at times the vein winds around the arteries. Varicosities in the vein result in the bulging protrusions that form the false knots (Figure 63).

Figure 63. Knots in the umbilical cord. The middle segment shows a *true* (figure of eight) knot; the upper segment shows two false knots, varicosities in the umbilical vein, red soft protrusions on the surface of the umbilical cord.

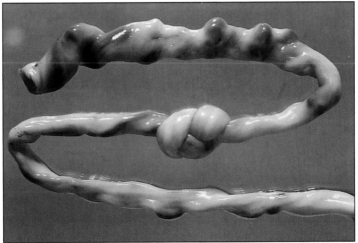

Fig. 63

Velamentous attachment of the cord

The attachment of the umbilical cord to the placenta varies in form and in location. Of these variations, the form of most importance is the velamentous (membranous) insertion, and the related anomaly, vasa previa. The other forms of cord attachment are mainly of statistical interest. The cord is inserted most often, not at the center, but eccentrically, between the center and the edge, in about 60 percent of placentas. Central insertion occurs in about 30 percent and marginal attachment in 10 percent.

Velamentous insertion of the cord, also known as membranous insertion, is the condition in which the cord is attached to the membranes at a distance from the placenta, with the cord vessels spread out, fan-like, on the amniotic surface between the edge of the placenta and the beginning of the cord (Figure 64). Velamentous insertion, relatively rare, occurring with about 1 percent of placentas, is more common with twins than with single gestations. Of itself this malformation of the cord is clinically innocuous, usually an incidental finding at delivery.

Figure 64. Velamentous insertion of the cord. The cord is attached to membranes at a distance from the edge of the placenta, with large vessels on the surface of the membranes bridging from the cord to the placenta.

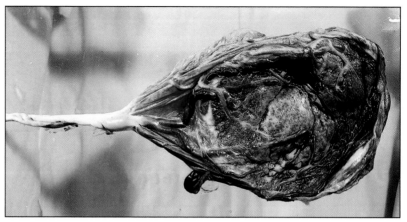

Fig. 64

Vasa previa

This abnormality poses a serious hazard for the fetus.

In this condition, with a velamentous insertion of the cord to the placenta, with the placenta low-placed, the exposed vessels in the membranous attachment pass over the internal os of the cervix. During labor, during dilatation of the cervix, the vessels are stretched and torn, causing hemorrhage into the amniotic sac and, later, with rupture of the membranes, hemorrhage externally. The bleeding is from the fetal circulation, from torn arteries in the membranous attachment, and leads to fetal exsanguination.

Vasa previa is extremely rare. Fetal mortality is over 50 percent.

Umbilical cord with two vessels

It is a fixed habit at delivery to examine and record the number of vessels in the transected umbilical cord. The presence of two vessels instead of three, by itself, is usually an incidental observation, a curiosity, with no apparent relevance pathologically.

The umbilical cord normally has three vessels, two arteries and one vein. As noted, in some instances the umbilical cord has two vessels, one artery and one vein.

Absence of one artery occurs in about 1 percent of singletons and much more often with twins, about 7 percent.

It is said to be associated with increased incidence of malformations; occurring by itself, as an incidental observation, this association is questionable. Single umbilical artery is, however, of quite consistent occurrence in cases of chromosome abnormalities, with trisomy, in association with multiple other obvious structural defects.

Amniotic sac abnormalities

Anatomy and physiology of the amniotic sac
Pathology of the amniotic sac
    Premature rupture
    Chorioamnionitis
    IUD present during pregnancy

The well-being of the fetus is directly linked to the physiologically intact structure and function of the amniotic sac and amniotic fluid. The amniotic sac and the amniotic fluid are subject to important pathologic conditions that adversely affect the fetus.

Anatomy and Physiology of the amniotic sac

The amniotic sac is usually alluded to as the "membranes."

The amnion is a thin tough transparent nonvascular sac containing amniotic fluid. The inner aspect of the amnion is lined with a simple skin-like layer of epithelium. Deep to this is a connective tissue layer. The amnion-chorion is applied to the uterine wall and covers the placenta and umbilical cord, becoming continuous with the skin of the fetus.

Pathologic conditions of the amniotic sac

The two main conditions affecting the amniotic sac are premature rupture of the membranes and chorioamnionitis, inflammation of the membranes.

Premature rupture of membranes

Premature rupture of membranes is of importance clinically and pathologically in two ways: (1) at times rupture triggers the development of chorioamnionitis, and (2) it is an important cause of premature delivery.

With premature rupture of the membranes, usually the leaking is slow and in some cases the leaking of the fluid stops, with apparent sealing off of the defect in the membranes. In other instances, cases near term, leaking continues but with little apparent harmful effect.

Chorioamnionitis following premature rupture of membranes varies in severity, at times is of minimal consequence, however at times leads to catastrophic infection of the fetus.

Premature delivery follows in about one-third of cases of premature rupture of membranes, and it is thought that the premature rupture is the event responsible for inducing the labor. Premature rupture of membranes occurring long before term is associated with high fetal-neonatal morbidity and mortality.

The cause of premature rupture in most cases is uncertain. It is thought that in some instances, with an ascending cervical infection, the inflammatory process reaches the membranes lying over the internal os, there weakening the membranes, causing premature rupture.

Some cases of premature rupture are due to incompetent cervix. The unsupported membranes, bulging through the prematurely dilated cervix, rupture.

At times with a footling breech presentation, the foot coming down first pushes through the membranes, through the cervix, into the vagina. Premature rupture at times occurs with hydramnios, probably due to increased pressure.

Chorioamnionitis

Chorioamnionitis, together with placental abruption, placenta previa, and placental infarction, is the fourth common important intrauterine complication of pregnancy.

Chorioamnionitis is an inflammation of the lining of the amniotic sac and the subjacent thin layer of tissue, the chorion (Figure 65). Chorioamnionitis is due to bacterial infection, most commonly *E. coli* or *staphylococcus*, corresponding to the flora usually present in the vagina.

At times, with chorioamnionitis, the infection, the inflammation, extends into subjacent placental tissue, placentitis.

Chorioamnionitis is an ascending infection with bacteria from the vagina and cervix reaching the chorion and amnion. The infection often occurs after premature rupture of membranes but also develops with membranes intact.

Chorioamnionitis is commonly observed in pathology examinations of placentas in as many as 10 percent.

In the more severe cases of chorioamnionitis, the diagnosis is evident in the delivery room, with the amniotic fluid cloudy and foul smelling.

The effects of chorioamnionitis are exercised on both the mother and the fetus. The mother, in advanced stages of the infection, develops leukocytosis and other symptoms of sepsis.

The fetus, bathed in the bacteria-infected amniotic fluid, likewise is endangered, exposed to intrauterine infection, to sepsis; at times this leads to fetal-neonatal meningitis. Aspiration of the infected amniotic fluid leads to intrauterine pneumonia.

IUD present during pregnancy

At times conception occurs in the presence of an intrauterine device (IUD). The presence of an IUD during pregnancy at times leads to intrauterine infection, sepsis, to premature labor, to vaginal bleeding, to placental abruption. However, the literature indicates that, for the most part, an IUD present during gestation remains innocuous and is expelled (often unanticipated) with the placenta at delivery.

Figure 65. Chorioamnionitis.
(a). Microscopic section. Amniotic
membrane over the upper surface;
underlying edematous chorion
heavily infiltrated with acute
inflammatory cells. Below are
elements of placenta, chorionic
villi. Premature rupture of
membranes 3 days before
delivery. Amniotic fluid cloudy,
purulent.

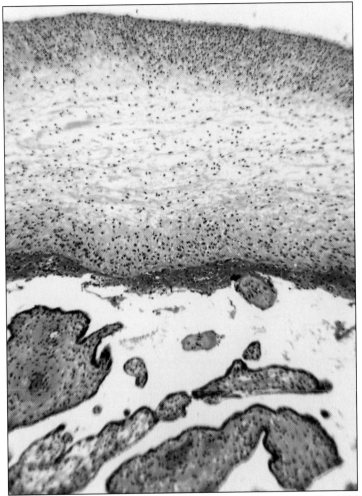

Fig. 65(a)

Figure 65(b). Acute inflammatory
reaction, with heavy infiltration of
polymorphonuclear leukocytes;
higher magnification of area of
inflammation in (a).

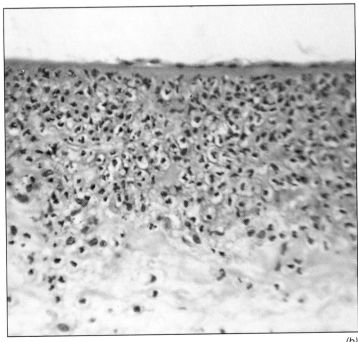

(b)

Amniotic fluid; conditions affecting the fetus

Oligohydramnios
    Potter's syndrome
Polyhydramnios

During the early stages of childbirth the amnion, the membranes, usually rupture and a quantity of amniotic fluid escapes.

Anatomy and physiology of the amniotic fluid

The average volume of amniotic fluid at term is about 1 liter. The amniotic fluid contains desquamated epithelial cells, lanugo (fine hair that covers the fetal body), vernix caseosa (the greasy substance covering the skin of the fetus).

The amniotic fluid provides a protective cushion for the freely floating fetus. In early pregnancy the fluid is formed as an active secretion of the amniotic membrane. Later in pregnancy fetal urine becomes the main source. The fetus swallows amniotic fluid during pregnancy. The fetus late in gestation increasingly aspirates and expels amniotic fluid from the respiratory tract. The amniotic fluid, being swallowed and aspirated, is then discharged as urine, is continuously recycled.

Pathology of the amniotic fluid

The amniotic fluid may be of decreased volume, oligohydramnios, or may be excessive, polyhydramnios.

Oligohydramnios

Illustrative Cases:
Case 19   *p. 276*
Case 44   *p. 339*

Oligohydramnios (*oligo-,* scanty; *-hydramnios,* amniotic water) is due either to a lack of production of amniotic fluid, or due to loss of fluid. Amniotic fluid is produced mainly by fetal urine. If there is hypoplasia or absence of kidney structure, as in Potter's syndrome, oligohydramnios results.

Very often, oligohydramnios is due to a "slow leak" of fluid, not recognized as such, at times mistaken for bladder incontinence by the mother, but is due to a small occult premature rupture of the membranes.

With oligohydramnios present, the cushioning effect of the amniotic fluid is lost. The body of the fetus is cramped together and there is risk of cord compression, fetal hypoxia.

Potter's syndrome

Illustrative Cases:
Case 19   *p. 276*
Case 44   *p. 339*

This is a genetic disorder presenting a unique association of ear malformations and kidney abnormalities. The ears are low-placed, overdeveloped, large, floppy. The renal abnormalities vary; kidneys are hypoplastic or absent, at times cystic. Other visceral abnormalities are usually present (Figure 176, page 277; Figure 350, page 340).

Polyhydramnios (hydramnios)

Illustrative Cases:
Case 13   *p. 264*
Case 14   *p. 268*

Polyhydramnios refers to excessive fluid in the amniotic sac. The volume of amniotic fluid at term is usually about 1,000 milliliters. Over 2,000 milliliters is considered polyhydramnios — but rarely is the opportunity at hand to measure the volume. The diagnosis is usually based on clinical impression. A mild degree of polyhydramnios is common and occurs in about 1 percent of pregnancies.

The cause of polyhydramnios is either excessive production of amniotic fluid or failure of amniotic fluid to be recycled by the fetus. Polyhydramnios occurs in cases with genetic defects, with twins, and is common with maternal diabetic conditions.

In cases of esophageal malformation, with obstruction, atresia, the fetus is unable to swallow amniotic fluid. Ordinarily amniotic fluid, produced mainly as fetal urine, is swallowed by the fetus and, thus, recycled. If the process of swallowing is interfered with, polyhydramnios results.

Anencephaly, in about 60 percent of cases, and frequently spina bifida cases, are associated with polyhydramnios; in these malformations, fluid escapes through the exposed meninges into the amniotic sac.

In cases of polyhydramnios the well-being of the fetus is adversely affected. Polyhydramnios is associated with increased fetal-neonatal mortality.

Fetal abnormalities causing hypoxia

Premature; with hypoxic complications
Postmature; postterm gestation, with hypoxic complications
Intrauterine growth retardation (IUGR); dysmaturity
    Ponderal Index
Fetal-neonatal anemia
Polycythemia

The fetus is affected not only by adverse gestational conditions as occur with maternal illness or placental abnormalities, but is also affected by adverse conditions that appear intrinsically in the fetus. These conditions are concerned with gestational age, prematurity and postmaturity, with manifestations of fetal nutritional deprivation, intrauterine growth retardation, and with the occurrence of fetal hematologic abnormalities, fetal anemia.

The gestational age, whether preterm or postterm, is not a factor in itself causing fetal damage.

Premature gestation; hypoxic complications

Prematurity per se is not a primary cause of hypoxic cerebral damage. However, a broad misconception persists that prematurity in itself causes brain damage.

The brain damage that often appears in the premature fetus is attributable to the immediate vulnerability of the premature fetus to injury, especially to hypoxic damage (page 13).

Premature labor exposes the fetus to severe injury. The same pathologic processes that trigger premature labor in the mother also are hazardous, hypoxia-producing processes affecting the fetus. Premature labor, miscarriage, is often preceded by acute illness, viral infection, toxemia—all processes damaging to the fetus (page 37). Damage to the fetus may be far advanced before the onset of the delivery process.

Once labor begins, the fragile immature fetus is subjected to physical injury as the fetus is forced through the birth canal. Hypoxic damage often occurs during delivery.

The premature newborn infant is susceptible to postnatal respiratory complications causing hypoxia, particularly recurrent episodes of apnea and bradycardia (page 105). The premature lung often develops hyaline membrane disease, respiratory distress syndrome (page 106).

The expressions "preterm" and "premature," although usually used synonymously, are in essence not the same. Preterm refers to time, the duration of the pregnancy. Premature is a biologic consideration of "ripeness," reflecting whether or not the appearance and performance of the newborn is consistent with the gestational age by date.

Maturity rating of the newborn

The level of development of the infant is assessed as the "maturity rating." In the first part of the maturity assessment, the neurologic responses, reflexes, are assessed; the more mature the infant is, the more complex, the more sophisticated, are the neurologic responses.

In the other part of the maturity rating, the physical features are assessed: skin texture, hair growth, development of the external ear, the breasts, and the external genitals, the pattern of the creases over the sole of the foot.

Body size is taken into account, but with reservations. Mothers with diabetic conditions produce babies that are inordinately large, macrosomic.

If the newborn infant is depressed, the maturity rating, the neurologic assessment, cannot be validly determined. In depressed infants, the reflex responses are reduced, skewing the result in the direction of lessened maturity.

Tocolytic agents

In times past it was the prevailing obstetric stance that, in cases of premature labor, it was necessary to halt the labor with tocolytic agents, to "try to put a few more weeks on the gestation." Effort to prolong the gestation, in unhealthy intrauterine circumstances, exposes the compromised fetus to mounting acute hypoxic damage. From a pathology perspective, plainly it is better to have the mother deliver and to hand the pediatrician a stable newborn, albeit less mature, than a somewhat more mature infant with manifest acute cerebral damage.

Postmature; postterm gestation, with hypoxic complications

The terms "**postmature**" and "**postterm**" are generally applied when the gestation extends beyond 42 weeks. The two terms are not synonymous however. Postterm is a time factor, an expression indicating that the duration of the pregnancy, based mainly on the date of the last menstrual period and on ultrasound assessment, is greater than 42 weeks. Postmaturity is a biologic factor, based on the physical features and neurologic findings of the newborn. Postmature infants show a level of development beyond that of the average term newborn.

Postterm pregnancy does not in itself cause fetal damage. Likewise, postmaturity is not, per se, a cause of fetal damage (page 39).

In cases of gestation lasting more than 42 weeks, the newborn infant is not necessarily postmature. An infant may be postterm, the product of a 43-week or longer gestation, but on physical and neurologic examination, present the pattern of a plainly average mature infant, not postmature. The reason for this circumstance: 40 weeks is the average length of time for the human fetus to become mature, but as in all things biologic, this figure is not applicable rigidly. As with apples on a tree, the fetus in most instances is "ripe" at an average time, at 40 weeks. For some, the fetus is organically ripe at less than 40 weeks; some require more than 40 weeks.

Accordingly, a newborn is properly assessed as less than mature, or more than mature, not by the length of pregnancy but according to the physical and neurologic status of the newborn, based not only on size but also on skin creases on the sole of the foot, hair and fingernail growth, skin, etc., and on the neurologic responses.

There are cases of pregnancy, at 40 weeks, in which the fetus in utero is in fact mature, but because of maternal factors not clearly understood, labor does not occur. Labor is delayed for three or four weeks. These infants, born at 43 plus weeks with physical features and neurologic function of a baby three or four weeks old, are both postterm and postmature. These infants show dry, peeling skin; the development of the external ear, the breasts, and the external genitalia are far advanced. The creases over the sole of the foot are deep and extend into the heel, indicating advanced maturity. Postmature infants usually have long hair and long fingernails.

The large size of a postmature fetus often causes dystocia, with prolonged labor, exposing the fetus to consequent physical and hypoxic injury.

Intrauterine growth retardation (IUGR); dysmaturity

In some cases, if the fetus has been exposed to prolonged adverse gestational processes, maternal illness, placental disorders, with deprivation of nutrition and oxygenation, the newborn infant, although showing physical and neurologic signs of maturity, is small and wizened, underweight, the pattern of dysmaturity. These deprived fetuses, newborn, often harbor old subacute hypoxic brain damage at birth. These enfeebled fetuses often do not tolerate the ordinary stress of labor and are born depressed.

Placental insufficiency, especially placental infarction, is at times the cause of IUGR. In some cases of IUGR, but rarely, placental "senescence" is evident, with the placenta small, indurated, and infiltrated with calcium deposits. In this circumstance, compromise of the postmature fetus is attributable to this placental disorder.

In infants who are postmature, but underweight, dysmature, it has been espoused that these fetuses "lose weight" during the period after 40 weeks because they "outgrew" the placenta. This concept is fictitious, without foundation; no one is able to weigh the fetus in utero at 40 weeks.

Dysmaturity varies in severity. Not only the brain but other organs may be affected. The thymus and adrenals, in most cases, are small, atrophied, reflecting prolonged intrauterine adverse conditions, deprivation.

Thymic atrophy, a gross reduction in size of the thymus, is a pathologic condition that reflects chronic deprivation, nutritional and infectious processes, affecting fetuses and newborn infants. Thymic atrophy occurs in cases of IUGR; the reduced size of the thymus is at times apparent in x-rays of the chest (Case 182, page 624; Case 212, page 694).

Most important pathologically is the subacute cerebral damage, silent at birth, that occurs with IUGR (page 24). Pathologically, this kind of latent subacute damage has been confirmed in the past in autopsy studies, observed in dysmature infants who die during delivery or soon after birth. In infants surviving, the latent cerebral damage ultimately is manifested as cerebral palsy and other cerebral disability. A high incidence of cerebral palsy in low birth weight infants is documented in the NIH Collaborative Perinatal Project (1965) and in previous studies.

Ponderal Index

The Ponderal Index is a measure of fetal nutrition and development. It is calculated as the weight in grams times 100, divided by the length in centimeters cubed (multiplied to the third power). The Ponderal Index is an indicator of the presence or absence of dysmaturity. A low Ponderal Index indicates IUGR, dysmaturity.

Fetal-neonatal anemia

Hematology studies
Causes of fetal-neonatal anemia
    Fetal-maternal transfusion syndrome
    Twin transfusion syndrome
    Erythroblastosis fetalis
        Hemolytic anemia
        Hydrops fetalis
        Hyperbilirubinemia
        Kernicterus
    Internal hemorrhage
        Intracranial hemorrhage
        Rupture of liver

Anemia often develops in the fetus, with the infant born pale and depressed. This anemia is often overlooked, its importance as a cause of intrauterine hypoxia not taken into account. Anemia in the fetus, in the newborn, as in the adult, causes hypoxia and debility. Prolonged anemia in the fetus leads to the accruing of hypoxic cerebral damage. Anemia making its appearance in the newborn requires immediate transfusion to prevent further hypoxic damage.

Hematology studies, newborn

The presence of anemia is indicated by the blood levels of hemoglobin, by the hematocrit, and by the red blood cell count (RBC).

Hemoglobin level measures the amount of hemoglobin in the blood (expressed as grams per 100 milliliters of blood). The hemoglobin in the red blood cells is the vehicle that carries oxygen through the body. A low hemoglobin level means anemia.

Hematocrit (*hem-*, blood; *-crit,* to separate) measures the volume of the red cells in the blood. This is determined by centrifuging a column of blood in a test tube: the height of the compacted blood at the bottom of the tube, expressed as a percentage of the height of the original column of blood, is the hematocrit. The hematocrit level and the hemoglobin level for the most part correspond, so that a low hemoglobin and a low hematocrit occur together.

The **red blood cell count (RBC)** is the third hematologic measurement of importance. The RBC indicates the number of red cells in a cubic milliliter of blood, expressed in millions. In the newborn, the RBC level is not relied on as much as the hemoglobin and hematocrit values.

The hematologic levels in the newborn are very high; this is normal, physiologic:
Hemoglobin level, 19.0 grams ± 2.2 grams (term)
Hematocrit 61 percent ± 7.4 percent (term)
RBC level 5.14 million ± 0.7 million (term)
(The hematologic levels for normal as given in laboratory sheets are for adults, and are not to be applied to the newborn. Normal ranges for adults: hemoglobin 14 grams ± 2 grams; hematocrit 44 percent ± 4 percent; RBC 5 million ± 0.8 million.)

The **white blood cell count (WBC)** (the number of white cells per cubic millimeter of blood) in the newborn is physiologically very high, in the range of 15,000 to 20,000 at term. (Normal for an adult is 7,000.) The high WBC level (normal) is often mistaken as a measure of sepsis. Determination of the white cell level is usually made by an electronic automated method of counting cells that includes the number of nucleated red cells present. It is important to carry out a laboratory procedure that determines the number of nucleated red cells present and to subtract this number from the electronically determined white cell count, to get the "corrected" WBC.

Nucleated red cells are present in the blood in newborn infants. Nucleated red cells are recorded as the number per 100 white blood cells. Normally, term infants have a range of 8 to 20 nucleated red cells per 100 white cells. At times, in the anemic fetus, newborn, the nucleated red cell count may rise to 300 or more.

Nucleated red cells in excessive number in the fetal blood mean there has been chronic fetal anemia. Red cells are produced in the bone marrow. In the early stage of formation, the young red cell in the marrow has a nucleus, a deep-staining structure in the center of the cell. As the red cell matures, the nucleus becomes smaller and finally is extruded before the red cell goes out into the blood circulation. If there is anemia, the bone marrow is stimulated to put out immature red cells, nucleated red cells. Accordingly, the presence of excessive nucleated red cells indicates chronic anemia. The increase of nucleated red cells in the blood takes time to develop; nucleated red cells in the blood indicate an anemia of long standing. Chronic anemia means chronic hypoxia.

Causes of fetal-neonatal anemia

The cause of anemia developing during fetal life, present at birth, in many instances is not clear. The anemia may be acute, of recent origin, as occurs following tearing of a short umbilical cord during delivery. More often the anemia is of chronic nature, with an intrauterine origin long before birth.

Fetal-maternal transfusion is being given increasing attention, thought to be a frequent cause of fetal-neonatal anemia. Likewise, with twins, anemia is common, due to pathologic processes in the twin transfusion syndrome. Erythroblastosis fetalis, once common as a cause of newborn anemia, is infrequent in the present day, attributable to preventive treatment.

Acute anemia in the newborn at times is due to internal hemorrhage. Massive intracranial bleeding and exsanquinating parturitional liver laceration that occur are acute processes, usually fatal.

Sepsis, the transmission of infection from the mother to the fetus, predisposes to anemia in the fetus, the newborn (Case 8, page 248; Case 34, page 316; Case 144, page 561).

Sickle cell disease is known to cause anemia in the mother and in the fetus, the newborn (Case 100, page 478).

Likewise, tearing of the umbilical cord during delivery leads to varying degrees of hemorrhage, with acute anemia.

Fetal-maternal transfusion syndrome: neonatal anemia

This syndrome results from the escape of large amounts of fetal blood into the maternal circulation. The transfer of fetal blood into the maternal circulation occurs to some degree in most, if not all, gestations. The amount of transfusion varies, but is severe in some instances. The cause, the pathogenesis, of the fetal-maternal transfusion process is associated with pathologic processes that damage elements of the placenta. The small blood vessels of the fetus present in the placenta are thin-walled and separated from the maternal blood vessels by a thin tissue layer (Figure 39, page 60). Damage to these placental vascular elements allows the blood to escape from the fetal vessels into the maternal blood.

In most cases of serious fetal-maternal transfusion, the exact cause is not clear. In some cases, defects in the placenta are thought to be due to direct trauma to the placenta, or to partial premature placental detachment, to focal infarcts in the placenta, or to other pathologic processes in the placenta. The diagnosis of fetal-maternal transfusion can be confirmed, and the amount of the transfusion quantified by laboratory tests, the acid-elution technique, by the Kleihauer procedure, performed on the mother's blood.

Twin (fetus-to-fetus) placental transfusion syndrome: fetal anemia

The fetal-placental circulation is primarily an independent, closed system. However, with twin gestation, at times there is a breakthrough, so that there may develop some degree of exchange of blood between fetuses, transfusion from one twin to the other through the placenta.

In monozygotic twins, fetus-to-fetus transfusion in some degree is thought to occur in almost all cases. With dizygotic twins, transfusion of substantial amount occurs in over 15 percent of cases.

In fetus-to-fetus transfusion syndrome, if the process becomes far advanced, the donor fetus is rendered small, underweight, and becomes anemic. The recipient twin becomes polycythemic, with elevated hematocrit, and becomes overweight, big (Figure 66).

Figure 66. Twin transfusion syndrome. Twins of unequal size, with the smaller twin being the donor and the larger twin being the recipient. (See Case 14, page 268.)

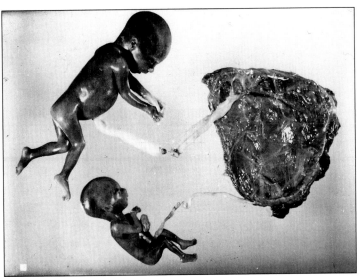

Fig. 66

The twin transfusion syndrome may begin early in gestation. Hypoxia develops in both twin fetuses.

In the small donor fetus, hypoxia is due to the anemia that develops. At times, the donor fetus dies if the process of exsanguination is rapid and ongoing. If the process is protracted, the donor fetus is often able to cope, able to compensate and maintain an adequate blood level.

The large plethoric recipient fetus, overloaded with an increased blood volume, goes into congestive heart failure, with resulting hypoxia. The fetus becomes bloated, with fluid accumulating in the tissues and body cavities.

Cerebral hypoxic damage that occurs with the placental twin transfusion syndrome at times is extensive. In my own experience I have observed a case of fetus-to-fetus transfusion, with one of the twins stillborn and, at autopsy, showing old brain damage and the surviving twin later developing cerebral palsy (Case 40, page 328) (Manterola, Towbin, and Yakovlev, 1966).

Erythroblastosis fetalis; Rh-incompatibility anemia

Erythroblastosis fetalis gains its name from the fact that the blood in affected infants has many primitive red cells, erythroblasts, nucleated red cells.

Erythroblastosis causes damage to the fetus and newborn through a sequence of pathologic processes: maternal-fetal blood Rh-incompatibility leads to hemolysis of fetal red cells, hemolytic anemia, with consequent heart failure, with bodily hypoxia, with hypoxic cerebral damage; hyperbilirubinemia, jaundice, results from the red cell hemolysis; the areas in the cerebrum previously damaged by hypoxia, areas of necrosis, become stained by the yellow bilirubin, producing the condition called "kernicterus."

Erythroblastosis fetalis, in times past, was one of the common causes of anemia at birth, occurring in about 1 percent of newborn, with over 50 percent being stillborn or dying soon after birth. Erythroblastosis produces profound changes in the body of the fetus, particularly affecting the blood-forming hematopoietic system, the liver, spleen, and ultimately the brain.

Infants surviving after erythroblastosis commonly develop cerebral palsy, predominantly the athetoid form, and other cerebral sequels, due to areas of hypoxic damage in the cerebrum.

In recent decades, with research studies defining the underlying causal factors, with development of precise prenatal serologic diagnostic tests, with treatment of the mother, the fetus can be protected and development of the disease in the fetus can be avoided, and the incidence in the newborn has been greatly reduced.

Hemolytic anemia in erythroblastosis fetalis

The manifestation that is elementary in erythroblastosis is anemia, due to the hemolysis of red cells in the blood and, as such, the disease was originally alluded to as "hemolytic disease of the newborn." Fundamentally the disease results from an incompatibility between the mother and fetus with respect to one or another of the blood group factors, usually the Rh factor. Although the fetal blood circulatory system through the placenta is independent, separate from the maternal circulation, the fact is that in most if not all gestations there is some breakthrough of fetal blood cells into the maternal blood. If the mother is Rh-negative and the fetus Rh-positive, there are built up in the mother's blood serum antibodies to the fetal red cells, antibodies that circulate through the placenta back to the fetus. The antibodies reaching the fetus cause hemolysis, disintegration of red cells, in the fetus and newborn.

The blood-forming tissues of the body, the hematopoietic system, the bone marrow, attempts to compensate for the red cell loss, for the anemia, by stepping up the formation of red cells; in this reactive process a large number of immature nucleated red cells, erythroblasts, are extruded from the bone marrow into the peripheral blood, giving the disease its name, "erythroblastosis."

Illustrative Cases:
Case 12   *p. 262*
Case 13   *p. 264*

Hydrops fetalis in erythroblastosis

The anemia that develops due to the hemolytic process varies from case to case. The anemia causes bodily hypoxia in the fetus (page 95). Hypoxia leads to myocardial weakening, to congestive heart failure. The fetus becomes edematous, bloated, hydropic. This is one of the main causes of hydrops fetalis (Figure 67a). The liver and spleen are greatly enlarged in erythroblastosis fetalis (Figure 67b). The placenta is usually enlarged (Figure 68).

Figure 67. Erythroblastosis fetalis; 34 weeks' gestation.
(a). Hydrops fetalis. Infant pale, anemic. Edema of the subcutaneous tissue, congestive heart failure with cardiac dilatation, hydrothorax, and ascites.
(b). Hepatosplenomegaly, characteristic of erythroblastosis fetalis. Abdominal organs exposed at autopsy. Liver occupies most of the abdominal cavity; enlarged spleen, dark red, in the lower portion of the abdomen.

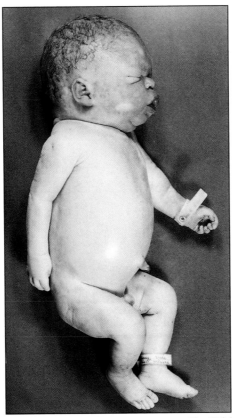
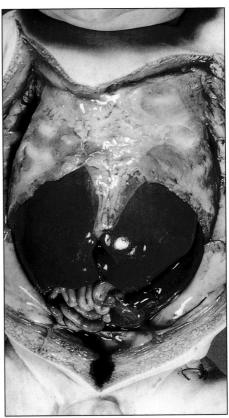

Fig. 67(a)   (b)

Figure 68. Placenta in a case of erythroblastosis fetalis; term. Weight of 1,160 grams, more than twice the weight of the average term placenta.

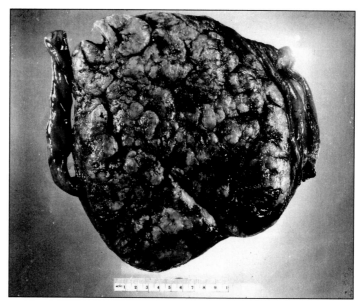

Fig. 68

Illustrative Cases:
Case 53   *p. 361*
Case 156   *p. 581*
Case 163   *p. 592*

Hyperbilirubinemia in erythroblastosis: jaundice

Hyperbilirubinemia refers to an increased level of bilirubin, a yellow pigment in the blood that comes from red cell breakdown, with the red-colored hemoglobin being converted to yellow bilirubin. Hyperbilirubinemia leads to jaundice, bile staining of the skin and other tissues.

Bilirubin pigment is cleared from the fetus in utero, removed by the placenta, so that in cases of erythroblastosis, the fetus, the infant, at delivery, usually is not jaundiced, but jaundice develops soon after birth.

Bilirubin levels reaching 12 to 20 milligrams postnatally are considered an indication for exchange transfusion. Bilirubin is normally present at low levels in the blood in infants and adults, at levels not perceptible outwardly as jaundice.

Jaundice, hyperbilirubinemia, *does* occur in conditions other than erythroblastosis.

Breast milk jaundice is a benign form of hyperbilirubinemia that occurs in about 1 in 200 breast-fed term infants. The jaundice is caused by a substance in the mother's milk that inhibits the breakdown and excretion of bilirubin in the infant. When breast feeding is stopped, the infant's bilirubin level soon decreases. This condition per se is not known to cause deleterious effects; it does not cause cerebral damage, does not lead to kernicterus.

Pathologically, jaundice develops neonatally with abnormalities of the liver. Jaundice occurs with infections, with cytomegalic viral disease, with sepsis in the newborn; jaundice occurs in infants with polycythemia.

Physiologic jaundice refers to the elevated bilirubin levels common postnatally, especially in premature infants. Neonates normally have a relatively high red cell count, high hemoglobin. The hemoglobin level gradually decreases during the postnatal period; this decline, associated with breakdown of red cells, causes an elevation of bilirubin, the breakdown product of hemoglobin. The infantile liver is often unable to handle the increase in bilirubin; bilirubin backs up in the body, stains the tissues, causes jaundice.

Kernicterus

The brain, in cases of erythroblastosis, as previously noted, shows focal areas of hypoxic infarctional damage, necrosis. With hyperbilirubinemia occurring in erythroblastosis, the necrotic foci become yellow stained; this is referred to as kernicterus (Figure 69).

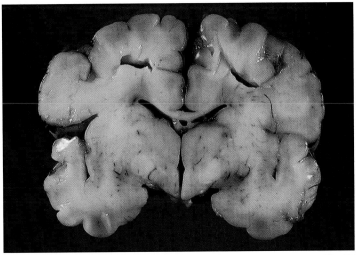

Figure 69. Kernicterus. Frontal section of cerebrum at autopsy showing focal areas of yellow coloration; edema of the brain. Premature birth at 34 weeks. Diagnosis of erythroblastosis. Infant lived 3 days, became jaundiced, developed abnormal neurologic signs.

Fig. 69

The term "kernicterus" originally was applied by German neuropathologists. In times past the basal ganglia were called basal nuclei. (In German, *kern* means nucleus; *-icterus* is Latin for jaundice.) Clinically, the problem of kernicterus is of broad concern in the interpretation of cases of cerebral palsy and other cerebral disability, cases with a history of neonatal hyperbilirubinemia.

Although kernicterus is in fact strictly an anatomic pathologic diagnosis, applied appropriately at autopsy in cases with the brain showing focal yellowing of the cerebrum, the term is currently used by clinicians as a diagnosis in sick newborn infants with hyperbilirubinemia, infants who develop neurologic signs postnatally, with poor reflexes, stiffness, lethargy, and respiratory distress. The diagnosis of kernicterus is made with the implication that the hyperbilirubinemia present *caused* the cerebral manifestations, *caused* cerebral damage in the infant.

Not taken into account, overlooked in such cases, are gestational hypoxia-producing complications that occurred, processes adverse to the fetus, to the newborn.

Accordingly, in cases of neonatal hyperbilirubinemia, cases that develop cerebral palsy, the question that arises is: Is the cerebral disability due to the effects of hyperbilirubinemia? Or, is the disability due to antecedent hypoxic damage incurred during early fetal life?

Most cases of erythroblastosis occur in prematures. In the premature cerebrum, hypoxia consistently causes damage to the periventricular structures, to the basal ganglia (pages 13, 185). Damage to the basal ganglia causes cerebral palsy (Chapter 3). It merits emphasis that in such cases of cerebral palsy, cases with a history of neonatal hyperbilirubinemia, the cerebral palsy is the consequence of antecedent early fetal hypoxic basal ganglia damage, unrelated to the hyperbilirubinemia.

There continue to be deep-seated misconceptions in the minds of clinicians, in pediatric literature, about the pathologic effects of hyperbilirubinemia and the pathogenesis of kernicterus.

Hyperbilirubinemia by itself does not cause cerebral damage. This has been proven in past neuropathology studies, in autopsy studies in humans, and in experimental animal studies. However, there remains in the clinical literature, expressed by pediatricians, misinformation about the effects of hyperbilirubinemia. What is not realized clinically is that jaundiced infants do not show pathologic changes in the brain unless there is antecedent and accompanying prolonged cerebral hypoxia. The hypoxia causes cerebral damage, areas of necrosis; the devitalized necrotic tissue secondarily becomes stained yellow by the bilirubin (bile) pigment.

Internal hemorrhage causing anemia in the fetus and newborn

Internal hemorrhage resulting from mechanical injury or hypoxic damage varies in severity. Massive hemorrhage as occurs at times with liver laceration, with hemoperitoneum, or at times with large intracerebral hemorrhage is usually rapidly fatal. Or the bleeding may be gradual, causing acute anemia with hypoxia, with the surviving newborn becoming increasingly pale, enfeebled, with gradually deteriorating vital function.

Intracranial hemorrhage

Extensive intracerebral hemorrhage occurs mostly in small premature fetuses and newborn, is due to hemorrhagic periventricular hemorrhage (page 15), and at times leads to acute anemia with hypoxia in surviving infants.

Intracranial hemorrhage is at times due to mechanical injury, to excessive molding during parturition, with dural venous laceration leading to subdural hemorrhage (page 131).

Liver injury: rupture, hemoperitoneum

Illustrative Cases:
Case 4   *p. 233*
Case 54   *p. 364*
Case 60   *p. 382*
Case 90   *p. 462*

Mechanical injuries of the liver incurred during parturition vary from minor blister-like subcapsular hematomas (Figure 70), to mangling lacerations involving entire lobes of the organ (Figure 71). Bleeding from a minor injury at times is slow, with anemia developing, with hypoxia. Hemorrhage in some cases is rapid, catastrophic, with exsanguination into the abdominal cavity; massive hemoperitoneum during parturition leads to stillbirth.

The causal mechanism in such liver damage is usually of intrinsic origin, the result of compression injury, crushing of the abdomen during descent of the fetus, in a manner analogous to intracranial damage consequent to excessive molding-compression of the head during delivery. With breech presentation, with the lower extremities flexed and pressing into the abdomen of the fetus, crushing injury of the bulky liver is prone to occur, especially if expulsion of the fetus is forceful and precipitous.

Especially vulnerable are the very young prematures; fatal crush injury usually occurs intranatally as the small fragile flexed fetus, breech first, is extruded through a rigid undilated cervix.

Affected infants present a distinctive external appearance — commonly a spindly pale (exsanguinated) premature infant without cyanosis, with a soft, slightly bulging belly, often with gray-blue discoloration of the skin about the umbilicus. This pale drawn appearance is in sharp contrast to the picture of edematous suffusion and cyanosis in the infant with terminal asphyxia.

The very large fetus is also vulnerable to rupture of the liver, particularly in cases of erythroblastosis and macrosomia.

The frequency of perinatal rupture of the liver is not generally realized. Well-documented studies of consecutive autopsies have revealed hepatic injury in up to 5 percent of stillbirths.

The effects of a liver injury may be delayed. Minor damage in the liver, a small tear with a sealed-off subcapsular hemorrhage, initially may remain occult, silent, with the newborn infant appearing well for a day or two, then suddenly becoming pale, going into shock, with the abdomen becoming distended, as the subcapsular hemorrhage ruptures, causing rapid bleeding into the abdominal cavity.

Figure 70. Liver damage incurred during delivery. The surface of the right lobe has a large, blister-like, subcapsular hematoma. Blood leaking from the lower edge of the hematoma with resulting hemorrhage into the abdominal cavity, hemoperitoneum. Spontaneous vaginal delivery, shoulder presentation; stillbirth, 22 weeks' gestation. View of abdominal viscera at autopsy.

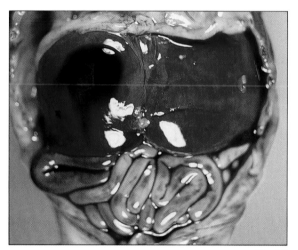

Fig. 70

Figure 71. Liver with crush laceration due to compression of the abdomen in a breech delivery through a partially dilated cervix. Right lobe of liver with a large jagged laceration, with resulting exsanguinating hemorrhage into the abdominal cavity, massive hemoperitoneum. Entrapment of after-coming head; stillbirth at 23 weeks' gestation. (Case 60, page 382.) View of the abdominal viscera at autopsy.

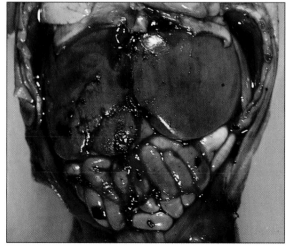

Fig. 71

Polycythemia; hyperviscosity syndrome

Polycythemia (*poly-*, many; *-cythemia*, cells in the blood) means there are excessive red cells in the blood. This condition, the opposite of anemia, paradoxically, also like anemia, causes hypoxia.

Polycythemia is diagnosed on the basis of elevated hemoglobin and hematocrit. The average hemoglobin level in the term newborn is 19 grams; average hematocrit is 61 percent. Hemoglobin concentration in excess of 22.0 grams or an hematocrit of more than 65 percent at any time during the first week of life should be considered evidence of polycythemia.

Two kinds of polycythemia occur:

Primary polycythemia. In the primary type, excessive red cells are formed pathologically, with the cause not known. This form of polycythemia occurs in adults.

Secondary polycythemia. In the secondary form, as occurs in the fetus and newborn, excessive red cell formation is triggered by the presence of hypoxia. (The Indians in the Andes have secondary polycythemia.)

During gestation, if the fetus is subjected to ongoing hypoxia due to hypoxia-producing maternal factors or placental disorders, a degree of polycythemia results. The red cells carry oxygen to the fetus; the increase in red cells in polycythemia is an effort to compensate, to increase oxygenation in the fetus.

When chronic hypoxia develops in the body, the bone marrow is stimulated to produce an increased output of red cells. The red cells that are pushed out into the blood are often immature, large, dark colored, and many are primitive and still contain a nucleus (nucleated red blood cells, NRBCs).

The effects of polycythemia are variable. The increased numbers of red cells in the blood cause thickening of the blood, the **hyperviscosity syndrome**. Hyperviscosity of the blood leads to sluggish blood flow in small vessels, to stasis-thrombosis, with consequent focal infarcts in tissues of the body. Focal infarcts occur in the kidney, intestines, skin, and in the brain, causing convulsions. Pulmonary compromise leads to cyanosis and dyspnea. Congestive heart failure occurs.

Polycythemia does not come on suddenly. Plainly, the presence of polycythemia at birth reflects prolonged intrauterine hypoxia, substantial evidence of ongoing chronic hypoxia in the weeks, months, prior to birth. The hypoxia-producing effects exercised by polycythemia on the fetus are continued in the newborn after delivery.

Postnatal hypoxia-producing conditions

Apnea
Hyaline membrane disease (HMD); respiratory distress syndrome
Meconium aspiration syndrome
Pneumothorax
Pneumonia
      Intrauterine origin
      Postnatal infection
DIC
Cardiac malformations causing hypoxia

Hypoxia beginning during intrauterine life is often increased, compounded, by tangential related complications developing after birth. These postnatal complications occur in prematurely born infants or in term infants previously compromised by intrauterine pathologic processes. Prematurity apnea, hyaline membrane disease, and meconium aspiration syndrome are significant examples of postnatal hypoxic complications.

Apnea as a cause of hypoxia in the newborn

Apnea means spontaneous arrest of breathing (*a-*, without; *-pnea*, breathing). Clinically, a period of arrest in respiration lasting 20 seconds or longer is regarded as an "apnea spell."

Three types of apnea are important in the newborn: apnea associated with prematurity, apnea associated with seizure activity, and apnea following injury to the spinal cord or brain stem during delivery.

Prematurity apnea

Illustrative Cases:
Case 126 *p. 530*
Case 136 *p. 546*
Case 189 *p. 638*

Cause of premature apnea. The cause of apnea in premature infants is not known. Apnea is a manifestation of malfunction of the respiratory control center in the brain. Apnea occurs spontaneously, automatically, and its occurrence in the premature cannot be controlled. There is no effective preventive treatment to deal with it, only resuscitation when it occurs. It is the most unyielding respiratory problem in premature infants.

Effects of apnea. Prolonged recurrent apnea causes hypoxia that directly affects the bodily functions. The heart, with the myocardium hypoxic, is immediately affected, leading to bradycardia; the slowing of the pump action of the heart compromises circulation, compounding the infant's hypoxia. Episodes of apnea with bradycardia are recorded clinically as "A and B" spells. Such spells are often prolonged and recurrent, with the infant becoming limp, unresponsive, and cyanotic.

The occurrence postnatally of recurring episodes of apnea is always an ominous matter. This clinical pattern often is the prelude to an accumulation of cerebral hypoxic damage leading to death. In my own pathology experience, in the investigation of premature cases with a clinical history of increasing apnea leading to death, the brain at autopsy consistently showed varying severity of hypoxic acute cerebral damage.

Premature infants who survive after prolonged recurrent apnea often develop cerebral palsy.

Seizure apnea

This kind of apnea occurs in mature newborn infants. The clinical pattern: a stable term infant, unexpectedly, has an onset of apnea spells and, with the apnea, seizure activity soon follows. Unlike the problem in the premature, the apnea spells cease when the seizures are treated and controlled.

Spinal cord and brain stem injury with apnea

Illustrative Cases:
Case 25   *p. 296*
Case 35   *p. 320*
Case 37   *p. 324*
Case 88   *p. 460*

With spinal cord or brain stem injury incurred during delivery, the primary effect is respiratory depression, apnea (page 138).

The apnea that follows neurologic damage tends to be a persistent respiratory depression, apnea that is sustained, not intermittent apnea spells.

Hyaline membrane disease (HMD); respiratory distress syndrome (RDS)

Illustrative Cases:
Case 45   *p. 343*
Case 54   *p. 364*
Case 55   *p. 366*
Case 56   *p. 368*
Case 57   *p. 373*
Case 189 *p. 638*

Hyaline membrane disease is a pathologic process that affects premature infants mainly. "Respiratory distress syndrome" is a clinical term, usually thought of as synonymous with HMD; however, this is not accurate; RDS is a preliminary diagnosis applied to premature infants having respiratory distress, cases that later may prove to have pneumothorax or other pulmonary problems, not HMD.

Many people know hyaline membrane disease as the disorder that killed Patrick Bouvier Kennedy, the premature son of President John F. Kennedy, 39 hours after his birth in 1963.

While appearing predominantly in premature infants, HMD does at times occur in mature infants, especially in cases with maternal diabetes.

Hyaline membrane disease compromises the function of the lung in a manner similar to pneumonia. The alveoli (air sacs) are clogged with pathologic material that hinders the transfer of oxygen to the blood. The term "hyaline membrane" (hyaline meaning glassy) refers to microscopic findings in the lung tissue, the alveolar sacs becoming lined with pink glassy-appearing membranes (Figure 72).

Hyaline membrane disease is due to the inadequate synthesis of the chemical "surfactant," produced in the fetal lung in increasing amounts as the gestational age of the fetus increases toward maturity.

Figure 72. Hyaline membrane disease, histologic section. Alveolar sac near the center shows a characteristic glassy pink membrane partially lining the inner surface of the alveolus; other alveoli with similar hyaline membranes. Premature at 33 weeks; intrauterine growth retardation, respiratory distress syndrome diagnosed; respiratory distress increased after birth; death at 36 hours.

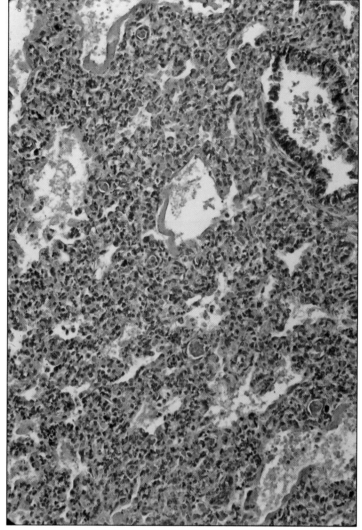

Fig. 72

The amount of lung surfactant at a given gestational age varies from case to case. Even prematures of 30 to 35 weeks' gestational age at times have inadequate surfactant and develop HMD, whereas preemies of younger gestational age at times appear to escape the effects of HMD.

Postnatally, with severe HMD present, there is consequent increasing bodily hypoxia leading to hypoxic cerebral damage, with periventricular hemorrhagic infarction and intraventricular hemorrhage. Cerebral matrix hemorrhage, not present at birth, at times develops in a period of days.

Hyaline membrane disease is usually very severe in small prematures and has a high mortality and morbidity. In affected prematures of less than 28 weeks' gestation, mortality reaches up to 80 percent.

Bronchopulmonary dysplasia (BPD)

Bronchopulmonary dysplasia is a syndrome of progressive pulmonary insufficiency that at times follows hyaline membrane disease. Infants with HMD usually gradually improve after three or four days. However, in some cases, with infants on positive pressure ventilation using high concentrations of oxygen, there is a worsening of the pulmonary condition due to the development of bronchopulmonary dysplasia.

Pathologically, the small branches of the bronchi in the lungs, the bronchioles, are affected. The lining mucosa of the bronchioles undergoes necrosis, followed by fibrosis, scarring of the bronchiolar walls, fibroplasia, with obliteration of the bronchioles. With increasing scarring of lung elements, respiratory function is reduced, and chronic hypoxia results.

The main causal process of BPD is presently thought to be oxygen toxicity. In affected infants there is an apparent high susceptibility of lung tissue to high concentrations of oxygen.

Meconium aspiration syndrome

Illustrative Cases:
Case 5   *p. 238*
Case 26   *p. 298*
Case 43   *p. 337*
Case 69   *p. 406*

This syndrome involves a sequence of physiologic and pathologic processes that begin during intrauterine life: meconium contamination of the amniotic fluid occurs; aspiration of the amniotic fluid by the fetus in some instances leads to meconium aspiration pneumonia.

Meconium staining of the amniotic fluid causes yellow to green discoloration of the amnionic membranes and placenta and cord (Figure 53, page 75, and Figure 73).

Figure 73. Meconium staining of the placenta and fetus. Amniotic fluid heavily stained with meconium. Loss of fetal activity for 1 day. Postmature; nuchal cord at delivery; stillborn; weight, 9 pounds.

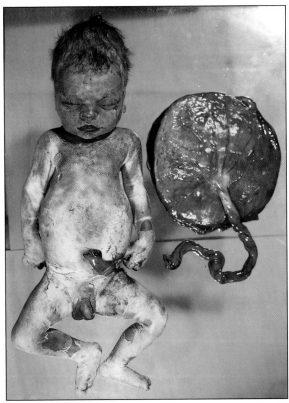

Fig. 73

Meconium amniotic fluid occurs due to bowel incontinence of the fetus. The anal sphincter opens and bowel content, meconium, is expelled into the amniotic fluid. This may occur early or late during labor.

Meconium amniotic fluid is loaded with desquamated debris from the fetus' skin and contains highly irritant enzymes from the fetal intestine. With aspiration, a chemical and foreign-body type pneumonia develops (Figure 74), a condition at times lethal.

Figure 74. Meconium aspiration pneumonia. **(a).** Histologic section; areas of pneumonia with lung alveoli containing acute inflammatory cells and aspirated pigmented skin squames. Lungs at autopsy were large, of firm ropy texture, mottled, with areas of gray-pink, dark red and purple.

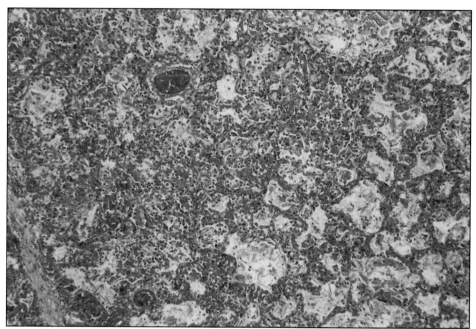

Fig. 74(a)

Figure 74(b). Brown meconium in lung alveoli. Histologic section under higher magnification; alveoli filled with aspirated brown-staining cellular debris. Clinical history of prolonged, complicated labor; amniotic fluid heavily meconium stained. Postnatal respiratory distress; infant lived 1 day.

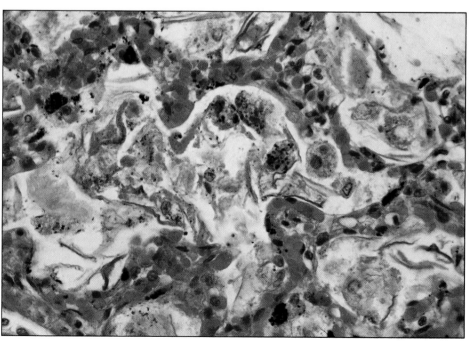

(b)

Meconium staining occurs in 10 to 20 percent of births and is very common in postterm deliveries.

Meconium staining at times occurs in cases of nuchal cord and other forms of intrauterine hypoxia-causing complications (Case 17, page 272). Meconium amniotic fluid occurs in circumstances other than hypoxia: compression of the abdomen, compression of the head. Meconium in the amniotic fluid, per se, is not a positive sign of fetal hypoxia, not an indication for early cesarean section.

The fetus *normally* aspirates amniotic fluid of varying amounts, that is, the fetus is known to have respiratory movements during intrauterine life, and ordinarily sucks in amniotic fluid — this is physiologic. However, during labor, *if the fetus is hypoxic*, the fetus is stimulated to go into vigorous respiratory action; the amount of amniotic fluid taken in is increased, and amniotic contents with meconium get drawn into the trachea and bronchi and, at times, into the lung substance.

Accordingly, the degree of meconium aspiration serves as an indicator, a gauge of the severity of intranatal hypoxia. If, during the intranatal period, the meconium is drawn deeply into the lung, it is indicative that severe fetal hypoxia was present prior to birth. If the infant at delivery has no meconium below the vocal cords, no deep aspiration, it is evidence that no inordinate fetal hypoxia was present intranatally.

Meconium staining of amniotic fluid is sometimes pointed to as an indication of intrauterine hypoxia. In this direction — does the absence of meconium reflect the absence of intranatal hypoxia?

The postnatal course following intrauterine meconium aspiration varies with the amount and consistency of the meconium and the depth of aspiration. If the meconium is thick, and if heavy deep aspiration has occurred, there is the problem first of mechanical obstruction of the tracheobronchial airways.

Pneumothorax

Pneumothorax, air in the thoracic cavity, air trapped between the lung and the outer thoracic wall, develops in 1 to 2 percent of neonates. The most frequent occurrence and the most severe degree of pneumothorax develops in depressed infants that require prolonged resuscitation and positive pressure ventilation after birth. A minor degree of pneumothorax may occur spontaneously in neonates and is often without symptoms, evident radiologically in infants who required no resuscitation at delivery.

The cause. In infants treated with positive pressure ventilation, the pressure exerted by the gas at times leads to overdistention of lung alveoli, causing rupture of the alveoli. Air escaping from the alveoli dissects into the interstitial connective tissue around the alveoli, forming clusters of small bubble-like cysts filled with air (interstitial emphysema). The air cysts at the pleural surface, rupturing through the pleura into the pleural cavity, give rise to pneumothorax (Figure 75).

The effect. Pneumothorax exerts its effect directly on the lung. With the trapped air steadily increasing and under mounting pressure, the lung becomes more and more compressed. The compression of the lung, the atelectasis, compromises respiration, compromises oxygenation of the infant, with the infant becoming increasingly cyanotic.

Tension pneumothorax can be relieved by appropriately inserting a tube through the chest wall into the pleural cavity.

If unrelieved, the pneumothorax, usually occurring tangential to other hypoxic perinatal complications, is commonly the terminal mechanism of injury superimposed on the newborn.

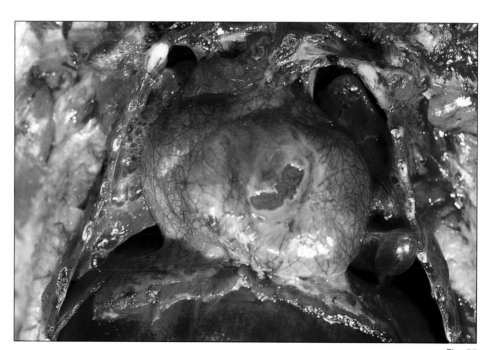

Figure 75. Pneumothorax. The pleural cavities are only partly occupied by lung structure. Surrounding the lungs are open spaces created by the pneumothorax process. The lung surface shows clusters of thin-walled air sacs formed by ruptured alveoli under pressure (interstitial emphysema). Infant born at 36 weeks' gestation, had grunting respirations and cyanosis. Infant was ventilated under pressure, failed to respond, and died at 24 hours. At autopsy pneumothorax was demonstrated, with lungs occupying about one-third of the thoracic cavities. Multiple visceral malformations were present. View of thoracic viscera at autopsy.

Fig. 75

Pneumonia in the fetus and newborn

Pneumonia, developing in the fetus, causes debility and sepsis in the newborn and additionally causes respiratory distress, hypoxia.

Pathologically, with pneumonia, the lungs are firm, consolidated. Microscopically, the air sacs, the alveoli, become filled with inflammatory cells, purulent exudate (Figure 76).

Bacterial infection of the lung in the newborn is of two types, differing in pathogenesis, differing in the time of origin: *intrauterine pneumonia*, with the infection contracted during fetal life, and *postnatal pneumonia*, with the infection incurred after birth. Whether the infection is incurred prenatally or postnatally, the pathologic effects are severe.

Intrauterine pneumonia

Illustrative Cases:
Case 78   *p. 434*
Case 79   *p. 437*
Case 80   *p. 440*
Case 144   *p. 561*

Bacterial infection of the lung in the fetus in most cases is the consequence of chorioamnionitis in the mother, premature rupture of membranes, with pneumonia resulting from aspiration of infected amniotic fluid by the fetus.

Maternal sepsis

The mother with chorioamnionitis often is clinically sick with fever, dehydration, leucocytosis, and other signs of sepsis prenatally. The fetus, infected, developing pathologic changes in the lung (Figure 76), is rendered septic. With the fetus surviving, the newborn infant is acutely depressed, with manifestations of sepsis, with compromise of vital function.

Pathologically, as noted, there is a direct relationship between chorioamnionitis and development of intrauterine pneumonia. With chorioamnionitis present, the fetus aspirates into the lungs amniotic fluid that is loaded with pathologic bacteria. From the lungs, the offending organisms invade the bloodstream; the resulting septicemia creates bodily sepsis.

Respiratory distress is present in the infant. With the pneumonic process in the lung exercising its effects immediately in the infant, pulmonary function, oxygenation of the infant, is reduced. The infant, in addition to being septic, is dyspneic, with labored respirations, and is cyanotic.

The diagnosis of pneumonia and sepsis is made bacteriologically and by x-ray. With bacteriologic cultures of the blood and tracheal aspirate, the most common bacteria found are streptococcus, staphylococcus, and coli organisms.

Intrauterine pneumonia frequently leads to stillbirth or newborn death early postnatally.

Figure 76. Pneumonia of intrauterine origin; microscopic section of the lung; above, alveoli filled with acute inflammatory cells, purulent exudate; in the middle portion of the illustration, a small bronchus likewise contains inflammatory exudate. Below, over-distended alveoli, the consequence of effort to ventilate the lung with positive pressure. Prenatally, rupture of membranes had occurred 2 months before delivery. Infant, dyspneic and cyanotic, died after 2 hours.

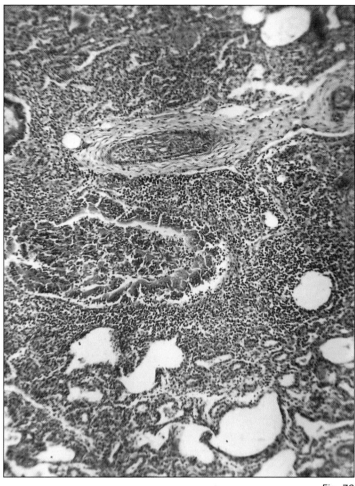

Fig. 76

Postnatal pneumonia

Illustrative Cases:
Case 7 *p. 244*
Case 8 *p. 248*

Infants that are in poor condition at birth, with intrauterine growth retardation and other intrauterine compromising conditions, are vulnerable to bacterial infection, commonly pneumonia. Varied types of bacteria produce pneumonia in the neonate, but the streptococcus, staphylococcus, and coli organisms are the most common causal agents. Chlamydia also can cause pneumonia in the neonate.

Bacterial pneumonia in the newborn due to postnatal infection is similar clinically to pneumonia of intrauterine origin, with manifestations of sepsis and respiratory distress developing, and similar radiologic and pathologic changes in the lung. Occurring postnatally in infants with other debilitating conditions, pneumonia often is the final contributing cause of death.

DIC (Disseminated intravascular coagulopathy)

DIC is a syndromic hematologic disorder that develops in newborn infants (and adults) in cases with antecedent ongoing illness, cases with debilitating disease complicated by acute stress. It occurs in cases of hyaline membrane disease, in depressed infants with intrauterine growth retardation, with sepsis, and with other stress conditions.

DIC, as it develops, is an hypoxia-producing process.

In the beginning stages of DIC, the thrombocytes (platelets) in the blood form conglutinations in blood vessels, causing thrombotic occlusion of vessels, giving it the name "disseminated intravascular coagulopathy." During the thrombotic process the platelets are "used up," consumed, leading to a low platelet count in the blood, thrombopenia. The loss of platelets predisposes to bleeding. Not only are platelets used up, but other blood elements that prevent bleeding are also diminished.

In the next stage of the sequence, with hemorrhage-preventing blood factors used up, bleeding develops at many sites, from the umbilical stump, in the urine, in the GI tract, in the lungs, and in the brain.

Anemia, resulting from blood loss, leads to mounting hypoxia with congestive heart failure.

Cardiac malformations causing postnatal hypoxia

With malformations of the heart causing hypoxia, the immediate effect on the infant is cyanosis, the "blue baby."

Pathologically, cardiac malformations vary in anatomical complexity and severity, ranging from the "acardiacus," a fetal body without a heart, to cases of infants born with latent defects that are long asymptomatic.

Cardiac hypertrophy is a common malformation in offspring of diabetic mothers.

Endocardial fibroelastosis is an unusual cardiac malformation in which there is opaqueness and thickening of the endocardial lining of the ventricles (Figure 183, page 283). The pathogenesis is unclear. At times, there are malformations in other organs.

The most common form of cardiac malformation is intraventricular defect, making up over 25 percent of cases. Atrial septal defect, persistent patent ductus arteriosus, and tetralogy of Fallot each account for about 5 to 8 percent of cases. It is not the province of the present consideration to detail the many forms of cardiac defects.

Cardiac malformations are of two causal types, genetic and induced.

Genetic malformations of the heart

Genetic malformations are inherited defects transmitted through defective genes or abnormal chromosomes (page 141). Over half of cases of trisomy 21, Down syndrome, have cardiac defects.

Induced malformations of the heart

Induced malformations are due to adverse gestational factors — such as exposure to intrauterine hypoxia, maternal illness, irradiation — occurring during embryonic or early fetal life and affecting the development of the organism (page 141). When the embryo or early fetus is exposed to a noxious process, those structures that are actively undergoing formation at that time are specifically highly susceptible to injury, with the consequence that, if the organism survives, it will have defects in the structures previously insulted.

At six to eight weeks of gestation, the embryonic heart is being formed. If an adversive intrauterine condition, an insult to the organism, occurs at this time, this predisposes to defective formation of the heart. It is of note that offspring of mothers with diabetic conditions have a high incidence of malformations, particularly abnormalities of the cardiovascular system.

Cardiac malformations of varying severity are diagnosed in about 1 percent of liveborn infants.

With the advent of surgical treatment of cardiac defects in recent times, there has been much improvement in the clinical status, the well-being and survival, of affected infants. In cases of complex malformations with hypoxia that cannot be ameliorated by treatment, hypoxic death occurs soon after birth. Infants with less severe anomalies that survive with ongoing hypoxia postnatally are prone to incur hypoxic visceral damage, cerebral hypoxic damage.

Infections Causing Fetal-neonatal Brain Damage

Bacterial meningitis
Viral infections
> **TORCH**
> **Influenza**
> **Cytomegalic viral disease**
> **Herpes simplex**
> **Rubella**
> **HIV (AIDS)**

Other fetal-neonatal infections
> **Toxoplasmosis**
> **Syphilis**
> **Chlamydia**

Certain pathologic bacteria and viral agents have a predilection for the brain, causing damage directly to the brain tissue. Of most importance are bacterial meningitis and cytomegalic viral infection of the brain.

Bacterial meningitis

Neonatal bacterial meningitis, although rare, occurring with an incidence of 4 cases per 10,000 live births, is important, having a high mortality rate and leaving surviving infants with brain damage, with sequels of mental retardation and blindness.

Meningitis in the newborn is caused predominantly by streptococci and coli organisms. In the pathogenesis of meningitis, the offending bacterial agent invades the bloodstream, producing the manifestations of sepsis in the infant. The invading bacteria, although present throughout the body, target the meningeal covering of the brain and cord. The infection spreads to the underlying surface of the brain, into the cerebral cortex, creating a meningoencephalitis, with damage to the cortex. The subarachnoid fluid at times becomes purulent.

Clinically the affected neonate presents manifestations of sepsis, with fever, lethargy, and with depression of vital functions. Infants develop bulging fontanelles due to edema and swelling of the brain. Stiffening, opisthotonos with bowing of the back, occurs due to inflammation around the spinal cord.

Diagnosis is made by the finding of positive bacteriologic cultures of the blood and spinal fluid. The spinal fluid at times is turbid; organisms often can be detected by direct bacteriologic examination of the spinal fluid.

With the inflammatory process present, nerve cells of the cortex are depleted; residual scarring of the cortex follows. The damage to the cortex leaves surviving infants with varying neurologic disabilities, often with mental retardation, seizures, blindness, or deafness.

Two distinct patterns of meningitis have been delineated with regard to source of infection and time of onset of meningitis:

Fetal-neonatal meningitis, with manifestations that appear within 48 hours of birth, is attributable to infection contracted during fetal life. In such cases there is at times a maternal history of intranatal sepsis — the consequence of premature rupture of membranes with chorioamnionitis. These infants usually also have pneumonia. Fetal-neonatal meningitis usually is marked by a fulminating course with high mortality of 50 to 60 percent.

Postnatal meningitis, with manifestations that appear several days after birth, is attributable to infection contracted from environmental contacts, from the mother or in the nursery. The clinical course is usually less severe than with fetal-neonatal meningitis; mortality is 10 to 20 percent.

Predisposing factors causing meningitis, in addition to maternal sepsis, are prematurity and intrauterine growth retardation of the fetus. Low birth weight term infants, weighing less than 2,500 grams (5 1/2 pounds), have an incidence of meningitis three times greater than infants weighing more than 2,500 grams.

Viral infections causing fetal-neonatal brain damage

Viral disease is second only to hypoxia in its importance as a cause of fetal-neonatal brain damage leading to lasting neurologic disability.

Of the viral diseases that affect the fetus and newborn — infections that damage the brain — of most concern has been cytomegalic viral disease. Increasing attention is presently directed to herpes infection and HIV infection in the fetus and newborn. Rubella infection causing intrauterine encephalitis is well known; however, in the present day with attention given to prevention, such cases are rare. Other viral infections are thought at times to be transmitted from the mother to the fetus and newborn, causing visceral disease, as occurs with neonatal myocarditis (Case 101, page 480).

TORCH

This is an acronym used to identify viral and viral-like agents that damage the embryo and fetus. (T, toxoplasmosis; O, other; R, rubella; C, cytomegalovirus; and H, herpes simplex.) Besides the TORCH agents, a host of other viruses have been implicated as causing damage to the embryo and fetus, including coxsackie virus, measles virus, and poliovirus.

Influenza

Influenza is a hazard to the mother and to the fetus. The virus of influenza does not infect the fetus; damage to the fetus is due to the hypoxia-producing effects of the mother's sepsis and fever. With acute illness in the mother, with fever, the metabolic oxygen requirements of the mother are sharply increased, leaving the fetus oxygen-deprived, hypoxic.

Pregnant women are highly susceptible to influenzal viral infection. Almost all women during pregnancy report periods of "the flu," or upper respiratory infections, with fever, prostration — illnesses that hang on for days, weeks. Influenza during the Asian flu epidemic at times resulted in fetal death; postmortem studies in these cases revealed hypoxic cerebral damage.

Cytomegalic viral disease (CMV)

Illustrative Cases:
Case 163   *p. 592*
Case 197   *p. 654*
Case 216   *p. 704*

Cytomegalic viral disease is increasingly recognized to be the most frequent, most serious, infection affecting the fetus and newborn. Generally overlooked in years past, CMV is now increasingly diagnosed in neonates. The laboratory diagnosis of CMV by culturing and specifically identifying the virus is difficult. New diagnostic methods using DNA probes are being introduced. Clinically the diagnosis can be made, with reasonable certainty, on the basis of the syndromic presence of persisting liver and spleen enlargement, hyperbilirubinemia, and platelet deficiency and other hematologic findings; neurologically there is persisting lethargy and weakness. This syndromic pattern with hepatosplenomegaly is unlike that caused by hypoxia.

In the pathologic process, the cytomegalic virus-infected cell develops a large red nuclear inclusion, and the nucleus and cytoplasm of the cell become enlarged (*cyto-,* cell; *-megaly,* large). Pathologically, the virus infects the liver, spleen, kidney, brain, and other organs.

Cytomegalic infection in the fetus is transmitted from the mother. CMV infection in women is of high incidence (50 to 70 percent of pregnant mothers have CMV antibodies serologically), but only in a small percent does the maternal infection become transmitted through the placenta and cause fetal-neonatal infection and organic damage during gestation. CMV is asymptomatic during gestation, and the diagnosis is not made prior to delivery. The importance of CMV disease in the newborn was generally overlooked in the past, and the diagnosis was missed clinically and pathologically. CMV, now considered the most frequent perinatal viral disease, is estimated to involve 8 per 1,000 births and to be responsible for brain damage in 1 per 1,000 births.

The damage to the brain is primarily in the deep periventricular structures affecting periventricular white matter and basal ganglia. This pattern of damage in the cerebrum is similar to the damage that occurs with hypoxic insult to the premature brain. The predilection of CMV for the deep cerebral strata is indicative of a pathologic process having origin in early premature fetal life, at a time when germinal matrix is present, tissue highly vulnerable to damage by hypoxia as well as by viral insult.

With the pathologic processes of CMV infection ongoing through intrauterine life, through the premature and maturing periods of the fetus, as with intrauterine hypoxic exposure, the damage extends to the cerebral surface, to the cortex, creating here a meningoencephalitis.

The deep cerebral damage, the necrotic tissue, absorbs calcium. In the newborn, and later, the presence of deep cerebral calcifications, demonstrated by x-ray, characterizes CMV disease in the brain.

Late clinical sequels, reflecting damage to periventricular structures, to basal ganglia, appear as spastic cerebral palsy, with ex vacuo hydrocephalus due to loss of periventricular tissue, and cortical manifestations of mental retardation, seizure disorder, deafness, and ocular disorders.

In cases of CMV disease with less severe cerebral damage, although without manifestations postnatally, infants may develop deafness and other subtle neurologic abnormalities in later infancy.

Clinically, in retrospective interpretation of cerebral palsy and other neurologic disabilities in infants, of importance in litigation, it is necessary to be mindful of CMV infection as a cause of cerebral palsy.

Years back, CMV was only of academic research interest, an entity that was unknown to most clinicians. Even though the characteristic hepatosplenic enlargement and other identifying findings of CMV disease were present, were detailed and described in the newborn hospital record, the diagnosis of CMV infection was not thought of, was not applied.

In cases of cerebral palsy, with recorded evidence of neonatal hepatosplenomegaly and related findings, it is pertinent to bring into consideration CMV disease as the cause of the cerebral palsy.

Herpes simplex infection causing fetal-neonatal brain damage

Fetal-neonatal herpes infection is being diagnosed with increasing frequency. This is due to a real increase in incidence and to a heightened awareness of the infection. In the adult, the epidemic increase of genital herpes in recent years is well known to doctors and the public; in the newborn, correspondingly, systemic herpes infection is an increasing problem. In the past, the diagnosis of herpes viral infection, clinically and pathologically, was often overlooked, both in adults and in the newborn.

Transmission of herpes simplex infection from the mother to the fetus at times takes place early in utero; however, in most cases the fetus is infected during delivery, during the descent through the birth canal.

Transplacental infection occurs in cases following active recent genital infection in the mother. In the fetus, organ involvement occurs, particularly affecting the brain. Fetal herpes is known to cause malformation, at times miscarriage, stillbirth. Surviving newborn usually show intrauterine growth retardation.

Intrapartum fetal infection is increasingly recognized to be the most frequent route of fetal infection with herpes simplex.

The incidence of maternal herpes during pregnancy is 1 to 2 percent. In cases of maternal infection with herpes virus, genital lesions may or may not be evident at parturition. The presence of overt genital lesions greatly increases the hazard for the fetus. Premature infants born of mothers infected with herpes, delivered vaginally, are at high risk.

Pathologic studies of cases of fetal-neonatal herpes viral disease reveal varying severity of involvement of the major organs; the lungs, liver, heart, and kidneys may be affected, showing focal areas of necrosis. In the brain, periventricular damage as well as cortical lesions occur.

Clinically, in affected newborn, the initial manifestations commonly are lethargy and convulsions. The syndrome of disseminated intravascular coagulopathy (DIC) occurs with the viral infection (page 114).

In infants who survive after neonatal herpes viral disease, the neurologic sequels include microcephaly, mental retardation, spastic motor disabilities, and seizure disorder.

In recent years, specific antiviral drugs have improved the prognosis for infected infants. Although other viral infections resist antiviral medication, two drugs, *acyclovir* and *vidarabine*, have proven effective in infants with herpes infection.

Rubella (German measles) encephalitis in the fetus and newborn

Maternal rubella infection during early pregnancy has devastating effects on the fetus. During the 1964 German measles epidemic in the United States, an estimated 40,000 infants were born with brain damage due to maternal infection, and an equal number of stillbirths occurred. In recent decades mass vaccination, routine immunization, has almost eradicated the disease in children and thereby reduced transmission of rubella to susceptible, nonimmunized pregnant women.

Prenatal routine serologic testing identifies pregnant women with low or no rubella titer, indicating that the mother is susceptible, that she does not have immunity through natural infection or vaccination. If the susceptible mother is exposed to German measles during the first 8 to 12 weeks of gestation, the fetus is at high risk for damage to the brain.

Pathologically, maternal infection during the early weeks of gestation damages the embryo and results in induced malformations, referred to as the "rubella syndrome" or "rubella embryopathy." The malformations are mostly of the brain, heart, and eyes.

With the pathologic processes of rubella infection continuing through the early months of gestation, destructive inflammation, necrosis of tissue, occurs in the liver, brain, and other organs. The cerebrum incurs meningoencephalitis of varying severity, with damage to the deep periventricular structures, the basal ganglia, and to the cortex.

Infected newborn infants usually are small, showing the effects of intrauterine growth retardation. The infants are anemic; liver and spleen are involved, hepatosplenomegaly; eye abnormalities, cataracts and microphthalmia, commonly are present at birth. Infants are depressed, hypotonic, and frequently have neonatal seizures.

In infants surviving, with infection having occurred during the first 8 weeks of gestation, as many as 85 percent will have detectable defects during infancy. Characteristically, there is microcephaly, mental retardation, spastic motor disability, blindness, and hearing loss.

HIV infection (AIDS); fetal-neonatal encephalopathy

As with AIDS in adults, the effects of the human immunodeficiency virus on the fetus and newborn vary over a broad range. The infection, transmitted in utero, may devastate the brain. In other cases, manifestations are long delayed or may never be apparent.

The pathologic effects of HIV infection present at birth often are obscured by other brain-damaging processes originating during gestation or postnatally. Gestation is commonly complicated by maternal cocaine or other drug abuse; commonly maternal nutrition is poor, with resulting pregnancy low weight gain.

Premature birth is frequent. Intrauterine growth retardation is evident in most HIV-infected infants. Frequently there is a superimposed cytomegalic viral or other infection.

Pathologically, in infected newborn infants with brain involvement, the process is progressive destructive encephalitis damaging the brain diffusely, the deep structures as well as the cortex. The blighted brain lags in growth, with resulting microcephaly developing during infancy. Calcifications of basal ganglia are at times demonstrable radiologically.

In cases with brain damage resulting from the HIV infection, neurologic manifestations may come on rapidly, or the disabilities may not appear until late in infancy or may be delayed for years. The neurologic disabilities are of a broad spectrum, often including intractable seizures, mental retardation, blindness, and spastic quadriplegia.

Other infections causing fetal-neonatal brain damage

In addition to the viral infections discussed here, a number of other agents, microorganisms, are known to infect the fetus, causing brain damage. Of these, toxoplasmosis, caused by the protozoan *Toxoplasma gondii*, and syphilis, caused by *Treponema pallidum*, are of significant incidence.

Toxoplasmosis as a cause of fetal-neonatal encephalitis

Fetal infection with *Toxoplasma gondii* is of importance in its incidence and severity, second only to cytomegalic viral infection. This protozoan parasite is transmitted to human adults via cysts in undercooked meat and via cat feces contaminated with the cysts. Most women have no toxoplasma antibody and are at risk for acquiring toxoplasma infection during pregnancy. Toxoplasmosis has been detected in up to 2 per 1,000 live births in the United States. Fetal infection is acquired transplacentally.

Pathologically the infection causes focal necrotizing meningoencephalitis with a predilection for the periventricular strata, causing periventricular infarction. Calcification occurs in areas of necrosis in the cerebrum. Periventricular inflammation around the aqueduct at times causes aqueductial obstruction, later resulting in hydrocephalus. In the fetus, eye structures are affected, causing chorioretinitis.

As with other intrauterine infections, the newborn infants are small, under-nourished, anemic. Hepatosplenomegaly occurs. The enfeebled infants often are stillborn or die soon after birth.

Surviving infants are severely mentally retarded and have motor manifestations of cerebral palsy and seizures. X-rays of the head reveal calcifications in the brain. Eye examination reveals chorioretinitis.

Syphilis; fetal-neonatal infection with nervous system sequels

In times past, before effective antibiotic treatment, syphilis was the most feared disease of the newborn. The infants (often misdiagnosed at delivery) were highly infective. Little could be done in the way of treatment.

Syphilis is caused by a spirochete, *Treponema pallidum*. This is a spiral bacterium difficult to demonstrate microscopically, difficult to culture. The spirochete crosses the placenta to the fetus after the twentieth week of pregnancy. Early prenatal diagnosis and treatment of the mother usually safeguards the fetus.

Fetal infection, syphilis in the newborn, is usually termed "congenital syphilis." The incidence has been much reduced as a result of prenatal maternal surveillance. However, there has been a resurgence of syphilis in recent years.

With intranatal gestational syphilis, stillbirth is common. Premature delivery occurs in up to 50 percent of cases. Often the newborn infants are small for gestational age.

All the tissues of the body are susceptible to damage by the spirochete of syphilis. In classic cases of congenital syphilis, the affected newborn have enlargement of the liver and spleen; the infants have florid rhinitis, called "snuffles," respiratory distress due to lung involvement, "pneumonia alba," and skin rashes. However, abnormal neurologic signs are uncommon in the neonate with syphilis. In newborn infected infants, examination of the spinal fluid consistently reveals a positive serology for syphilis. The infection of the nervous system consists of a latent subacute meningoencephalitis. Neurologic manifestations, however, are usually long delayed, for years.

The bodily manifestations, the stigmata of congenital syphilis, that appear in childhood are characteristic. Blindness develops due to interstitial keratitis. Destruction of nasal bones, with depression of the ridge of the nose, produces the "saddle nose." Scars, "rhagades," develop in the skin at the edges of the mouth. Notched teeth are a classic sign of congenital syphilis.

Late nervous system manifestations mainly reflect cortical damage, due to the ongoing meningoencephalitis. Mental retardation and epilepsy develop.

Chlamydia infection

Chlamydia disease, due to the organism *chlamydia trachomatis*, is common among unmarried women pregnant for the first time. Stillbirth and neonatal death occur ten times more often among chlamydia-infected women than among uninfected controls.

Physical Injury of the Nervous System in the Fetus and Newborn

External abnormalities of the head consequent to parturition
Subdural hemorrhage
Spinal cord and brain stem injury

Physical injury present in the newborn in most instances is due to intrinsic forces that impact on the fetus during parturition.

External abnormalities about the head — caput succedaneum, cephalohematoma, and molding — are common. Forceps marks, abrasions of the skin, appear at times following the application of low forceps. More important, with difficult parturition, cerebral subdural hemorrhage and at times spinal cord and brain stem injury occur.

The hazards confronting the fetus mount to a climax during the hours of labor. Birth is the most endangering experience to which most individuals are ever exposed. The perinatal period has a death rate greater than any other time of life. The birth process, even under optimal controlled conditions, is a traumatic, potentially crippling, event for the fetus. Compressed and forced through the birth canal, the fetus is subjected to rapid, often turbulent, bodily alterations. Often the borderline between what is physiologic and what is pathologic is not distinct. Although all parts of the body are vulnerable to mechanical injury during birth, the most sensitive target proves to be the structures of the nervous system. Particularly for the premature fetus — unready and fragile, expressed through a physiologically unprepared, unrelaxed birth canal — parturitional injury is an imminent threat.

In a broad view, the occurrence of brain damage in the newborn, its incidence and significance, has in the past often been presented in the literature in an obscure, inaccurate manner. Despite increasing information from the laboratory, old misconceptions regarding "birth injury" continue to be transmitted in the medical and lay literature.

External abnormalities of the head consequent to parturition

Forceps application; "forceps marks"
Fractures of the skull
Caput succedaneum
Cephalohematoma
Molding of the head

During passage through the birth canal, in cases with cephalic presentation, the head undergoes changes evident externally at delivery; commonly there is a caput succedaneum, at times a cephalohematoma, and usually some degree of molding. In assessing intracranial injury in the newborn, it is important that these external abnormalities of the head, their causes and pathologic significance, be understood. The presence of a large caput succedaneum or a prominent degree of molding does not automatically mean there is associated intracranial injury.

Forceps application; "forceps marks"

Forceps application to the head as a cause of brain damage continues to be a subject of clinical dispute. It has been concluded by some that the application of obstetric forceps, even low-outlet forceps, crushes the head, causing acute brain damage that later leads to cerebral palsy and other chronic cerebral disability. This clinical interpretation still is conveyed at times despite pathology investigations, autopsy studies, that indicate there is no substantial basis linking the use of low forceps to acute brain injury.

Low forceps application at times leaves "forceps marks," abrasions about the head. Such surface marks are common, not reflective of internal trauma.

No doubt the hasty or faulty application of forceps may cause direct cranial damage. However, the forceful employment of forceps, combined with excessive traction, usually causes damage, not directly to the cranium, but indirectly to the spinal structures and brain stem.

The use of high forceps and midforceps, common in times past, was a hazard for the mother and the fetus. Laceration of the cervix and vagina occurred, with dangerous hemorrhaging. Damage to the head of the fetus occurred with deformation of the head, with skull fracture and intracranial lacerations. In the present day, such head injuries are avoided by resorting to cesarean section.

Fracture of the skull

Extensive fractures of the skull incurred during delivery of the fetus are rare in present-day obstetrical practice. The infrequency of skull injury in the fetus during delivery is largely due to the elasticity and compressibility of the soft cranial bones, to the ease with which they can override one another at their broad, loose sutures.

Indentation of the calvarium

This is the most common traumatic lesion of the skull. The injury, sometimes called a "depressed fracture," is not a fracture at all, but merely an indentation of the wall of the calvarium, appearing as a depression in the cranium, usually 3 to 4 centimeters wide (Figure 77). Indentations are the result of flicking inward of the flexible resilient plate of bone, like depressing the side of a ping-pong ball.

Most commonly the deformity is produced as the head is pulled under the promontory of the pelvis during a breech or forceps extraction. The deformity of the skull in most cases is easily corrected, and the lesion is usually without complications. With indentation, at times tearing of small blood vessels between the dura and the overlying bone occurs, with the formation of a localized epidural hematoma.

Figure 77. Indentation of the calvarium ("depressed fracture" of the frontal bone). Note the associated persisting downward displacement of the frontal bone and the overriding of the parietal bone.

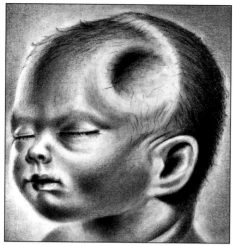

Fig. 77

Caput succedaneum

Illustrative Cases:
Case 18   *p. 274*
Case 27   *p. 301*
Case 64   *p. 391*
Case 203 *p. 669*

This is an area of boggy swelling that forms in the scalp over the presenting part of the head in cephalic presentations. The elevated, rounded area of the caput succedaneum corresponds to the portion of the scalp surface that is exposed within the opening of the dilated cervix during labor. Pathologically, the scalp in the area of the caput is swollen to three or four times its normal thickness and is suffused with edematous hemorrhagic fluid (Figure 78). The circumscribed area of edema and congestion is due to local interference with circulation produced by the close embrace of the rigid cervical ring; this local swelling and edema of the scalp is similar to that which occurs distal to a tourniquet on a limb.

The location of the caput succedaneum is such that it adds to the elongation-distortion that develops with the process of parturitional cranial molding. Most commonly, the caput occurs asymmetrically over the crown of the head, in the parietal region, in association with vertex presentations. With breech presentations, analogous swelling and hemorrhagic discoloration occur over the buttocks and scrotum or labia. With brow presentation, the swelling occurs over the frontal area and forehead, and in face presentation the eyelids, cheek, and nose are edematous and reddened.

Postnatally the caput succedaneum gradually diminishes, often disappearing during the first day after birth. The presence of a large caput, consequent to a protracted labor with strong uterine contractions, although not of direct bearing neurologically, does signify that injury to dural and other intracranial structures may be anticipated.

Figure 78. Caput succedaneum. **(a).** At birth, head showing localized prominence over the left posterior region forming a caput. Prolonged labor with cervix completely dilated at 11 hours. Intranatal death.

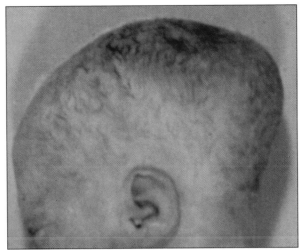

Fig. 78(a)

Figure 78(b). Incision of the caput succedaneum at autopsy. Cut surface showing gelatinous hemorrhagic edematous thickening forming the caput succedaneum.

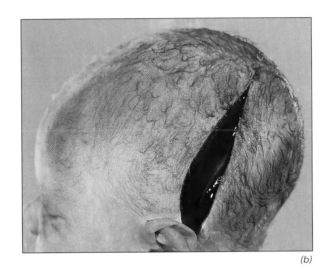

(b)

Figure 78(c). Caput succedaneum formation; section through the head showing a circumscribed thickening in the scalp due to edema and hemorrhage in the soft tissue of the scalp, creating a caput succedaneum.

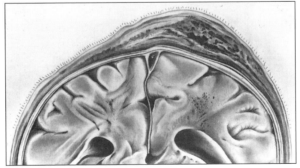

(c)

With brow presentation a caput succedaneum forms over the forehead (Case 22, page 286).

In cases of face presentation, with the face protruding foremost into the cervix, a caput succedaneum forms over the face, resulting in diffuse red edema over the forehead, eyes, face, and chin (Figure 79).

With breech presentation, the buttocks, pushing forward through the birth canal, forms the equivalent of a caput succedaneum over the buttocks area (Figure 80) (Case 4, page 233).

Figure 79. Face presentation; the reddened edematous "caput" over the face. Term pregnancy. Loss of fetal heart tones during labor. Difficult midforceps delivery; intranatal death.

Figure 80. Breech presentation with area of reddening over the buttocks, analogous to a caput succedaneum. 24 weeks' gestation; loss of fetal heart tones during labor.

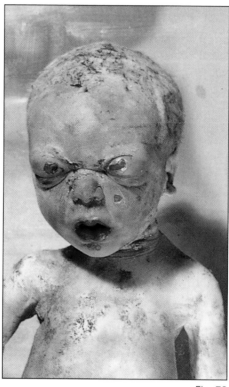 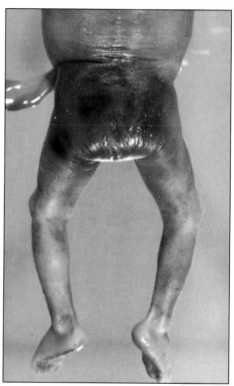

Fig. 79   *Fig. 80*

Cephalohematoma

Cephalohematoma is a localized accumulation of blood, a hematoma, deep to the scalp, between the bone surface and the periosteum (Figure 81). The periosteum, the fibrous sheath normally tightly adherent to the outer surface of the skull bone, becomes detached in the formation of the cephalohematoma. The difference between caput succedaneum and cephalohematoma: The caput is an extravasation of edema fluid and blood *through* the scalp soft tissue; the cephalohematoma is an extravasation of blood *under* the scalp. Unlike caput succedaneum, variably located on the head, cephalohematoma is confined to the periosteal sheath of a single bone, commonly the right parietal bone, and never crosses a suture line.

Cephalohematoma is a rare condition occurring in less than 1 percent of newborns, and varies in size from a centimeter to golf ball proportions.

Cephalohematoma is generally considered to be due to mechanical trauma: during labor, with the cyclic uterine contractions, the presenting surface of the fetal head is subjected to forward and backward movements and compression against the sides of the birth canal. The friction of this repeated tangential traction and recoil, it is thought, causes loosening and avulsion of the periosteum, tearing blood vessels and leading to hematoma formation.

Cephalohematoma is a more serious lesion than caput succedaneum. The hematoma swelling often tends to increase during the first day or two after birth, as more and more blood accumulates, but it gradually recedes in subsequent weeks as the blood is absorbed.

Although exerting no direct effect on the underlying brain, cephalohematoma, like caput succedaneum, reflects a difficult parturition, and at times its presence is immediately overshadowed by concomitant major intracranial hypoxic or mechanical injury.

Figure 81. Cephalohematoma over the right parietal bone. **(a).** External appearance of cephalohematoma.

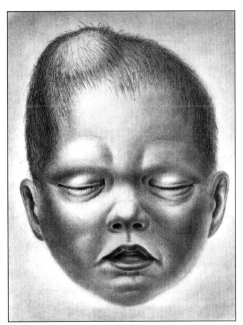

Fig. 81(a)

Figure 81(b). Frontal section through the involved region of the head, through the hematoma over the right parietal bone; the extravasation of blood is confined to the subperiosteal stratum.

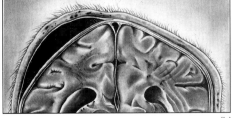

(b)

Molding of the head

Molding of the head, changes in the shape of the fetal head, from a rounded ball to an elongated football shape, is the consequence of the lateral compression exerted on the fetal head in its passage through the birth canal (Figure 82).

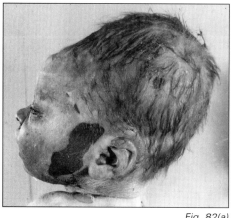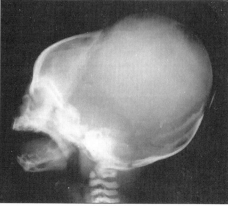

Fig. 82(a)   *(b)*

Figure 82. Molding of the head; maternal cephalopelvic disproportion. Postmature at 43 weeks; newborn weight, 4,000 grams (9 pounds). Intranatal death, early maceration. **(a).** Severe vertical molding. **(b).** X-ray of the head corresponding to (a) showing molding, with parietal bone overlapping the frontal and occipital bones.

The plastic changes of the head in molding are possible because of the softness of the bone and because the broad, loose sutural connections permit displacement and overlapping or overriding of the individual skull bones (Figure 83). Overriding is usually most conspicuous over the parietal region, one parietal bone being tucked under the other, but commonly it also involves the parietal bones in conjunction with the frontal or occipital bones.

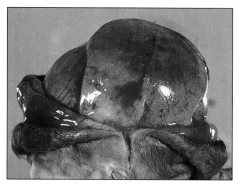

Fig. 83

Figure 83. Molding of the head with overriding of the skull bones; parietal bone overriding the frontal and occipital bones. Autopsy examination: scalp flaps rolled back to expose the molding displacement of the skull bones.

The shape of the molded head, the pattern of the distortion and the direction of the elongation, is determined primarily by the position of the fetal head as it becomes engaged and traverses the birth canal. Vertical elongation of the head, the most common form of molding, occurs with vertex presentations; the face and forehead are compressed and flattened (Figure 84).

Figure 84. Vertical molding of the head. Arrows indicate force of lateral compression exerted on the head during the descent through the birth canal, causing elongation of the head.

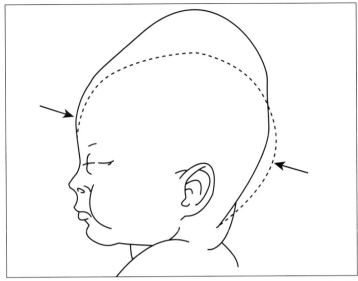

Fig. 84

Molding of some degree occurs regularly in cephalic delivery, with the oversize fetal head — positioned as the forward element — penetrating, dilating, overcoming the circumferential resistance of the birth canal. In the newly born infant, the elongation of the head caused by molding usually is further increased and exaggerated by the presence of a caput succedaneum.

Molding is often viewed as a physiologic part of the process of parturition, a mechanism that allows delivery of the relatively oversize head through the tight pelvic conduit. Pathologically it is of concern because the forces that bring it about may also produce intolerable stress and damage to intracranial structures. There is no doubt that severe parturitional distortion of the fetal head, excessive molding, imposes strain on the dural structures, and that the resulting stretching and tearing of the dura and its venous channels leads to subdural hemorrhage.

Subdural hemorrhage due to dural-venous laceration

Clinically, in the past, in infants with neurologic signs after birth, often the diagnosis of subdural hemorrhage was applied empirically, almost automatically, routinely, and generally in error, as ultimately shown at autopsy. In recent years there has been increasing cognizance of the predominance of hypoxic brain damage, rather than subdural hemorrhage, as the main cause of postnatal neurologic disability.

Subdural hemorrhage appears as an extravasation of blood between the surface of the brain and the apposing dura lining the inner aspect of the skull.

The dura, in addition to lining the inner aspect of the skull, forms two fibrous sheets, septa, that extend into the cranial cavity. The tentorium is a horizontal tent-like structure spread over the upper surface of the cerebellum, separating the cerebellum from the posterior part of the cerebrum that lies above. The other dural sheet, the falx, is a midline septum between the cerebral hemispheres.

Incorporated into the dural septa, at their edges, are large venous channels that receive the veins that drain the brain.

Pathogenesis of subdural hemorrhage; dural-venous laceration. Tearing of the dural septa, tearing of the venous channels, causes subdural hemorrhage. Dural-venous laceration is mainly endogenous in origin, in most cases occurring intranatally during active labor in the descent through the birth canal. The immediate causal mechanism is directly related to parturitional molding of the fetal head. During delivery, with molding, the taut tentorium and falx, tightly attached to the cranial bones, are forced to adjust to the altered, elongated shape of the head; in the fetus, the dural sheets, stretching across the cranial cavity like guy wires, resist excessive change in the shape of the head. If molding is protracted and severe, or if it occurs suddenly, the fibrous dural septa, subjected to intolerable tension and strain, give way, split, and tear as shown in Figure 85. Stretch-tearing of the tentorium and other dural structures results in rupture of the venous sinuses within the dura and avulsion of the attached bridging veins from the brain—with the consequent subdural hemorrhage.

Figure 85. Subdural hemorrhage, pathogenesis. View of the intracranial dural structures, the falx cerebri above and the tentorium spreading downward. Stretch injury consequent to vertical molding elongation distortion of the head; characteristic laceration of the tentorium at its attachment to the falx, penetrating the dural venous blood sinus; resulting subdural hemorrhage.

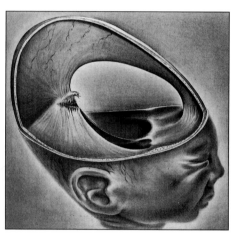

Fig. 85

Causal factors clinically contributing to subdural hemorrhage are: (1) Macrosomia; with the large head of the macrosomic fetus subjected to excessive molding, stretch-tearing of the dural structures results. (2) Precipitous labor; with the head unmolded, forced rapidly through the birth canal, the dural structures subjected to sudden stress, stretch and tear. (3) Breech presentation; delivery of the aftercoming head often is difficult, traumatic, especially in prematures; the aftercoming head, unmolded, is forced through a rigid incompletely dilated cervix. This is a hazard, resulting in tentorial laceration with posterior fossa subdural hemorrhage.

With cephalic presentation, during descent the head is gradually molded, reducing the head circumference, facilitating passage of the head through the birth canal. In contrast, with breech birth, the aftercoming head remains unmolded, with a relatively large circumference. This is conducive to intracranial stress, with resulting tentorial stretch-tear, with posterior fossa subdural hemorrhage.

Two patterns of subdural hemorrhage in the neonate are of concern: posterior fossa subdural hemorrhage and cerebral subdural hemorrhage.

Figure 86. Posterior fossa subdural hemorrhage, the consequence of tentorial laceration. Accumulation of blood leads to rapidly fatal compression of the brain stem.

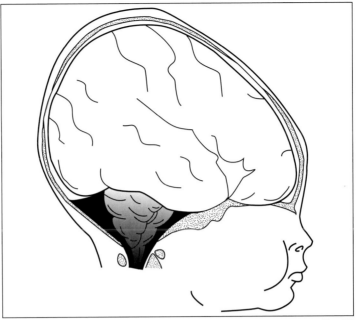

Fig. 86

Figure 87. Cerebral subdural hemorrhage occurring as a thin film over the upper surface of the cerebrum. Excessive cranial molding; bleeding follows stretch and tear of bridging veins attached to the superior sagittal dural venous sinus.

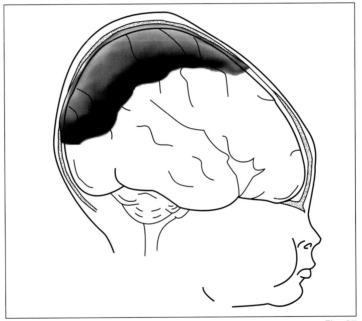

Fig. 87

Posterior fossa subdural hemorrhage

Posterior fossa subdural hemorrhage is almost always fatal. The accumulation of blood in the posterior fossa, usually the consequence of a tear at the junction of the falx and tentorium near the attachment of the vein of Galen, results in lethal compression of the brain stem (Figures 85 and 86).

Cerebral subdural hemorrhage

The cerebral form, with blood over the convexity of the hemispheres, occurs mainly at term and, although common, is usually mild. With molding of the head during labor, the bridging veins between the medial superior aspect of the cerebrum and the superior sagittal sinus become stretched and may tear. Bleeding in this area is usually limited to a thin film of blood forming over the cerebrum (Figure 87).

Breech delivery

Breech presentation, with the fetus flexed, with the buttocks directed downward toward the cervix, is a hazard to the fetus in two ways. In breech deliveries endogenous spinal injury is relatively frequent. Damage is commonly present in the lower thoracic, lumbar, and sacral segments and is attributable to hyperflexion of the spine during descent of the fetus. In other cases of breech delivery, spinal injury may be of exogenous obstetrical origin, due to traction or manipulation in extracting the aftercoming head.

Breech birth also is a cause of liver compression, liver laceration (page 102).

Spinal cord and brain stem injury

Forms of injury
>   **Spinal fracture and dislocation**
>   **Spinal epidural hemorrhage**
>   **Brain stem injury**

Causes
Effects

Physical injury to the spinal cord and brain stem due to excessive forceful obstetrical processes is rare in the present day.

In decades past, when the use of high forceps with axis traction was acceptable obstetric practice, pathologically, at autopsy, cases of spinal cord and brain stem injury were common, observed in up to 10 percent of newborn deaths.

In present day obstetric practice, forceful forceps delivery is avoided, with resort increasingly to cesarean section in complicated births.

Forms of injury

Spinal cord and brain stem injuries present in the neonate vary in pattern and severity.

Spinal fracture-dislocation; cord laceration

In the most severe form, the spinal cord incurs lacerations, at times transectional tears. Fracture of the spine with dislocation of vertebrae occurs in some cases due to excessive traction at delivery. The vertebral bodies become separated one from another, with the cord stretched and torn (Figure 88).

Figure 88. Fracture dislocation of spine present at birth. View of the thoracic cavity with viscera removed at autopsy. Excessive traction during delivery; stillbirth. As shown, cervical vertebrae are separated, pulled apart; transectional tear of the cord.

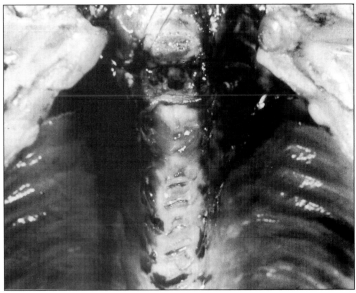

Fig. 88

Spinal epidural hemorrhage

Spinal epidural hemorrhage is the commonest form of spinal injury in the newborn. The lesion, although it often does not appear of lethal character, is of importance in that its presence is an indication that the cord and other spinal structures have been exposed to trauma. At autopsy, in cases with extensive epidural bleeding, the cord, when exposed, appears mired in gelatinous hemorrhagic material (Figure 89).

Figure 89. Spinal injury; spinal epidural hemorrhage. At autopsy, view of the posterior aspect of the body cavity, viscera removed. The vertebral canal has been opened, removing the column of vertebral bodies and the spinal cord; a thick layer of gelatinous epidural hemorrhage in the thoraco-cervical portion of the canal. Precipitous delivery of a premature infant in a primipara. Infant apneic at birth, survived 4 hours.

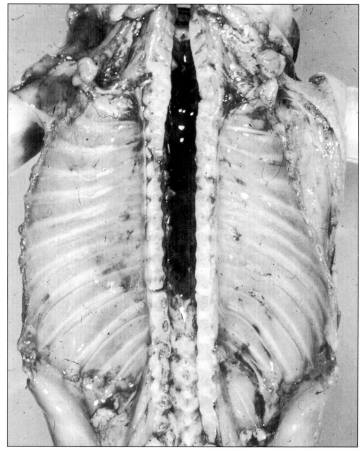

Fig. 89

In cases of neonatal epidural spinal hemorrhage, damage to the neighboring spinal structures varies. At times with epidural hemorrhage there occurs grossly visible avulsion of spinal nerve roots and laceration of the meninges (Figure 90).

Figure 90. Spinal cord injury. Epidural hemorrhage associated with laceration of the dura and damage to the substance of the cord. Premature infant of 37 weeks' gestation, lived 16 hours; respiratory depression and hypotonia.

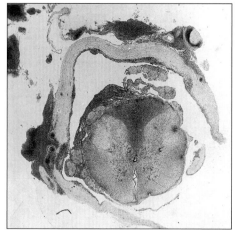

Fig. 90

Brain stem injury

Brain stem damage is at times found in conjunction with stretch injury of the spinal cord. Forceful traction tends to produce compression injury of the brain stem, the medulla being drawn down and herniated into the foramen magnum. The brain stem, throttled in the foramen, suffers laceration injury as well as compression (Figure 91). The cerebellum, lying posteriorly, impaled on the edge of the foramen magnum, may be severely damaged as the surface structures grind against the base of the skull and are torn (Figure 92).

Figure 91. Laceration of the brain stem incurred during delivery. Transection of the brain stem at the level of the fourth ventricle. Laceration and hemorrhage of the cerebellar peduncles on each side of the fourth ventricle. Complicated breech extraction with difficulty delivering the aftercoming head. Infant apneic, cyanotic, hypotonic; death after 2 hours.

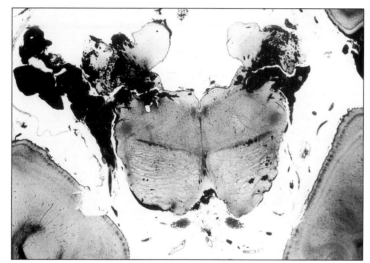

Fig. 91

Figure 92. Brain stem injury with damage to the cerebellum. Hemorrhagic laceration, fragmentation, of the ventral surface of the cerebellar hemispheres. Damage due to excessive traction at delivery. Damage to the ventral portion of the cerebellum related to the margins of the foramen magnum. Delivery of term infant with high forceps; forceps slipped and reapplied. Infant apneic, ventilated at birth; death after 4 hours. Autopsy revealed spinal injury as well as cerebellar injury.

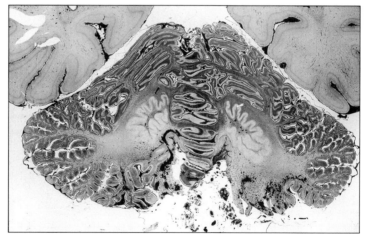

Fig. 92

Causes of spinal cord and brain stem injury

Spinal cord injury is due to causal processes that are endogenous or exogenous.

Endogenous causes are pathologic conditions present prior to labor or early in labor that cause spinal injury in the fetus. Malposition, causing hyperextension or hyperflexion of the fetus, is the major factor in endogenous spinal injury (Hellström and Sallmander, 1968). In some cases of unrelieved abnormal cephalic presentations, with brow presentation (Case 22, page 286) and with face presentation (Figure 79, page 128; Case 178, page 616), and at times in breech or transverse presentation, with persisting hyperextension or hyperflexion, the resulting narrowing of the spinal canal and compression of the cord, especially at the foramen magnum, reduces the cord segment to a gelatinous paste.

Exogenous forces are the cause of most spinal cord and brain stem injury, injury resulting from excessive force applied obstetrically during delivery. Forceful longitudinal traction — particularly when combined with flexion, hyperextension, or torsion of the spinal axis — has been considered the most important cause of neonatal spinal and brain stem injury. Two basic mechanical components are involved: stretch injury and compression injury. Stretch injury occurs when excessive traction is applied on the trunk to obtain the aftercoming head in breech delivery. It also may occur with excessive forceps traction in cephalic presentation.

Effects of spinal cord and brain stem injury

Apnea is the prime symptom of spinal cord and brain stem injury. The clinical pattern of neonatal spinal injury as characterized in the old German literature pictured the newborn infant *"mit Herzschlag aber nicht atmend,"* with heartbeat but not breathing. The direct effects of neonatal spinal cord and brain stem injury appear in three main clinical groups.

In the first group, death occurs rapidly during labor or soon after birth, the consequence of intolerable injury to vital regulatory centers in the brain stem and upper cord. In infants who survive initially, central respiratory depression, punctuated by periods of apnea, is often complicated terminally by superimposed peripheral pulmonary respiratory distress due to hyaline membrane disease or pneumonia.

The second group comprises infants who survive for long periods, often years, with crippling neurologic defects directly due to spinal injury present at birth. Disability may range from the transient and mild to permanent paraplegia. As has been pointed out, there must exist a large number of instances of perinatal injury of mild degree, with minimal neurologic symptoms, in children who are awkward or spastic, that are relegated to the category of cerebral palsy. In cases of spinal injury at birth in which minimal damage to the cord and nerve roots occurs, clinically there may result corresponding neurologic defects affecting limbs, diaphragm, or other parts. Damage to the cranial nerve nuclei or nerve roots associated with brain stem trauma at birth may be a causal factor in facial diplegia, extraocular muscle imbalance, and other cranial nerve deficits in children.

The third group of cases comprises newborn infants with spinal injury who, secondarily, suffer cerebral hypoxic damage. Respiratory depression and systemic hypoxia imposed at birth by spinal injury may result in widespread hypoxic devastation of the cerebrum. The effects of the superimposed cerebral damage may prove far more crippling than those of the primary spinal injury; infants so blighted may ultimately manifest symptoms of mental retardation, cerebral palsy, epilepsy, and other neurologic disorders.

Malformations of the Nervous System

Pathogenesis of malformations
Malformations; basic types
  Genetic microcephaly
  Macrocephaly
  Chromosome-linked malformations
  Cerebral dysplasias
  Neural tube defects
  Obstructive hydrocephalus

Malformations of the nervous system, relatively rare in occurrence, are of great variety. Basic patterns, as presented here, are of relevance in clinical practice.

Malformations, pathologically, are *formative* defects, abnormalities in organ structure due to primary defects in formation originating in embryonic or early fetal life. In this context, excluded are defects in structure consequent to breakdown of tissue, *encephaloclastic* damage, incurred during intrauterine life. The interpretation of malformations, clinically and pathologically, is encumbered by ambiguity in classification and terminology. In this direction, especially confusing is the use of the term "congenital."

"Congenital malformation," a term widely used, is of variable interpretation. Literally, it means a deficit existing before birth, seemingly inclusive of inborn genetic abnormalities *and* abnormalities due to encephaloclastic damage (breakdown of structures previously well formed, damage acquired during fetal life). However in common usage medically, "congenital" has come to mean inborn defects, exclusive of acquired encephaloclastic defects. Because of its equivocal connotation, the term "congenital defect" will not be applied here in classifying nervous system malformations.

Pathogenesis of nervous system malformations

Inborn defects
  Genetic
  Chromosomal
Induced defects (embryonic)

With regard to causation, malformations are of two basic types: **inborn,** due to defective genes or abnormal chromosomes, and **induced,** due to abnormalities acquired by the embryo.

Inborn malformations: genetic, chromosomal

In times past, inborn defects, of hereditary nature, were recognized by their familial occurrence. The experiments of Mendel elaborated mechanisms of hereditary defects. In recent times advances in chromosome analysis have provided insight into intrinsic mechanisms of a broad group of inborn malformations. Current molecular genetic techniques probe deeply into basic pathogenesis of inborn defects.

Genetic causes of malformations

Genes are the component parts that make up chromosomes. Gene-linked abnormalities are the result of defective genes present in the chromosomes.

The number of genes in the 23 pairs of chromosomes in each human cell is estimated to be between 50,000 and 100,000. The introduction of modern molecular genetic research techniques has made possible the location of genes on chromosomes: Over 1,000 human genes have been located. Applying these advances, linkage can be made between bodily abnormalities and specific genes.

Genetic malformations are transmitted through abnormal genes. Abnormal genes may be inherited, contributed by one or both parents. Or the abnormal gene may arise through mutation, the conversion of a normal gene to an abnormal gene.

Gene abnormalities account for a vast variety of structural disorders, such as familial microcephaly, and metabolic abnormalities, such as phenylketonuria (PKU), that cause mental retardation.

Chromosomal causes of malformations

Chromosome-linked malformations are due to abnormalities in chromosomes in the cells of the body. There may be a less than normal number of chromosomes or an excessive number, or there may be defects in the form of the chromosomes.

Induced malformations (embryonic): causes

Illustrative Case:
Case 185 *p. 630*

Induced malformations originate when the cells of the embryo are exposed to noxious processes, with the result that parts of the embryo develop abnormally. Induced malformations of the nervous system and other structures occur with maternal disease, particularly diabetes, and with maternal exposure to irradiation or infection. If the embryo survives, the fetus will have defects corresponding to the abnormal cellular parts of the embryo.

In many cases the cause of a malformation is uncertain, with differentiation between genetic and induced etiology problematic. Certain malformations, in some instances, are genetic, in other cases are induced. For example, it appears that anencephaly in some instances is genetic, appearing repeatedly in a family. In other cases, anencephaly is conclusively an induced abnormality following exposure to noxious processes during the beginning of gestation.

Malformations: basic types

Selected types of malformations are presented, correlated with pathogenesis.

Genetic microcephaly; microcephaly vera

Illustrative Case:
Case 102   *p. 484*

This is a cerebral malformation, a genetic abnormality transmitted down through families, with one or both parents microcephalic and the offspring microcephalic. These microcephalic people in common reference are called "pin-heads." All are mentally retarded.

These familial cases are considered to be *microcephaly vera,* true microcephaly, in contrast to the small head of infants with Down syndrome or the microcephaly in infants consequent to brain damage originating during fetal life with failure of the damaged brain to grow after birth. Microcephaly vera, in addition to its occurrence in families, may occur as an isolated case independently, without apparent genetic influence.

Figure 93. Microcephaly vera. The forebrain, the cerebrum, is small; miniaturization of the cerebrum is accented by the normal-size cerebellum. An 11-year-old with noticeably small head; severe mental retardation with hyper-activity. Neurologic examination with no significant abnormalities; no motor abnormalities; no seizure disorder. At autopsy, the weight of the brain, 520 grams, approximately 50 percent of average for the age. The length of the cerebrum, about 75 percent of average. On section, the brain showed a somewhat simplified convolutional pattern; the deep structures, the white matter, the basal ganglia, and the ventricles, were of normal appearance.

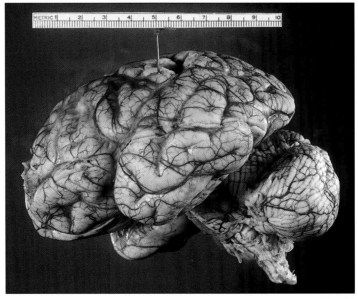

Fig. 93

Anatomically, in cases of microcephaly vera, the cerebrum is small, a miniature of a normal brain externally (Figure 93); in the cut sections, the structures are small but of ordinary configuration. Microscopically no tissue abnormality is evident.

Genetic microcephaly varies in degree. Mental retardation generally corresponds to the degree of smallness of the head, of the brain, and ranges from mild to severe.

In many individuals with marginal microcephaly, with mental retardation, the causal factor is overlooked.

There are many cases of familial mental deficiency in which the brain shows no abnormality studied grossly and microscopically. There are cases in which the brain specimen of a severely retarded child, the offspring of retarded parents, studied thoroughly in the laboratory, applying all present-day state-of-the-art methods of pathology investigation, reveals no abnormalities. The implication persists, however, that there is present an underlying organ abnormality in the brain tissue, an abnormality not yet demonstrable. It is likely that some cases fall into the group of unrecognized marginal microcephaly.

Genetic microcephaly is to be distinguished from encephaloclastic microcephaly, the failure of the brain to grow due to early fetal damage to deep cerebral structures (page 31).

Macrocephaly (Megalocephaly)

Illustrative Cases:
Case 230 *p. 729*
Case 233 *p. 734*

A much enlarged head at birth characterizes this condition. This brain abnormality is a form of malformation, a true hyperplasia of the brain. In this condition the heavy brain is well proportioned in all its parts and without microscopic alteration. The weight of the brain in megalocephaly varies, from 1,600 grams and more. Because of the large head, the condition is often initially misdiagnosed as hydrocephaly. Clinically, although intellect may be unimpaired, usually there is mental retardation.

Chromosome-linked abnormalities

Down syndrome
Trisomy D
Trisomy E
Sex-chromosome syndromes
    Klinefelter syndrome
    Turner syndrome
    Fragile-X syndrome

The demonstration in 1956 that human cells have 46 chromosomes was the first step in establishing the link between chromosome abnormalities and related defects in body structure. Two years later, in 1958, the first chromosome-linked disorder in humans was demonstrated with the discovery that in Down syndrome there was an excess of cell chromosomes, 47 instead of the normal 46.

Chromosomes are complex packages of genes contributed equally by the mother and father. Of the normal 46 chromosomes in human cells, there are 22 pairs of *somatic* chromosomes (linked to specific body structures) and separately the *sex* chromosomes X and Y. Half of the somatic chromosomes come from the mother and half from the father, so that in each pair of somatic chromosomes, one chromosome is contributed by each parent.

The sex chromosomes occur in pairs as XX or XY, with XX for the female and XY for the male. A male inherits a single X chromosome from his mother and a Y chromosome from his father, whereas a female gets an X from each parent.

The chromosome pattern, with the chromosomes separated out, is referred to as the karyotype. As seen in Figure 94, the somatic pairs have been sorted out according to size and form and have been assigned the numbers 1 to 22. In Down syndrome, with 47 chromosomes, the extra member was found to be like the chromosomes in pair number 21 (Figure 95). Accordingly, the abnormal chromosome pattern in Down syndrome is designated trisomy 21, meaning there are 3 somatic chromosomes at the 21 location.

Figure 94. Karyotype, normal human pattern; 46 chromosomes; chromosome pairs numbered consecutively, 1 to 22, together with male Y and female X chromosomes.

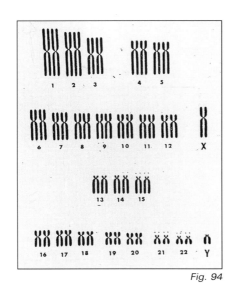

Fig. 94

Figure 95. Trisomy 21; Down syndrome karyotype, 47 chromosomes; extra chromosome at the 21 location.

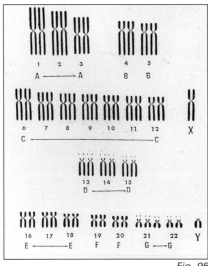

Fig. 95

Many of the chromosome pairs are similar, one with another; it was found expedient to place similar pairs in groups and, beginning with the largest chromosomes, to designate the groups as A to G (Figure 95). Thus Down syndrome, trisomy 21, is also referred to as trisomy G, and trisomy 13 is referred to as trisomy D.

Chromosomal abnormalities affect not only somatic chromosomes but also sex chromosomes. Defects in the X chromosome characterize the fragile-X syndrome; this commonly results in mental retardation.

Chromosome-linked abnormalities of the brain, clinically, are consistently associated with mental deficiency and other defects in motor and sensory function, and at times with psychiatric problems.

Cause and incidence of chromosome-linked disorders. The elementary cause of chromosome-linked disorders, in many aspects, remains undetermined. An important causal factor is associated with advanced maternal age. For example, the incidence of trisomy 21, Down syndrome, with mothers below the age of 30 is about 1 in 1,000 pregnancies; at 40 years the incidence is about 1 in 100 pregnancies. Similarly, the incidence of other chromosome-linked abnormalities rises with advanced maternal age.

Regarding the etiology, it is thought that with advancing age the ovary yields ova with chromosomes defective in number and form. Abnormal chromosomes from sperm are known to contribute to the occurrence of Down and other syndromes. With regard to paternal age, it is not clear whether the factor of advanced paternal age is associated with abnormal chromosomes contributed by sperm.

The overall incidence of chromosome-linked abnormalities is approximately 1 in 200 live births. Severely defective fetuses usually die during early fetal life and are aborted; chromosome abnormalities are said to occur in over 60 percent of early spontaneous abortions.

With chromosome disorders, all the structures of the body are susceptible to defective formation. In most major chromosome disorders that affect the bodily structures, the brain almost always is significantly compromised.

Down syndrome; trisomy 21 (G)

Illustrative Cases:
Case 18 *p. 274*
Case 223 *p. 719*
Case 227 *p. 725*

Down syndrome is by far the most frequent chromosome-linked disorder found in the general population. It is also of special interest because it was the first abnormal chromosome pattern identified in the human. As previously noted, in Down syndrome there are 47 chromosomes, with the extra chromosome at location 21 of the somatic chromosome pairs; accordingly, Down syndrome is called trisomy 21.

The incidence of Down syndrome in live births overall is about 1 in 800. As with other chromosome abnormalities, the incidence increases with the age of the mother, being less than 1 in 1,000 with young mothers and mounting to 1 in 32 births in mothers over the age of 45.

Microcephaly of moderate degree, but noticeable, is characteristic. The head tends to be rounded. The brain in most cases (adult) is small, weighing about 1,000 grams (normal adult brain weight, 1,200 grams). The brain is shortened, with blunted frontal and occipital poles. The cerebral convolutional pattern appears simplified, with broadened convolutions and lacking tertiary sulci (Figure 96).

Microscopically, in Down syndrome, in cases of younger age, the brain shows no specific abnormalities.

Figure 96. Down syndrome. Rounded contour of the cerebrum with blunting of the frontal poles. Convolutions large, of simplified pattern. **(a).** Superior view of cerebrum. **(b).** Lateral view.

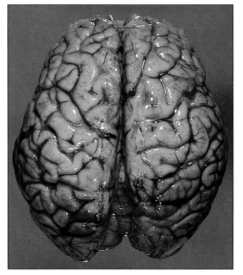
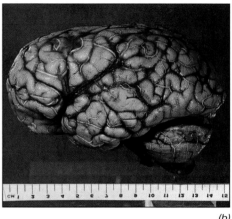

(b)

Fig. 96(a)

Cardiac defects, mainly septal defects, occur in about 50 percent of cases of Down syndrome. Defects of the intestinal tract are common.

The external bodily characteristics of persons with Down syndrome, in addition to small head and short stature, typically include slanting eyes, with facial features of an Oriental appearance (Down syndrome was called mongolism in times past.) The hands are small, with short stubby fingers. The main crease on the palm of the hand is single and transverse instead of two split lines, and is referred to as the simian crease, in that the single crease is like that found in the ape (Figure 97). Hypotonia and hyperextensibility of the joints are commonly present. A high arched palate and misshapen ears are characteristic. The eyes show speckling of the iris, Brushfield spots. The tongue is large and thick.

Mental retardation is the outstanding neurologic abnormality with Down syndrome. The degree of mental retardation varies. Most people with Down syndrome are considered moderately retarded, with an IQ of around 50. Overall, Down syndrome accounts for about 10 to 15 percent of moderately retarded people in the general population. Down syndrome affects about 1 in 1,000 children.

Importantly, however, persons with Down syndrome with advancing age have a predisposition to develop Alzheimer's disease (Case 223, page 719). Rapidly developing personality changes occur, with increasing hostility and further loss of intellect. In such cases, the brain microscopically shows senile plaques and neurofibrillary tangles, changes typical of Alzheimer's disease.

Figure 97. Simian crease of the palm in Down syndrome, a single transverse crease, differing from the normal pattern of two segments arising from each side that diverge in midpalm.

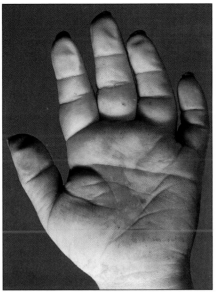

Fig. 97

Trisomy 13 (D)

Illustrative Case:
Case 41 *p. 330*

In most cases, trisomy D results in stillbirth. Among live births, the incidence is about 1 in 10,000. Clinically, there are multiple severe malformations of the brain and other viscera, incompatible with survival.

The cerebral malformations that characterize trisomy D are **holocephaly** (*holo-,* whole, combined), a cerebrum with a single ventricle due to failure of the forebrain to divide into two lateral ventricles; and **arrhinencephaly** (*a-,* without; *-rhinencephaly,* olfactory brain), absence of the olfactory lobes and tracts.

Severe facial deformities occur with the cerebral abnormalities, including fusion of the eyes (cyclopia), abnormalities of the nose, and cleft lip and palate. Visceral abnormalities occur, commonly cardiac defects. Skeletal defects occur, at times polydactylism and syndactylism.

With severe cerebral malformations there is corresponding neurologic compromise. Few live long enough to show mental retardation.

The trisomy 13 (D) karyotype is shown in Figure 95, page 144.

Trisomy 18 (E)

This syndrome occurs in about 1 in 10,000 live births, preponderantly affecting females.

A great variety of cerebral abnormalities occur with trisomy 18, including malformation of the cerebral convolutions and abnormalities of the brain stem. Visceral abnormalities occur.

Fewer than 1 percent survive the first decade, with survivors profoundly retarded in mental and motor function.

Sex-chromosome syndromes

An abnormal number of X and Y chromosomes occur in Klinefelter syndrome, Turner syndrome, and other similar syndromes. Abnormality in the structure of the X chromosome, of broad occurrence, characterizes the fragile-X syndrome.

Mental deficiency occurs consistently in the sex chromosome syndromes, often complicated by psychiatric disorder.

Klinefelter syndrome (47, XXY)

This abnormality occurs in about 1 in 800 males; those affected have an extra X chromosome. Klinefelter syndrome accounts for about 1 percent of mentally retarded persons; the IQ ranges around 50. Severe psychosocial disorders, appearing in early childhood, often precede the bodily abnormalities that characterize Klinefelter syndrome — eunuchoid physique, hypogenitalism, tall stature. No consistent cerebral dysplasias occur with Klinefelter syndrome.

Turner syndrome (45, X)

Turner syndrome, with a chromosome pattern of a single X sex chromosome, occurs in about 1 in 5,000 female infants. Abnormal bodily features include webbing of the neck, stunted growth, and lack of development of breast and other secondary sex characteristics. The failure of sexual maturation is linked to ovarian insufficiency; ovaries are very small, fibrotic.

Mental retardation occurs consistently, usually of mild degree.

Malformation of the cardiovascular and urinary tract are frequent; however the brain shows no morphologic abnormalities.

Fragile-X syndrome

In this syndrome there are localized defects in the X chromosome. This syndrome is very common, and as a cause of mental retardation it is thought to be second only to Down syndrome.

With reference to Figure 94, the X chromosome is seen to have two short arms and two long arms. Fragmentation, breaking away of one or both long arms of the X chromosome creates the pattern of the fragile-X syndrome.

Fragile-X syndrome, like Down syndrome, is estimated to affect 1 in 1,000 children. In fragile-X syndrome, there is a predisposing heredity factor, with more than one child in a family being affected.

Fragile-X syndrome, being due to an abnormality of the male sex chromosome X, occurs predominantly in males. However an attenuated form of the syndrome appears in females. Girls who inherit a faulty X chromosome from their father appear to be protected from the deleterious effects by the normal X chromosome inherited from their mother.

Clinically, fragile-X syndrome is characterized by a triad: moderate mental retardation; dysmorphic facial features, with a long narrow face; and genital abnormalities, commonly with enlarged testes. Behavior difficulties, with hyperactivity and emotional instability, are often a greater problem than the mental deficiency.

Neuropathologic studies are few and have revealed no consistent brain abnormalities.

Cerebral dysplasias

Heterotopias
Schizencephaly
Malformation porencephaly
Lissencephaly
Macrogyria

The cerebral dysplasias (*dys-*, poorly; *-plasia*, formed) are a heterogenous group of malformations in which there is an apparent arrested development of major parts of the cerebrum, especially the cortex, with resulting disorder in the anatomic pattern of the cerebrum.

The basic pathogenesis has to do with faulty development of the cerebral cortex. The cortex is derived from cells in the germinal matrix (page 4). Beginning in the embryo and then early in fetal life, germinal cells in the periventricular zones appear to migrate outward, to the surface, to form the cortex. The migrating cells form wave-like strata in the midzones of the cerebral wall, between the germinal matrix deposits centrally and the cortex at the surface (Figure 98).

Figure 98. Migration of germinal matrix cells through the cerebral wall toward the cortex. Section through the cerebrum; fetus of 16 weeks' gestation. As shown here, in the cerebral wall, between the germinal matrix (located periventricular) and the forming cortex, there are wave-like strata, maturing neuronal elements, migrating from the germinal matrix toward the cortex.

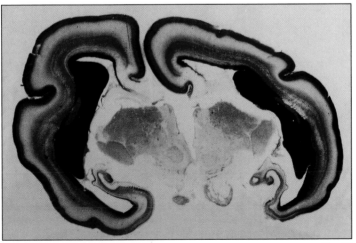

Fig. 98

Four main forms of cerebral dysplasia are heterotopias, malformation porencephaly, lissencephaly, and macrogyria.

Heterotopias

Heterotopias (*hetero-,* different; *-topia,* place) are ectopic "islands" of cortex that develop deep in the cerebral wall, in the midst of white matter (Figure 99). These islands of cortical tissue apparently derive from clusters of stranded migrating germinal matrix cells that fail to reach the cortex.

Figure 99. Heterotopic islands of cortex in the cerebral white matter. Cerebral convolution, upper right, with many clustered islands of cortical gray tissue in the convolutional white matter.

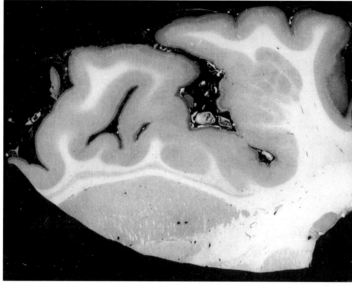

Fig. 99

Schizencephaly

Illustrative Case:
Case 219   *p. 710*

In this malformation the cerebrum presents a deep cleft extending transversely over the cerebral hemispheres. From the surface of the cleft, ectopic deposits of cortical tissue extend deeply into the underlying white matter.

Malformation porencephaly

Porencephaly refers to the presence of a porus, a cavitation, in the wall of the cerebrum. Malformation porencephaly (Figure 100), of rare occurrence, pertains to a defect in the development of the cerebrum, a localized agenesis of the cerebral wall. This is in contrast to encephaloclastic porencephaly (Figure 101), the result of severe damage to an area in the cerebral wall, with the devitalized tissue becoming absorbed, leaving a loculated cavitation lined with scar tissue (page 28).

Malformation porencephaly appears as a through-and-through opening in the cerebral wall (Figure 100a) representing a defect in the genesis of the cerebrum. In contrast to encephaloclastic porencephaly in which the cavity is lined with scar tissue, malformation porencephaly, is identified by the presence of a vestigial cortical lining that extends into the porus from the surface (Figure 100b).

The interpretation of the pathology of porencephaly presented here is one commonly applied. However, in the literature there is broad variation in the differentiation between encephaloclastic and malformation porencephaly.

Figure 100. Malformation porencephaly. The patient in this case was hemiplegic from the time of birth, with spasticity in the right arm and leg. In addition to developmental retardation, there was severe impediment of speech. **(a).** The lateral view of the left side of the cerebrum shows a through-and-through cavitation that extends from the surface and communicates with the lateral ventricle. At autopsy the defect was covered by an arachnoidal membrane.

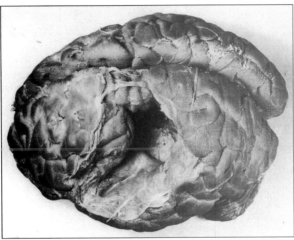

Fig. 100(a)

Figure 100(b). Section through the cerebrum at the level of the porencephaly. Of significance, identifying the abnormality as a malformation, is the ingrowth of cortical tissue into the cavitation, evident at the upper and lower lip of the porus.

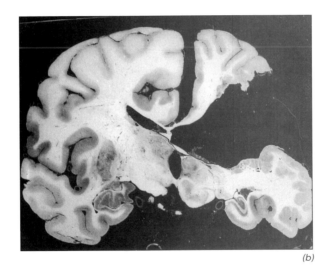

(b)

Figure 101. Encephaloclastic porencephaly. A large cavitation in the wall of the left cerebrum; the cystic structure is loculated, crisscrossed by residual strands of scar tissue. Infant with severe spasticity and developmental retardation.

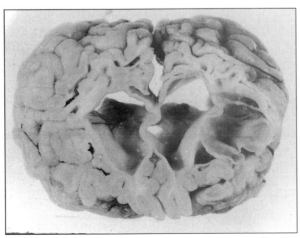

Fig. 101

Lissencephaly

Illustrative Case:
Case 225   *p. 722*

Lissencephaly (*lissen*-, smooth; -*cephalon*, brain) is a brain with a smooth surface, with few or no convolutions (Figure 102). The lissencephalic brain resembles the premature brain of a 17-week-old fetus (Figure 103).

Recent studies have revealed that lissencephaly in some cases is due to a chromosomal abnormality, a defect in chromosome 17 (Dobyns et al., 1993).

Figure 102. Lissencephaly. Superior view of the brain. Microcephalic 8-year-old with severe mental deficiency, sensory defects, spasticity. Brain weighed 800 grams (normal, 1,100 grams). The cerebrum, externally smooth with only a few sulci, resembled the cerebrum of a 17-week-old fetus.

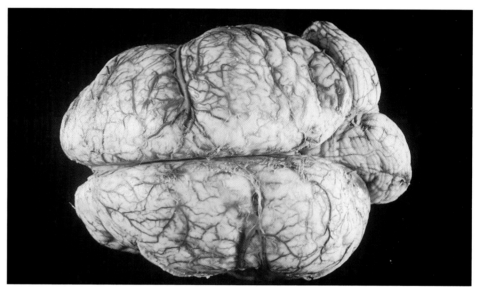

Fig. 102

Figure 103. Fetal brain of 17 weeks' gestation, with smooth cerebral surface.

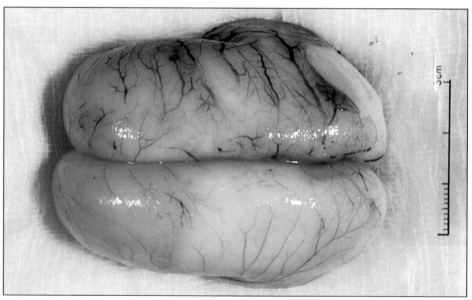

Fig. 103

Microscopically, in the lissencephalic cerebrum the rudimentary cortex is made up of haphazardly scattered neuronal elements. This dysplasia forms as a result of faulty, inadequate, migration of germinal cells to form the cortex. With the arrest of cortex development, convolutions fail to form, resulting in the lissencephalic smooth cerebrum.

Macrogyria

Brains with macrogyria have only a few oversize cerebral convolutions; this represents another form of compromised cortex development, with arrest of convolution formation (Figure 104).

Figure 104. Macrogyria, most prominent in the frontal region. Superior view of the brain. 10-month-old infant, severe developmental retardation, muscular twitchings, little motor control. Brain weighed 750 grams. Microscopically the pattern of the frontal cortex poorly defined, with neurones distributed in a disorderly fashion.

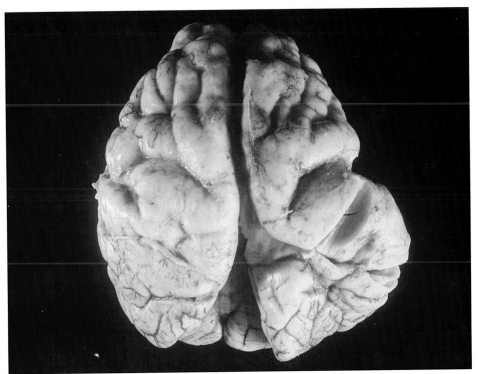

Fig. 104

Clinically, cases of cerebral dysplasias are relatively rare, but cases do appear in small numbers among the population of mentally retarded persons. The head size is reduced, with obvious microcephaly. These infants are essentially unresponsive to their environment. Mental deficiency and defective motor function are of severe degree in cases of cerebral dysplasia.

Neural tube defects

Anencephaly
Spina bifida

The nervous system develops from a *thickened plate* of ectoderm on the surface of the embryo (Figure 105). By infolding of the ectodermal neural plate, the *neural groove* is formed. Later, with closure of the groove, the *neural tube* is formed. The neural tube has a lining of germinal matrix cells that later contribute to the neuronal elements of the nervous system. The central canal persists in the spinal cord and, in an analogous manner, in the brain as the ventricular system.

Figure 105. Embryonic development of the nervous system. **(a).** Ectodermal neural plate. **(b).** Infolding of the neural plate to form the neural groove. **(c).** Closure of the neural groove to form the neural tube.

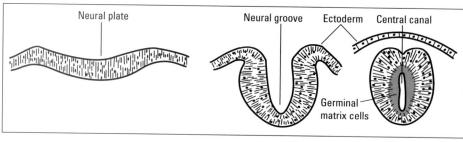

Fig. 105(a,b,c)

Neural tube defects occur due to failure of the neural tube to close normally. The two main types of neural tube defects are anencephaly and spina bifida, in their various forms.

Neural tube defects have a multifactorial etiology, in some instances being of genetic familial nature, in other instances occurring as isolated cases. Experimentally, in laboratory animals, neural tube defects have been induced by exposure to various chemical agents early in pregnancy.

Neural tube defects vary in incidence, with a prevalence rate of 1.0 percent in Northern Ireland; in North America the incidence is about 0.1 percent. Genetic factors must contribute to these differences in incidence.

Anencephaly

Most anencephalics die soon after birth, and although anencephaly has no immediate relevance to problems of chronic cerebral disability, this malformation is presented to demonstrate a most severe form of cerebral malformation (Figure 106).

Anencephaly involves the derivatives of the most anterior portion of the neural tube. The cranial bones are missing; the exposed base of the skull is covered with hemorrhagic structureless gelatinous tissue. The brain stem and cerebellum in some cases are spared, permitting the infant to live briefly.

Anencephaly, with absence of the cerebrum, is essentially an all-or-none defect, with no intermediate variants.

Figure 106. Anencephaly. **(a).** Facial features showing characteristic protruding eyes, large flat nose, and large irregular ears. **(b).** Upper surface of the head; absence of cerebral tissue; skull bones covered with remnants of thin stringy vascular gelatinous tissue. Mother was 39 years old. Gestation was 36 weeks. Infant lived briefly.

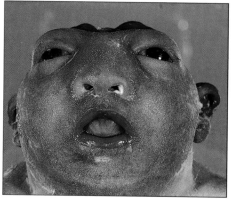
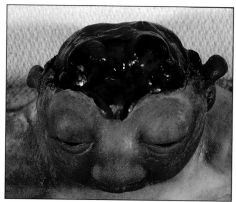

Fig. 106(a)   (b)

Spina bifida; meningomyelocele

Illustrative Case:
Case 226   *p. 724*

Spina bifida in its most severe form, referred to as rachischisis (*rach-*, spine; *-schisis*, split), appears as an open groove over the midposterior of the back, with the defect lined with soft gelatinous tissue (Figure 107a).

Figure 107(a). Rachischisis, the most severe form of spina bifida; associated with anencephaly. The spinal canal lies open, covered with hemorrhagic stringy fibrous tissue; absence of spinal cord. Pregnancy was associated with polyhydramnios. Infant of 34 weeks' gestation lived 14 minutes. **(b).** Meningomyelocele. Red, hemorrhagic, tumor-like mass on the back, over the spine; a protrusion of meningeal and spinal cord tissue through a defect in the posterior portion of the spinal canal.

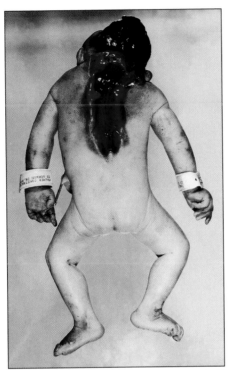
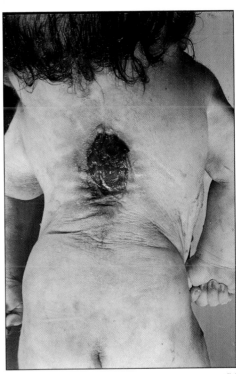

Fig. 107(a)   (b)

Spina bifida is due to faulty closure of the spinal portion of the neural tube (Figure 105b).

Meningomyocele is a variant of spina bifida resulting from defective closure of a segment of the neural tube, allowing herniation of meningeal and spinal cord tissue, appearing in the form of a soft tumor-like mass over the spine (Figure 107b).

Lesser forms of spina bifida consist of defects in the lower vertebrae, but no bulging mass, with the defect masked externally by a midline dimple in the skin or a tuft of hair over the lower spine.

With spina bifida, with the cord tethered in the spinal canal at the level of the defect, ultimately, with growth of the child, the traction effect on the cord may lead to impaction of the brain stem at the foramen magnum, causing interference with cerebrospinal fluid circulation and the development of hydrocephalus, the Arnold-Chiari syndrome.

Obstructive hydrocephalus (aqueductal obstruction)

Illustrative Cases:
Case 101   *p. 480*
Case 184   *p. 628*
Case 226   *p. 724*
Case 228   *p. 726*

Obstructive hydrocephalus (Figure 108) is due to blockage of the outflow of cerebrospinal fluid from the ventricles. Commonly the impediment is at the aqueduct of Sylvius in the midbrain, aqueductal narrowing, stenosis, or aqueductal atresia, complete closure of the channel, with consequent enlargement of the lateral and third ventricles. At times the obstruction is at the foramina of the fourth ventricle or there is blockage in the subarachnoid space interfering with circulation of the cerebrospinal fluid.

Figure 108. Hydrocephalus; origin during intrauterine life. Gradual enlargement of the head after birth. Malformation of the heart present, patent ductus arteriosus. At age 6 years, IQ of 30. **(a).** The enlarged head, 26 inches (66 centimeters] in circumference (average at 6 years, 52 centimeters). Child had difficulty balancing the large heavy head. 6 years old.

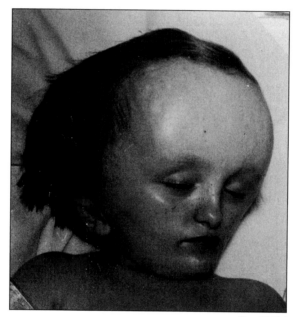

Fig. 108(a)

Figure 108(b). Hydrocephalus. Brain specimen in case shown in (a). The cerebrum converted to a flabby bag-like structure. Externally, convolutions broadened and flat. Cerebral walls thinned, of 3 to 6 centimeters in thickness. Pathologically, the hydrocephalus was apparently due to aquaductal obstruction; whether genetic or induced, was unclear.

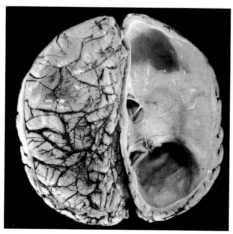

(b)

During the development of obstructive hydrocephalus, the backup of fluid in the ventricles is under pressure; in the cerebrum the periventricular strata are compromised, the cerebral white matter gradually destroyed, leaving the ventricles enlarged, the cerebral walls thinned, and, on the surface, the convolutions flattened. The head becomes increasingly enlarged consequent to the ballooning of the cerebrum.

Occlusion of the aqueduct leading to obstructive hydrocephalus is of two distinct causes pathologically:

Malformation stenosis of the aqueduct, developing in embryonic life. The aqueduct is formed from a segment of neural tube (Figure 105); the narrowed aqueduct is in essence a malformation of the neural tube.

Acquired obstruction of the aqueduct is due to impaction of the opening of the aqueduct by blood clot and cellular fragments, debris cast off from periventricular hemorrhagic infarctions. This type of aqueductal occlusion acquired during fetal life is referred to on page 17, and is not directly relevant to the present consideration of formative defects.

The neurologic effect of hydrocephalus basically depends on the amount of cerebral substance lost, with mild hydrocephalus evoking mild mental retardation and other functional neurologic loss. Hydrocephalus with enlargement of the head present at birth occurs in 1 to 2 per 1,000 pregnancies.

Other Visceral Damage Associated with Nervous System Damage in the Fetus and Newborn

All the organs of the body in the fetus and newborn are susceptible to hypoxic and mechanical injury. Plainly the brain is the organ most vulnerable to injury.

Pathologic studies reveal that at autopsy in cases with hypoxic damage to the brain, commonly there is analogous hypoxic damage in the kidney, adrenal, or other viscera. The degree and distribution of the damage is generally related to the severity of the hypoxic exposure. Diffuse damage to parenchymal cells may be more or less evenly spread through the organ; in a given case, widespread neuronal damage may be present in the cerebrum, together with tubular necrosis in the kidneys and fatty metamorphosis in liver cells and in myocardial fibers. Focal hemorrhagic infarcts frequently appear as small scattered lesions, minute infarcts, hemorrhagic extravasates in the form of petechiae, on the pericardium and in the thymus and other viscera (Figure 109).

Figure 109. Hypoxic focal hemorrhagic infarcts (petechiae) of thymus. Term pregnancy; decreased fetal movements day before delivery (fetus in coma). Evidence of fetal distress during labor. At autopsy, congestive heart failure with hydrothorax.

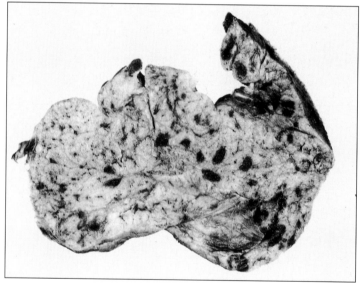

Fig. 109

In some cases, a major portion of an organ may be infarcted, at times whole-organ infarction occurs (Figures 110 and 111).

Figure 110. A case of multiple visceral hypoxic infarction. **(a).** Massive cerebral infarction. **(b).** Intestinal infarction. Maternal history of hypertension; gestation of 32 weeks; diminished fetal activity in the last two weeks; fetal heart tones present day before delivery. Placenta showed multiple large infarcts.

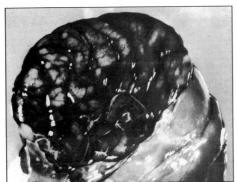

Fig. 110(a)

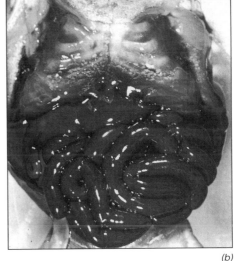

(b)

Figure 111. Lung infarct in a premature newborn. Increasing respiratory distress postnatally; death at 3 days; congestive heart failure. **(a).** Left lung, at autopsy; left lower lobe firm and dark red. **(b).** Corresponding longitudinal section of lung showing thrombosis of large vein and infarction of lower lobe.

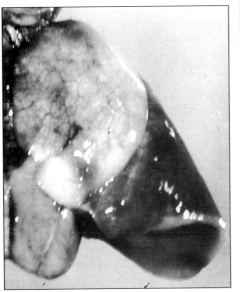

Fig. 111(a)

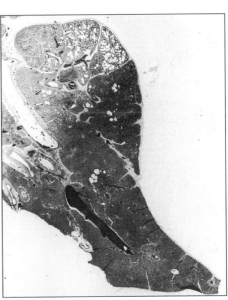

(b)

Mechanical injury to the structures of the fetus during birth, at times life threatening, as with spinal injury and crush injury of the liver, often imposes secondary hypoxic sequels. As discussed on page 138, spinal injury with resulting respiratory depression leads to bodily hypoxia, with hypoxic cerebral damage. Mechanical crush injury to the liver, with laceration of the liver, leads to intra-abdominal hemorrhage with consequent acute anemia, with hypoxia (page 102).

References and Additional Reading

Bolognese, R. J., R. H. Schwartz, and J. Schneider (1982). *Perinatal Medicine*. Baltimore: Williams & Wilkins.

Brand, M. M., and A. Bignami (1969). The effects of chronic hypoxia on the neonatal and infantile brain. *Brain* 92: 233–254.

Cohen, M., and U. Roessmann (1994). *In utero* brain damage: relationship of gestational age to pathological consequences. *Dev Med Child Neurol* 36: 263–270.

Collaborative Perinatal Project (1965). (Collaborative Study of Cerebral Palsy, Mental Retardation and Other Neurologic and Sensory Disorders of Infancy and Childhood). Research Profile No. 11. National Institutes of Health, Bethesda, Maryland, Public Health Service Publication No. 1370. Washington, D.C.: U.S. Government Printing Office. (The National Institutes of Health in 1959 formulated the Collaborative Perinatal Project, a study of 50,000 pregnant women and their offspring. Postmortem investigations of neonatal deaths were done. Detailed neuropathologic studies were carried out in the Neurology Department of Harvard Medical School.)

Csermely, H. (1972). Perinatal anoxic changes of the central nervous system. *Acta Paediatrica Academiae Scientiarum Hungaricae* 13: 293–299.

Dobyns, W. B., O. Reiner, R. Carrozzo, and D. H. Ledbetter (1993). Lissencephaly. *JAMA* 270: 2838–2842.

Ellis, W., B. W. Goetzman, et al. (1988). Neuropathologic documentation of prenatal brain damage. *Am J Dis Child* 142: 858–866.

Freeman, J. M., ed. (1985). *Prenatal and Perinatal Factors Associated with Brain Disorders*. NIH Publication No. 85–1149. Washington, D.C.: U.S. Government Printing Office.

Gossey, S., M. C. Golaire, et al. (1982). Cerebral, renal and splenic lesions due to fetal anoxia and their relationship to malformations. *Dev Med Child Neurol* 24: 510–518.

Gruenwald, P. (1951). Subependymal cerebral hemorrhage in premature infants, and its relation to various injurious influences at birth. *Am J Obstet Gynecol* 61: 1285–1292.

Hallervorden, J. (1949). Über eine Kohlenoxyvergiftung im Fetalleben mit Entwickkungsstörungen der Hirnrinde. *Allgemeine Zeitschrift für Psychiatrie und Psychisch-Gerichtliche Medizin* 124: 289–298.

Hellström, B., and U. Sallmander (1968). Prevention of cord injury in hyperextension of the fetal head. *JAMA* 202: 1041–1044.

Kalbag, R. M., and A. L. Woolf (1967). *Cerebral Venous Thrombosis*. London: Oxford University Press.

Larroche, J. C. (1968). Nécrose cérébrale massive chez le nouveau-né. *Biol Neonate* 13: 340–360.

Latham, D., G. W. Anderson, and N. J. Eastman (1954). Obstetrical factors in the etiology of cerebral palsy. *Am J Obstet Gynecol* 68(1): 91–96.

Macgregor, A. R. (1946). The pathology of still-birth and neonatal death. *Br Med Bull* 4: 176.

Malamud, N., H. H. Itabasi, et al. (1964). An etiologic and diagnostic study of cerebral palsy. *J Pediatr* 65: 270–293.

Manterola, A., A. Towbin, and P. I. Yakovlev (1966). Cerebral infarction in the human fetus near term. *J Neuropathol Exp Neurol* 25: 479–488.

Mayes, L. C., M. Granger, et al. (1993). Neurobehavioral profiles of neonates exposed to cocaine prenatally. *Pediatrics* 91: 778–783.

Mills, J. L., et al. (1993). Moderate caffeine use and the risk of spontaneous abortion and intrauterine growth retardation. *JAMA* 269: 593–597.

Nelson, K. B., and J. H. Ellenberg (1986). Antecedents of cerebral palsy. *N Engl J Med* 315: 81–86.

Neuburger, F. (1934). Fall einer Intrauterinen Hirnschädigung nach Leucht-gasvergiftung der Muter. *Beitr Gerichtl Med* 13: 85–95.

Niswander, K. R. (1983). Labor and operative obstetrics: Asphyxia in the fetus and cerebral palsy. In Pitkin, R. M., Zlatnik, F. J., eds., *The Year Book of Obstetrics and Gynecology*. Chicago: Year Book Medical Publishers. Pp. 106–124.

Okazaki, H. (1983). *Fundamentals of Neuropathology: Perinatal Nervous System Damage and Malformations*. New York and Tokyo: Igaku-Schoin.

Pritchard, J. A., P. C. MacDonald, and N. F. Gant, eds. (1985). *Williams Obstetrics*. Norwalk, Conn.: Appleton-Century-Croft.

Sander, C. H. (1980). Hemorrhagic endovasculitis and hemorrhagic villitis of the placenta. *Arch Pathol Lab Med* 104: 371–373.

Schwartz, P. (1961). Birth injuries. In *Pathology of the Nervous System*. New York: McGraw-Hill.

Stanley, F., and E. Alberman (1984). *The Epidemiology of the Cerebral Palsies*. Philadelphia: J. B. Lippincott.

Taylor, E. S. (1976). *Beck's Obstetrical Practice and Fetal Medicine*. Baltimore: Williams & Wilkins.

Towbin, A. (1968). Cerebral intraventricular hemorrhage and subependymal matrix infarction in the fetus and premature newborn. *Am J Pathol* 52: 121–140.

——— (1969). Cerebral hypoxic damage in the fetus and newborn. *Obstet Gynecol Surv* 24: 628–632.

——— (1970a). Central nervous system damage in the human fetus and newborn. *Am J Dis Child* 119: 529–542.

———— (1970b). Central nervous system damage in the premature related to the occurrence of mental retardation. In C. R. Angle and E. A. Bering, Jr., eds. *Physical Trauma as an Etiological Agent in Mental Retardation. Proceedings of a Conference on the Etiology of Mental Retardation, Omaha, Nebraska; 1968.* National Institute of Neurological Diseases and Stroke. Washington, D.C.: U.S. Government Printing Office. Pp. 213–239.

———— (1971). Organic causes of minimal brain dysfunction: Perinatal origin of minimal cerebral lesions. *JAMA* 217: 1207–1214.

———— and G. L. Turner (1972). Norwood Project: Placental studies. Unpublished.

———— (1977). Trauma in pregnancy: Injury to the fetus and newborn. In Tedeschi, C. G., Eckert, W. G., Tedeschi, L. G., eds., *Forensic Medicine.* Philadelphia: W. B. Saunders. Pp. 436–486.

———— (1978). Cerebral dysfunctions related to perinatal organic damage: Clinical-neuropathologic correlations. *J Abnorm Psychol* 87: 617–635.

———— (1978). Obstetric factors in fetal-neonatal visceral injury. *Obstet Gynecol* 52: 113–124.

———— (1986). Obstetric malpractice litigation: The pathologist's view. *Am J Obstet Gynecol* 155: 927–935.

Vogt, C., and O. Vogt (1920). Zur Lehre der Erkrankungen des striären Systems. *J Psychol Neurol* 25: 627–846.

Volpe, J. J. (1979). Intracranial hemorrhage in the newborn: Current understanding and dilemmas. *Neurology* 29: 632–635.

———— (1987). *Neurology of the Newborn* (Second ed.). Philadelphia: W. B. Saunders. Page 217.

Yakovlev, P. I. (1970). Whole brain serial histologic sections. In C. G. Tedeschi, ed., *Neuropathology: Methods and Diagnosis.* Boston: Little, Brown.

———— and R. K. Rosales (1970). Distribution of the terminal hemorrhages in the brain wall in stillborn prematures and nonviable neonates. In C. R. Angle and E. A. Bering, Jr., eds. *Physical Trauma as an Etiological Agent in Mental Retardation. Proceedings of a Conference on the Etiology of Mental Retardation. Omaha, Nebraska; 1968.* National Institute of Neurological Diseases and Stroke. Washington, D.C.: U.S. Government Printing Office. Pp. 67–78.

Young, E. F., and C. B. Courville (1962). Central softening of the cerebral hemispheres in the newborn. *Clin Pediatr* 1: 95–102.

2 The Depressed Brain-Damaged Newborn: Clinical-Pathologic Correlations

Newborn neurologic assessment
    Postdelivery performance of the newborn
        Acute cerebral damage present
        Subacute cerebral damage present
    Fontanelles: condition
    Imaging studies of the brain
    Decreased fetal activity
    Monitoring of the fetus
    Meconium staining
    Apgar score
    Acidosis
    Hypoglycemia
    Apnea
    Seizure activity
    Neurologic depression due to medication
    Spinal fluid examination, xanthochromia

Late neurologic sequels in infants born with cerebral damage
    Acute cerebral damage present at birth: sequels
        Premature newborn: sequels
        Mature newborn: sequels
    Subacute cerebral damage present at birth: sequels

Newborn depression: misdiagnosis of causation

Newborn neurological assessment

For the neurologist in assessing a case with apparent brain damage present at birth, a case with outcome of cerebral palsy and other neurologic conditions, the fact that the newborn was depressed and had to be resuscitated is a major factor in the interpretation of causation.

Was the depression of the newborn due to acute fresh brain damage incurred during labor and delivery? Or was the infant's condition the result of adversive gestational processes originating long before birth, with the fetus chronically enfeebled, unable to cope with the stress of labor and delivery, with the fetus, the newborn, depressed at delivery?

Investigators in the past evolved evidence that the underlying brain damage in cases of cerebral palsy originated in early fetal life. This was the opinion voiced by the German school of neuropathology, by Sigmund Freud, (Freud, 1897) and others. (Freud is usually remembered as the generator of the psychoanalytic school of clinical psychiatry. It is not generally known that he was an experienced investigative neurologist.) Freud did extensive research in the causation of cerebral palsy. He concluded that, in infants in poor condition at delivery, often the depression of vital function was due, not to damage incurred during labor and delivery, but was attributable to prenatal deprivation and enfeeblement, due to damage incurred during early fetal life.

Recently, Nelson (1988), in reviewing the interpretations of Freud and others, commented, "The balance of current evidence appears to be tilting toward Freud's point of view." Research studies, from the NIH Collaborative Perinatal Project and from other investigations, provide evidence that depression of the newborn at delivery often is due, not to intranatal hypoxia, but is the result of chronic fetal deprivation, to fetal damage, enfeeblement, originating during early intrauterine life (Niswander, 1983; Nelson and Ellenberg, 1987; Towbin, 1987; Ellis, Goetzman, and Lindenberg, 1988).

In the present day, clinically, in the evaluation retrospectively of a case of cerebral palsy, much attention may be directed to the fetal monitoring records, meconium staining, acidosis, and other tangential findings considered significant. However, experience dictates that the most substantial basis for interpreting the nature of the neurologic depression in the newborn is not the details of the delivery but the *performance of the newborn after birth,* in the hours after delivery.

Postdelivery performance of the newborn

Consideration of the infant's postdelivery performance provides information that indicates when the manifest brain damage was incurred, information as to whether the brain damage was acute, recent, or subacute, old.

Depression of vital function in the newborn at delivery has two distinctive causal mechanisms (Towbin, 1987). In one group, the underlying pathogenesis is related to *acute* cerebral damage incurred during labor and delivery. In the other group, the depression is primarily due to the presence of old, *subacute* cerebral damage incurred weeks or months prior to labor, with the previously compromised, enfeebled fetus unable to tolerate the ordinary stress of labor and delivery.

The two types of depressed newborn, those with acute cerebral lesions and those with subacute lesions at birth, are different with regard to gestational background events, different with regard to pathologic changes in the brain at birth, and different with regard to postnatal course (Table 4). In both groups, the clinical picture, the state of depression during the first few minutes, in the first hour, may be similar. In the subsequent hours and days, in the early months of life, the clinical pattern is different.

Table 4.

ASSESSMENT OF NEUROLOGIC DEPRESSION IN THE NEWBORN

Postnatal performance: Two clinical patterns

Infants born with **acute** brain damage compared to infants with **subacute** brain damage

ACUTE BRAIN DAMAGE IN THE NEWBORN
(Damage incurred during labor and delivery)

PREGNANCY PERIOD	*DELIVERY*	*POSTNATAL PERIOD*
Normal pregnancy until labor.	During delivery– Complications cause acute hypoxic brain damage.	After delivery– Infant stays depressed. Postnatal days– Infant kept in ICU many days, limp, comatose, depressed.

SUBACUTE (OLD) BRAIN DAMAGE IN THE NEWBORN
(Damage incurred in early fetal life)

PREGNANCY PERIOD	*DELIVERY*	*POSTNATAL PERIOD*
Pregnancy initially normal. Early in pregnancy, complications. Fetus incurs hypoxic brain damage. Damaged fetus survives. Period of fetal "recovery." Fetus enfeebled. Brain damage becomes subacute, old.	During delivery, fetus stressed.	At delivery– Newborn infant with transient depression. Soon improved, becoming stable, responsive, active, first day.

Acute cerebral damage present at birth: postdelivery performance of the newborn

Infants harboring acute brain damage show it. They are severely depressed at delivery. The acute damage is frequently caused by an obvious catastrophic hypoxia-producing complication, such as an entangled, compressed umbilical cord around the fetus' neck. If prolonged, such complications result in acute, stroke-like hemorrhagic damage in the brain. CT studies show evidence of cerebral swelling (pages 32 and 168). At autopsy, the damage is recognized pathologically as being of acute infarctional nature and freshly formed (Figure 8, page 11; Figure 9, page 12; Figure 11, page 13; Figure 12, page 13).

The newborn infant with extensive acute cerebral damage in most cases dies soon after delivery. Those that survive remain depressed for days, comatose, and then lethargic, often with episodes of respiratory arrest. These infants often require prolonged intensive care, with hospitalization extending for weeks. In cases with unremitting depression of vital function, systemic and neurologic deterioration and death occur after a period of days or weeks.

Subacute cerebral damage present at birth: postdelivery performance of the newborn

Newborn infants at times harbor cerebral damage that is old, pathologically *subacute*, damage due to adversive hypoxia-producing processes during fetal life, damage incurred weeks, months before birth. In these cases with subacute cerebral damage, neurologic depression of the newborn infant is usually present, generally of a transient nature. With the fetus compromised, enfeebled by gestational complications during intrauterine life, surviving marginally, often the fetus cannot tolerate the ordinary stress of labor and delivery and is born with a low Apgar score. However, once delivered, the surviving newborn with old, subacute brain damage tends to respond early, and within hours the infant may be out in the regular nursery, breathing on its own, responsive and active. If the newborn infant shows the effects of severe chronic intrauterine deprivation, is dysmature, anemic, or if the infant incurs complications soon after delivery, postnatal depression may be protracted.

Although most infants harboring subacute cerebral damage are born depressed, in some instances the infants have good Apgar scores and initially show no evidence of brain damage. It is the onset of seizures, sudden and unexpected, during the first day, that signals the possibility of brain damage; ultrasound and CT studies in the infants often confirm the presence of cerebral lesions, far advanced, subacute. It is of importance clinically to note that these infants do not have signs of acute cerebral damage, do not have evidence in the CT scans of cerebral swelling, do not have bulging fontanelles (pages 33 and 168).

In pathology studies of infants born with subacute brain damage who are stillborn or die soon after birth, at autopsy the brains of these infants show cerebral lesions that are recognized pathologically as being of some age, subacute (Figure 23, page 24; Figure 24, page 25).

Although well known to neonatal pathologists (Hallervorden, 1949; Brand and Bignami, 1969; Ellis, Goetzman, and Lindenberg, 1988; Towbin, 1977), the occurrence of subacute cerebral damage in the newborn is not generally realized by clinicians, by neonatologists, pediatricians, and neurologists. Accordingly, clinicians are prone to ascribe newborn depression to intranatal events. However, the clinical literature is also coming to be aware of the syndromic occurrence of the deprived, enfeebled, subacutely brain-damaged fetus who does not tolerate the superimposed stress of labor and delivery, shows fetal monitor abnormalities, and at delivery the newborn is neurologically depressed.

The occurrence of subacute cerebral damage, present at birth, is due to pregnancy complications that exert a damaging effect on the fetus. In reviewing the prenatal history, often there are evident pregnancy complications — maternal chronic illness or episodes of acute illness, vaginal bleeding — occurring weeks or months before labor. Maternal illness reverberates directly on the fetus; the resulting effect, the common denominator, is oxygen deprivation, fetal hypoxia. If adversive conditions for the fetus are prolonged, not only is there oxygen deprivation, with accumulation of subacute hypoxic cerebral damage, but there is also nutritional loss, with IUGR, intrauterine growth retardation.

Infants born with subacute damage, although depressed at birth, soon improve, and, unless seizures or other postnatal complications develop, the babies are usually discharged from the hospital during the first week.

In assessing the neurologic status of the newborn infant, in addition to the performance of the infant, two other clinical observations provide direct evidence of the presence or absence of acute fresh brain damage: the condition of the fontanelles and imaging studies, ultrasound and CT or MRI studies of the brain.

Fontanelles

The fontanelles, the palpable "soft spots" on the baby's head, contribute information regarding intracranial and bodily processes. Ordinarily, the fontanelles are flat and have a soft to firm feel.

With acute pathologic processes affecting the brain, the fontanelles become bulging and tense (Figure 112).

Acute pathologic processes affecting the brain, like meningitis and acute hypoxic damage, cause the brain to "soak up" fluid, to become edematous. With edema, the brain becomes swollen and pushes against the pliant yielding fontanelles, causing bulging of the fontanelles. The absence of bulging fontanelles is substantial evidence ruling out acute fresh hypoxic damage in the newborn infant.

Figure 112. Fontanelles in the newborn. **(a).** View of the fontanelles from above; on the left, the larger anterior fontanelle (soft spot); on the right, at the crossing of the sutures, the narrow posterior fontanelle. **(b).** Side view, with the fontanelles flat, soft, in the normal infant. **(c).** Bulging fontanelles, tense, in infants with cerebral edema, cerebral swelling.

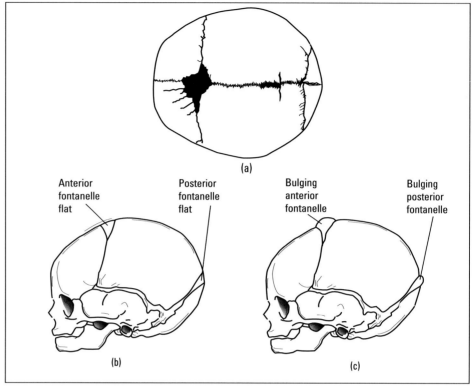

Fig. 112(a,b,c)

In a newborn infant, the findings of CT scan evidence of cerebral lesions and absence of bulging fontanelles provide substantial confirmation that the cerebral damage is subacute.

Imaging studies of the brain

Ultrasound and CT studies of the newborn brain provide visible evidence regarding the presence or absence of acute cerebral damage, evidence based on the appearance of the cerebral lateral ventricles, the large chambers deep within the cerebrum containing cerebrospinal fluid. In imaging studies of the brain, normally, the lateral ventricles are patent, plainly visible (Figures 30 and 31, page 32). When the brain has acute fresh cerebral damage, the brain becomes edematous, swollen, and the ventricles become compressed; the CT scan indicates this — ventricles are not visible (Figures 32 and 33, page 32). Accordingly, in CT studies the positive evidence of acute cerebral damage is obliteration of the ventricles. If ventricles are patent in the CT scan or the ultrasound image, it is conclusive evidence that there is no cerebral edema, no cerebral swelling, no acute fresh cerebral damage (Case 119, Figure 449, page 519; Case 131, Figure 457(b), page 539; Case 176, Figure 488, page 613; Case 236, Figure 554, page 741).

Although the CT scan rules out the presence of acute cerebral damage, it does not rule out the presence of old, subacute, cerebral damage latently accrued weeks or months before birth.

In a comprehensive neurologic assessment of the newborn infant, in addition to the postnatal progress of the infant, taken into account are details of the mother's pregnancy course, the events of labor and delivery, together with laboratory and other relevant information. Attention is directed to clinical factors regarding fetal activity, fetal monitoring, meconium staining, Apgar score, and other physical and laboratory findings in the case. In this, it is important to correlate underlying pathologic processes related to the clinical findings.

Decreased fetal activity

Decreased fetal activity reflects enfeeblement of the fetus. The loss of fetal activity is known as the "fetal alarm signal." Fetal kicking may be a better indicator of fetal health than the heart beat (Sadovsky and Yaffe, 1973). Pathologic gestational processes have an adversive effect on the fetus, exercising their pathologic effects during intrauterine life, rendering the fetus hypoxic and weakened.

Pathologically, there are two main causes of decreased fetal activity:

1) *Acute* hypoxia-producing intrauterine complication, such as cord compression with a tight nuchal cord, developing over a period of days, leading to rapidly increasing fetal hypoxia with associated collapse of vital function, paralysis of the fetus — loss of fetal activity.

2) *Chronic* intrauterine compromise, with fetal deprivation, intrauterine growth retardation, gradual fetal enfeeblement, fetal exhaustion, loss of fetal activity.

Monitoring of the fetus

During complicated labor attention becomes focused on the fetal monitor record. Electronic fetal monitoring yields records that at times are equivocal, problematic. Clinically, abnormalities in the monitor record are commonly thought to mean fetal hypoxia, and at times are translated to mean acute brain damage is going on. This is an interpretive exaggeration, pathologically not valid.

Monitor records show what the fetal heart rate is: normal, increased (tachycardia), or decreased (bradycardia). Abnormalities in heart rate reflect myocardial exhaustion.

Essentially, two pathologic processes can cause fetal bradycardia as it appears in electronic fetal monitoring: (1) When the fetus is chronically compromised during intrauterine life and enfeebled, the fetus may not be able to tolerate the stress of labor and decompensates, becomes bradycardic. The bradycardia is not due to inordinate hypoxia. (2) When a fetus, previously healthy, is subjected to sudden acute hypoxia during labor, as occurs with massive placental detachment, bradycardia that develops is due to the direct effect of oxygen deprivation on the muscle of the heart (page 8).

Meconium staining of amniotic fluid

Meconium staining occurs in 10 to 20 percent of births and is very common in postterm deliveries. Meconium in the amniotic fluid, per se, is not a positive sign of fetal hypoxia, is not an indication for early cesarean section.

Meconium amniotic fluid occurs due to bowel incontinence of the fetus. The anal sphincter opens and bowel content, meconium, is expelled into the amniotic fluid. This may occur early or late during labor. It may occur with hypoxia, but not always. Meconium staining occurs in circumstances other than hypoxia: compression of the fetal abdomen, compression of the fetal head.

Clinically, when meconium staining of the amniotic fluid appears during labor, it is sometimes considered to be a sign of fetal hypoxia. In this direction, does the absence of meconium reflect an absence of hypoxia?

Meconium staining itself is a poor predictor of outcome. In clinical studies of meconium-stained infants weighing over 2,500 grams at birth, 99.6 percent did not later have cerebral palsy (Freeman and Nelson, 1988).

Apgar score

The immediate postnatal condition of the newborn infant is clinically evaluated by the Apgar score, originated by Virginia Apgar in 1953. Five bodily functions are assessed: heart rate, respiration, muscle tone, reflex irritability, color (pink, pale, cyanotic). Each function is graded as 0 (absent), 1, or 2 (good function). Accordingly, a total score of 10 reflects a healthy newborn. A score of 5 or less indicates that the infant is substantially depressed. The Apgar score is recorded at one minute and five minutes after birth.

The Apgar score is not a dependable indicator of antecedent intranatal hypoxia, and is not a valid indicator of the presence of acute hypoxic damage in the newborn. A low Apgar score does not automatically mean there has been intranatal hypoxia. In many cases, a low score is reflective of a chronically compromised, enfeebled fetus, enfeebled due to intrauterine pathologic processes, a fetus unable to cope with the stress of labor.

The one-minute Apgar score is not substantial; most authorities disregard the one-minute score. During the first 60 seconds of the newborn's life, the delivery staff is occupied with regular routine handling of the infant, tying the cord, aspirating, cleaning. There is no precise measurement of the heart, respiration, and reflexes during the first minute. This is done reasonably at five minutes.

The Apgar score, as with the monitor record, is not an accurate predictor of neurologic outcome (Freeman and Nelson, 1988).

Acidosis

Acidosis, in infants as in adults, has many causes. Low blood pH makes its appearance in acutely compromised newborn, hypoxic during the intranatal period, as well as in enfeebled low birth weight infants chronically compromised during intrauterine life. Also, significantly, many "good" newborn infants, with good Apgar scores, have a transient low blood pH. Plainly, a low pH does not automatically mean intranatal hypoxia has occurred.

Animal studies have shown that the fetus during intrauterine life has a low blood pH, a physiologic acidosis. A transient carryover of the fetal low blood pH does not, per se, indicate a pathologic condition.

Recent clinical studies have shown that, as with a low Apgar score and meconium staining, acidosis in the newborn has little predictive value as to neurologic outcome (Freeman and Nelson, 1988).

Hypoglycemia

Often much attention is focused on the finding of a low blood sugar level in a depressed newborn, and often it is pointed to as a cause of newborn brain damage. However there is substantial clinical and pathologic evidence that hypoglycemia per se does not cause neurologic damage. The opinion that hypoglycemia is a cause of newborn brain damage, although often stated in the literature, is erroneous.

In assessing the neurologic compromise of infants found to have low blood sugar, often overlooked are adversive gestational factors, such as maternal illness, infection, anemia, intrauterine growth retardation, factors that are substantial in causing fetal-neonatal compromise.

The immature fetus is physiologically maintained in a hypoglycemic state. Primate studies, in the rhesus monkey, and studies with other mammals, reveal that the blood level of the fetus in midgestation normally averages 20 milligrams percent and does not rise to adult levels until near term (Dawes, 1968). Reasonably, this applies to the human fetus and newborn as well. Premature infants are commonly hypoglycemic, often with very low blood glucose levels, and this does not render them neurologically damaged. The factor of neonatal hypoglycemia as a cause of newborn brain damage is much overstated.

Newborn infants, mature as well as premature, are refractory to hypoglycemia. Hypoglycemia is known to be common in newborns, demonstrated clinically in series of cases taken at random in well newborn infants. The presence of hypoglycemia would generally go undetected unless the infant has perinatal problems — and has blood chemistry studies done — and low blood glucose is registered, incidentally.

Apnea in the newborn: neurologic connotations

The onset of apnea in a newborn does not connote the presence of acute brain damage.

Apnea in the newborn at times is due to spinal cord injury (page 106).

Apnea means a cessation of breathing for 20 seconds or more. Apnea is common in premature infants; the cause is not clear. Apnea episodes occur in over 50 percent of prematures (page 105).

Apnea in the mature newborn is relatively rare. Apnea episodes that occur in mature newborn infants usually prove to be the antecedent of seizure activity, with the apnea followed by frank seizure activity. Subsequent seizures are commonly associated with periods of apnea.

Seizure activity: early postnatal onset

The occurrence of seizures in the newborn period does not automatically make it certain that the underlying cerebral damage was incurred during labor and delivery. There is increasing clinical opinion that when seizures appear soon after birth, the process is not attributable to acute intranatal asphyxial brain damage, but rather, the cause must be sought in pathologic processes, brain damage, prior to birth (Chapter 5).

It is well known that epilepsy commonly occurs after brain damage involving the cerebral cortex. Pathologically, the brain lesion forms a seizure-generating (epileptogenic) focus in the cortex. The epileptogenic lesion can be incurred in the fetal brain antenatally, weeks or months before birth. In the premature fetus, brain damage beginning deep in the cerebrum (causing cerebral palsy) may extend to the cortex, causing epilepsy and mental retardation, and other cortical disabilities.

With damage originating deep in the cerebrum and extending to the cortical surface, with the fetus surviving to term, the lesions in the cortex become subacute and are capable of causing seizure activity soon after birth. (Seizures are known to occur even before birth, in utero; fetal seizures are marked by episodes of in utero hyperactivity, in cases that postnatally, soon after birth, develop seizure activity.)

Neurologic depression due to (anticonvulsant) sedation

Infants previously stable and active that unexpectedly develop seizures require sedation with anticonvulsants. Phenobarbital is given in high dosage, medication that per se depresses neurologic function. Often the depressing effect of the anticonvulsant medication is overlooked and the newborn's depressed state is erroneously attributed to acute brain damage.

Spinal fluid examination; xanthochromia

Spinal fluid examination is usually done in newborn infants that are depressed or develop seizures.

Two main purposes in examining the spinal fluid in the newborn are:

(1) In the diagnosis of infection, meningitis, by bacteriologic studies of the fluid. With infection, the fluid, normally clear, colorless, and watery, becomes turbid.

(2) In the diagnosis of intracranial hemorrhage.

Blood in the spinal fluid may be due to fresh, acute intracranial damage, or it may be due to old, subacute damage. The presence of blood does not automatically mean there has been recent brain damage; old subacute cerebral damage often continues to be hemorrhagic, oozing blood into the spinal fluid. (**Traumatic tap:** At times the spinal fluid is bloody due to blood escaping into the fluid from torn blood vessels, damaged by the spinal tap needle in penetrating the spinal canal.)

Xanthochromia: Spinal fluid that has a yellow discoloration is referred to as xanthochromic (*xantho-,* yellow; *-chromia,* color).

The finding of xanthochromic spinal fluid, fluid drawn soon after birth, is of major importance in defining the time of incurrence of the cerebral damage. Xanthochromia is due to the presence of *old* hemorrhagic damage in the brain.

With hemorrhage in the brain, with blood escaping into the spinal fluid, red cells become lysed, broken down. The hemoglobin from the red cells first gives the spinal fluid a pink color. The hemoglobin gradually degenerates, forming a yellow pigment that gives the spinal fluid a yellow color — xanthochromia. (Just like a hemorrhagic black and blue bruise in the skin gradually becomes yellow-green after a period of time.) This change in color takes many days, and it continues to be present for weeks and months when there is an old hemorrhagic lesion in the brain.

Subacute lesions tend to ooze blood into the cerebrospinal fluid for a long time. In such circumstances, in addition to xanthochromia, the fluid contains some red blood cells.

The finding of xanthochromic spinal fluid soon after birth is of direct importance in assessing cases of newborn infants with manifest evidence of brain damage. The finding of xanthochromic spinal fluid soon after birth indicates damage that is old, subacute, incurred a period of time before birth, not during labor and delivery.

Late neurologic sequels in infants born with brain damage

The late neurologic sequels of neonatal *acute* cerebral damage and *subacute* cerebral damage are different.

Acute cerebral damage present at birth: neurologic sequels

The late effects of acute cerebral damage in surviving infants depends on the gestational age at birth.

Premature newborn: If the newborn infant is immature, premature at less than 34 to 35 weeks' gestation, acute hypoxic damage will target germinal matrix and adjoining basal ganglia and periventricular white matter, with the surviving infant developing cerebral palsy. If the deep cerebral damage extends through the cerebrum to the cortex, there will be cortical manifestations, mental retardation, seizure disorder, and at times psychopathy.

Mature newborn: Acute hypoxia in the mature fetus and newborn, as in the adult, causes damage to the cerebral cortex rather than the basal ganglia. Therefore, surviving infants are subject to the development of cortical manifestations of mental retardation and epilepsy and other cortical disability.

Subacute cerebral damage present at birth: neurologic sequels

In the first months after birth, infants with subacute lesions may appear to have good neurologic function. After a few months, however, delays in motor function and other abnormal neurologic findings become manifest.

Subacute cerebral damage present in the term newborn has its origin during early premature fetal life (page 166). In the premature fetus, hypoxia primarily damages the deep cerebral structures, extending to the neighboring basal ganglia, and at times extending through the cerebral hemispheric wall to the cortex. When gestation is carried to term, the cerebral damage becomes subacute, varying in severity — at times minimal and at times extensive, with involvement of deep and cortical structures (Figure 23, page 24; Figure 24, page 25). When affected infants with deep and cortical damage survive, they are subject to the development of basal ganglia dyskinesias of cerebral palsy, as well as superimposed cortical manifestations of mental retardation and epilepsy.

Newborn depression: misdiagnosis of causation; erroneous birth records

Despite the accumulated clinical and pathology research data that demonstrate otherwise, neonatology and pediatric hospital resident doctors, in cases of depressed newborn, continue to record almost automatically the initial diagnosis of "depression due to intranatal hypoxic cerebral damage." As Niswander points out, however, while various unfavorable events may occur during delivery, it does not automatically make certain that these events cause cerebral damage, newborn depression, and cerebral disability (Niswander, 1983).

In cases of newborn depression, often overlooked, not taken into consideration, is the fact that obvious pregnancy complications adversive to the fetus had occurred, that the depression of the newborn was attributable to chronic intrauterine enfeeblement of the fetus.

Once the diagnosis of depression due to intranatal hypoxic damage is imprinted in the infant's record, that diagnosis *sticks,* and in the years that follow, pediatricians and neurologists will be given to understand that the child, now with cerebral palsy, suffered intranatal hypoxia. In cases of cerebral palsy that come to litigation, this initial recorded diagnosis of intranatal hypoxia often becomes an important issue.

References and Additional Reading

Apgar, V. (1953). A proposal for a new method of evaluation of the newborn infant. *Curr Res Anaesth* 32: 260.

Brand, M. M., and A. Bignami (1969). The effects of chronic hypoxia on the neonatal and infantile brain. *Brain* 92: 233–254.

Dawes, G. S. (1968). *Foetal and Neonatal Physiology.* Chicago: Year Book Medical Publishers.

Ellis, W., B. W. Goetzman, and W. E. Lindenberg (1988). Neuropathologic documentation of prenatal brain damage. *Am J Dis Child* 142: 858–866.

Freeman, J. M., and K. B. Nelson (1988). Intrapartum asphyxia and cerebral palsy. *Pediatrics* 82: 240.

Freud, S. (1897). *Infantile Cerebral Paralysis,* R. A. Lassin, trans. Reprint, Coral Gables, Fla.: University of Miami Press, 1968.

Hallervorden, J. (1949). Uber eine Kohlenoxyvergiftung im Fetalleben mit Entwickkungsstörungen der Hirnrinde. *Allgemeine Zeitschrift für Psychiatrie und Psychisch-Gerichtliche Medizin* 124: 289–298.

Nelson, K. B. (1988). Perspectives on the role of perinatal asphyxia in neurologic outcome. Pages 3–10 in the *Proceedings of a Symposium on Perinatal Asphyxia* held on October 26, 1988, at Toronto, Ontario, by the American Academy for Cerebral Palsy and Developmental Medicine and by the Canadian Medical Protection Association.

——— and J. H. Ellenberg (1987). The asymptomatic newborn and risk of cerebral palsy. *Am J. Dis Child* 141: 1333–1335.

Niswander, K. R. (1983). Labor and operative obstetrics. Asphyxia in the fetus and cerebral palsy. In R. M. Pitkin and F. J. Zlatkin, eds., *The Year Book of Obstetrics and Gynecology.* Chicago: Year Book Medical Publishers.

Sadovsky, E., and H. Yaffe (1973). Daily fetal movement recording and fetal prognosis. *Obstet Gynecol* 41: 845–850.

Towbin, A. (1977). Trauma in pregnancy: Injury to the fetus and newborn. In Tedeschi, C. G., Eckert, W. G., Tedeschi, L. G., eds., *Forensic Medicine.* Pp. 436–486. Philadelphia: W. B. Saunders.

——— (1978). Cerebral dysfunctions related to perinatal organic damage: Clinical-neuropathologic correlations. *J Abnorm Psychol* 87: 617–635.

——— (1986). Obstetric malpractice litigation: The pathologist's view. *Am J Obstet Gynecol* 155: 927–935.

——— (1987). The depressed newborn: Pathogenesis and neurologic sequels. *Perinatology Neonatology* 11: 16–18.

——— and G. L. Turner (1978). Obstetric factors in fetal-neonatal visceral injury. *Obstet Gynecol* 52: 113–124.

3 Cerebral Palsy: Pathogenesis

Neurologic aspects of cerebral palsy

Neuroanatomic and neurophysiologic basic factors in cerebral palsy

Causation: cerebral palsy pathogenesis
    Acute hypoxic cerebral damage
    Subacute hypoxic cerebral damage
    Chronic pattern of cerebral palsy

Transition of cerebral damage: acute to subacute to chronic forms

Cerebral palsy as a time marker

Cerebral palsy is a neurologic disorder characterized by defective fine motor control, a dyskinesia (*dys-*, abnormal; *-kinesia*, motor). Three main forms of dyskinesia occur in cerebral palsy: hypertonia (spasticity), hypotonia (the "floppy" infant), and athetosis (involuntary, purposeless movements). These patterns of dyskinesia are usually intermixed in a person with cerebral palsy, with one type or another predominating; thus, in spastic cerebral palsy there is usually an element of hypotonia in a part of the body, or athetosis. The neurologic disorder is not evident at birth; manifestations of the disability appear in early infancy. The disability is nonprogressive after infancy. Infants with cerebral palsy, in most cases, show more than one nervous system disability. Commonly there is some degree of mental retardation, at times seizure disorder.

Despite the common occurrence of cerebral palsy in the general population — there are estimated to be more than half a million cases in this country — many people have no idea what cerebral palsy looks like in a person affected. As to pathogenesis, extremely few people, questioned, have a valid notion about the cause of cerebral palsy. This is true even among doctors.

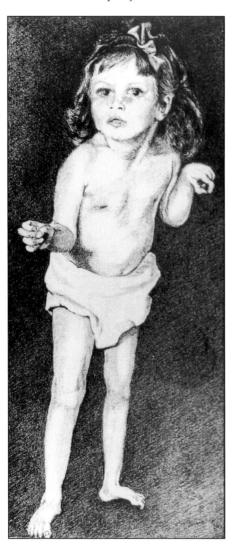

Figure 113. A child with cerebral palsy. (Drawing by F. W. Klutzow)

Typical cases of spastic cerebral palsy can be observed on any busy street. Characteristics of cerebral palsy are illustrated in Figure 113 — a child walking stiffly, knock-kneed with a "scissor gait" or at times walking on a wide base, feet apart, with hands moving artlessly about, wiggling purposelessly, with face grimacing, mouth drooling, with speech difficult, slow, drawn out in a monotone.

Pathology studies of the brain in cerebral palsy, studies of the structural changes, were infrequently carried out in the past. In 1920, the Vogts showed that the essential damage in the cerebral palsy brain was in the deep structures of the cerebrum, in the basal ganglia. Also consistently in the cerebrum there was decreased white matter with enlargement of the ventricles (Figure 114).

For over a hundred years one of the classic questions in neurology, in the field of cerebral palsy, has been: When is the brain damage in cerebral palsy incurred? During labor and delivery? Or is the brain damage incurred prenatally, during fetal life, weeks, months, before birth?

Figure 114. Cerebral palsy, spastic quadriplegia; brain specimen showing characteristic chronic lesions. Basal ganglia on the left with an area of destruction, cavitation; overall decrease in the white matter around the ventricles, "ex vacuo hydrocephalus." Specimen from an 8-year-old: in addition to spastic cerebral palsy, the child had mental retardation and epilepsy.

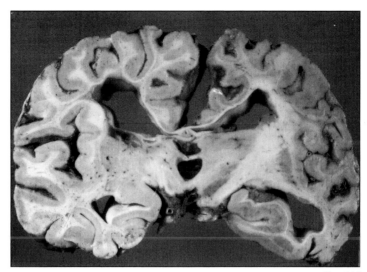

Fig. 114

The idea that cerebral palsy was due to hypoxic brain damage incurred at term during the process of birth, during labor and delivery, was imprinted in the medical literature in the pioneer study by William John Little, in a clinical presentation to the Obstetrical Society of London in 1861 (Little, 1861). Historically, cerebral palsy became known as Little's disease.

Other observers, neurologists and neuropathologists, subsequently evolved evidence that the underlying brain damage in cases of cerebral palsy originated in early fetal life, the consequence of hypoxia-producing pregnancy complications, maternal illness, placental disorders. This was the opinion voiced by the German school of neuropathology, by Sigmund Freud (Freud, 1897) and others. (Freud, known best for his psychoanalytic studies, also was a neurologist and neuropathologist. In his early years, 1885 to 1897, he published widely in the German medical literature, particularly with reference to infantile cerebral palsies.)

Freud opposed the concepts of Little, that cerebral palsy resulted from brain damage incurred at term, during birth. Freud concluded that, in infants in poor condition at delivery, often the depression of vital function was due not to damage incurred during labor and delivery, but to prenatal deprivation and enfeeblement, *due to damage incurred during fetal life.* Nelson (1988) in reviewing the interpretations of Little and Freud, commented, "The balance of current evidence appears to be tilting towards Freud's point of view." Mounting research evidence, from the NIH Collaborative Perinatal Project and from other studies — clinical research as well as pathology studies — supports Freud's interpretation.

The question — When was the damage incurred? — has an important bearing in obstetric malpractice litigation in cases of cerebral palsy. Despite current research information to the contrary, the diagnostic opinion of many present-day neonatologists and pediatric neurologists remains wedded to the original views of Little, that cerebral palsy is due to acute brain damage incurred during labor and delivery, commonly in infants born at term. These clinicians base their interpretations on such findings as low blood pH values, acidosis, widely accepted as the "gold standard" indicator of acute hypoxic damage incurred during birth. As Nelson indicates, current research data reveal that fetal monitor abnormalities, low pH, and a low Apgar score are poor predictors of acute brain damage, damage that leads to cerebral palsy. Rather, it is evident that cerebral damage that leads to cerebral palsy is incurred during early fetal life, is present in a latent subacute form at birth, with manifestations of brain damage making their appearance as cerebral palsy in the early months of infancy.

"Cerebral palsy" is sometimes implied to be a catch-all, "wastebasket" diagnosis. This is not warranted. In a given case — taking into account the pathogenesis, the characteristic evolution of clinical manifestations, the common neurologic findings — it is plain that cerebral palsy is a specific clinical entity.

Neurologic aspects of cerebral palsy

The clinical sequence of manifestations in the development of cerebral palsy, the natural history of the disorder, is characteristic. Often the pregnancy record of the mother indicates the occurrence of complications, maternal illness or other pathologic processes that compromise the immature fetus. In cases in which the immature fetus has incurred brain damage due to gestational complications, and has survived through the gestation, the fetus is born at term. However, very often in cases of cerebral palsy there is a history of premature birth. In the past, prematurity was recognized as a causal factor (even by Shakespeare, in *Richard III*). Clinically, cerebral palsy has been called the disease of prematurity.

Cerebral palsy cannot be diagnosed at birth. There are no specific abnormal reflexes or other neurologic signs that signify cerebral palsy in the newborn. In early infancy, the baby may be "floppy," hypotonic. But as the affected baby goes through the first few weeks and months, the mother notices a retardation in motor activity. At three to four months, distinct neurologic abnormalities become apparent on clinical examination. The pediatrician finds that the infant is now hypertonic. Reflexes are "hyperactive." This refers to the knee jerk reflex: flexing the knee and tapping the tendon below the knee causes the leg to spring forward; a normal reflex is 1+ to 2+, hyperactive reflexes are 3+ or 4+. The other reflex usually recorded is the ankle reflex: flexing the foot and tapping the Achilles tendon causes the foot to jerk downward. Clonus is usually noted; extending the leg and flexing the foot quickly toward the shin causes the foot to oscillate rapidly backward and forward when the test is positive. The plantar reflex (Babinski test) consists of stroking the sole of the foot from heel to toe; normally, the toes tend to clench; in the abnormal response, the toes flare out, are "upgoing."

This group of neurological reflexes, when abnormal, are indicators of **basal ganglia** damage, present in the development of cerebral palsy. At about 6 to 12 months, in affected infants the diagnosis of cerebral palsy can be made. The head circumference gradually falls below normal, to the lower percentiles, microcephaly. Follow-up CT scan studies of the brain reveal enlargement of the ventricles, the chambers in the cerebrum; this pathologic condition is called **ex vacuo**

hydrocephalus, reflecting loss of deep cerebral tissue; often there are cystic changes in the cerebral walls and, at times, calcium deposits in the deep structures of the cerebrum.

Eye problems are common in cerebral palsy, especially strabismus (cross-eyedness), due to imbalance of the muscles that control movement of the eyeballs. Speech disorders frequently are a major handicap for people with cerebral palsy; the compromise of fine motor control affecting muscles of the tongue and face present a mechanical hindrance in articulating consonants and in maintaining voice tone. The act of swallowing is often affected, due to involvement of the muscles of the mouth that initiate swallowing; choking on food and aspiration of food material is an ongoing hazard, at times lethal, in infants with cerebral palsy.

Clinical patterns in cerebral palsy

Cerebral palsy is a dyskinesia, a disorder of fine motor control, a disorder of motor tone. Dyskinesias are essentially disorders of the basal ganglia.

Three main forms of dyskinesia occur in cerebral palsy, reflecting basal ganglia damage: hypertonia, hypotonia, and athetosis.

Hypertonicity. Spastic quadriplegia is the term commonly applied when all four limbs are spastic, hypertonic, usually the lower limbs more than the upper. In cases termed diplegia, spasticity is limited mainly to the legs. Spasticity in cases of cerebral palsy, present over the years, leads to contractures, with joints becoming fixed in place, immovable, with wasting of unused musculature. Contractures can to some degree be prevented, ameliorated, by physiotherapy and by surgery. Spinal curvature deformities, kyphosis and scoliosis, often develop due to imbalance in the degree of muscle pull on parts of the spinal column.

Hypotonicity. This refers to cases of cerebral palsy with neurologic manifestations of reduced muscle tone, floppiness.

Athetosis. This is characterized by manifestations of involuntary, purposeless movements, with facial grimacing.

These patterns of dyskinesia are usually intermixed, with one type or another predominating; thus, in spastic cerebral palsy there is usually an element of hypotonia and/or athetosis. This reflects the common location of the cerebral lesion, in the basal ganglia.

The severity of cerebral palsy varies in affected children.

Minimal forms of cerebral palsy often go unrecognized, undiagnosed, and affected children are viewed simply as "awkward children." Many of these cases are examples of organic **minimal brain dysfunction** (Chapter 7). Clinical assessment commonly reveals a history of complicated gestation or premature birth, and a precise neurologic examination may reveal evidence of organicity, the presence of neurologic soft signs, minimal abnormal reflexes, athetoid movements, reflecting latent minimal brain damage.

The majority of cases of cerebral palsy are of intermediate severity; these are people who get about, are seen on the street, with "scissor gait," grimacing; often they are athetoid, mentally retarded. However, in some instances mentation apparently is not affected; many of these people are of average mentality, or more, some becoming professors, doctors, lawyers.

In its severest form, affected individuals are rendered helpless, with inexorable contractures, and become wheelchairbound or bedfast.

Infants with cerebral palsy often show more than one disability. Commonly, there is mental retardation and seizure disorder. These separate disabilities reflect damage to specific, different, parts of the cerebrum: cerebral palsy being due to deep (basal ganglia) damage; mental retardation, epilepsy, psychopathy being due to surface cerebral damage, to the cortex.

A comprehensive neurologic assessment is a *sine qua non* in assessing cases of cerebral palsy, particularly in cases brought to litigation. It is inadequate to characterize the disability simply as cerebral palsy. It must be made clear, in detail, the pattern and degree of functional disability.

Hemiplegic (asymmetrical) cerebral palsy

Illustrative Cases:
Case 103   *p. 485*
Case 132   *p. 540*
Case 139   *p. 552*
Case 200   *p. 661*
Case 216   *p. 704*

Hypoxic damage that occurs in the deep strata of the premature brain is at times asymmetrical (Figure 17, page 17). In infants surviving, the sequelant effect, the cerebral palsy dyskinesia that develops, is asymmetrical, affecting one side of the body more than the other side.

Neuroanatomic-neurophysiologic factors in cerebral palsy

The brain, like other organs in the body, has specific functions, many functions. Essentially, each neurologic function is related anatomically to a particular structure in the brain. The two main parts of the human brain are (1) the forebrain, the cerebrum, occupying most of the cranial cavity, that mediates basic sensory, motor, and intellectual processes in man, and (2) the brain stem, located in the lower posterior part of the cranial cavity, the structure with regulatory centers that control elementary vital functions such as respiration and cardiac action.

Basic anatomic structures of the cerebrum are shown in Figure 1, page 4.

The cerebrum, forming two symmetrical hemispheres, each with a central ventricle filled with cerebrospinal fluid, is covered with membranes, the meninges. The arachnoid, one of the meninges, a webby sheet, is separated from the brain surface by the subarachnoid space, containing cerebrospinal fluid. Surrounding the arachnoid is the thick fibrotic dura.

The surface of the cerebrum, forming convolutions, has a thin outer layer of "gray matter," the cortex, containing nerve cells. The cortex over the frontal region of the cerebrum is concerned with mentation; damage here results in deficient intellect, mental retardation, and at times results in distortion of intellect, psychopathy.

The middle portion of the cortex over the convexity of the cerebrum is the "motor cortex," concerned with control of voluntary motion of the body. Damage to the motor cortex results in paralysis, loss of motor function of the affected part.

The posterior portion of the cerebral cortex is sensory, concerned with tactile sensation, hearing, vision, and other receptive processes. Thus, damage to the posterior pole of the cerebral surface, the visual cortex, leads to "cortical blindness."

Scars in the cortex are known to cause seizure disorders.

The "white matter" of the cerebrum, a thick layer deep to the cortex, is composed of bundles of delicate conduction fibers, streaming from nerve cells in one part of the brain to another, forming a network of thick interlacing cable-like "nerve tracks."

Basal ganglia, commonly referred to as the "extrapyramidal system," are deposits of gray matter, large aggregates of nerve cells, bordering each cerebral ventricle near the base of the cerebral hemispheres (Figure 1, page 4). The basal ganglia regulate, modify, body movements, adjusting and smoothing out fine motor function. Basal ganglia damage results in dyskinesia, disturbance in body kinetics. The two common forms of dyskinesia are cerebral palsy, due to damage to the cerebral basal ganglia, manifest in infancy, and parkinsonism, due to damage to basal ganglia in the brain stem, occurring mainly in old people.

Germinal matrix (Figure 3, page 5), present only in the premature, immature cerebrum, is another cerebral structure of immediate importance in the present consideration, in analyzing the pathogenesis of cerebral palsy. Germinal matrix tissue lies along the lining of the cerebral ventricles and is composed of primitive cells, seed cells, contributing to the genesis of basal ganglia and other developing neuronal structures in the brain. Germinal matrix is of a transitional nature, present only in the premature, immature cerebrum, not present in the adult. The germinal matrix gradually becomes attenuated, used up, and is no longer present in the cerebrum after 35 weeks of gestation.

Causation: cerebral palsy pathogenesis

The causes of cerebral palsy as projected in the past, based mainly on clinical concepts, were speculative. Misconceptions remain deeply rooted in lay and medical thinking today. For example, the notion still persists that cerebral palsy can result from crushing of the fetal head with obstetric forceps, a claim often heard in obstetric malpractice suits. This concept regarding obstetric forceps trauma is out of a time past, an anachronism long disproved in pathology studies.

Clinically, it was realized a long time ago that basic information about the pathogenesis of cerebral palsy, about the causal mechanisms, could be obtained only at its origin, through pathology studies of fetal-neonatal acute cerebral damage and by correlating the findings with neuropathology studies in infants who develop cerebral palsy and related cerebral disabilities.

The opportunity to comprehensively study the pathogenesis of fetal-neonatal brain damage presented itself in the Collaborative Perinatal Project (1965) conducted by the NIH. This was a nationwide study of over 50,000 pregnancies and their outcome, carried out in 15 medical centers. In the cases of fetal and newborn death, autopsies were performed and correlated with the clinical data, with concern particularly to damage to the brain. Although the pathology information that was derived was widely imprinted in the medical literature, much of this information has not penetrated clinical thinking, so that interpretations of the pathogenesis of fetal-neonatal brain damage and sequelant cerebral palsy presented by clinicians still reflect the state of knowledge of decades past.

The interpretation of the pathogenesis of cerebral palsy presented here is based on principles of elementary pathology established by research workers in the past, particularly research information that evolved in the NIH Collaborative Perinatal Project. These facets of information, these basic principles of pathology, form the foundation for the present interpretation and are presented in the following overview:

1. The brain is a biologic machine organized so that each part governs a specific function — the frontal lobe, intellect; the posterior of the cerebrum, vision. Given an assessment of the neurologic functional disability in an infant, the corresponding damaged part of the brain can be identified.
2. The neurologic disorder in cerebral palsy, the dyskinetic defect in motor coordination, is due to damage in a certain specific part of the brain, the *basal ganglia,* located deep in the brain.
3. This deep cerebral damage is due to hypoxia and occurs consistently, specifically, only in the immature, premature brain, during fetal life or in the premature newborn.
4. Complications, with hypoxia, at term (mature) delivery do not cause deep cerebral damage; at term, hypoxia causes surface (cortical) cerebral damage.
5. Maternal illness and other gestational complications during pregnancy, exercising an hypoxia-producing effect on the fetus, cause cerebral damage.

6. If the fetus incurs acute cerebral damage during early fetal life, and survives to term, the infant is born bearing subacute cerebral damage.

7. Deep cerebral damage incurred in the premature, immature, fetal period at times extends to the cerebral surface, to the cortex. Pertinently, surface cerebral damage that occurs with hypoxia at term does not extend inward to the deep cerebral structures, does not affect the basal ganglia.

Basal ganglia damage

The link between lesions of the basal ganglia and clinical dykinesias was defined by the German school of neuropathology, by the Vogts in 1920. Neuropathologists subsequently have confirmed this relationship between the deep cerebral structures, the basal ganglia and periventricular white matter, and the occurrence of cerebral palsy (Crome, 1972; Malamud, Itabasi, et al., 1964; Towbin, 1960).

Acute hypoxic cerebral damage in the newborn

To understand the pathogenesis of cerebral palsy, it is of fundamental importance to recognize the occurrence of the two basic patterns of fetal-neonatal hypoxic cerebral damage: hypoxia causes *deep* damage in the premature, immature cerebrum. In the mature cerebrum, hypoxia causes surface *cortical* damage (Figure 10, page 12).

The predisposition of the premature fetal brain to incur hypoxic damage in the deep cerebral structures, in the persisting germinal matrix, in the basal ganglia and periventricular white matter, was defined by research pathologists in the past (Gruenwald, 1951; Banker, 1961; Schwartz, 1961; Yakovlev and Rosales, 1970; Larroche, 1972; Csermely, 1972; see also page 14 of this volume).

In contrast to the deep location of cerebral lesions in the premature fetus, studies have shown that in the mature fetus and newborn, hypoxic damage in the cerebrum is localized mainly in the surface strata, in the cortex (Csermely, 1972; Larroche, 1972; see also page 13 in this volume). Experimentally, likewise, hypoxia at term in the guinea pig causes cortical damage (Windle, Becker, et al., 1944). These past observations, defining two patterns of hypoxic cerebral damage in the newborn with reference to gestational age, were confirmed in studies in the NIH Collaborative Perinatal Project (Towbin, 1968, 1970a, 1970b, 1977).

The specificity in location of fetal-neonatal acute cerebral hypoxic damage — deep in the premature and cortical at term — is influenced by three biologic factors, all related to gestational age: the presence or absence of germinal matrix tissue, the momentum of local organogenesis, and the early development of the deep vascular elements in the premature cerebrum (Towbin, 1968, 1970a, 1970b).

As previously pointed out, in the premature fetus and newborn, damage to the deep structures of the cerebrum, when severe, in some instances extends outward through the cerebrum to the surface, affecting the cerebral cortex and, in addition to cerebral palsy, leads to cortical disabilities of mental retardation, epilepsy, or blindness, in infants surviving (page 17).

Pertinently, however, as pathology studies have shown, surface damage at term does not penetrate inward, does not affect the basal ganglia, does not lead to cerebral palsy (Figure 22, page 22).

In most cerebral palsy cases the central question is — *when* did the brain damage occur? During labor and delivery? Or did it originate during early fetal life? Or during the postnatal period?

The occurrence of problems during labor and delivery does not automatically make certain that there is a causal relationship between these events in the intranatal period and the later development of cerebral disabilities in the offspring.

In analyzing pathogenesis, it is requisite that consideration be given to complications adverse to the fetus that occurred during the pregnancy, such as maternal illness, placental disorders, fetal-neonatal anemia. Maternal illness during pregnancy directly affects the maternal-placental-fetal complex, compromising the fetus. Pathologically, the underlying process exercises its effects through the common denominator of intrauterine hypoxia (Courville, 1971; Csermely, 1972; Towbin, 1968; Windle, Becker, et al., 1944). The severity of the maternal illness does not necessarily correspond to the degree of fetal damage. A mild maternal illness may prove disastrous for the fetus; at other times the fetus seems to escape manifest damage. Pregnancy illness — dangerous for the fetus — often is minimized, overlooked, often goes unreported by the mother, and is not likely to be recalled in testimony years after the pregnancy.

The wide spectrum of gestational complications, maternal, placental, and other pathologic processes that adversely affect the well-being of the fetus, are considered in detail on page 35.

Subacute hypoxic cerebral damage in the newborn

Gestational hypoxia-producing complications at times result in fetal death, miscarriage, with the autopsy revealing hypoxic cerebral damage. But this is not an all-or-none process. The intrauterine pathologic process, occurring in the premature period, may prove sublethal, causing acute cerebral damage, with the fetus surviving. If the gestation then goes to term, the acute cerebral lesions gradually become *subacute,* undergoing "healing" with scarring (Figure 23, page 24; Figure 24, page 25).

In the case presented on page 24, the mother was hospitalized two months before delivery with pneumonia and vaginal bleeding. The infant, born at term, died on the first day. The brain at autopsy showed far-advanced old cerebral infarctional damage, thick broad patches of pale necrotic tissue in the deep periventricular layers of the cerebrum (Case 47, page 348).

The diagnosis clinically of the presence or absence of subacute cerebral damage in the newborn, the differential diagnosis between acute and subacute cerebral damage, is based — not on problems that may have occurred during labor and delivery — but is determined primarily by the postnatal performance of the newborn infant (Chapter 2).

The fetus — previously enfeebled by hypoxic injury during the premature period, bearing **subacute** cerebral damage at term — often does not tolerate the ordinary stress of labor, with the result that fetal monitor abnormalities appear, and the infant is born depressed, with a low Apgar score. Usually, however, the infant responds to treatment in the delivery room and is soon stable, responsive, and active, and has a short hospital stay.

In contrast, in infants with **acute** hypoxic cerebral damage present at birth, the postnatal course is different from that of subacute cases. With acute brain damage present, the infants are depressed at birth and remain unstable, limp, comatose, in the intensive care nursery, for prolonged periods, and are discharged only after weeks of hospitalization.

In infants with subacute cerebral damage, neurologic manifestations are subliminal during the early weeks of infancy. The presence of such subclinical cerebral damage, present, but latent, at birth, accounts for cases of cerebral palsy that develop in infants born at term. However, in light of current pathology information, it does not mean that the cerebral damage was imprinted at the time of the term birth.

The fact that newborn infants at times harbor latent subacute lesions in the brain, while well known to neonatal neuropathologists, is not generally realized by neonatologists, pediatricians, and neurologists. Accordingly, clinicians are prone to ascribe manifest brain damage to intranatal causes.

Subacute cerebral lesions, in surviving fetuses and newborns, gradually become quiescent, with the devitalized tissue gradually being absorbed, forming cavitations, or the areas damaged are converted to scar tissue. These changes are present in brain specimens in cases that survive for months and years, cases clinically with manifestations of cerebral palsy (Figure 114, page 179).

In times past, the cause of cerebral palsy, the pathogenesis of the lesions in the brain, was unclear, a subject of speculation clinically. Current pathology studies, in the context presented here, indicate the transition of acute hypoxic cerebral damage in the fetus and newborn, to subacute damage, and to the chronic lesions in the brain in cerebral palsy.

Chronic pattern of hypoxic cerebral damage in cerebral palsy

The brain in cases of cerebral palsy shows distinctive gross pathologic changes (Figure 2, page 4; Figure 26, page 27; Figure 114, page 179). The anatomic structures in the cerebrum that are mainly affected are the basal ganglia, the periventricular white matter, and the ventricles. Characteristically, the basal ganglia show scarring, at times calcium deposits and cavitations; periventricular white matter is decreased, at times showing focal or diffuse cystic damage. The loss of periventricular tissue results in enlargement of the ventricles, **ex vacuo hydrocephalus.** These structural changes in cerebral palsy, for the most part are readily evidenced in CT and MRI studies (Figure 35, page 34; Figure 37, page 35).

The structural damage in the brain in cerebral palsy is reflected outwardly in the development of microcephaly. Microcephaly, smallness of the head and the brain, commonly makes its appearance during the first year, often with the head circumference falling below the fifth percentile. Enlargement of the brain depends on the growth, the thickening, of the deep layers of the cerebrum. Failure of the brain to grow in cases of cerebral palsy reflects profound damage to the deep cerebral structures, with consequent growth stasis, microcephaly.

The commonly expressed opinion by clinicians, that when the head is of normal size at birth, it is evidence that the brain was undamaged prenatally, is a speculative, erroneous concept. Pathology studies have shown that the newborn brain at times has far-advanced chronic damage, with the head of normal size.

CT scans and MRI studies, imaging studies, contribute substantial information in assessing cerebral palsy; these radiologic procedures have limitations, however. CT scans show shadows, black, gray, and pale translucent areas. Scans can accurately diagnose the size of ventricles and the presence of blood, calcifications, and cysts. The radiologist, on the basis of scans, cannot make pathologic tissue diagnoses, except for speculative interpretations. Cerebral tissue at times has far-advanced devastation, but of a form not grossly visible. Damage with diffuse loss of nerve cells often is not evident to the naked eye, and can be diagnosed only microscopically. Accordingly, it cannot be expected that radiologic studies, ultrasound, CT, MRI scans, would validly diagnose the presence or absence of such tissue damage. Accordingly, in cases in which the brain scans reveal no changes in the basal ganglia or cortex, there may in fact be much damage, scarring, and nerve cell depletion. In cases of cerebral palsy, the basal ganglia, grossly and on CT scan and MRI, may appear unchanged, but microscopic examination shows devitalized tissue. A CT scan interpretation that says no changes are evident in the cerebral structure does not mean there is, for sure, no damage in the tissue.

The transition of cerebral damage —acute to subacute, to the chronic forms in cerebral palsy

In the pathology laboratory, the pathogenesis of cerebral palsy is demonstrated anatomically by step-by-step transitional studies correlating patterns of acute deep cerebral lesions in newborn infants, with cases having corresponding subacute lesions, and then correlating the lesions in these cases with the characteristic deep chronic lesions in cases of cerebral palsy. The transition of the patterns of deep cerebral damage, from acute to subacute to the chronic forms, is illustrated in Figure 115. The nature of the lesions in all three stages is the same pathologically, all being of infarctional nature, differing only in age — acute, subacute, chronic.

Figure 115. Correlation of analogous cerebral lesions indicating transition from acute deep hypoxic cerebral damage in a premature newborn infant to subacute deep hypoxic cerebral damage to chronic deep cerebral periventricular damage.
(a). Periventricular hypoxic acute hemorrhagic infarction, appearing as black blotchy areas deep in the cerebrum. **(b).** Pale, devitalized periventricular patches, the subacute stage of hypoxic damage. **(c).** Chronic pattern of damage, the residue of cerebral damage following early fetal hypoxia; loss of periventricular structures with contraction and scarring of tissue, with consequent enlargement of ventricles; pattern of cerebral damage in cerebral palsy.

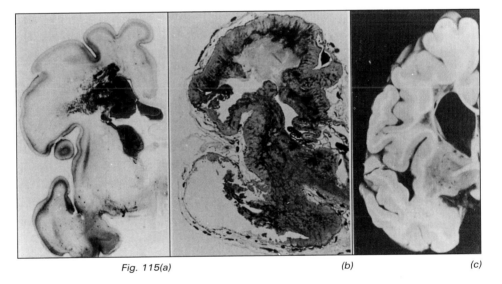

Fig. 115(a)   *(b)*   *(c)*

The concept that cerebral palsy occurs due to hypoxic complications at term delivery remains deeply ingrained in medical thinking (Paneth, 1986). Clinicians point to the large number of cases of cerebral palsy in infants delivered at term. Despite substantial clinical and pathologic evidence to the contrary, cerebral palsy in infants delivered at term is often erroneously attributed to negligent obstetric care during delivery. In such cases of term delivery, cases reported as an "uncomplicated pregnancy," often overlooked is a history of maternal illness, vaginal bleeding, or other early gestational hypoxia-producing complications adversive to the premature fetus.

There is mounting current research information, in both pathology studies and clinical statistical surveys, that indicates that cerebral palsy is not caused by intranatal hypoxia at term (Nelson and Ellenberg, 1986; Nelson, 1988; Niswander, 1983).

Cerebral palsy–a time marker

The fact that cerebral palsy does *not* occur as a result of hypoxia at term is of broad importance clinically.

In most cases of brain-damaged infants, clinically the main question is — When did the brain damage occur? During labor and delivery? Prenatally, a long time before birth? Postnatally? The preponderance of such problem cases deals with infants born at term who develop cerebral palsy.

Cerebral palsy has long been known as "the disease of prematurity." Cerebral palsy is due to hypoxic brain damage incurred by premature newborn infants or, more often, incurred during fetal life due to gestational complications. The development of cerebral palsy in infants born at term indicates (1) that cerebral damage occurred during fetal life due to intrauterine hypoxia-producing pathologic processes, processes often overlooked, and (2) that the cerebral damage is not attributable to the events of delivery at term.

In studies of the pathogenesis of cerebral palsy, it is well established that cerebral palsy is due to damage to deep structures in the cerebrum, damage to the basal ganglia, and that this form of damage occurs specifically only in the premature immature fetus (or premature newborn) prior to 35 weeks' gestation.

In this direction, in defining retrospectively the time of incurrence of the cerebral damage, the presence of cerebral palsy indicates a time factor, a time marker. This time factor, applied in the assessment of cerebral palsy infants born at term, establishes that the underlying brain damage was incurred weeks, months, before the time of birth.

References and Additional Reading

Banker, B. Q. (1961). Cerebral vascular disease in infancy and childhood. *J Neuropathol Exp Neurol* 20: 127.

Collaborative Perinatal Project (1965). (Collaborative Study of Cerebral Palsy, Mental Retardation and Other Neurologic and Sensory Disorders of Infancy and Childhood). National Institutes of Health, Bethesda, Md. Public Health Service Publication No. 1370. Washington, D.C.: U.S. Government Printing Office.

Courville, C. B. (1971). *Birth and Brain Damage.* Pasadena, Calif.: Margaret F. Courville.

Crome, L. (1972). *Pathology of Mental Retardation.* Baltimore: Williams and Wilkins.

Csermely, H. (1972). Perinatal anoxic changes of the central nervous system. *Acta Paediatr Academiae Scientiarum Hung* 13: 293–299.

Ellis, W., B. W. Goetzman, et al. (1988). Neuropathologic documentation of prenatal brain damage. *Am J Dis Child* 142: 858–866.

Freud, S. (1897). *Infantile Cerebral Paralysis,* L. A. Rassin, trans. Reprint, Coral Gables, Fla.: University of Miami Press, 1968.

Gruenwald, P. (1951). Subependymal cerebral hemorrhage in premature infants, and its relation to various injurious influences at birth. *Am J Obstet Gynecol* 61: 1285.

Larroche, J. C. (1968). Nécrose cérébrale massive chez le nouveau-né. *Biol Neonate* 13: 340–360.

——— (1972). Post-haemorrhagic hydrocephalus in infancy: Anatomical study. *Biol Neonate* 20: 287.

Little, W. J. (1861). On the influence of abnormal parturition, difficult labour, premature birth, and asphyxia neonatorum on the mental and physical condition of the child, especially in relation to deformities. *Lancet* 2: 378–379.

Malamud, N., H. H. Itabasi, et al. (1964). An etiologic and diagnostic study of cerebral palsy. *J Pediatr* 65: 27–293.

Manterola, A., A. Towbin, and P. I. Yakovlev (1966). Cerebral infarction in the human fetus near term. *J Neuropathol Exp Neurol* 25: 479–488.

Nelson, K. B. (1988). Perspectives on the role of perinatal asphyxia in neurologic outcome. Pages 3–10 in the *Proceedings of a Symposium on Perinatal Asphyxia* held on October 26, 1988, at Toronto, Ontario, by the American Academy for Cerebral Palsy and Developmental Medicine and the Canadian Medical Protective Association.

——— and J. H. Ellenberg (1986). Antecedents of cerebral palsy. *N Engl J Med* 315: 81–86.

Neuburger, F. (1934). Fall einer Intrauterinen Hirnschädigung nach Leuchtgasvergiftung der Muter. *Beitr Gerichtl Med* 13: 85–95.

Niswander, K. R. (1983). Labor and operative obstetrics: Asphyxia in the fetus and cerebral palsy. In Pitkin, R. M., Zlatnik, F. J., eds., *The Year Book of Obstetrics and Gynecology*. Chicago: Year Book Medical Publishers. Pp. 106–124.

Paneth, N. (1986). Birth and the origins of cerebral palsy. *N Engl J Med* 315: 124–126.

Schwartz, P. (1961). *Birth Injuries of the Newborn: Morphology, Pathogenesis, Clinical Pathology and Prevention*. New York: Hafner.

Takashima, S. (1970). Studies on vascular architecture and cerebral vascular diseases of the newborn infants. *Fukuoko Acta Med* 61: 376.

Towbin, A. (1960). *The Pathology of Cerebral Palsy*. Springfield, Ill.: Charles C Thomas.

———— (1968). Cerebral intraventricular hemorrhage and subependymal matrix infarction in the fetus and premature newborn. *Am J Pathol* 52: 121–140.

———— (1970a). Central nervous system damage in the human fetus and newborn. *Am J Dis Child* 119: 529–542.

———— (1970b). Central nervous system damage in the premature related to the occurrence of mental retardation. Pages 213–239 in the *Proceedings of a Conference on Physical Trauma as an Etiological Agent in Mental Retardation* held October 13–16, 1968 at Omaha, Nebraska, by the National Institute of Neurologic Diseases and Stroke.

———— (1977). Trauma in pregnancy: Injury to the fetus and newborn. In Tedeschi, C. G., Eckert, W. G., Tedeschi, L. G., eds., *Forensic Medicine*. Philadelphia: W. B. Saunders. Pp. 436–486.

———— (1986). Obstetric malpractice litigation: The pathologist's view. *Am J Obstet Gynecol* 155: 927–935.

———— (1987). The depressed newborn: pathogenesis and neurologic sequels. *Perinatology Neonatology* 11: 16–18.

———— and G. L. Turner (1978). Obstetric factors in fetal-neonatal visceral injury. *Obstet Gynecol* 52: 113–124.

Vogt, C., and O. Vogt (1920). Zur Lehre der Erkrankungen des striaren Systems. *J Psychol Neurol* 25: 627–846.

Windle, W. F., R. F. Becker, et al. (1944). Alterations in brain structure after asphyxiation at birth. *J Neuropathol* 3: 224–238.

Yakovlev, P. I., and R. K. Rosales (1970). Distribution of the terminal hemorrhages in the brain wall in stillborn prematures and nonviable neonates. In C. R. Angle and E. A. Bering, Jr., eds. *Physical Trauma as an Etiological Agent in Mental Retardation: Proceedings of a Conference on the Etiology of Mental Retardation. Omaha, Nebraska; 1968*. National Institute of Neurological Diseases and Stroke. Washington, D.C.: U.S. Government Printing Office. Pp. 67–78.

Mental Retardation Due to Brain Damage Present in the Newborn

4

Causes of mental retardation

Mental retardation, in a large number of cases, is due to damage to the cerebral cortex, damage incurred during fetal-neonatal life. This form of mental retardation is commonly referred to as organic mental retardation. Considering that there is a host of other causes of mental retardation disorders — chromosome disorders, congenital disorders, metabolic disorders, infectious diseases, trauma — it is not possible to define what percentage of mental retardation is due to organic damage or what percentage is due to various other causes.

Commonly, in cases of mental retardation the defect is coupled with some degree of motor disability characteristic of cerebral palsy, and the diagnosis of psychomotor retardation is applied clinically. At times the retarded child also has a seizure disorder (Chapter 5) or presents a behavior disorder, psychopathy (Chapter 6).

In cases of organic mental retardation, in analyzing the pathogenesis of the underlying damage, it is necessary to take into consideration relevant basic brain anatomy and physiology: In the nervous system there is a direct relationship between structure and function; damage to a specific part of the brain leads to a corresponding specific functional disability. Conversely, the presence of a specific clinical disability reflects the location of the part of the brain that is damaged. For example, the frontal lobe of the cerebrum relates to the function of intellect; damage to the surface (cortex) of the frontal lobe leads to deficient mentation, mental retardation, or to a distortion of mentation, psychopathy, behavior disorders. Damage to the deep structures of the cerebrum, to the basal ganglia, causes cerebral palsy (Chapter 3).

Hypoxia as a cause of mental retardation

In the newborn, damage present in the cerebrum, in most cases, is due to hypoxia, consequent to complications during gestation or delivery, complications that compromised the oxygen supply of the fetus and newborn.

Hypoxic exposure of the fetus and newborn does not cause brain damage indiscriminately through parts of the brain. Location of hypoxic cerebral damage is governed by the gestational age at the time of the hypoxia-producing complication (Figure 10, page 12). In the **premature** fetus or newborn, prior to 35 weeks of gestational age, hypoxia causes damage specifically to deep cerebral structures, to basal ganglia; this leads to cerebral palsy in surviving infants. In the premature fetus and newborn, hypoxic cerebral damage, originating in the deep cerebral structures, at times extends outward to the cerebral cortex, with mental retardation developing superimposed on cerebral palsy in infants surviving (page 17).

In the **mature** fetus and newborn, hypoxia at times causes damage to the cerebral cortex. In the mature fetus and newborn, the hypoxic damage affecting the cerebral cortex does not penetrate to the deep cerebral structures, does not cause cerebral palsy (page 22).

Term infants at times are born harboring cerebral hypoxic damage that is of subacute form, pathologically old, incurred weeks or months before birth, damage that is clinically latent at birth. In surviving infants, the damage becomes chronic pathologically, with the infant clinically developing mental retardation, or other disability, months or years after birth.

In analyzing cases of organic mental retardation, in a child with manifest brain damage, with psychomotor retardation, with mental retardation and cerebral palsy, often the central question is, when was the brain damage incurred? In the prenatal period, weeks or months before birth? At term, during labor and delivery?

In a given case, with a child having both mental retardation and cerebral palsy, it is pertinent to take into account the fact that the presence of cerebral palsy indicates damage to deep cerebral structures, to basal ganglia, damage known to occur specifically in the premature period (page 13); hypoxia at term does not cause deep cerebral damage, does not cause cerebral palsy (Towbin, 1970, 1978; Niswander, 1983; Nelson and Ellenberg, 1986). Accordingly, the presence of cerebral palsy in a child with mental retardation is a **time marker,** dating the time of incurrence of the underlying brain damage in the premature period (page 190).

Mental retardation is usually gauged according to IQ. An IQ of 70 is considered mild, borderline retardation. An IQ of 50 to 70 is considered moderate mental retardation and corresponds to a mental age (MA) of 7 to 10 years. An IQ of 20 to 50 is considered severe retardation, with an MA of 3 to 6 years. Profound mental retardation includes those with an IQ of 0 to 10, with an MA of 0 to 2 years.

It is not the province of the present volume to present all the varied and rare causes of mental retardation. The more common causes will be dealt with here.

Hypoxic brain damage accounts for many, probably most, cases of severe and profound mental retardation, especially cases that also have serious motor disability, cerebral palsy. Cases of profound retardation, characterized by the institutionalized "crib cases," require total, around-the-clock care.

Perinatal hypoxia varies in severity and results, correspondingly, in varied degrees of cerebral damage. The conclusion emerges that a large percent of cases of mild and moderate mental retardation are the consequence of fetal-neonatal hypoxia. There is no way of clinically identifying all these cases; the precise incidence of mild and moderate mental retardation due to fetal-neonatal hypoxia remains undetermined. There is no doubt, however, that this is a very large group, contributing to a large percentage of the mental retardation in the general population.

Chromosome disorders as a cause of mental retardation

In assessing cases of mental retardation, two common forms of chromosome disorder come into consideration: Down syndrome and fragile-X syndrome.

Down syndrome

Down syndrome (trisomy 21) is the most frequently identified chromosome disorder causing mental retardation (page 146). Down syndrome results in a moderate level of retardation in most cases. Down syndrome comprises about 15 percent of cases of retardation found in the population of state institutions for the mentally retarded. The general public, unaware of fetal-neonatal hypoxia as a cause of mental retardation, is led to believe, through television and other media presentations, that Down syndrome is the usual, typical form of mental retardation.

The bodily characteristics, the facial features of Down syndrome are usually evident in the delivery room, with the diagnosis being confirmed by the standard laboratory chromosome studies. Infants with Down syndrome, in addition to having abnormal facial features, usually have other structural abnormalities, involving the skin (the simian line of the hands, a deep transverse palmar crease), the hands, and other skeletal structures. About 40 percent of Down syndrome infants have congenital malformations of the heart.

It is of some importance to note that many persons with Down syndrome live to the age of 50 or more. With aging, the brain in Down syndrome undergoes degenerative changes of Alzheimer's disease; these persons require increasing custodial care (page 146).

Fragile-X syndrome

Fragile-X syndrome (page 148) is a chromosome abnormality associated with mental retardation, usually of mild to moderate degree, and is apparently very common, of high incidence in the general population, estimated to affect 0.1 percent of children. The laboratory diagnosis of the fragile-X defect is complicated and requires a special test procedure, not just the standard chromosome analysis done for Down syndrome cases. If only the standard chromosome analysis is done, and reported as normal, this is not conclusive; the special fragile-X test procedure must be done.

Malformations of the brain causing mental retardation

The term "malformation," applied pathologically, refers to defective development of a body structure, originating in the embryo, resulting in a stunting or distortion of the structure (page 140). The term does not apply to defects of a body structure due to injury, consequent to damage to a fetal structure previously normally formed. For example, it does not apply to encephaloclastic damage to the brain, to breakdown with scarring and cavitation, that occurs following hypoxic damage during fetal life.

Malformations are of two types with regard to cause — genetic and induced.

Genetic malformations

Genetic malformations are inherent defects transmitted through abnormal genes, and at times appear in a familial pattern (page 141).

Induced malformations

Induced malformations are structural defects caused by adversive factors, drugs, infections, or other noxious (teratogenic) agents affecting the fertilized ovum or embryo, compromising orderly development of the embryo (page 141). The noxious intrauterine process, the teratogenic causal agent, is often obscure, undetected, latent.

Malformations of the brain are of great variety, and are usually associated clinically with severe or profound mental retardation.

Microcephaly

Illustrative Case:
Case 102   *p. 484*

Microcephaly, smallness of the head (brain) of an infant, is a factor that often comes to attention during assessment of organic mental retardation. There are two kinds of microcephaly — **microcephaly vera** (primary microcephaly) and **encephaloclastic** (secondary) microcephaly. Microcephaly vera, true microcephaly, refers to a malformation, genetic or induced, in which the brain is small because the organ, from embryonic life on, failed to grow (page 142). Encephaloclastic microcephaly, in contrast, refers to cases in which a small head is due to damage incurred during fetal life, with scarring and cavitation, with consequent failure of the brain to grow. This form of microcephaly is commonly present in children with cerebral palsy (page 188).

Macrocephaly

Illustrative Cases:
Case 230   *p. 729*
Case 233   *p. 734*

This condition refers to an inordinately large size of the brain, associated clinically with mental retardation (page 143).

Hydrocephaly

Illustrative Case:
Case 235   *p. 738*

Hydrocephalus refers to enlargement of the cerebral ventricles. The head, correspondingly, becomes enlarged.

Two forms of hydrocephalus occur:

Obstructive hydrocephalus. In this type of hydrocephalus the ventricular enlargement results from a blockage of the cerebrospinal fluid circulation in the brain (page 156). The blockage is usually due to a narrowing, a stenosis, of the aqueduct through which the cerebrospinal fluid circulates, obstructive hydrocephalus. Pathologically, in many cases the stenosis appears to be a formative defect.

Ex vacuo hydrocephalus. This form of hydrocephalus is due not to a congenital defect but to enlargement of the cerebral ventricles consequent to destruction of deep periventricular cerebral tissue (Figure 26, page 27; Figure 114, page 179). The damaged brain fails to grow; consequently, the head is not enlarged but, paradoxically, often is small, microcephalic. This condition occurs with cerebral palsy and is easily defined with CT scan of the head.

Metabolic disorders

Metabolic disorders in the newborn associated with mental retardation are varied, with over 75 types having been identified. PKU (phenylketonuria) is the most common type; others are rare. Metabolic disorders are inborn, genetically transmitted. PKU is the cause of approximately 2 percent of cases of severe mental retardation. The disorder is presumptively identified at birth by a routine urine spot test. Approximately 1 in 14,000 newborns have a positive test. PKU infants, typically blond and blue-eyed, appear normal at birth. In suspected cases, the diagnosis is confirmed by blood tests that measure the level of phenylalanine in the blood. Treatment with low phenylalanine diets, instituted early, appears to be beneficial in some cases.

Infectious diseases, newborn

Infectious diseases are a significant cause of brain damage present in the newborn, causing sequels of mental retardation and other lasting cerebral disabilities (Remington and Klein, 1983). In the human fetus and newborn, of increasing importance are two infectious processes, *E. coli* bacterial meningitis and cytomegalic viral (CMV) disease (page 116).

Bacterial infection

Bacterial infection of the nervous system, in the form of meningitis (inflammation of the meninges, the membranous coverings of the brain) is reported to occur in 0.4 per 1,000 births, with the causal organism being *E. coli* (*Escherichia coli*) or beta hemolytic streptococcus in approximately 65 percent of cases. The clinical picture is that of sepsis, with lethargy, fever, seizures; bodily stiffness, arching of the back (opisthotonos) is characteristic. An increase in the white cell count of the blood, leucocytosis, occurs. Diagnosis is made by examination of the cerebrospinal fluid, obtained by spinal tap. Often the fluid is frankly cloudy. Laboratory examination of the spinal fluid reveals an increased number of white cells; protein level is elevated; sugar level is decreased. Bacteriologic culture of the spinal fluid and blood (there is usually an accompanying septicemia, a bloodstream infection) is done to identify precisely the causal organism, so that appropriate antibacterial medication can be given. Culture reports of "no growth," must be interpreted with reservation. In newborn babies, especially in small premature infants, often it is difficult to obtain adequate specimen to send to the laboratory for culture; frequently false-negative results are reported.

Pathologically, in meningitis the inflammation in the covering meninges extends to the adjacent brain surface, to the cortex. It is this inflammatory damage of the cortex that precipitates the acute neurologic abnormalities and causes the cortical *sequels of mental retardation, epilepsy, behavior disorders,* and other lasting neurologic disability. In some cases adhesions form between the meninges and the cortical surface, causing interference with cerebrospinal circulation and consequent obstructive hydrocephalus (page 116).

Viral disease

Viral disease is increasingly considered to be of importance as a cause of fetal-neonatal brain damage and as a cause of lasting neurologic disability stemming from birth — second only to hypoxia.

Cytomegalic viral disease (CMV)

Illustrative Cases:
Case 163   *p. 592*
Case 197   *p. 654*
Case 216   *p. 704*

Cytomegalic viral disease is recognized to be the most frequent, most serious, infection affecting the fetus and newborn (page 118). Generally overlooked in years past, CMV is now increasingly diagnosed in neonates. The laboratory diagnosis of CMV by culturing and specifically identifying the virus is difficult. Clinically the diagnosis can be made, with reasonable certainty, on the basis of the syndromic presence of persisting liver and spleen enlargement, hyperbilirubinemia (jaundice), and platelet deficiency, and other hematologic findings; neurologically there is persisting lethargy and weakness. This syndromic pattern is unlike that caused by hypoxia and other fetal-neonatal pathologic processes.

The infection is caused by one of the five known herpes viruses that occur in man. In the pathologic process, the cytomegalic virus-infected cell develops a large red nuclear inclusion, and the nucleus and cytoplasm of the cell become enlarged (*cyto-,* cell; *-megaly,* large). Pathologically, the virus infects the liver, spleen, kidney, brain, and other organs.

The damage to the brain is primarily in the deep periventricular structures (periventricular white matter and basal ganglia) in locations simulating hypoxic damage. The pathologic process is ongoing through the premature and mature periods of fetal life and postnatally. In some cases, calcifications are evident in radiologic studies of the brain. Late clinical sequels consist of microcephaly of varying severity, often with dilated ventricles (ex vacuo hydrocephalus), with manifestations of mental retardation, spastic cerebral palsy, deafness, and ocular disorders.

Cytomegalic viral infection in the fetus is transmitted from the mother. CMV infection in women is of high incidence (50 to 70 percent of pregnant mothers have CMV antibodies serologically) but only in a small percent does the maternal infection become transmitted through the placenta and cause fetal-neonatal infection and organic damage during gestation. CMV infection is asymptomatic during gestation, and the diagnosis is not made prior to delivery. The importance of CMV disease in the newborn was generally overlooked in the past and the diagnosis was missed clinically and pathologically. CMV disease, now considered the most frequent perinatal viral disease, is estimated to involve 8 per 1,000 births and to be responsible for brain damage in 1 per 1,000 births.

The importance of cytomegalic viral disease in obstetric malpractice litigation lies in being able to define retrospectively, with reasonable medical probability, the latent presence of this brain-damaging neonatal disease. Years back, CMV was only of academic research interest, an entity that was unknown to most clinicians (and still is to many). Even though the characteristic hepatosplenic enlargement and other identifying findings of CMV disease were present, were detailed and described in the newborn hospital record, the diagnosis was not thought of, was not applied. In cases brought to litigation five or ten years after birth, as commonly occurs today, cases in which the pathogenesis is enigmatic, cases in which hypoxia as a causal mechanism is open to question — it is important that the hospital record of the newborn infant be carefully analyzed for written evidence of the presence of hepatosplenomegaly and other clinical findings that identify a latent infection of CMV disease.

The occurrence of other viral infections, such as rubella, that cause fetal-neonatal encephalitis is well known; such cases are episodic, rare.

Toxoplasmosis

Infection with *Toxoplasma,* a protozoan parasite, is widespread (page 122). Cases of overt neonatal infection lead to chronic sequels of mental retardation, epilepsy, and other neurologic defects, together with specific defects (chorioretinitis).

Trauma

Obstetric injury was in times past thought to be a common cause of acute brain damage in the newborn, leading to mental retardation and other neurologic disability. However, recent pathology studies have shown that intracranial damage due to physical causes is rare in the present day (Towbin, 1970). In the past it was contended the obstetric forceps caused crushing of the head that led to acute brain damage. Despite the fact that there is no basis pathologically for this contention, this anachronism is still sometimes conveyed by clinicians.

Tumors causing brain damage in the newborn

Illustrative Case:
Case 116 *p. 512*

Neoplastic growths occur in the newborn, rarely; they are usually teratomas (highly malignant cancerous tumors composed of a variety of epithelial and mesodermal elements). Vascular tumors, hemangiomatosis malformations, are progressive neoplastic growths having origin during fetal life, becoming manifest soon after birth. In surviving children, damage to brain structures due to tumor growth results in mental retardation, epilepsy, and other cerebral disabilities.

References and Additional Reading

Crome, L. (1972). *Pathology of Mental Retardation.* Baltimore: Williams and Wilkins.

Nelson, K. B., and J. H. Ellenberg (1986). Antecedents of cerebral palsy. *N Engl J Med* 315: 81–86.

Niswander, K. R. (1983). Labor and operative obstetrics: Asphyxia in the fetus and cerebral palsy. In Pitkin, R. M. and F. J. Zlatnik, eds., *The Year Book of Obstetrics and Gynecology.* Chicago: Year Book Medical Publishers.

Remington, J. S., and J. O. Klein (1983). *Infectious Diseases of the Fetus and Newborn Infant.* Philadelphia: W. B. Saunders.

Towbin, A. (1970). Central nervous system damage in the human fetus and newborn. *Am J Dis Child* 119: 529–542.

———— (1978). Cerebral dysfunctions related to perinatal organic damage: Clinical-neuropathologic correlations. *J Abnorm Psychol* 87: 617–635.

———— (1987). Neuropathologic correlates. In D. E. Tupper, ed., *Soft Neurological Signs.* New York: Grune & Stratton, Inc. Pp. 157–178.

Volpe, E. P. (1971). *Human Heredity and Birth Defects.* New York: Pegasus.

Warkany, J., R. J. Lemire, et al. (1981). *Mental Retardation and Congenital Malformations of the Central Nervous System.* Chicago: Year Book Medical Publishers.

5

Seizure Disorders Due to Cerebral Damage in the Fetus and Newborn

Seizure patterns

Biologic causal factors

Seizures in the newborn; two patterns of seizure onset
    Delayed (late) onset
    Early onset

At times, the first portent of trouble in a newborn, the first sign of brain damage, is the unexpected occurrence of seizures in the postnatal period. The question then arises: When was the brain damage incurred? Intranatally, during labor and delivery? Prenatally, even weeks or months before birth? Or postnatally? The answer lies in the correlation of the clinical and pathologic factors in the case.

Plainly, the occurrence of seizures in a newborn infant does not automatically make it certain that the underlying cerebral damage was incurred during the processes of birth.

Seizure patterns

In the neurologic assessment of an infant, at birth and in later years, specific seizure patterns are referred to clinically. In older infants, and in children and adults with epilepsy, the common types of seizures include:

Tonic-clonic seizures (grand mal) consist of a rapidly recurring series of convulsions, with alternating phases of stiffening of the body (tonic) followed by a period of shaking (clonic), with the convulsions followed by a period of unconsciousness.

Petit mal seizures are episodes of spacing out lasting one to thirty seconds, with loss of motor activity, occurring several times a day; petit mal is common in older infants and children but is not recognized in the newborn.

Status epilepticus is a form of severe epilepsy with seizures, persisting for hours and days, resistant to treatment with anticonvulsant medication.

Newborn infants rarely have organized generalized tonic-clonic seizures. Prematures, especially, have unpatterned forms of seizures. The common forms of seizure activity in newborn infants are characterized as "subtle seizures," consisting variously of repetitive blinking of the eyes, sucking movements of the mouth with drooling, spastic posturing of the trunk and limbs, arching of the back, and bicycling, pedaling motions of the legs. Clonic movements occur, with rhythmic jerking of a limb. At times, seizure activity is preluded by episodes of apnea, "seizure apnea."

Fetal seizures are known to occur. The human fetus may manifest seizure activity during the last part of gestation. This is recognized clinically, with the mother reporting the sudden onset of an episode of fetal hyperactivity followed by a period of loss of fetal activity. EEG studies of the human fetus have been carried out; cases with abnormal fetal EEG findings have been reported with the occurrence of convulsions postnatally in these cases.

Myoclonic seizures, a form appearing in older infants, consist of recurring sudden twitching of muscle groups, jerking movements of an extremity or other part of the body.

Jitteriness is a state of tremulousness, very common in the newborn and is not a seizure disorder. Jitteriness is stimulus sensitive; seizures are not. Jitteriness is essentially a self-limited condition, usually lasting three or four days.

Biologic causal factors in seizure disorders

Seizure disorders are the product of two causal factors: (1) the hereditary factor, the predisposition to the disorder, and (2) the organic factor, brain damage, the presence of an epileptogenic lesion in the cerebral cortex (Scholz and Hager, 1956).

The **hereditary** factor involved in the pathogenesis of epilepsy refers to the intrinsic susceptibility of a person to the disease. Anyone, everyone, can be made to have a seizure, such as a convulsion induced by electric shock. Clinically, however, it is apparent that, given the same circumstances, some individuals will develop seizures while others will not.

The **organic** factor is concerned with seizures brought on by brain damage, by the presence of an epileptogenic lesion. In the newborn, in most cases, this is due to antecedent hypoxic cortical damage.

In neuropathology studies of the brain in cases with seizure disorder, at times the causal lesion is grossly visible; however, often the epileptogenic focus cannot be readily identified, even microscopically. The natural history of neonatal seizure disorder and the subsequent development of chronic epilepsy, follows a syndromic pattern: (1) hypoxia-producing complications during intrauterine life or postnatally result in (2) the imprinting of *acute damage* in the cerebral cortex; this is followed by (3) a *latent* silent interval, without seizures, during which the cerebral lesion may "quiet down" and form scars; the latent period is followed by (4) the *onset of seizures* triggered by exposure to stress.

In adults, in a person with chronic epilepsy, seizures are usually triggered by physical exertion, by mental stress, or by acute illness, such as an infection with fever. In the newborn with brain damage, the seizure-triggering mechanism often is physical, the stress of labor and delivery.

Seizure disorder in the newborn: two patterns of seizure onset

As indicated in Table 5, in the newborn, two patterns of seizure disorder occur with regard to the time of onset. In one group, onset of seizures is delayed for a day or more after birth. In the other group, seizures have their onset early on, during the first day. Of direct importance is the question — was the seizure activity due to **acute** cerebral damage incurred during birth, or was the seizure triggered by an old, **subacute,** cortical lesion incurred during intrauterine life, long before birth?

In analyzing seizures in the newborn, in determining whether the seizure-causing cerebral damage is acute, fresh, incurred during birth, or subacute, old, incurred long before birth, two factors require consideration: (1) **the postnatal clinical performance** of the newborn and, relative to this, (2) **the time interval between birth and the onset** of seizure activity.

Table 5.

Two Patterns of Neonatal Seizures: Delayed-Onset Group Compared to Early-Onset Group

	Delayed onset of seizures	Early onset of seizures
Gestational history	Uncomplicated pregnancy	Pregnancy complications adversive to the fetus; maternal acute and chronic illness; placental disorders
Labor and delivery	Perinatal hypoxia-producing complications	No major hypoxia-producing processes present
Patterns of damage in the cerebrum	Acute cortical hypoxic cerebral damage	Subacute cerebral damage extending from deep structures (basal ganglia) out to the cortex
Fetal monitor record	Abnormal, reflecting acute hypoxic complication	At times abnormal, reflecting intolerance of previously damaged and weakened fetus to the stress of labor
Immediate postdelivery condition	Severe protracted newborn depression; to NICU	Transient newborn depression; improved, stable; to regular nursery
Postnatal course, first day	Prolonged depression; comatose; no seizure activity	Stable after transient depression; active and alert for hours prior to (unexpected) onset of seizures
Seizure onset	Delayed until after 24 hours, until beginning of clinical improvement	Early onset, seizures often within hours after delivery
Hospitalization, duration	Prolonged NICU care; hospitalization for weeks	Relatively brief hospitalization
Late neurologic sequels	Cortical manifestations, mental retardation, epilepsy; no cerebral palsy	Dyskinetic manifestations (basal ganglia) of cerebral palsy; cortical manifestations of mental retardation and seizure disorder

Delayed-onset of neonatal seizures; in newborn infants with acute hypoxic cerebral damage

Acute hypoxic cerebral damage is present in newborn infants consequent to hypoxia-producing complications such as placental abruption or tight nuchal cord or tight umbilical cord knot. If the newborn is mature, at term, the acute hypoxia damages the cerebral cortex. If the newborn is premature, damage occurs in the deep cerebral structures and often extends to the cerebral surface, to the cortex (page 17).

The postnatal performance of an infant with delayed seizures, with *acute* hypoxic cerebral damage incurred during the hours of labor and delivery, is characteristic: The newborn infant is limp, comatose, has a low Apgar score, with a delayed cry, with depressed respiration, cyanosis, congestive heart failure — and the infant remains in this depressed state for days, requiring long intensive care, long hospitalization. Seizures in the affected unresponsive infant in such cases usually are not manifest soon after birth but appear after a latent period, as the baby improves, gradually coming a day or more after delivery. As described by Volpe (1975), in newborn infants with primary hypoxic damage incurred at birth, "At approximately 24 hours of age the infant often becomes less depressed and associated with this change in level of consciousness, seizures usually appear."

Early-onset neonatal seizures; in newborn infants with subacute hypoxic cerebral damage

The infants in this group are born with latent, old, subacute damage, cerebral lesions that are clinically silent. These infants may be depressed at delivery but soon respond and usually are in good condition, stable, alert, and active, in the hours after birth. The postnatal performance of the infants in this group differs from that described in infants that have acute fresh brain damage, infants that remain depressed and comatose for prolonged periods. The clinical course of infants with old subacute cerebral lesions is often compromised by the sudden unexpected onset of seizures, early during the first day.

In these infants, of direct importance is the question — When was the cerebral damage incurred? Was the seizure activity due to *acute* cerebral damage incurred during birth, or was the seizure triggered by an old *subacute* cortical lesion incurred during intrauterine life, long before birth?

It is increasingly realized that at times infants are born harboring subacute, old, cerebral damage that triggers seizures. Subacute cerebral damage is the result of gestational hypoxia-producing complications, affecting the premature, immature, fetus. Maternal, placental, and umbilical cord complications, adversive to the fetus, may come on gradually, beginning weeks or months before delivery, with the compromised fetus surviving, marginally, to term.

The damage, pathologically, is at first of acute nature; if the fetus survives, matures, the cerebral damage becomes subacute ultimately, with the disintegrating tissue forming scars and cavitations.

The actual occurrence of latent subacute cerebral lesions in the newborn, while well known to neonatal neuropathologists, is not generally realized by clinicians, by neonatologists, pediatricians, and neurologists. Accordingly, clinicians are prone to ascribe manifest brain damage in the newborn to an intranatal cause. In this direction, seizures postnatally are usually attributed, often erroneously, to hypoxic cerebral damage having origin during labor and delivery. However, there is increasing clinical opinion that when seizures appear soon after birth, the process is not attributable to an acute intranatal asphyxial brain damage, but rather, the cause must be sought in pathologic processes, brain damage, prior to birth.

Postseizure (postictal) depression. Seizures in the newborn, whether due to acute or to subacute cerebral damage, cause neurologic depression. Seizures in the newborn, as in the adult, have a shocking effect on the body, referred to as the postictal state (*ictus* meaning a blow), causing lethargy, at times coma. With the onset of seizures, the neurologic status of the infant tends to deteriorate.

Medication-sedation depression. In treatment of the seizure, the neurologic status of the infant is, necessarily, further depressed by the medication. In order to control the seizure activity, phenobarbital is administered — medication that depresses the neurologic status of the infant. Clinicians commonly overlook the depression-producing effects of phenobarbital given to newborn infants and mistakenly ascribe the infant's lethargy to intranatal hypoxic damage. However, subsequently, after the seizures are controlled and the phenobarbital level is reduced, the infant improves, becoming more active and alert.

References and Additional Reading

Keegan, K. A., Jr., F. Waffarn, and E. J. Quilligan (1985). Obstetric characteristics and fetal heart rate patterns of infants who convulse during the newborn period. *Am J Obstet Gynecol* 153(7): 732–737.

Legido, A., R. R. Clancy, and P. H. Berman (1991). Neurologic outcome after electroencephalographically proven neonatal seizures. *Pediatrics* 88(3): 583–596.

Levine S. C., P. Huttenlocher, M.T. Banich, and E. Duda (1987). Factors affecting cognitive function of hemiplegic children. *Dev Med Child Neurol* 29: 27–35.

Scholz, W., and H. Hager (1956). Epilepsy. *Handbuch des Speziellen Pathologischen Anatomie und Histologie: Nervensystem.* Berlin: Springer-Verlag.

Vargha-Khadem, F., E. Isaacs, et al. (1992). Development of intelligence and memory in children with hemiplegic cerebral palsy: The deleterious consequences of early seizures. *Brain* 116: 315–329.

Volpe, J. J. (1975). Neurologic disorders. In G. B. Avery, ed., *Neonatology.* Philadelphia: J. B. Lippincott. Page 754.

Psychopathy: Behavior Disorders Related to Fetal-Neonatal Brain Damage

6

Illustrative Cases:
Case 105   *p. 490*
Case 148   *p. 570*

In the clinical assessment of a manifestly brain-damaged child, in some cases the history and the neurologic and psychologic evaluation of the child indicate the presence of behavior problems varying in type and severity. The psychologic problem may be severe, of the nature of autism (profound withdrawal from social contact), or one of lesser degree, in the nature of "minimal brain dysfunction," with hyperactivity, inattention, and bizarre behavior (Chapter 7). The link between brain damage and consequent cerebral dysfunction — loss of intellect and psychiatric disorders — is well documented in clinical and neuropathologic studies, as in the development of major psychoses in children after recovery from encephalitis and in cases of chronically brain-traumatized "punch-drunk" veteran prize fighters.

In the field of pathology, in the study of disease mechanisms, there is an axiom: An organ damaged by a pathologic process can manifest two types of handicap — **reduction** of function and/or **distortion** of function. Applied here, with reference to the brain, damage to the cortex of the frontal lobes of the cerebrum causes reduction of intellectual function, mental retardation, and, at times, distortion of intellectual function, psychopathy — both disabilities stemming from the same pathologic process.

Cerebral damage in the newborn leads to four main chronic neurologic disabilities — the tetralogy of cerebral palsy, epilepsy, mental retardation, and psychopathy. The underlying cause of the cerebral damage in most of these cases is fetal-neonatal hypoxia, less often, infectious disease (Chapter 1). An affected child may have one or more of these four major cerebral disabilities. At times, as the child grows older, the main disability takes the form of a behavior problem. The combination of mental retardation and psychopathy is of frequent occurrence. Over 20 percent of retardates have significant psychiatric disturbances (Towbin, 1989); clinically, the term "dual diagnosis" is commonly applied to cases with mental retardation and psychiatric disturbance.

Many clinical and pathological studies have underscored the relationship between gestational complications and the subsequent development of behavior disorders in children (Strauss and Lehtinen, 1947; Pasamanick, Rogers, and Lilienfeld, 1956; Bender and Faretra, 1961; Taft and Goldfarb, 1964; Whittam, Simon, and Mittler, 1966; Torrey, Hersh, and McCabe, 1975; Towbin, 1978, 1989).

In children who develop behavior disorders consequent to brain damage present at birth, the clinical record, the developmental history, is characteristic. The mother usually reports that the infant does not nurse well, does not sleep well, is a "whiny baby," and later is described as a nervous child. Problems are precipitated in the early school years, commonly with reports of impulsiveness, tantrums, hyperactivity, and varied deviant behavior.

Neurologic examination commonly reveals a constellation of minor nervous system abnormalities, *soft signs* — abnormal reflexes, defects in balance, in motor and sensory function, abnormal EEG, abnormal CT scans of the brain (Towbin, 1987). Very often these neurologic findings, as well as positive findings in the psychometric assessments, such as the Bender-Gestalt and the Halstead-Reitan test battery, present evidence of organicity, meaning that the manifest cerebral abnormalities are due to structural defects in the brain, to brain damage.

In neuropathologic studies, the link between fetal-neonatal hypoxic cerebral damage and the development of mental retardation, psychopathy, and other developmental disabilities is demonstrated in transitional forms of brain damage, by relating anatomically acute cerebral lesions in the newborn to analogous subacute lesions in infants with neurologic manifestations that live for a brief period and in turn relating these subacute patterns of damage to old chronic scar lesions found in brain specimens in cases of mental retardation, psychopathy, and other cerebral disabilities (Towbin, 1978).

The following is an example of a major psychotic disability that occurred in a case with a clinical history of a complicated delivery. Pregnancy was at term; after prolonged labor, cesarean section was resorted to. The mother noted no abnormalities during infancy, but during the early school years, the child was described as "nervous" by her teachers; she was withdrawn from regular school because of emotional disturbances. She had difficulty in learning to read and was considered moderately retarded. She developed increasing personality changes, with periods of fantasy and delusions, and was institutionalized at 18 years of age with a diagnosis of schizophrenia. Physical examination revealed slight spasticity of the left extremities, with hyperactive reflexes. She remained institutionalized; death occurred at age 42. Neuropathologic study of the brain revealed cerebral cortical scarring (Figure 116), a lesion consistent with damage incurred at birth.

Figure 116. Major psychosis in a case with a history of complicated birth; birth by cesarean section after prolonged labor. The right frontal lobe of the cerebrum shows circumscribed old scarred infarctional lesion, a depressed area of contracted distorted convolutions near the midline, a lesion consistent pathologically with damage incurred at birth.

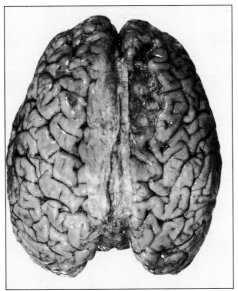

Fig. 116

With regard to the correlation of clinical and pathologic details presented in this case, certainly this is an unusual example. In such case studies of cerebral disability stemming from birth, the effort in the pathology laboratory to identify a causal lesion, in many, if not most cases, is not fruitful, probably mainly due to technical limitations.

It merits note that structural abnormalities of the brain, cases of malformation, chromosome disorders, in some instances are clinically marked by psychiatric behavior. Down syndrome, in cases reaching advanced age, commonly develop psychiatric manifestations of Alzheimer's disease (Case 223, page 719).

As is evident in clinical practice, psychiatric disorders have many causal factors, with organic processes, cerebral damage, being but one — and, in a cross-sectional sense, its incidence and significance are problematic. The relationship between a complicated gestation and birth and the subsequent development of a behavior disorder in a child may be significant; however, in a given case, the possible cause-and-effect relationship needs to be viewed with reservation.

References and Additional Reading

Bender, L., and G. Faretra (1961). Pregnancy and birth histories of children with psychiatric problems. *Proceedings of the Third World Congress of Psychiatry* 2: 1329–1333.

Craft, M. (1969). Mental disorder in the defective: A psychiatric survey among in-patients. *Am J Ment Defic* 63: 829–834.

Pasamanick, B., M. E. Rogers, and A. M. Lilienfeld (1956). Pregnancy experience and the development of behavior disorder in children. *Am J Psychiatry* 112: 613–618.

Strauss, A. A., and L. A. Lehtinen (1947). *Psychopathology and Education of the Brain-Injured Child.* New York: Grune & Stratton.

Taft, L. T., and W. Goldfarb (1964). Prenatal and perinatal factors in childhood schizophrenia. *Dev Med Child Neurol* 6: 32–43.

Torrey, E. F., S. P. Hersh, and K. D. McCabe (1975). Early childhood psychosis and bleeding during pregnancy. *J Autism Dev Disord* 5: 287–297.

Towbin, A. (1971). Organic causes of minimal brain dysfunction: Perinatal origin of minimal cerebral lesions. *JAMA* 217: 1207–1214.

——— (1978). Cerebral dysfunctions related to perinatal organic damage: Clinical-neuropathologic correlations. *J Abnorm Psychol* 87: 617–635.

——— (1987). Neuropathologic correlates. In D. E. Tupper, ed., *Soft Neurological Signs.* New York: Grune & Stratton, Inc. Pp. 157–178.

——— (1989). Behavior disorders of mentally retarded persons, the dually diagnosed: Factors of pathogenesis. *J Clin Psychol* 45: 910–918.

Whittam, H., G. B. Simon, and P. J. Mitler (1966). The early development of psychotic children and their siblings. *Dev Med Child Neurol* 8: 552–560.

Minimal Brain Dysfunction Due to Brain Damage in the Fetus and Newborn

7

Premature brain: minimal hypoxic damage

Mature brain: minimal hypoxic damage

The syndrome of minimal brain dysfunction describes the large group of infants, children, and adolescents within our population who have behavioral disorders often accompanied by learning defects, reading inability, hyperactivity, and motor disturbances described as inordinate awkwardness, or abnormal neurologic findings and electroencephalograph irregularities. Many individuals with the diagnosis of attention deficit disorder (ADD), slow learners, often with behavioral problems, are really people with minimal brain damage. Individually, in affected children, the syndrome is of vexing importance. Characteristically, with the disorder making its appearance in the classroom, concern is transmitted in an all-too-familiar sequence from the teacher to the parent, to the family doctor, to the specialist, the psychiatrist, and the social worker. The course of the condition in many instances remains intractable (Clements, 1966; Connors, 1967; Towbin, 1971).

Minimal brain dysfunction is estimated to affect over 3 million children in this country.

In a major portion of cases, it is evident that minimal brain dysfunction is known to be due to hypoxic brain damage incurred during fetal life or postnatally.

A host of other conditions affecting the neonatal central nervous system — genetic, metabolic, infectious, and toxic agents — are thought to contribute to the occurrence of minimal brain dysfunction, and, although much less frequent, these causal factors often claim broader emphasis than do the effects of hypoxia, the process that underlies the bulk of neonatal neuropathologic case material.

Mechanical injury, in addition to hypoxic damage, occurs in the fetus, present in the newborn. Spinal cord and brain stem damage of varying severity occurs (page 134). Sublethal minimal spinal cord injury, in infants surviving, results in minor neurologic disability. Children with such disability, with this form of minimal neurologic dysfunction, are sometimes mistakenly considered to have "mild cerebral palsy" or are regarded as "clumsy children" (Ford, 1966).

Although all the structures of the body are vulnerable to hypoxic injury during gestation and delivery, the most sensitive target proves to be the brain. Hypoxic brain damage is imprinted in the fetus and newborn when complications occur during pregnancy and delivery (page 105). Complications due to maternal illness, placental disorders, umbilical cord entanglements with compression exercise their damaging effects through the common denominator of fetal-neonatal oxygen deprivation, hypoxia. Postnatally, in the newborn, hypoxia is often due to antecedent brain damage, damage that compromises respiratory function. Apnea, episodic arrest of respiration, is particularly common in the premature infant. Cerebral hypoxic damage in the newborn at times is due to pulmonary complications, to respiratory distress syndrome (hyaline membrane disease), pneumonia, or pneumothorax.

Hypoxic injury in the fetus and newborn is not an all-or-none process. Acute cerebral lesions present at birth are of a wide range of severity. Anatomic-pathologic studies of the brain in fetuses and infants dying in the postnatal period demonstrate that damage to the brain ranges from diffuse damage to minor focal lesions. Hypoxic complications during pregnancy and delivery vary in degree and duration. Severe, unremitting hypoxia leads to fetal or neonatal death. With less severe episodes of hypoxia, brain damage of a lesser extent occurs and the fetus may survive, harboring subacute, old, "healed" lesions in the brain (page 24).

Minimal cerebral damage, changes of minor severity, are commonly evident pathologically in the newborn. Clinically, however, the occurrence in the newborn of subclinical minimal cerebral damage and the subsequent minor dysfunction in children is not widely recognized.

What is the pathogenesis of hypoxic cerebral damage, the step-by-step bodily changes that occur from the onset of oxygen deprivation to the time that acute damage is imprinted in the brain? Hypoxia leads to a consistent sequence of bodily changes in consecutive stages, with each stage precipitating the next (Table 1, page 7). Hypoxia causes weakening of the heart muscle, myocardial fatigue, with resulting "backward" heart failure. Backward heart failure results in blood being dammed back in the venous system of the body. Venous stasis with thrombosis occurs. Venous thrombosis leads to infarctional damage, focal and diffuse, devitalization of cerebral tissue with hemorrhage. Pathologically, the lesion may be massive, analogous to stroke damage in the adult. More often the lesions are circumscribed, small.

Two basic patterns of hypoxic cerebral damage occur in the human fetus and newborn (Figure 117): In the **premature** fetus and newborn, prior to 35 weeks' gestation, hypoxic damage occurs primarily in the deep periventricular strata of the cerebrum, affecting the deep layers of white matter and adjoining basal ganglia. In the **mature** fetus and newborn, the primary target for hypoxic damage is the cerebral cortex. The localization of cerebral damage, deep in the premature, cortical at term, is not a random occurrence but is based on specific biologic factors (page 14). The main determining factor is the presence or absence of germinal matrix tissue.

Figure 117. Two basic patterns of hypoxic cerebral damage, related to gestational age. In the premature, damage originates in the deep cerebral strata; infants surviving develop manifestations of cerebral palsy. At term, in the mature cerebrum, damage is limited to the cortex; infants surviving develop cortical disabilities of mental retardation and epilepsy.

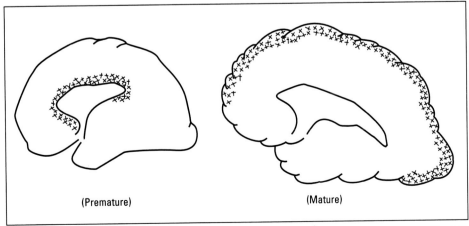

(Premature)   (Mature)

Fig. 117

Premature brain: minimal hypoxic damage

Minimal hypoxic cerebral damage of two forms appears in the premature, deep damage affecting the germinal matrix, and periventricular leucomalacia (Figures 118a and b).

Deep cerebral damage. In the premature brain in the deep periventricular stratum of the cerebrum there are thick deposits of embryonic tissue, germinal matrix, bulging into the ventricles (page 14). The deposits of germinal matrix are depots of "building material," required for future formation of the basal ganglia and other deep neuronal assemblies and for the development of the cerebral cortex. The germinal matrix tissue gradually is used up as the brain matures, and is almost gone in the mature brain.

The matrix tissue, soft and friable, is manifestly vulnerable to hypoxia and readily undergoes infarctional disintegration. Damage in the germinal matrix spreads by adjacency to the neighboring basal ganglia and white matter.

Minimal forms of deep cerebral damage begin in the premature cerebrum as small focal areas of devastation in the deep deposits of germinal matrix (Figure 118a); on the right, the germinal matrix (the thick dark pad of tissue bulging from the inner aspect of the hemispheric wall into the ventricular space) shows a pale, longitudinal patch of necrosis, infarctional damage, with a minute thrombus-filled vein at its center.

Figure 118a. Minimal hypoxic cerebral damage, premature infant. Cerebrum showing persisting germinal matrix tissue; the pad-like germinal deposits are deeply located, attached to the inner surface of the hemispheric walls, and bulge into the lower lateral portion of the ventricle space on each side. Matrix deposits show minimal hypoxic infarctional lesions, more pronounced on the right, appearing as irregular, pale patches of necrosis; thromboses in small veins in the matrix. History of spontaneous delivery at 32 weeks' gestation due to premature detachment of the placenta; infant lived 2 days. Autopsy revealed infarctional damage in other organs in addition to the brain.

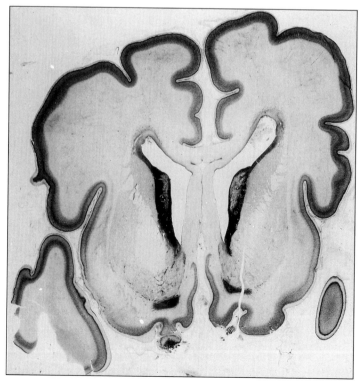

Fig. 118a

Periventricular leucomalacia (page 18). In the premature brain, in addition to lesions in the matrix deposits, small areas of necrosis may appear in the deep white matter around the ventricles, focal periventricular leucomalacia (*leuco-*, white; *-malacia*, softness), in the nature of microinfarcts (Figure 118b) (Banker and Larroche, 1962).

Figure 118b. Periventricular leucomalacia, appearing as focal lesions, cloud-like islands of necrosis in the cerebral white matter. Premature birth at 34 weeks of gestation.

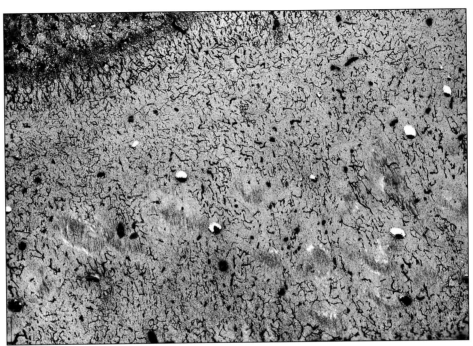

Fig. 118(b)

Minimal hypoxic lesions in the deep cerebral structures are of frequent occurrence in the premature, being evident at autopsy almost universally in infants at 7 months' gestation. In laboratory studies in the Collaborative Perinatal Project, in postmortem examination of 140 premature newborn infants of 22 to 35 weeks' gestation, deep cerebral infarctional damage of severe to moderate degree was present in 48 percent of the cases (Towbin, 1970). Significantly, in the other 52 percent of cases, acute hypoxic changes of minimal form were present, often with the lesions scattered diffusely through the germinal matrix and adjoining tissue.

The natural growth and development of the fetal brain requires that the germinal matrix tissue be adequate and undamaged. Hypoxic damage in the germinal matrix and deep white matter, even though the lesions appear minute, imposes an irrevocable loss of *anlage* "building material" and an erosion of maturing tissue, creating a lasting handicap. These small acute infarcts are the precursors of subacute and chronic lesions.

Mature brain: minimal hypoxic damage

During fetal life, as the brain matures and the germinal matrix decreases, the cerebral cortex becomes the target for hypoxic damage, resulting in damage of varying pattern and severity.

Cortical damage of minimal nature occurring in the term fetus and neonate is commonly of cellular order, with varying number of cells injured and eliminated. The cortex becomes punctuated by shrunken, deeply staining neurones that appear singly or in clusters, as demonstrated in Figure 119.

Figure 119. Minimal hypoxic neuronal damage; histologic section of cortex. In the upper part of the illustration, shrunken, darkened, damaged neurones with obliteration of fine intracellular architecture. In contrast, below, are intact neurones with preserved intracellular detail, with nuclei and nucleoli.

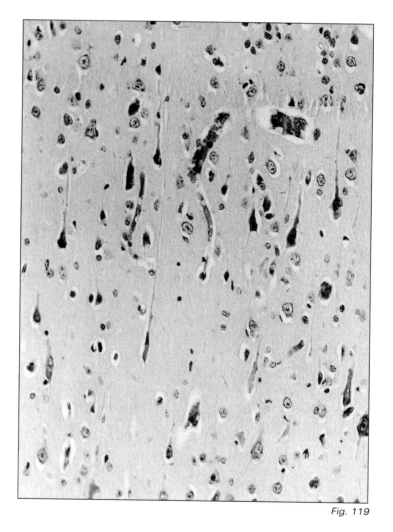

Fig. 119

In the term fetus and neonate, with exposure to hypoxia protracted, the cortex may develop focal, patchy devastation (Figure 120). In infants surviving, the small islands of damaged cortical tissue are repaired by gliosis, with resulting focal areas of surface scarring and contraction. Such hypoxic lesions may lead to functional central nervous system disturbances manifest in later years.

Figure 120. Focal cortical hypoxic cerebral damage; section through frontal lobe convolutions. Cortex well differentiated, with well-defined laminar architecture (term gestation). In the middle portion of the illustration the cortex shows patchy confluent pale areas of hypoxic infarctional necrosis. Mature stillborn infant; severe intrauterine hypoxia with fetal death prior to onset of labor, due to retroplacental hemorrhage (premature detachment of placenta from uterine wall).

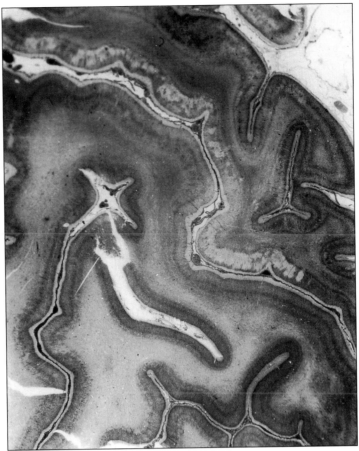

Fig. 120

In infants with perinatal injury that survive, with sublethal cerebral damage, the acute lesions, whether minor or extensive, gradually "quiet down," become **subacute,** old, and ultimately undergo healing, leaving scars and cavitations.

It is a basic axiom in pathology that when an organ is damaged, the severity of the damage determines the degree of the consequent functional defect manifested. In the newborn, as in the adult, and as in the laboratory in experimental animals, there is essentially a direct correlation between the degree of brain damage present and the severity of the resulting functional disability. Massive lesions in the brain generally cause major loss of function. Lesser lesions, "small bites," cause lesser signs and symptoms. Small lesions, depending on their location, may be occult, latent, clinically silent; in other instances, small lesions manifest their presence by evoking minor neurologic abnormalities, "soft signs" (Towbin, 1987). The conclusion is inescapable: Minor lesions (minimal cerebral damage present in the newborn) contribute to the occurrence of sequelant minor functional disability, to manifestations of minimal brain dysfunctions.

Fetal and neonatal damage results not only in the reduction of cerebral nervous system function but also in the distortion of such function. Clinically, in addition to the three commonly recognized sequels of neonatal brain damage — mental retardation, cerebral palsy, and epilepsy — attention is being focused on a fourth, behavioral disorders in children with history of prematurity or other neonatal complications.

Variability of the clinical pattern of minimal brain dysfunction in children can be correlated pathologically with the diversity in distribution of damage that occurs in the newborn brain. In the fetus and newborn, all portions of the brain are vulnerable to injury, with some parts being biologically more susceptible than others, with the site of the injury varying with gestational age. As in the adult, and as observed in the laboratory in experimental animals, the clinical abnormalities that develop following brain damage in the newborn depend on the specific *location* of the lesions in the brain. Perinatal damage to the cerebrum in the precentral region leads to motor defects; lesions in the frontal lobe are related to disorders of mentation; lesions at other sites result in corresponding defects in sensory or other functions and at times to manifestations of epilepsy.

Latency in the occurrence of clinical symptoms is common with brain damage in adults, with the outward effects being obscured, delayed, often surfacing months or years after the time of the brain injury. Analogously, brain damage present in the newborn may remain latent, silent, for years, with neurologic signs and symptoms appearing later in childhood and adolescence as manifestations of minimal brain dysfunction.

Clinically, the latent occult effects of minimal cerebral damage aren't generally realized. When cerebral damage occurs, loss of neurologic function may be transient, to a greater or lesser degree. With acute cerebral damage, with the center of the lesion devitalized and the surrounding margin of tissue compromised by edema and inflammation, loss of function is maximum. With survival, the devitalized center, being unable to regenerate, becomes contracted and scarred. In the periphery of the lesion, the pathologic changes are largely reversible, so that, in time, much of the function returns. Commonly, the effects of such damage, small lesions that are minimized and sublimated, may become neurologically undemonstrative. This does not erase their presence, their significance. *Return of function may be considered "within normal limits," but this does not take into account the subtle loss of versatility and acumen previously possessed, prior to the cerebral damage.*

Gestation and birth form an inexorable leveling mechanism; with the brain marred at birth, the potential of performance may be reduced from that of a genius to that of a plain child, or less. The damage may be slight, imperceptible clinically, or it may spell the difference between brothers, one a dexterous athlete and the other "an awkward child."

Substantially, it is said, all of us have a touch of mental retardation, cerebral palsy, or other blight — some more, some less — the endowment pathologically of gestation and birth. The full significance of neonatal brain damage, the broad impact of its late effects, its influence not only on the newborn and the young but also on adult neuropsychiatric mechanisms, has not yet been fully explored. In studies of older children and young adults with behavioral disturbances, dropouts and delinquents, observers have pointed out the high incidence of prematurity and other perinatal complications and the presence of "organicity," neurologic indications of residual cerebral damage in these older individuals. It is evident that adults, even in later years, may continue to manifest cerebral dysfunction due to remote cerebral scars, lesions incurred in the fetal-neonatal period.

References and Additional Reading

Banker, B. Q., and J. C. Larroche (1962). Periventricular leucomalacia of infancy. *Arch Neurol* 7: 386–410.

Clements, S. D. (1966). *Minimal Brain Dysfunction in Children, National Institute of Neurological Diseases and Stroke monograph 3.* Public Health Service publication 1415.

Connors, C. K. (1967). The syndrome of minimal brain dysfunction: Psychological aspects. *Pediatr Clin North Am* 14: 749–766.

Denhoff, E. (1965). Bridges to burn and build. *Dev Med Child Neurol* 7: 3–8.

Ford, F. R. (1966). *Diseases of the Nervous System in Infancy, Childhood, and Adolescence.* Springfield, Ill.: Charles C. Thomas.

Pasamanick, B., and A. M. Lilienfeld (1955). Association of maternal and fetal factors with development of mental deficiency. 1. Abnormalities in the prenatal and paranatal periods. *JAMA* 159: 155–160.

Rosen, E. J. (1969). Behavioral and emotional disturbances associated with cerebral dysfunction. *Appl Ther* 11: 531–543.

Towbin, A. (1969). Mental retardation due to germinal matrix infarction. *Science* 164: 156–161.

——— (1970). Central nervous system damage in the fetus and newborn. *Am J Dis Child* 119: 529–542.

——— (1971). Organic causes of minimal brain dysfunction: Perinatal origin of minimal cerebral lesions. *JAMA* 217: 1207–1214.

——— (1978). Cerebral dysfunctions related to perinatal organic damage: Clinical-neuropathologic correlations. *J Abnorm Psychol* 87: 617–635.

——— (1987). Neuropathologic correlates. In D. E. Tupper, ed., *Soft Neurological Signs.* New York: Grune & Stratton, Inc. Pp. 157–178.

——— (1989). Behavior disorders of mentally retarded persons, the dually diagnosed: Factors of pathogenesis. *J Clin Psychol* 45: 910–918.

Case Studies

A Case of **_Massive asymmetrical periventricular cerebral hemorrhagic infarction in a 1-day-old infant prematurely born at 35 weeks of gestation._**

Premature rupture of membranes occurred and spontaneous labor developed. The mother was diabetic. The infant appeared edematous at birth and was in respiratory distress; toward the end of the first day he showed sudden rapid deterioration, became unresponsive, and died. Necropsy revealed congestive heart failure with congestion of the liver, spleen, and kidneys; hyaline membrane disease of the lung was present; the pancreas showed islet hyperplasia. The brain showed prominent congestion of the superficial veins.

The brain specimen showed asymmetrical massive hemorrhagic infarctional damage of the deep structures of the cerebrum (Figure 121). On the left, hemorrhagic infarction extended through the wall of the cerebral hemisphere. The germinal matrix on both sides also showed hemorrhagic infarction. Within the hemorrhagic debris lining the ventricle, dilated veins with thromboses were evident (page 11).

Significantly, in this case the zone of necrosis in the cerebral wall was more extensive than the area of hemorrhage, indicating that the primary nature of the lesion was infarctional, and the hemorrhagic suffusion secondary. Leakage of blood into the lateral ventricle, intraventricular hemorrhage, was also present.

Periventricular infarction in the fetus and newborn is essentially a bilateral process, generally affecting both sides about equally. At times, however, the damage appears mainly on one side, as in this case. Infants surviving, correspondingly, have disability mainly on one side and are usually diagnosed as hemiplegic cerebral palsy.

Figure 121. Massive asymmetrical periventricular hemorrhagic infarction of the cerebrum. Frontal whole-brain section showing an extensive hemorrhagic infarction of the periventricular white matter on the left and also hemorrhagic infarction of the germinal matrix deposits on both sides. The necrosis of the hemispheric wall on the left extends beyond the hemorrhagic zone, out to the surface of the cerebrum. Hemorrhage extends inward from the deep infarction into the ventricle, intraventricular hemorrhage.

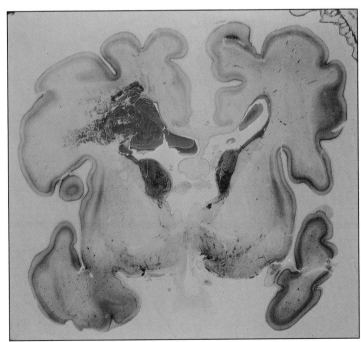

Fig. 121

A Case of   *Minimal periventricular (germinal matrix) hemorrhagic infarction in a premature infant of 32 weeks' gestation who lived 2 days.*

The infant in this case, of 32 weeks' gestation, weighed 3 pounds 4 ounces and lived 2 days. The placenta showed evidence of premature separation. Terminally, the infant developed respiratory complications, of both central and peripheral nature. The autopsy revealed visceral congestion and multiple thrombotic and embolic vascular occlusions; the portal vein contained a thrombus, and the entire small intestine was infarcted. The superficial cerebral veins were moderately congested. Pulmonary embolism was found. Hyaline membrane disease was evident histologically.

Histologic section of the cerebrum through the frontal region (Figure 122a) shows a mound of deeply staining matrix tissue on the lower lateral aspect of each ventricle. Within the matrix are patches of pale necrotic tissue — areas of hemorrhagic infarction (page 14; page 220). Veins in the matrix are distended, contain thromboses (Figure 122b).

Figure 122(a). Small hemorrhagic infarcts in the periventricular germinal matrix tissue. The germinal matrix, blue-staining deposits at the lower lateral aspect of the ventricles, show tan hemorrhagic patches of infarcted tissue. Infant of 32 weeks' gestation; lived 2 days.

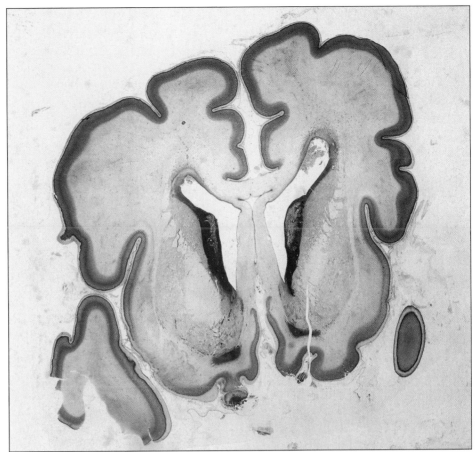

Fig. 122(a)

Figure 122(b). Higher magnification of the periventricular portions of the cerebrum. In the areas of germinal matrix infarctional devastation, small veins are evident, distended with thrombus material.

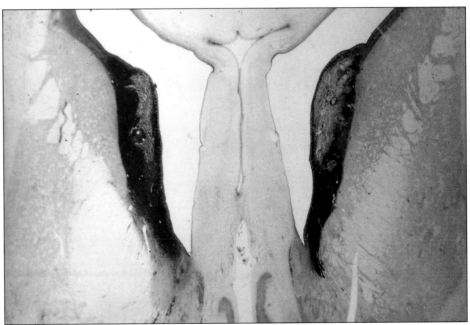

(b)

A Case of   *Periventricular hemorrhagic infarction in a premature infant.*

The infant, born at 35 weeks of gestation, suddenly developed respiratory distress and stopped breathing.

At autopsy the cerebral ventricles showed periventricular hemorrhagic infarctional necrosis (page 15). The ventricles were filled with blood (Figure 123).

Correlating the clinical and pathologic facets in this case: Premature infants often are born harboring periventricular infarcts under the lining of the ventricles in the germinal matrix and neighboring white matter, lesions that are clinically silent, latent; affected infants at first appear in good condition. In such circumstances, in some cases, the infarcts become suffused, distended, with blood; blood ruptures through the lining of the ventricles, creating massive intraventricular hemorrhage. As in this case, the affected infant, previously in good condition, precipitously decompensated, became apneic and died.

Figure 123. Periventricular hemorrhagic infarctional necrosis. Premature brain; midfrontal section through the brain specimen. The ventricles are lined with ragged bloody necrotic tissue. At autopsy, blood filled the cerebral lateral ventricles and extended into the third ventricle.

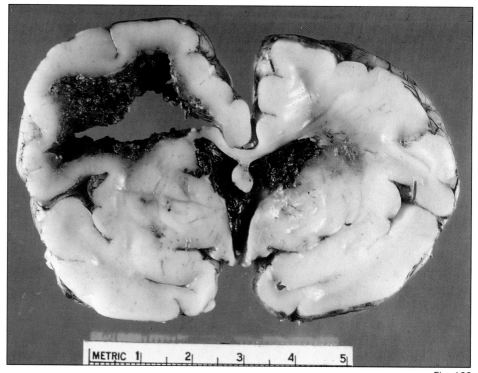

Fig. 123

A Case of   *Premature placental detachment; breech birth; liver injury and intracranial injury, subdural hemorrhage.*

With the pregnancy at 24 weeks, vaginal bleeding and uterine contractions developed. The fetal heart was audible early in labor. With rupture of the membranes, bloody amniotic fluid escaped. Full breech presentation was present. Birth was vaginal with breech extraction. Intrauterine death had occurred during labor.

At delivery, premature placental detachment was evident, with a large retroplacental hemorrhage present.

The placenta (Figure 124) showed extensive adherent retroplacental hematoma accumulation, some brown and leathery, old. A portion of the placental plate was thinned, compressed, by retroplacental hematoma deposits that became detached during delivery of the placenta (page 66).

The placenta showed focal infarction (Figure 125). Pathologically, there is a link between placental infarction and retroplacental hemorrhage; retroplacental hemorrhage at times is due to bleeding that originates in necrotic infarcted placental tissue (page 71).

The stillborn infant was cyanotic (Figure 124). The head appeared large and was rounded; with breech birth, with the buttock of the fetus advancing foremost, dilating the rigid birth canal, the aftercoming head remains rounded, is not subjected to molding.

The body of the infant showed the effects of the full breech presentation (Figure 126). The buttocks, the part of the body foremost in the descent of the fetus through the birth canal, showed severe edema and reddening, changes analogous to the formation of a caput succedaneum in a cephalic birth (page 128).

At autopsy, the liver showed a large subcapsular bleb (Figure 127); under the bleb was a laceration of the liver, a crush injury. The liver damage is attributable to compression of the abdomen by the fetus' flexed lower extremities, occurring as the fetus was propelled through the tight birth canal (page 102). The abdomen showed hemoperitoneum (Figure 127); blood had escaped from the liver injury into the abdomen (Figure 128).

The large unmolded aftercoming head (like the abdomen, compressed during labor) showed intracranial damage, subdural hemorrhage (Figure 129). The falx was torn from its attachment anteriorly and adjoining dural veins were torn, with consequent subdural hemorrhage over the cerebrum (page 134).

The cerebellar hemispheres showed surface lacerations and subarachnoid hemorrhage (Figure 130).

Figure 124. The newborn infant and placenta with retroplacental hemorrhage. The maternal surface of the placenta shows adherent deposits of red gelatinous blood clot, recent retroplacental hematoma, evident over the lower third of the surface; some portions of the hematoma were leathery and brown, pathologically indicating that this part of the retroplacental hematoma was old, chronic, had developed weeks before labor. The surface of the placenta in the upper right third shows a broad crater-like thinning of the placental mass caused by compression of the spongy placental plate by retroplacental hemorrhage, hematoma deposit previously present, loosened during delivery of the placenta. The stillborn infant was cyanotic. The proportionately large head was round, not molded, being an aftercoming head in a breech delivery.

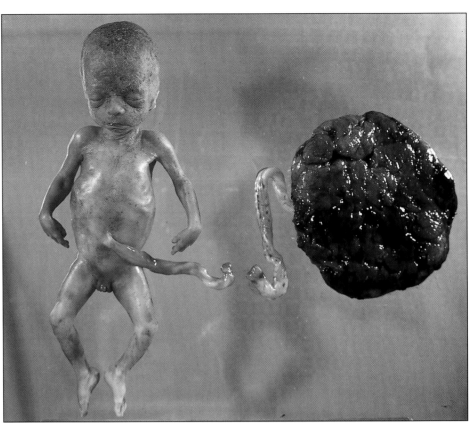

Fig. 124

Figure 125. Placental infarct. A section through the thin portion of the placenta; circumscribed and confluent pale areas of devitalized infarcted tissue.

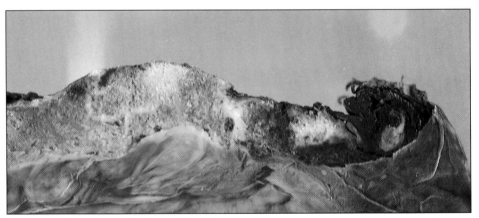

Fig. 125

Figure 126. Frank breech presentation. The illustration indicates hyperflexed position of the fetus in this case during delivery. The buttocks, the part of the fetus advancing foremost down the birth canal, wedging its way through the rigid cervix, became red and edematous. The flexed lower extremities, squeezed against the abdomen by lateral compression exerted on the fetus in its passage down the birth canal, caused damage to the liver in this case (Figure 127).

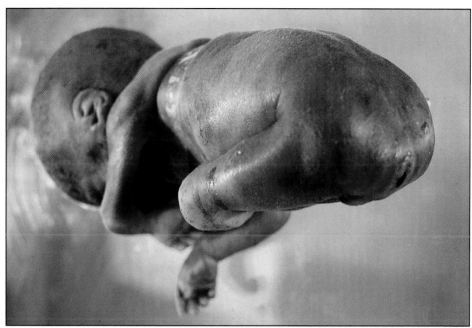

Fig. 126

Figure 127. Compression laceration of the liver with bleb formation. (As shown, the liver at autopsy brought forward to expose the liver damage.)

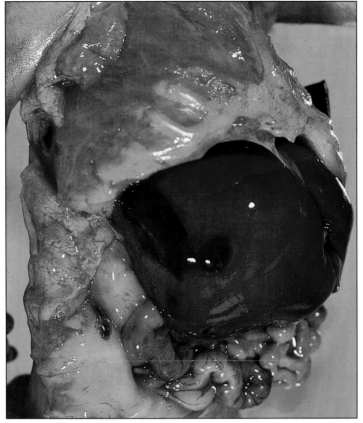

Fig. 127

Figure 128. Hemoperitoneum. Blood oozing from the liver laceration, from the subcapsular bleb, with copious free blood in the abdomen.

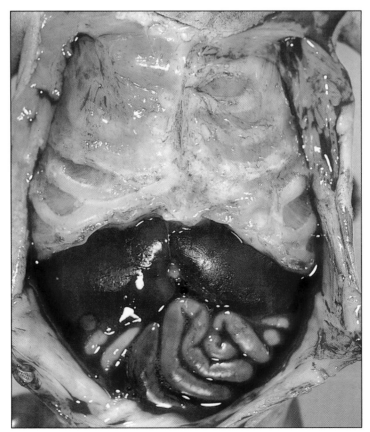

Fig. 128

Figure 129. Subdural hemorrhage. At autopsy, the bones of the skull removed from above, exposing a lake of subdural blood over the cerebrum.

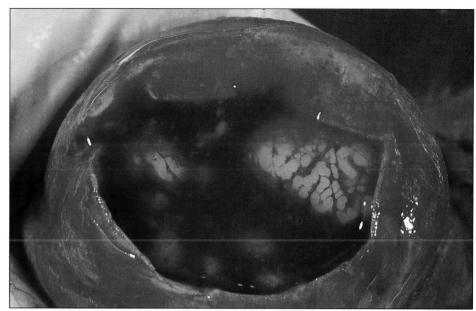

Fig. 129

Figure 130. Cerebellum showing surface injury of both hemispheres, with subarachnoid hemorrhage.

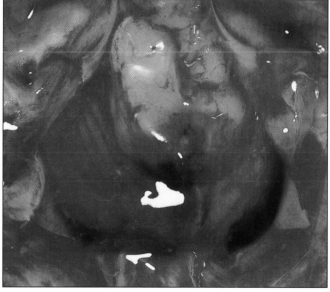

Fig. 130

A Case of   *Meconium aspiration pneumonia; macrosomia; maternal familial diabetes.*

This was a difficult forceps delivery of a term macrosomic, 10-pound baby (Figure 131). The mother had a familial history of diabetes. Macrosomia (*macro-*, large; *-somia*, body) occurs commonly in offspring of mothers with overt or latent diabetes (page 48).

Labor was prolonged. The amniotic fluid was heavily stained with thick brown meconium.

At birth the infant was cyanotic, limp, and severely depressed. Increasing respiratory depression developed. X-ray of the chest showed evidence of meconium aspiration pneumonia. Death occurred at 23 hours.

Severe cyanosis was evident at autopsy. The lungs were large, mottled, and purple (Figure 132a). The lung tissue was of a ropy, rubbery character. The cut surface of the lung was dark red with a light brown tinge (attributable to aspirated meconium). The lungs, microscopically, showed meconium pneumonia (page 108); the lung tissue presented many inflammatory cells containing meconium (Figure 132b); as seen in Figure 132c, some of the alveolar sacs in the lungs are filled with aspirated brown meconium-stained scaly material, desquamated debris from the meconium-stained skin (Figure 132c).

Spinal injury, spinal epidural hemorrhage was present (Figure 133), attributed to the difficult forceps delivery of the big fetus (page 135).

The brain was edematous and congested (Figure 134a), the consequence of hypoxic congestive heart failure. The cerebral cortex, microscopically, showed prominent neuronal hypoxic damage (Figure 134b), reflective of the terminal systemic hypoxia imposed by the meconium pneumonia.

Figure 131. Macrosomic 10-pound baby born of a mother with a family history of diabetes.

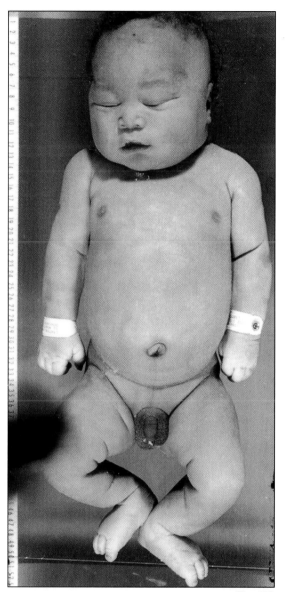

Fig. 131

Figure 132(a). Lungs, aspiration pneumonia; lungs mottled red and purple, of doughy ropy texture; thoracic viscera viewed at autopsy.

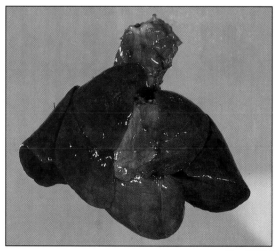

Fig. 132(a)

Figure 132(b). Meconium pneumonia; microscopic section of the lung showing infiltration of inflammatory cells; some cells with heavy deposits of brown meconium.

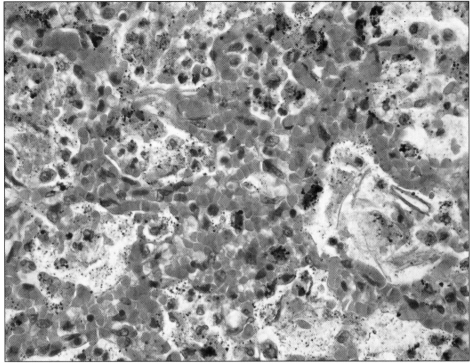

Fig. 132(b)

Figure 132(c). Lung alveolar sacs filled with meconium and squames, scaly desquamated debris from the meconium-stained skin; microscopic section of the lung, high magnification.

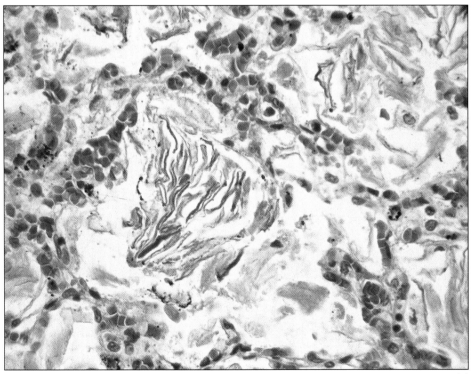

(c)

Figure 133. Spinal epidural hemorrhage; spinal injury related to the difficult forceps delivery of the macrosomic fetus. The spinal canal, as viewed at autopsy; the spinal cord, lifted aside, exposing a thick collection of epidural blood extending through the cervical and upper thoracic segments.

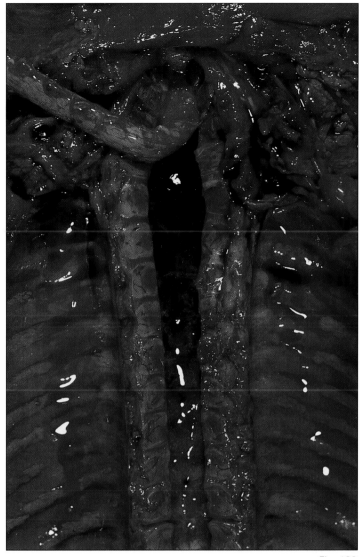

Fig. 133

Figure 134(a). Brain, edematous, swollen, congested. (The two irregular white streaks on the cerebral surface are artefacts, tears incurred in the autopsy dissection.)

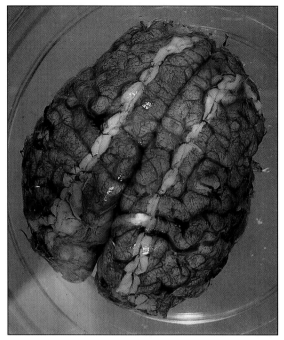

Fig. 134(a)

Figure 134(b). Nerve cell hypoxic damage, cerebral cortex; microscopic section of the cerebral cortex. Damaged cells are shrunken and darkened, in contrast to neighboring preserved nerve cells with cellular architecture intact, with the cell bodies showing clear cytoplasm and distinct nuclei.

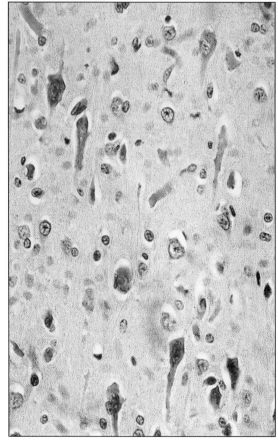

(b)

A Case of *Massive hemorrhagic infarction of one side of the cerebrum in a premature fetus.*

Gestational age was 27 weeks. The delivery was complicated by a compound presentation, with one arm presenting with the vertex of the head. At delivery, prolapse of the umbilical cord and excessive bleeding occurred. The infant was stillborn. The placenta showed retroplacental hemorrhage.

Autopsy revealed spinal injury, with laceration of the spinal cord; this was correlated with the history of the complicated compound presentation. The brain showed prominent congestion of superficial veins on gross examination. The whole-brain histologic section (Figure 135) showed massive cerebral infarction was present on one side (page 15). On the other side of the cerebrum, the vena terminalis, the main vein draining the deep strata of the cerebrum, was filled with a thrombus (page 11). In sections of the cerebrum at a deeper level, intraventricular hemorrhage was present. Histologic study revealed that the infarctional process affected not only the matrix and adjoining white matter of the forebrain but also the basal ganglia.

Figure 135. Massive asymmetrical infarction of the cerebrum. Premature brain of 22 weeks' gestation. Whole-brain horizontal section, stained with hematoxylin-eosin. On the left, the entire cerebral hemisphere is destroyed by a venous hemorrhagic infarction. Thrombosis of veins as occurs in such cases is demonstrated in this section of the brain. On the right, a large cerebral vein located on the lateral aspect of the ventricle is dilated and occluded by thrombus.

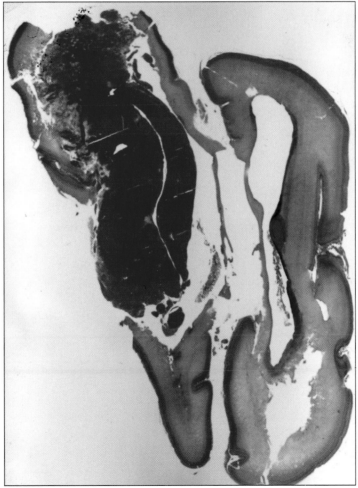

Fig. 135

A Case of **Postnatal pneumonia in a dysmature (IUGR) premature infant.**

Premature labor developed in this mother, who had a history of two previous miscarriages. The duration of the pregnancy, based on available clinical information, was uncertain. The gestational age was estimated to be 31 weeks or more, based on the physical appearance of the infant, the mature facial features, advanced development of the ears, the head hair and, at autopsy, based on the level of development of the brain and other organs.

The infant at birth was severely depressed but responded to care and became "very active."

The infant presented a graphic picture of dysmaturity, a long skinny baby with a large head (Figure 136). The baby weighed 1 pound 2 ounces (506 grams). (The average weight at 30 weeks' gestation is 1,300 grams.) This was an obvious example of intrauterine deprivation, intrauterine growth retardation (IUGR) (page 94).

The infant was supported with oxygen and fed by stomach tube.

The infant gradually weakened, with increasing periods of apnea. She developed an area of inflammation, reddening, around the stump of the umbilicus, acute omphalitis. She showed subtle seizure activity prior to death on the fourth day.

At autopsy, congestive heart failure was evident, with a greatly dilated heart occupying a large portion of the chest cavity (Figure 137). The body organs were congested. The thymus and adrenals were small, atrophied, evidence of chronic intrauterine compromise of the fetus.

Microscopic study of the tissue at the root of the umbilical cord showed severe acute purulent inflammation, acute omphalitis (Figures 138 and 139).

The lung, microscopically, in some parts, showed small bronchi filled with amorphous material (aspirated) with purulent exudate, with the surrounding lung alveoli filled with pus, a pattern of aspiration pneumonia (Figure 140). The aspiration apparently occurred when the enfeebled infant, fed by tube, vomited and aspirated.

Figure 136. Dysmaturity; newborn infant of 30 to 31 weeks gestation, with a long skinny body, characteristic of dysmaturity, intrauterine growth retardation (IUGR). Weight was 506 grams (average at 30 weeks, 1,300 grams). The baby presented physical features of advanced maturity, based on facial features, well developed ears, black growth of head hair. Infant lived 4 days.

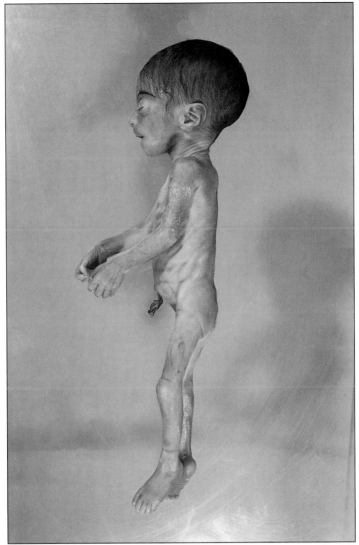

Fig. 136

Figure 137. Autopsy showed manifestations of heart failure, with the enlarged dilated heart filling much of the thorax.

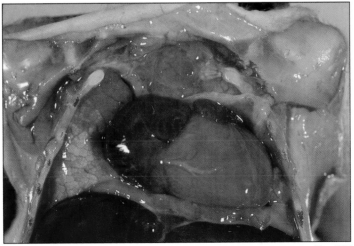

Fig. 137

Figure 138. Acute omphalitis. The area around the umbilical stump became inflamed, reddened. Microscopic section postmortem showed acute suppurative inflammation of the tissue at the root of the umbilical stump.

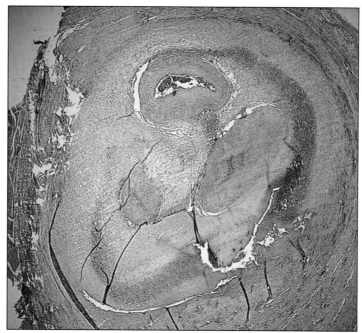

Fig. 138

Figure 139. Section of lung showing aspiration pneumonia. The small bronchial structures in the center are filled with aspirated amorphous material and purulent exudate. The infant had been fed by tube and apparently had vomited and aspirated (Figure 140).

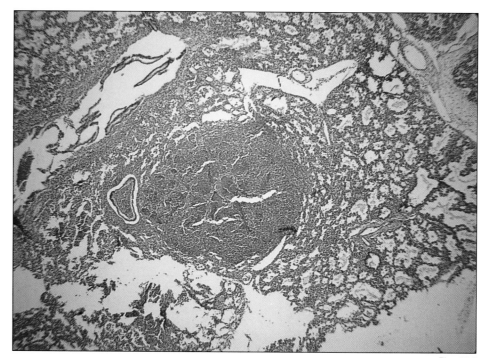

Fig. 139

Figure 140. Aspirated material in the lung, with associated inflammation, exudate.

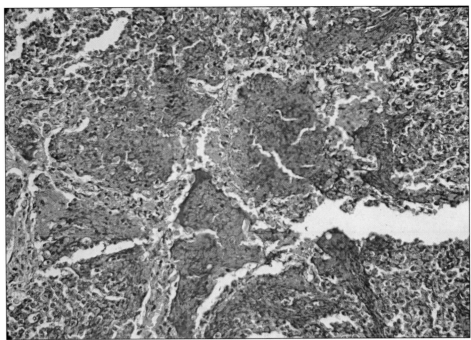

Fig. 140

A Case of   ***Postnatal pneumonia and anemia developing in a dysmature (IUGR) term infant.***

The mother had episodes of recurrent fever with skin rash.

The mother went into spontaneous labor at term. Evidence of fetal distress appeared and an emergency cesarean section was done. The amniotic fluid was meconium stained.

At birth, the infant was flaccid and cyanotic during the first 20 minutes.

The placenta at delivery had an adherent retroplacental hematoma (Figure 141). The placenta was small, weighed 460 grams. Placental calcification was present, reflecting placental insufficiency (page 76). The maternal surface showed diffuse speck-like points of calcium deposition (Figure 142).

The placenta showed chorioamnionitis.

The newborn infant was small, dysmature, weighed 4 pounds 9 ounces, reflecting intrauterine growth retardation. He was pale (Figure 141), anemic, and required transfusion.

He remained in poor condition, with fever, increasing cyanosis, and respiratory difficulty prior to death on the third day.

The main finding at autopsy was the presence of fulminating bacterial pneumonia, with abscess formation (Figures 143, 144, 145). Bacterial cultures of the lungs yielded a gram-negative organism, *Pseudomonas aeruginosa*.

This case presents the clinical pathologic sequence of placental premature senescence, with calcification, placenta insufficiency, leading to fetal deprivation, intrauterine growth retardation. The newborn, anemic and enfeebled, developed a bacterial respiratory infection that proved fatal. The infection may have been contracted during fetal life, related to the mother's febrile illness or to the chorioamnionitis. Or, the infection in this debilitated newborn may have been incurred in the days after birth.

Figure 141. Pale, anemic infant. Placenta with retroplacental hematoma.

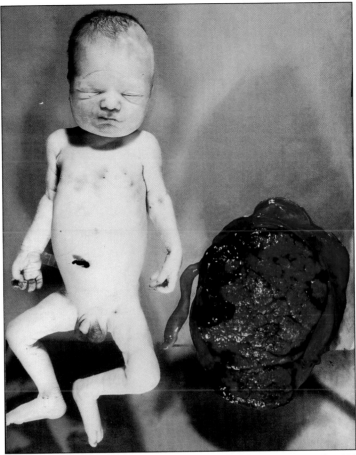

Fig. 141

Figure 142. Placental calcification; portion of the maternal surface showing speckled yellow points of calcification.

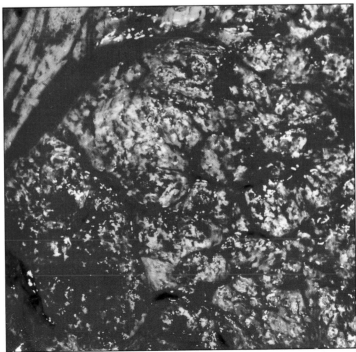

Fig. 142

Figure 143. Lung abscess; close-up photograph of the lung surface showing an area of yellow inflammatory exudate overlying a large abscess of the lung.

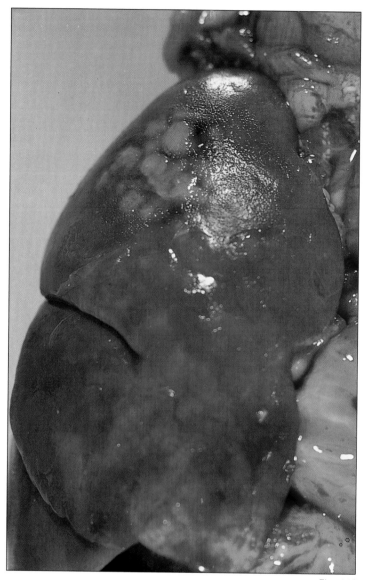

Fig. 143

Figure 144. Histologic section of the lung; confluent areas of abscess formation and diffuse pneumonia (Figure 145) (hematoxylin-eosin stain).

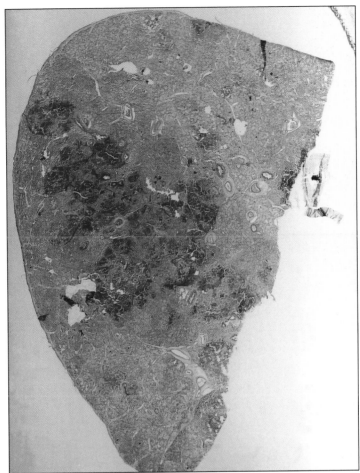

Fig. 144

Figure 145. Photomicrograph of the section of area of pneumonia in the lung, with inflammatory exudate in the alveoli (hematoxylin-eosin stain).

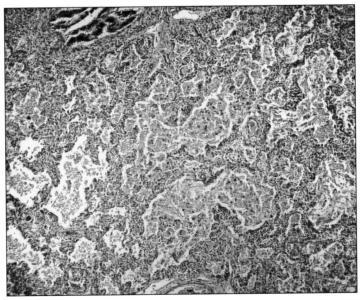

Fig. 145

A Case of   *Precipitous birth; small newborn; death due to subdural hemorrhage and spinal injury, with associated severe acute congestive heart failure.*

Pregnancy was near term. The mother reported she had felt "sick" the week before delivery.

After the onset of contractions, labor developed rapidly over a period of two hours. The second stage of labor was short, with delivery occurring precipitously. Thick meconium was present.

Fetal heart had been audible 10 minutes before birth. The newborn infant appeared lifeless, limp, cyanotic, and failed to respond to resuscitation.

Three major pathologic processes were evident at autopsy: (1) hypoxic congestive heart failure (page 8), (2) posterior fossa subdural hemorrhage (page 133) and (3) spinal injury.

Heart failure of acute severe degree was evident, with the enlarged dilated heart occupying the thoracic cavity (Figure 146); the large veins entering the heart were congested, distended with blood. The lungs were dark red, congested. Characteristic of acute congestive heart failure, the liver and spleen were enlarged (Figure 147). The brain was congested and edematous, showing flattening of the surface of the cerebral convolutions (Figure 148).

The head externally showed a caput succedaneum, indicating that there had been a substantial period of labor, that the head had been subjected to the forces of parturition. There was little molding of the head.

At autopsy the cerebrum had a thin layer of subdural blood over the outer surface. The brain stem was surrounded with free blood; about 4 milliliters of blood was in the posterior fossa (Figure 149). This form of intracranial hemorrhage is due to stretching and tearing of dural and venous structures around the brain stem.

Examination of the spinal structures showed free blood around the cord, in the subdural and epidural space (Figure 150).

Pathologically, the findings intracranially and in the spinal structures were attributable to mechanical injury, the consequence of a forceful precipitous birth (page 41).

Figure 146. Congestive heart failure; enlarged dilated heart; engorged veins leading to the heart. Precipitous delivery; hypoxic newborn death.

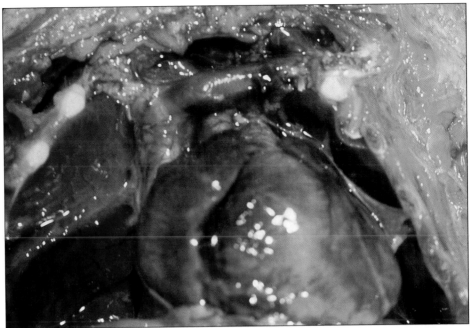

Fig. 146

Figure 147. Enlargement, congestion, of the liver. The spleen, at the lower right, likewise is greatly enlarged, congested.

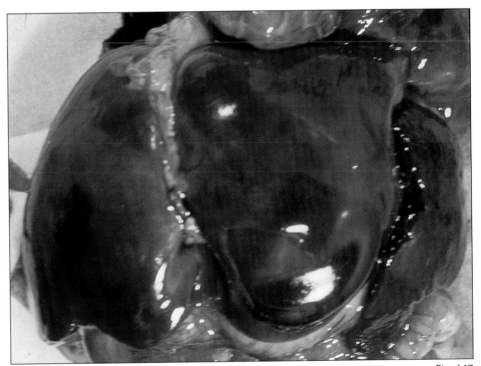

Fig. 147

Figure 148. Cerebral edema, with flattening of surface of the convolutions, the consequence of hypoxic congestive heart failure.

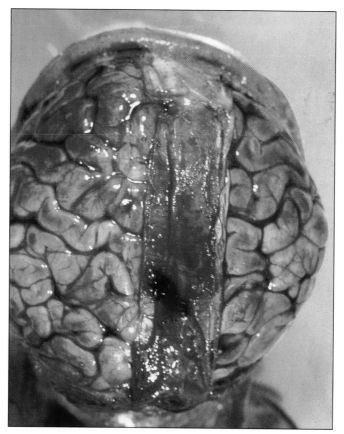

Fig. 148

Figure 149. Posterior fossa occupied by 4 milliliters of (subdural) blood.

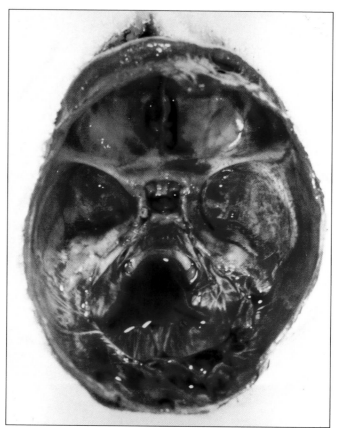

Fig. 149

Figure 150. Spinal injury, subdural and epidural hemorrhage, due to forceful and precipitous delivery.

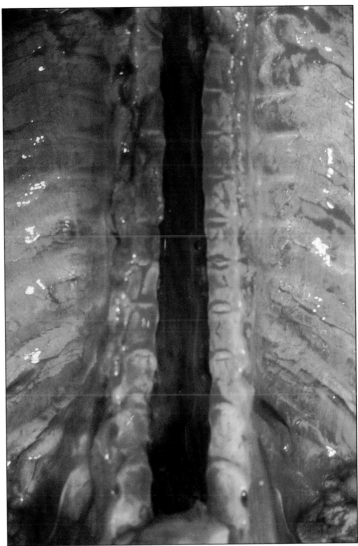

Fig. 150

A Case of   *Prolapse of the umbilical cord. Stillborn premature with cerebral hemorrhagic infarction; intraventricular and subarachnoid hemorrhage.*

Spontaneous rupture of membranes occurred at 22 weeks of gestation. Leaking of amniotic fluid began 2 days before delivery. Mother developed fever of 102 degrees. Prior to delivery, vaginal examination revealed a loop of prolapsed pulsating umbilical cord in the vagina (page 80). The prolapsed segment of the cord was hemorrhagic, necrotic (Figure 151).

The infant was stillborn.

The placenta examined after delivery pathologically showed chorioamnionitis (Figure 152), the consequence of the premature rupture of membranes; the mother's prenatal fever is attributable to the chorioamnionitis.

At autopsy the fetus showed congestive heart failure, with dilated heart (Figure 153), hydrothorax, and enlarged liver, with congestion of the viscera. The brain was congested and showed deep cerebral venous hemorrhagic infarction with intraventricular hemorrhage (Figure 154a) and subarachnoid hemorrhage (Figure 154b).

Figure 151(a). Prolapsed loop of umbilical cord extending down from the fetus and placenta. Above the prolapsed loop a gauze tie indicates level of the cervical os. **(b).** Umbilical cord prolapse; close-up view. Portion of the cord in the lower part of the illustration shows hemorrhagic discoloration of the prolapsed segment. Portion of the cord in the upper part of the illustration is pale and flattened, the result of compression in the pelvis.

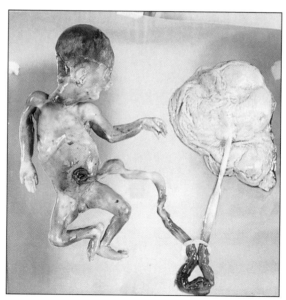
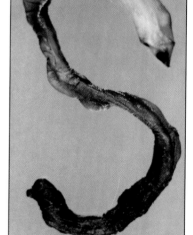

Fig. 151(a)   (b)

Figure 152. Chorioamnionitis; histologic section of the placenta. Amniotic surface above, placental elements below. Infiltration of acute inflammatory cells in the amnion and in the deeper layers.

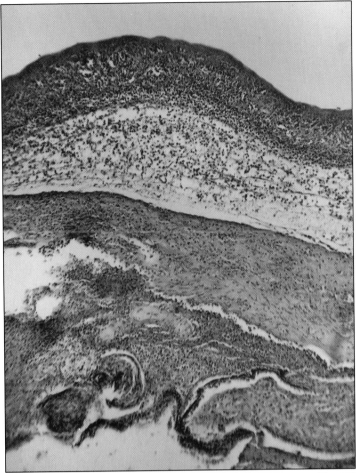

Fig. 152

Figure 153. Heart in congestive heart failure, distended with blood.

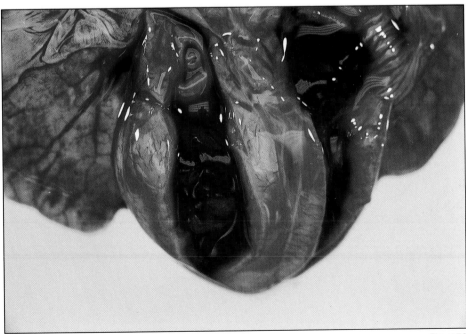

Fig. 153

Figure 154(a). Cerebral hemorrhagic infarction of deep cerebral structures, with hemorrhage extending into lateral ventricles. Frontal section of brain.

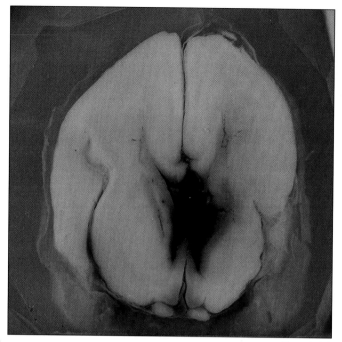

Fig. 154(a)

Figure 154(b). Subarachnoid hemorrhage around the brain stem and upper spinal cord, from the fourth ventricle, through the foramina of Luschka and Magendie, into the subarachnoid spaces, forming a thick cake of blood around the brain stem.

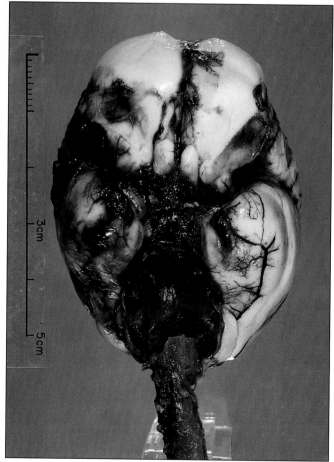

(b)

A Case of

A complicated breech presentation, with prolapse of an arm; premature rupture of membranes; chorioamnionitis.

This case demonstrates a basic pathologic sequence, beginning with a complicated breech presentation (in this case, a prolapsed limb protruding through the cervix) with premature rupture of membranes, with subsequent chorioamnionitis, maternal sepsis, and birth of a small depressed infant dying in congestive heart failure.

The mother had a poor reproductive history, with two of her three previous pregnancies ending with miscarriage.

The mother was admitted at 23 weeks of gestation, in active labor, with leakage of amniotic fluid. Uterine contractions continued during the following day; the mother developed sepsis, with fever of 106 degrees. After a prolonged labor lasting over 24 hours, the small depressed infant was delivered.

Delivery was complicated by a compound breech presentation, with prolapse of the right arm, protruding downward, alongside of the breech, through the cervix. Figure 155 shows the effects of the breech presentation, with circumscribed edema and redness of the buttocks, in the form of a caput succedaneum. The right forearm and hand, prolapsed with the breech presentation, were edematous and reddened.

With the prolapsed arm penetrating downward into the cervix, premature rupture of the membranes had occurred; the membranes, the amniotic sac, were infected, with resulting severe chorioamnionitis (Figure 156).

As a consequence of the chorioamnionitis, the mother developed sepsis with high fever.

The newborn infant, surviving the complicated birth, was deeply depressed, and expired after 6 hours in congestive heart failure.

At autopsy the organs were congested. In the thorax the large veins entering the heart were engorged. Likewise the right atrium was distended with blood (Figure 157). The subcutaneous tissues were edematous. These postmortem findings of congestive heart failure form the final chapter in this pathologic sequence beginning with the compound breech presentation.

Figure 155. Edema and mottled red discoloration of the buttocks and of the right forearm and hand, representing a form of caput succedaneum in this compound breech-arm presentation. Prolapse of the right arm occurred during the descent of the fetus in the birth canal. The edema and congestion of the buttocks and arm are analogous to the circumscribed edematous swelling of the scalp that occurs as a caput succedaneum in cephalic presentation.

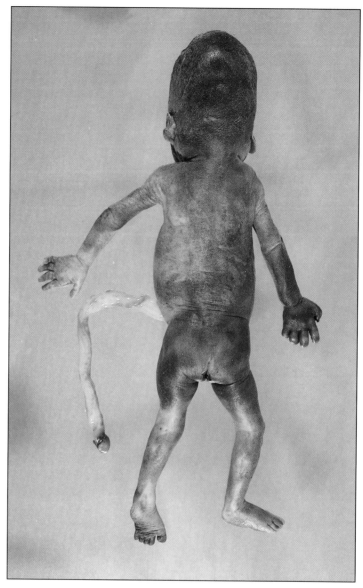

Fig. 155

Figure 156. Chorioamnionitis. The histologic section shows the amniotic surface of the placenta, diagonally across the field, coated with a thick layer of purulent inflammatory exudate. Below and to the left are the chorionic villi of the placenta.

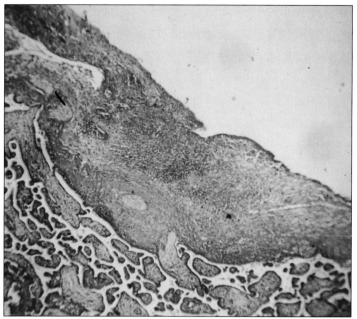

Fig. 156

Figure 157. Congestive heart failure; distention of the right atrium and of the large veins of the mediastinum entering the heart.

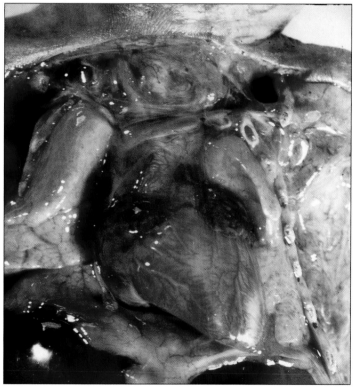

Fig. 157

A Case of   *Erythroblastosis fetalis; hydrops; intrauterine death.*

Erythroblastosis occurs with Rh-negative mothers bearing an Rh-positive fetus (page 98). Hydrops, with the fetus becoming ballooned with a great accumulation of edema fluid, is the most severe form of erythroblastosis fetalis. As in this case, most hydropic fetuses die in utero.

The mother in this present case was Rh-negative. She had had three previous deliveries; the offspring, as often occurs with Rh-negative mothers, did not have manifestations of erythroblastosis.

The present gestation was at term. On admission to the hospital, fetal death was diagnosed. It was evident that the fetal death had occurred a day or more previously. Considerable difficulty was encountered in delivering the oversize stillborn infant. During delivery large areas of skin slipped away, were denuded. The body of the infant was very large and edematous; weight was 11 pounds (Figure 158).

At autopsy, ascites was present; the abdomen contained 200 milliliters of watery fluid. Hydrothorax and hydropericardium were present. Characteristic of erythroblastosis, there was hepatosplenomegaly (Figure 159). The enlarged liver extended 3 centimeters below the costal margin. The spleen was approximately three times the average size. The body viscera were congested and edematous.

Characteristic of erythroblastosis fetalis, the placenta was large, edematous, boggy, over three times the average weight.

In erythroblastosis, in the common form, with the Rh-negative mother bearing an Rh-positive fetus, fetal Rh-positive red blood cells escape into the mother's circulation, causing the mother to develop antibodies to the fetal cells. The antibodies in the mother's blood serum are transferred through the placenta to the fetus, causing hemolysis of the fetus' red cells. The red cell hemolysis leads to jaundice; with destruction of the fetus' red cells, the fetus becomes anemic. Anemia causes heart failure in the fetus. With increasing congestive heart failure, the fetus becomes edematous, creating fetal hydrops, as in the present case.

Figure 158. Hydrops fetalis in a case of erythroblastosis fetalis. Intrauterine death; skin slipping, denuded areas, occurred during difficult delivery of this oversize, edematous,11-pound stillborn infant.

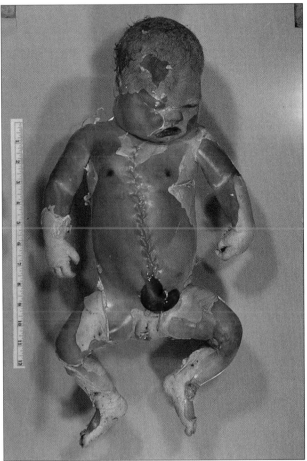

Fig. 158

Figure 159. Liver and spleen enlargement in this case. Hepato-splenomegaly is characteristic of erythroblastosis fetalis.

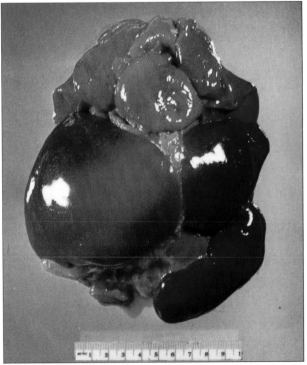

Fig. 159

A Case of   *Erythroblastosis fetalis with hydrops.*

The mother had had two previous pregnancies, both ending in stillbirth. The present pregnancy was at 34 weeks. During the last 3 weeks prior to admission to the hospital, there had been rapid abdominal enlargement. Diagnosis of polyhydramnios was made (page 91). The fetus had become less active. The baby was delivered by cesarean section.

At birth, the infant was large and edematous (Figure 160), presenting the characteristic hydrops form of erythroblastosis fetalis (page 99).

The mother and the baby were both blood type O. Studies of the Rh factors revealed the mother was CDe-ce; the baby's Rh factors were CDE-ce. The erythroblastosis was attributed to sensitization of the mother by E. A Coombs test on the baby's blood was positive.

The newborn infant's condition was poor. He was anemic. An exchange transfusion was done soon after birth, but the infant died an hour after birth.

The placenta (Figure 161) was large and edematous, weighed 850 grams, over two times the average weight of the placenta at 34 weeks.

The baby weighed 6 pounds 7 ounces (average weight at 34 weeks is 4 pounds 8 ounces). At autopsy there was extreme edema of the body. The skin was pale. On incising the skin, watery fluid oozed from the water-logged subcutaneous tissue.

Changes of congestive heart failure were present. Hydropericardium was present (Figure 162). The pericardial sac contained 20 milliliters of fluid. Each pleural sac contained 15 to 20 milliliters of fluid. The abdomen contained 50 milliliters of ascitic fluid. The heart was enlarged, dilated, distended with blood (Figure 163).

The liver and spleen were enlarged (Figure 164). The liver weighed 200 grams, twice the average weight of the liver at 34 weeks of gestation; likewise the spleen, weighing 25 grams, was three times the average weight for 34 weeks.

This case demonstrates the characteristics of the hydrops form of erythroblastosis fetalis, presenting severe edema, anemia, congestive heart failure with ascites, hydrothorax and hydropericardium, and the enlargement of the liver and spleen.

Figure 160. Hydrops form of erythroblastosis fetalis. Severe bodily edema. Pale skin reflects the severe anemia present.

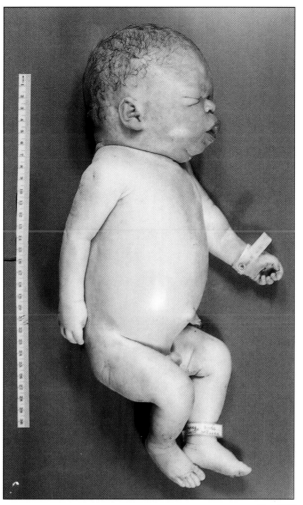

Fig. 160

Figure 161. Placenta, characteristic of erythroblastosis fetalis, is enlarged, with a weight of 840 grams, twice the average weight for 34 weeks.

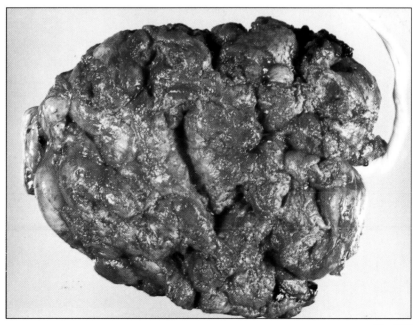

Fig. 161

Figure 162. Hydropericardium evident at autopsy, together with ascites and hydrothorax present.

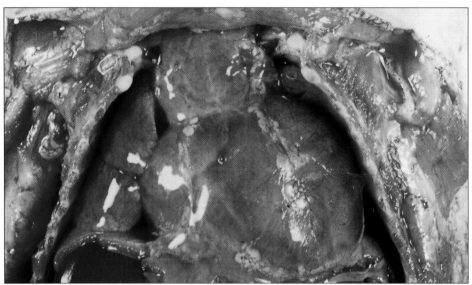

Fig. 162

Figure 163. Heart large, dilated, in congestive heart failure.

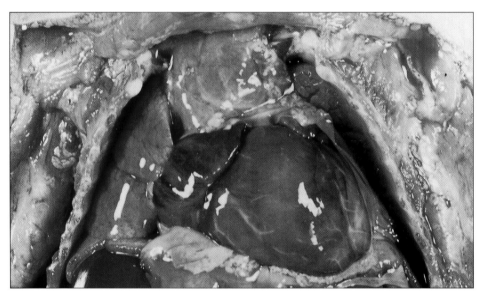

Fig. 163

Figure 164. Liver and spleen enlarged, characteristic of erythroblastosis fetalis.

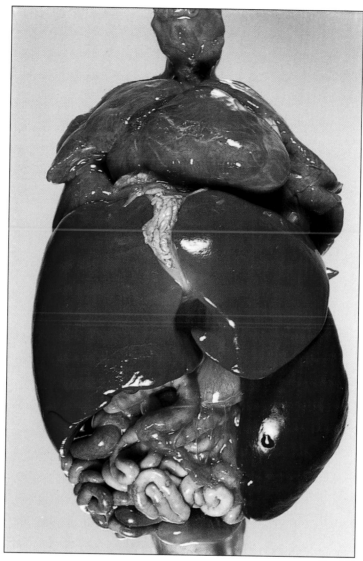

Fig. 164

A Case of   *Twin transfusion syndrome; premature twins of unequal size.*

Spontaneous labor occurred at 20 weeks of gestation. The mother's abdomen had increased greatly during the previous week, polyhydramnios. The abdomen was about the size of a 9-month pregnancy. Fetal heart tones were audible at the time of admission. The abdomen was tense, and when the membranes ruptured, about a gallon of clear yellow fluid escaped. Polyhydramnios is common in twin pregnancy.

At birth, the twins were of unequal size (Figure 165).

The larger twin, born first, weighed 520 grams; this weight is excessive for the gestational age (average weight at 20 weeks is 316 grams). The smaller infant weighed 160 grams.

The larger infant lived briefly. Prior to death, spontaneous movements of the infant were present. The infant was deeply cyanotic. At autopsy, findings of congestive heart failure, with ascites, were present.

The smaller infant was lifeless at delivery.

The placenta was of excessive size (Figure 165). A thin partition membrane separated the placental surface into two unequal portions; the membrane was delicate, transparent, characteristic of monochorionic diamniotic placentas.

Research studies, injecting the placental blood vessels, have demonstrated that in twin gestations having one placenta, most, if not all, placentas have vascular anastomoses of varying extent, causing fetal-fetal transfer of blood.

In this case, although the placenta was not investigated to demonstrate the vascular anastomoses, this is a classic example of the transfusion syndrome outcome, with one twin being large, plethoric, in congestive heart failure, and with the lesser twin underweight, showing intrauterine deprivation (page 97).

Figure 165. Twin gestation, placental transfusion syndrome. Larger twin, the recipient, weighed 520 grams, was cyanotic, edematous, in congestive heart failure with abdomen distended due to ascites. Small twin, donor, weighed 160 grams. The placenta, edematous and disproportionately large, characteristic of twin transfusion syndrome.

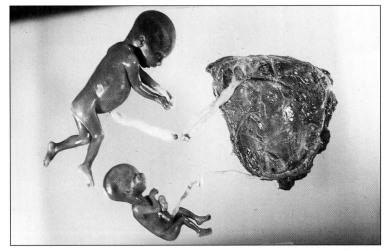

Fig. 165

A Case of *Teenage primiparous pregnancy, maternal anemia, manifestations of prediabetes, with macrosomic offspring; toxemia; premature placental detachment; stillbirth at 37 weeks.*

In this 16-year-old primipara, chronic fetal compromise occurred due to maternal anemia, manifestations of latent prediabetes (family history of diabetes), with excessive weight gain and fetal macrosomia. Toxemia and hypertension occurred during the last weeks of pregnancy. Placental detachment occurred in the hours prior to delivery.

Fetal death is attributable to the accumulated adverse effects of the mother's gestational medical problems.

The infant in this case was macrosomic, LGA (large for gestational age). The newborn weight was 7 pounds 4 ounces (3,262 grams), in the eightieth percentile. The average weight at 37 weeks of gestation is 2,800 grams. Accordingly, the baby was 460 grams, 1 pound, overweight. Macrosomia in offspring is commonly the first sign of latent prediabetes in the mother (page 48).

Regarding the retroplacental hemorrhage, there was no rupture into the amniotic sac; the mother did not collapse, did not go into shock (page 68). In cases of abruption, if the hematoma is present for a protracted period prior to fetal death, the placenta becomes indented by the retroplacental hematoma and at delivery shows a dished-out deformity of the maternal surface. The placenta in this case did not show this deformity. The implications are that the retroplacental hemorrhage was a late event, with the retroplacental hematoma in large measure accumulating after fetal death.

A Case of   *Nuchal cord occurring in early fetal life;*
retroplacental hemorrhage.

Nuchal cord is usually thought of as a complication that happens in term cases, around the time of delivery. The present case demonstrates that nuchal cord at times originates in early fetal life, contributing to fetal death. In other circumstances the nuchal cord, originating early, may remain in place, becoming hypoxia-producing at term (page 84).

In the present case, gestation was at 20 weeks. Episodes of vaginal bleeding occurred during the last month.

The birth was precipitous, breech. A tight nuchal cord was present. The infant was stillborn. When the nuchal cord was removed, the neck showed a pale ring, the imprint left by the tight nuchal cord (Figure 166).

The fetus was deeply cyanotic, due to the nuchal cord. Tightening of the nuchal cord leads to cord compression, compromising blood circulation through the cord, causing fetal hypoxia. The cord showed the effects of compression and the interference with cord circulation; the middle portion of the cord, the segment previously encircling the neck, was thin, mottled, while the proximal segment, attached to the fetus, was thick, edematous, discolored, with engorged blood vessels (Figure 166); the segment of the cord distally, attached to the placenta, was contrastingly narrow, pale.

In this case, a second major factor pathologically was the presence of a large retroplacental hematoma, tightly attached to the maternal surface. Most of the hematoma was old. Vaginal bleeding that occurred in this pregnancy is attributable to the old, ongoing retroplacental hemorrhage (page 68).

The autopsy revealed changes of hypoxic congestive heart failure, the consequence of the nuchal cord and the retroplacental hemorrhage.

Of incidental interest, the fetus showed the effects of the breech birth, an edematous dark red caput succedaneum over the buttocks (Figure 167).

Figure 166. Nuchal cord; early fetal death. Pale ring around the neck, the imprint of the nuchal cord. The middle portion of the cord (the part that had encircled the neck) thin, mottled; the segment proximal, toward the fetus, showing effects of circulatory obstruction, is thick, edematous, engorged; the distal segment of the cord, pale and narrow. Massive retroplacental hematoma. The left side of the placenta shows the cup-like amniotic sac with cord entering it. The hematoma, attached externally to the maternal surface, shows, in the lower mid portion, a circumscribed, deep red clot; most of the retroplacental clot firm and dark red-brown, pathologically old. The retroplacental hemorrhage, beginning long before delivery, gave rise to vaginal bleeding during the pregnancy.

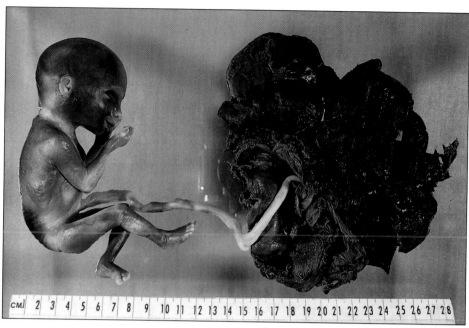

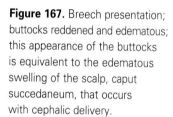

Fig. 166

Figure 167. Breech presentation; buttocks reddened and edematous; this appearance of the buttocks is equivalent to the edematous swelling of the scalp, caput succedaneum, that occurs with cephalic delivery.

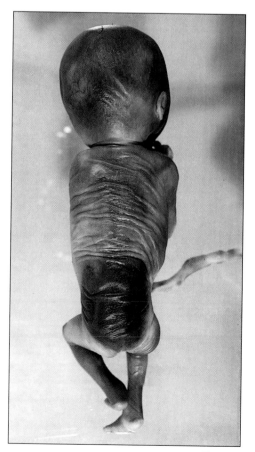

Fig. 167

A Case of   *Nuchal cord; long cord; intrauterine death.*

The pregnancy was at term. Gradual loss of fetal activity was noted during the 2 days prior to delivery. The infant was stillborn, slightly macerated. At delivery a loop of umbilical cord was wound tightly around the neck (page 83). The tight umbilical cord (Figure 168) had left a pale imprint, a deep groove, around the neck (Figure 169).

With the nuchal cord, the part around the neck becomes compressed; circulation through the cord is obstructed. The effect of this circulation compromise is evident in Figure 168; with blood flow from the fetus toward the placenta obstructed, the proximal segment of the cord, attached to the fetus, is edematous, thick, dark red; in contrast, the distal part of the cord, toward the placenta, was unaffected.

The fetus was edematous, with bodily changes of congestive heart failure.

At delivery, the amniotic fluid was dark green meconium stained; the placenta was meconium stained (Figure 170). Meconium staining apparently related to the hypoxic state of the fetus.

The umbilical cord was very long, 115 centimeters (45 inches) (Figure 171). The average length of the cord at term is 50 centimeters (20 inches). An excessively long cord is a risk factor for the fetus; often the long cord becomes entangled around the limbs, or the neck, as a nuchal cord. The long cord present in this case was the underlying cause of the fetal death.

Figure 168. Nuchal cord; loss of fetal activity prior to delivery. Obstruction of circulation through the cord; resulting edema and congestion of the segment of cord attached to the fetus.

Figure 169. Neck showing pale imprint caused by the tight nuchal cord.

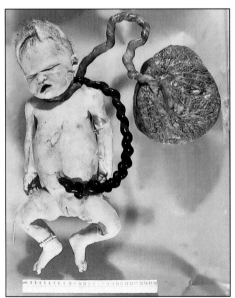

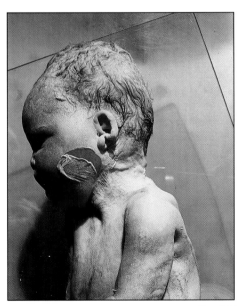

Fig. 168   *Fig. 169*

Figure 170. Meconium staining of the placenta.

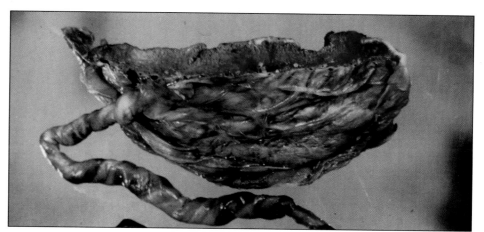

Fig. 170

Figure 171. Long cord malformation, 115 centimeters (average length at term, 50 centimeters).

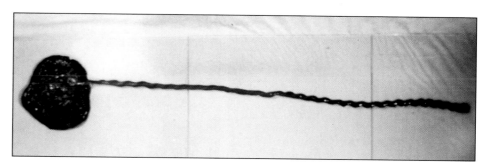

Fig. 171

A Case of **Caput succedaneum; Down syndrome.**

A prominent caput succedaneum was present at delivery (Figure 172). The mother stated that fetal movements had been absent for 1 day. At delivery the umbilical cord was wound around the neck three times, tightly, accounting for the intrauterine death. Maceration of the skin was present.

Down syndrome was diagnosed at delivery. The term infant weighed 2,260 grams, was dysmature, small for gestational age. The head viewed posteriorly was asymmetrical, with a bulging soft prominence on the right, a caput succedaneum (page 126); at autopsy, incision through the prominence revealed an edematous hemorrhagic thickening of the scalp, characteristic of a caput (Figure 173).

Down syndrome abnormalities were evident in the infant. Characteristic of Down syndrome, the palmar surface of the hands showed a transverse crease, a simian line (Figure 174). The fingers were short, stubby, deformed; similarly the toes were deformed. As commonly occurs in Down syndrome, the heart showed a septal defect, an opening in the septum between the right and left ventricles.

Figure 172. Caput succedaneum evident as a bulging distortion over the right occipital area. Clinically the infant was known to have died in utero prior to delivery; slipping of the skin, the denuded area, was a postmortem change.

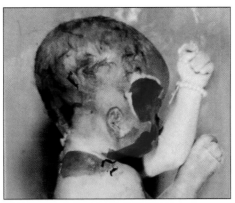

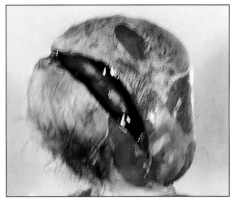

Fig. 172

Fig. 173

Figure 173. Incision of the soft, bulging caput; edematous hemorrhagic tissue through the thickened layers of the scalp, a pattern characteristic of caput succedaneum.

Figure 174. Down syndrome abnormality of the hand: transverse crease (the simian line), stubby distorted fingers, characteristic of Down syndrome. (Postmortem skin slipping.)

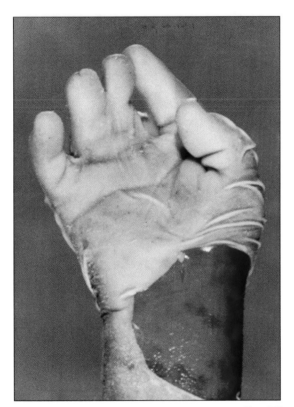

Fig. 174

A Case of   *Prolapse of the umbilical cord; renal agenesis*
             (Potter's syndrome) and oligohydramnios.

A loop of prolapsed umbilical cord was found in the vagina, protruding from the still tightly contracted cervix, as illustrated diagrammatically in Figure 175. As indicated, presentation was breech.

Oligohydramnios, a lack of amniotic fluid, was present (page 90). The gestation was at 33 weeks. The infant was stillborn. Fetal death in this case was due to hypoxia, to compression of the prolapsed umbilical cord, with consequent compromise of the umbilical cord circulation (page 81).

As seen in Figure 176, the ears of the baby were low-placed, large, and dysmorphic, indicating Potter's syndrome (page 91).

Maceration present, patchy denuding of the skin, was consistent with fetal death having occurred about one day previously, corresponding to the time of loss of fetal activity noted by the mother the day before admission.

Autopsy revealed bodily changes of hypoxic congestive heart failure, with venous congestion of the viscera and with hydrothorax (Figure 177).

Most significantly, the postmortem examination revealed renal agenesis, no vestige of kidney structure. This was plainly related pathologically to the oligohydramnios, to the lack of amniotic fluid, noted previously.

Amniotic fluid is mainly the product of urine excreted by the fetus. Accordingly, with renal agenesis, as in this case, there results oligohydramnios. With absence of the amniotic fluid cushion, the fetus is compressed, causing pressure deformation of the feet (Figure 178).

This case is a classic example of Potter's syndrome, the occurrence of kidney agenesis linked genetically with abnormal structure of the external ears, ears that are low-placed in the sides of the face, ears that are large and appear floppy.

Figure 175. Prolapse of the umbilical cord. Oligohydramnios, a paucity of amniotic fluid, with the amniotic membrane close around the fetus.

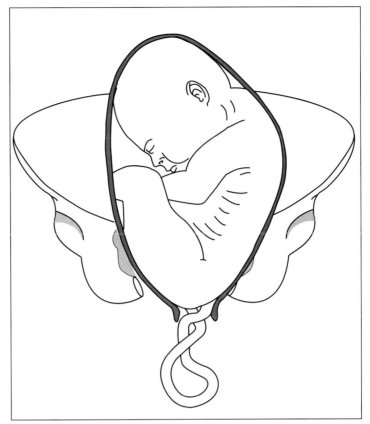

Fig. 175

Figure 176. Low-placed, large, floppy ears (the classic appearance in Potter's syndrome). Maceration, patchy denuded skin areas, reflective of recent intrauterine death.

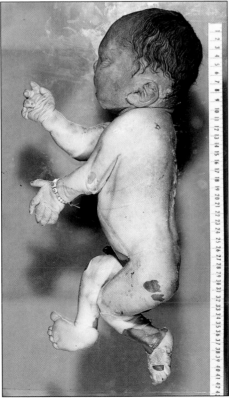

Fig. 176

Figure 177. Hydrothorax; manifestation of congestive heart failure in this case.

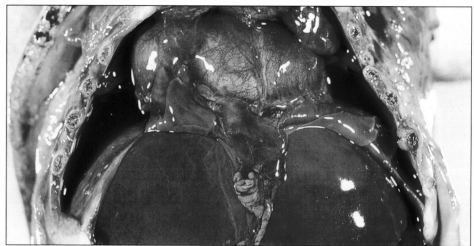

Fig. 177

Figure 178. Deformation of the feet in this case of oligohydramnios. The absence of amniotic fluid, loss of the amniotic cushion, results in pressure deformation of the feet.

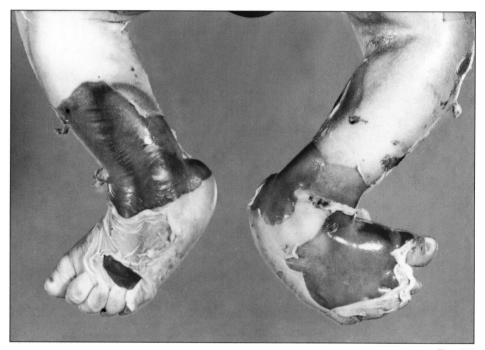

Fig. 178

A Case of   *Acute congestive heart failure with hydrops, with massive ascites; suspected Coxsackievirus infection.*

This case was a baby of 36 weeks' gestation. The mother said she had been treated for urinary tract infection during the pregnancy. She was a multipara, with two previous deliveries that were slightly premature. In the present case, presentation was cephalic and delivery was vaginal.

The newborn infant was in stable condition at birth.

The infant weighed 1,966 grams (4 pounds 7 ounces), was underweight, dysmature (average weight at 36 weeks' gestation is 2,600 grams).

During the first day the infant developed respiratory distress with retractions. However, early on day 2 he improved, with good color; x-ray of the chest showed clear lung fields. Toward the end of day 2 he developed respiratory distress and deteriorated rapidly; he developed acute congestive heart failure, became hydropic, with massive ascites, and died precipitously (page 9).

Although this was a dysmature underweight newborn, the cause of sudden acute cardiorespiratory failure, the cause of death, was obscure clinically.

At autopsy the baby was edematous and cyanotic (Figure 179). The baby's weight was 2,140 grams (4 pounds 12 ounces), an increase of almost 1/2 pound over the birth weight, attributable to edema. The abdomen was greatly distended.

The subcutaneous tissue on incision was very edematous. The distended abdomen was due to massive ascites (Figure 180). The pericardial sac was large, dilated, distended with fluid, hydropericardium. The heart was dilated, distended with blood (Figure 181).

The body organs showed severe venous congestion. The liver and spleen were enlarged. The brain was edematous and congested (Figure 182). These autopsy findings pathologically are the picture of acute congestive heart failure.

The lungs, microscopically, showed cellular thickening of the alveolar walls, and many alveolar spaces contained hyaline material, pathologically characteristic of viral pneumonia. Clinically it was suggested that this was a case of Coxsackievirus infection.

In cases of newborn Coxsackievirus infection, the source of the infection is usually obscure. The mother may or may not have had symptoms of a viral infection.

Coxsackie disease in newborn infants, as described in the literature, is characterized by a sudden onset of symptoms, with the infant presenting rapid cardiorespiratory decompensation, developing dyspnea, edema, ascites, and cyanosis.

This clinical pattern was present terminally in the infant in this case, and taking into account the pathology findings at autopsy and the microscopic findings in the lung tissue, the conclusion emerges that this was a case of viral infection, probably Coxsackievirus disease.

Figure 179. Infant who died with acute congestive heart failure, showing cyanosis, severe edema, abdominal distention (due to ascites).

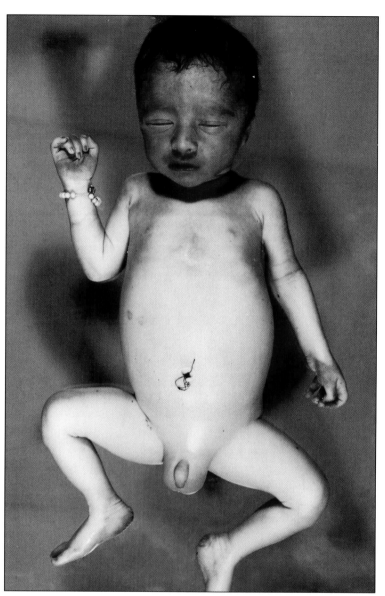

Fig. 179

Figure 180. Demonstration of the severity of the ascites: 100 millimeters of fluid collected from the abdomen.

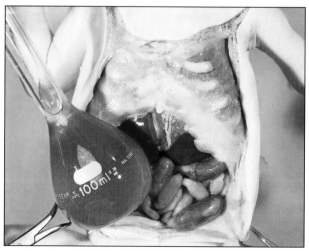

Fig. 180

Figure 181. Heart, distended with blood, in cardiac failure.

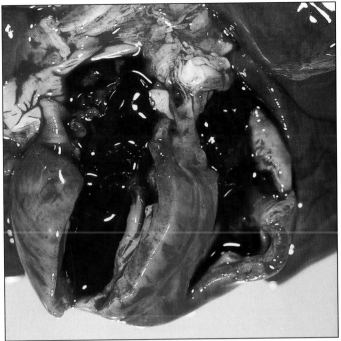

Fig. 181

Figure 182. Brain, congestion and edema due to congestive heart failure.

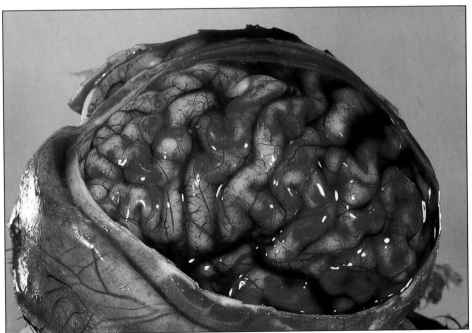

Fig. 182

A Case of   *Endocardial fibroelastosis in a newborn; congestive heart failure; hydrops fetalis.*

This was a severely edematous hydropic newborn.

The duration of this pregnancy was 27 weeks. The mother developed polyhydramnios. Presentation was double footling breech. The mother was admitted with premature rupture of the membranes, in active labor. The infant was stillborn. The amniotic fluid was clear.

One of the outstanding findings at autopsy was in the heart, the abnormal appearance of the endocardium lining the ventricles (Figure 183). The endocardium was leathery, thick, characteristic of endocardial fibroelastosis (page 114).

The effects of the congestive heart failure were evident in the body, in addition to the hydrops, with edema and congestion of the viscera.

At autopsy, severe hydrops was present (Figures 184 and 185), with the abdomen distended with ascites, the head and arms turgid with edema.

The distended abdomen contained 150 milliliters of clear amber ascitic fluid (Figure 186). Hydrothorax and hydropericardium were present (Figure 187).

The placenta likewise was large and boggy, edematous, with watery fluid oozing freely from the organ. The placenta weighed 660 grams, more than twice the average size of the placenta at 27 weeks (Figure 184). The placenta showed edematous chorionic villi and focal chorioamnionitis.

The etiology of endocardial fibroelastosis is obscure. Its occurrence is usually sporadic, but a familial incidence had been reported. Some cases are thought to be due to viral infection.

Figure 183(a). Endocardial
fibroelastosis; lining of the
ventricles is opaque, thickened,
leathery.

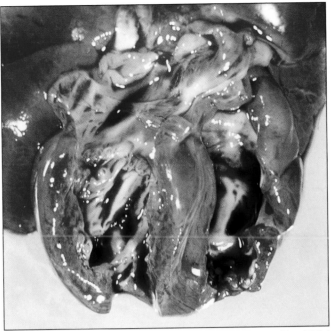

Fig. 183(a)

Figure 183(b). Endocardial
fibroelastosis, microscopic
appearance. Section through
the rounded trabecular muscles
on the inner aspect of the left
ventricle. The surface layer of
the trabecular muscles, the
endocardium, is irregularly
thickened, characteristic of
endocardial fibroelastosis.

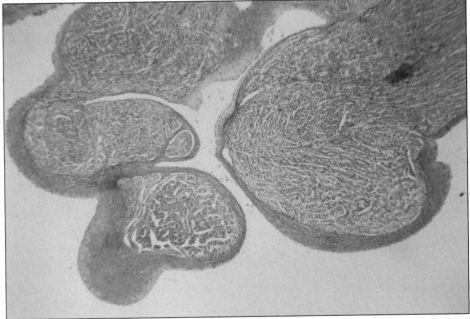

(b)

Figure 184. Hydrops fetalis in a case of endocardial fibroelastosis. Abdomen distended (ascites). Subcutaneous edema of the face and extremities. Placenta large and edematous.

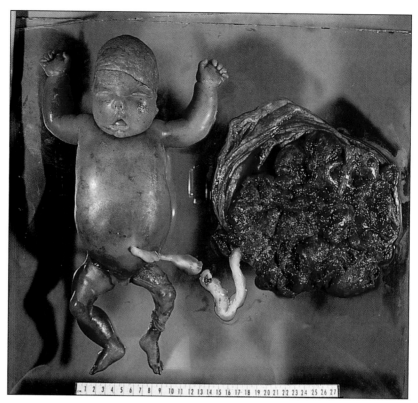

Fig. 184

Figure 185(a). Side view. **(b).** Severe subcutaneous edema; hydrops fetalis.

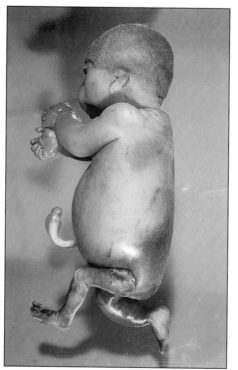

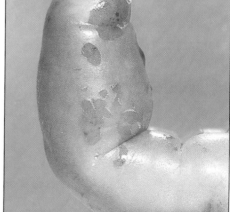

Fig. 185(a)   *(b)*

Figure 186. Ascites. Abdomen with 150 milliliters of clear amber watery fluid; hydrops fetalis. (View of abdomen at autopsy.)

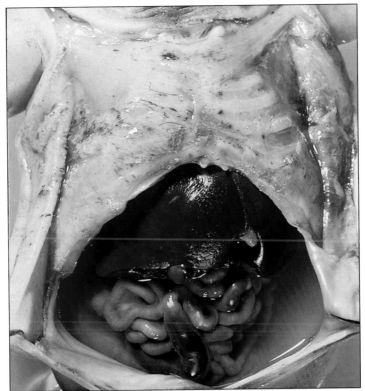

Fig. 186

Figure 187. Hydropericardium and cardiomegaly. The enlarged heart seen in the fluid-distended pericardial sac.

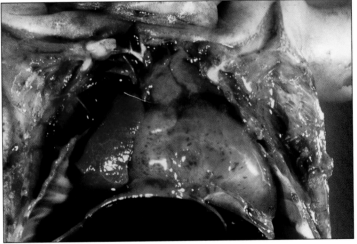

Fig. 187

A Case of   ***Brow presentation; spinal injury; intrauterine growth retardation.***

The delivery was complicated by a brow presentation that persisted for a long period; ultimately the brow presentation converted to vertex presentation, and the fetus delivered vaginally.

Heavy meconium staining of the amniotic fluid was present.

The newborn showed the effects of the initial brow presentation with severe edema and congestion, with livid discoloration of the forehead and frontal scalp (Figure 188). This edematous swelling is analogous to a large caput succedaneum occurring over the posterior of the head in a prolonged vertex delivery.

The newborn infant remained flaccid with little vital function, and died after 50 minutes.

Maternal factors adverse to the fetus had occurred during this gestation. The mother was obese, had hypertension, and had had an episode of pneumonia, had been febrile, during the first trimester. Later in the pregnancy she had had recurrent viral infections, influenza. The adverse gestational factors manifestly impacted on the fetus, on the newborn.

The newborn was dysmature, showing intrauterine growth retardation (IUGR). This was a term gestation, with the newborn weighing 4 pounds 15 ounces. The infant was long (20 inches) and thin, characteristic of dysmaturity, with little subcutaneous tissue (Figure 188).

The infant, with vital function compromised, died in congestive heart failure (page 8). The heart was enlarged, dilated, distended with blood (Figure 189). The viscera were congested. The brain was congested, edematous, swollen, showing flattening of the cerebral convolutions (Figure 190). The effect of the hypoxic congestive heart failure was evident in the cerebrum; small periventricular hemorrhagic infarcts were apparent in the cerebrum (Figure 191).

At autopsy, spinal injury was evident, with severe spinal epidural hemorrhage (Figure 192). The spinal injury, affecting spinal cord function, was of intrinsic etiology, attributable to distortion, hyperextension, of the spinal axis during the period of the brow presentation. The spinal injury was the cause of the limpness, the paralysis, of the newborn infant (page 135).

Pathologically, two main causal factors contributed to the newborn's death. First, the adverse maternal gestational factors of obesity and acute illnesses resulted in an enfeebled dysmature infant. Second, the complicated delivery, the brow presentation, resulted in stress on the spinal structures, with consequent spinal epidural hemorrhage, injury affecting cord function, leading to compromise of vital function and death in congestive heart failure.

Figure 188. Brow presentation, with the presenting part of the head, the brow and frontal area, showing severe edema and congestion, changes of the nature of a caput succedaneum. Intrauterine growth retardation, term gestation; weight 4 pounds 15 ounces. Infant long and thin with little subcutaneous tissue (dysmaturity).

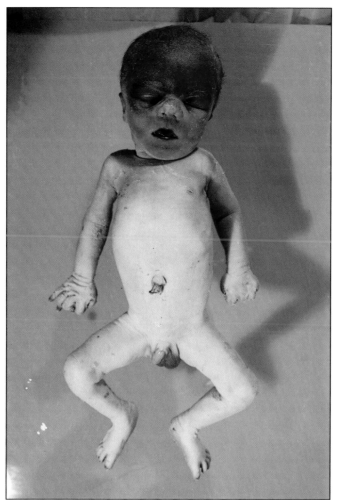

Fig. 188

Figure 189. Congestive heart failure; heart and large veins engorged, distended with blood.

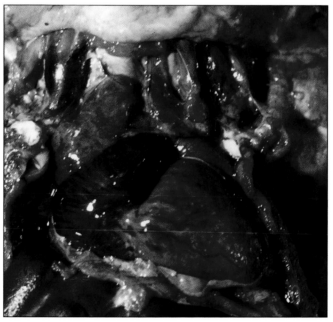

Fig. 189

Figure 190. Cerebral congestion, edematous swelling, with flattening of the convolutions; the effect of congestive heart failure.

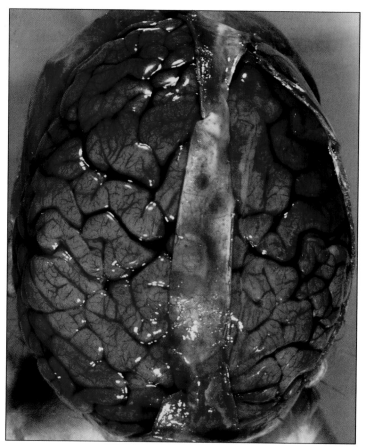

Fig. 190

Figure 191. Small periventricular hemorrhagic infarcts in the cerebrum; subacute lesions reflecting chronic adversive gestational factors, intrauterine growth retardation. Frontal section of brain.

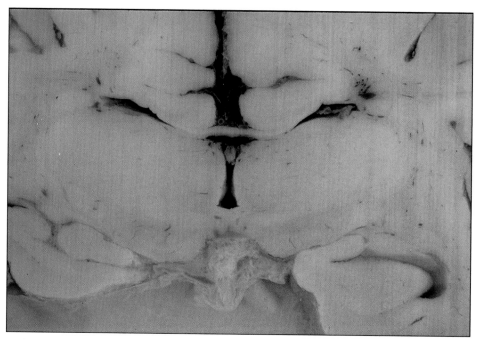

Fig. 191

Figure 192. Spinal epidural hemorrhage. **(a).** At autopsy, vertebral column removed, spinal cord removed, exposing a thick deposit of epidural blood on the posterior aspect of the spinal canal.
(b). Spinal cord; surface of the dura with deposits of epidural blood.

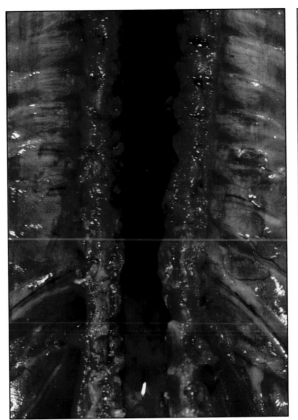

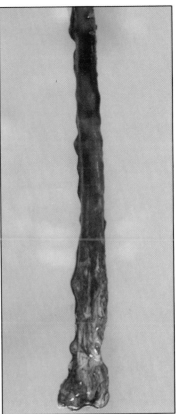

Fig. 192(a)

(b)

A Case of   *Congestive heart failure in a dysmature premature newborn; intrauterine device (IUD) present at delivery.*

Gestation was at 28 weeks. Premature rupture of membranes had occurred 4 weeks before delivery; the mother had had fever; she was treated with antibiotics and improved.

An IUD was recovered during delivery.

Delivery was spontaneous, vaginal. Amniotic fluid was clear.

The placenta, microscopically, showed chorioamnionitis.

The infant in poor condition at birth, lived for 1 1/2 hours. The weight was 1 pound 6 ounces (618 grams) (the average for 28 weeks is 1,000 grams), a low birth weight for the gestational age. The baby appeared undernourished, dysmature (Figure 193).

The head was elongated, molded, and there was a caput succedaneum, indicating that the fetal descent through the rigid, unrelaxed birth canal had been slow and difficult.

At autopsy, visceral changes of congestive heart failure were evident (page 8). The heart was large, dilated, and distended with blood (Figure 194). The brain was congested and edematous (Figure 195).

The thymus and adrenals were atrophied, reflecting prolonged intrauterine deprivation, dysmaturity (page 94).

The chorioamnionitis is attributable to the presence of the IUD and to the premature rupture of the membranes long before delivery. This intrauterine circumstance was adverse to the well-being of the fetus, born dysmature, enfeebled, succumbing after birth in congestive heart failure.

Figure 193. Dysmature, emaciated, low birth weight infant of 28 weeks' gestation. Premature rupture of membranes 4 weeks before birth; IUD and chorioamnionitis present at birth. Molding elongation of the head; caput succedaneum present.

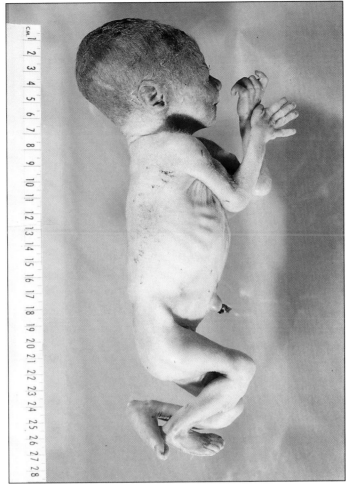

Fig. 193

Figure 194(a). and (b). Large dilated heart, reflecting terminal cardiac failure.

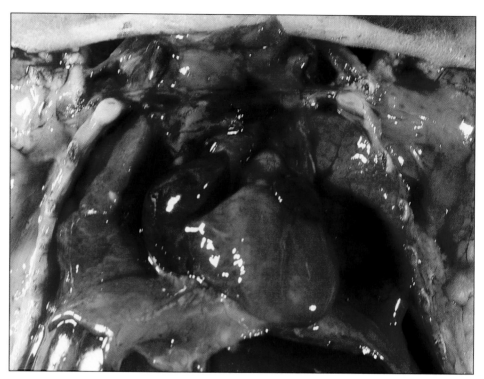

Fig. 194(a)

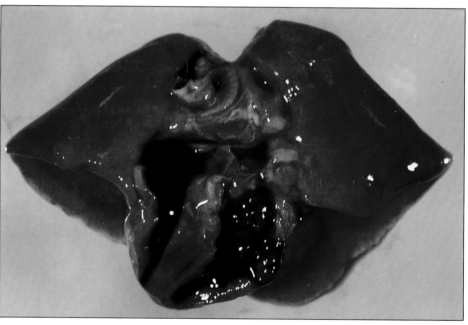

(b)

Figure 195. Edema and congestion of the brain, due to congestive heart failure.

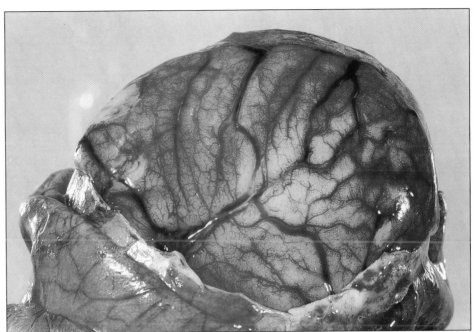

Fig. 195

A Case of   *Fetal death due to placental disease; hemorrhagic endovasculitis.*

This pregnancy was at term. The mother stated that fetal activity had gradually decreased and was absent during the 2 days before admission to the hospital.

On admission, fetal heart sounds were absent. Fetal death was diagnosed.

Regarding the cause of the fetal death, the mother had problems during this pregnancy, problems adversive to fetal well-being. She had gained weight excessively, reflecting a metabolic imbalance, and had episodic hypertension and albuminuria; she had had vaginal bleeding reflecting placental disease. Although these were contributory, the main cause of fetal death, with reasonable medical probability, was placental disease. The placenta was small, evidencing placental insufficiency. The placenta, microscopically, showed a chronic process of hemorrhagic endovasculitis (Figures 196 and 197).

Regarding the hemorrhagic endovasculitis (HEV), this is a pattern of pathologic changes, observed microscopically, affecting the blood vessels, the arteries, of the placenta (page 74). The vessel walls are thickened (medial and intimal hyperplasia), with narrowing of the vascular channels. Thrombosis of vessels occurs. There is evidence of perivascular hemorrhage.

HEV has been reported as common among stillborn infants and liveborn infants who are small for their gestational age.

The cause of HEV has not been established. There is evidence of viral infection (inclusion bodies) and other infections in some cases.

The inflammatory changes in the placenta are of chronic nature, adversely affecting the fetus over a prolonged period.

The mother had intermittent bleeding during midpregnancy, reflecting the presence of retroplacental hemorrhage (confirmed at delivery) that compromised placental function.

These placental pathologic processes were latent, clinically silent, processes for which doctors cannot be held culpable.

The fetus showed the effects of intrauterine deprivation, decreased fetal activity, reflecting the processes that ultimately caused intrauterine death.

Figure 196. Hemorrhagic endovasculitis. The histologic section through the placenta shows a small blood vessel with perivascular hemorrhage, characteristic of hemorrhagic endovasculitis.

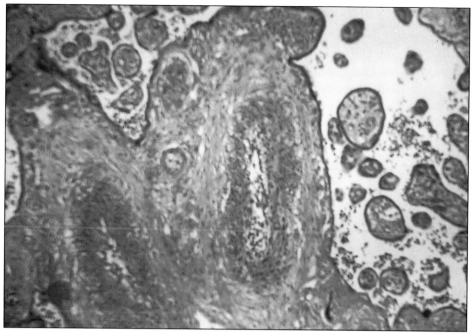

Fig. 196

Figure 197. Hemorrhagic endovasculitis; a small blood vessel showing characteristic inflammatory changes in the vessel lining (endothelium); the endothelial cells are edematous, ballooned out; obliteration of the lumen.

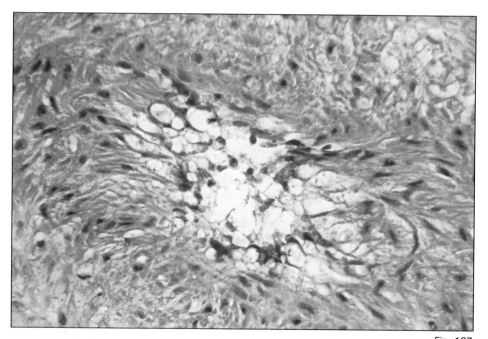

Fig. 197

A Case of   *Spinal injury leading to respiratory death.*

This was a teenage pregnancy; the mother was a primipara who had been hospitalized prior to labor for treatment of hypertension.

As often occurs in young primiparas, labor was prolonged; this was a cephalic vaginal delivery with low forceps extraction.

The infant was apneic at birth, cyanotic, in poor condition, limp. Respirations were delayed and irregular. During the 5 hours of survival there were recurrent episodes of cardiorespiratory collapse.

The main finding at autopsy was severe spinal epidural hemorrhage (page 135); a thick extravasation of blood was present on the posterior aspect of the spinal canal through the cervical and thoracic portions (Figure 198).

This pattern of damage, spinal epidural hemorrhage, affects the neighboring spinal cord, causes spinal shock, compromising function of vital centers in the cervical cord governing cardiac and respiratory function, resulting in apnea.

At autopsy the organs of the body showed the effects of cardiac failure, were severely congested, especially the brain (Figure 199).

Microscopically the cerebral cortex showed hypoxic neuronal damage (Figure 200), with affected neurones shrunken and deep-staining histologically.

Of interest was the finding in the cerebrum of an old lesion in the left cerebrum (Figure 201), an area of brown discoloration, a subacute focal infarct, reflective of an hypoxic episode during early intrauterine life.

This case demonstrates the clinical-pathologic link between the occurrence of a complicated delivery and consequent spinal injury, with the cervical cord affected, causing compromise of cardiac and respiratory function, leading to hypoxic damage to the viscera, to the brain, with hypoxic neuronal damage evident in the cerebral cortex.

Figure 198(a). Spinal epidural hemorrhage; the column of vertebral bodies removed, exposing the spinal canal and cord. Blood appears deep in the canal, behind the spinal cord in the epidural space. A complicated delivery with prolonged labor; forceps delivery.

(b). Spinal epidural hemorrhage. The cord removed; thick deposit of blood posteriorly in the canal, in the epidural tissue, extending from the cervical level to the midthoracic level.

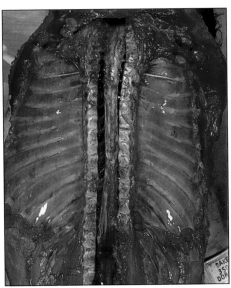

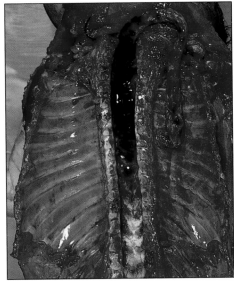

Fig. 198(a)   *(b)*

Figure 199. Brain showing severe congestion and edematous flattening of the surface of the cerebral convolutions, the effects of congestive circulatory failure.

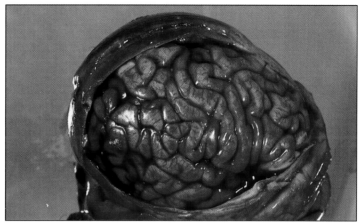

Fig. 199

Figure 200. Neuronal hypoxic damage. Histologic section of motor cortex; damaged nerve cells shrunken, elongated, deeply staining; surviving neurones, biologically more durable, appear with large clear-staining nuclei, and with central nucleoli.

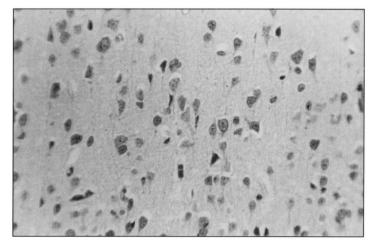

Fig. 200

Figure 201. Subacute focal periventricular (hemorrhagic) infarct in the left cerebrum, appearing as a small area of tan discoloration (tan coloration due to breakdown of hemoglobin).

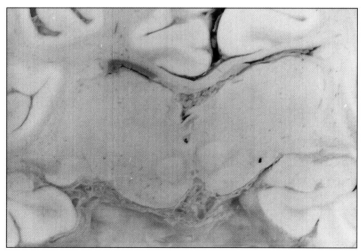

Fig. 201

A Case of **Nuchal cord; intrauterine hypoxia with meconium aspiration and congestive failure.**

The mother was admitted at 42 weeks of gestation in "false labor" and was discharged. She was readmitted a week later; decreased fetal activity had occurred. Fetal death was diagnosed at this time, at 43 weeks. At delivery, a tight nuchal cord was present (page 83). Amniotic fluid was meconium-stained (page 75). The infant and the placenta were meconium-stained (Figures 202, 203).

At autopsy the head showed molding and a caput succedaneum (Figure 202), indicating that the fetus was subjected to labor while still alive.

Changes of congestive failure were present (Figure 204). Watery fluid, ascites, was present in the abdomen, and hydrothorax was present. The heart was dilated; body organs were congested.

Meconium aspiration was evident at autopsy (page 108). The lung, examined microscopically, showed heavy accumulations of squames (scales of desquamated cells from the skin surface) (Figure 205). Some of the squames were meconium stained.

Correlation of the clinical-pathologic sequence: The presence of a caput succedaneum and molding of the head indicated that the fetus, while still alive, had been subjected to labor. Loss of fetal activity is attributable to intrauterine hypoxia brought on by the tight nuchal cord, by compression of the cord. Intrauterine hypoxia, when present, causes stimulation of the respiratory center in the fetus' brain; this triggers increasing respiratory movements by the fetus. The fetus aspirates quantities of amniotic fluid containing meconium and meconium-stained squames desquamated from the meconium-stained skin. Terminally, the hypoxic fetus developed congestive heart failure.

Figure 202. Meconium staining; caput succedaneum and molding of the head. Tight nuchal cord present at delivery, removed.

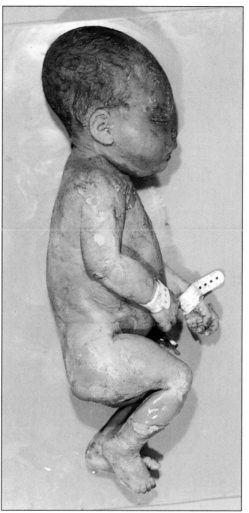

Fig. 202

Figure 203. Meconium staining of the fetal surface of the placenta.

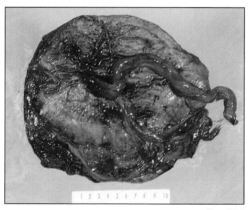

Fig. 203

Figure 204. Congestive heart failure with cardiac dilatation, ascites, and hydrothorax.

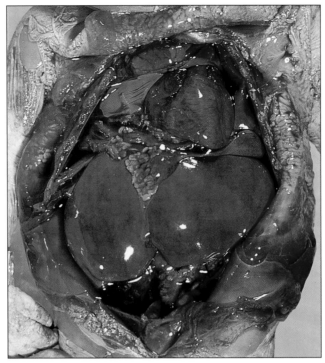

Fig. 204

Figure 205. Lung tissue, microscopic section. Alveolar spaces with accumulation of meconium-stained squames (scales desquamated from the skin surface and aspirated).

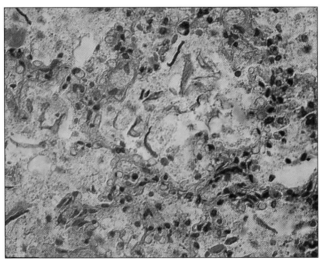

Fig. 205

A Case of   *Premature rupture of membranes. Newborn death; congestive heart failure; old, subacute, periventricular infarction with intraventricular hemorrhage; multiple visceral infarcts.*

Premature rupture of membranes occurred 2 weeks before labor. Gestation was at term. At delivery, nuchal cord was present, wrapped around the neck two times tightly. Labor lasted over 20 hours; there was severe molding of the head and a caput succedaneum (Figures 206, 207).

At delivery the infant was severely depressed, pale, limp, and unresponsive. The infant improved but on the third day became increasingly apneic and expired.

At autopsy, the caput succedaneum evident externally as an area of boggy softening of the scalp, on incision revealed a layer of edema and hemorrhage (Figure 207).

Congestive heart failure was evident, with cardiac enlargement and dilatation (Figure 208), and congestion of viscera. Venous engorgement of the lungs and adrenals led to focal infarcts in these organs (page 158). Figure 209 shows lung infarction; Figure 210 shows adrenal infarction.

The brain was edematous, swollen. The brain stem, the cerebellum, showed a heavy deposit of subarachnoid blood (Figure 211).

The examination of the deep structures of the brain specimen revealed prominent deposits of periventricular hemorrhage and intraventricular hemorrhage (Figure 212). Extension of the intraventricular hemorrhage into the subarachnoid space accounted for the blood around the brain stem.

The tan color of the periventricular lesions, due to the presence of disintegrating hemoglobin pigment, indicates that these cerebral hypoxic lesions were old, subacute, with origin during fetal life, long before the time of birth.

Figure 206. Molding of the head; elongation of the head.

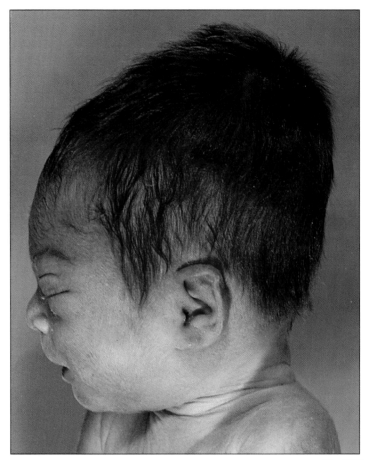

Fig. 206

Figure 207. Molding of the head with overlapping of the frontal bone. The scalp has been reflected, exposing an area of edema and hemorrhage in the scalp, a caput succedaneum.

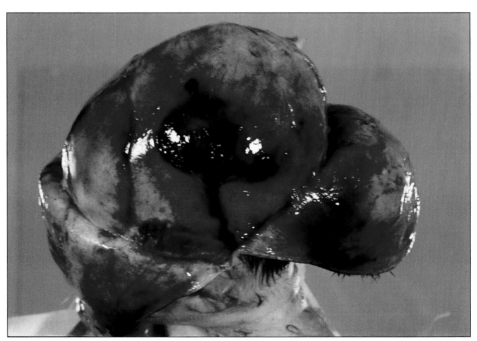

Fig. 207

Figure 208. The heart, in congestive heart failure. **(a).** Enlargement of the heart, especially the right atrium and ventricle.

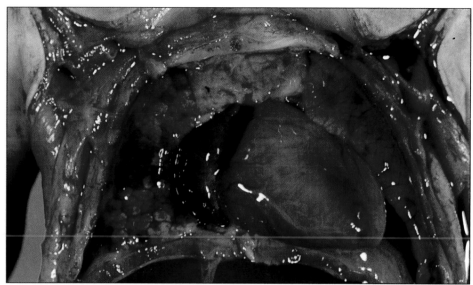

Fig. 208(a)

Figure 208(b). Heart, dilated, distended with blood.

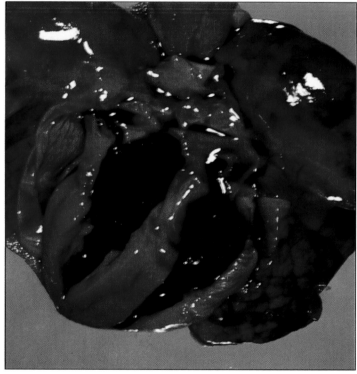

(b)

Figure 209. Lung with infarction in the lower lobe. Longitudinal section of the lung (microscopic section) showing hemorrhagic infarction in the lower lobe.

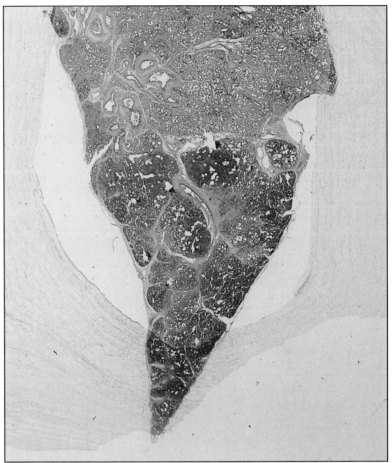

Fig. 209

Figure 210. Adrenal with focal infarction. Microscopic section showing areas of necrosis and marginal hemorrhage.

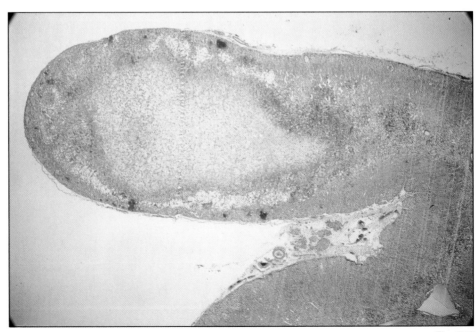

Fig. 210

Figure 211. Subarachnoid hemorrhage around the brain stem, cerebellum; blood source from intraventricular hemorrhage (Figure 212). Cerebral edema resulting from hypoxic congestive heart failure; flattening of the surface of the convolutions due to edematous swelling.

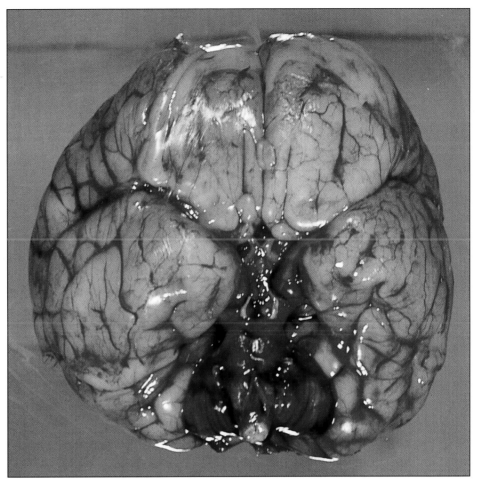

Fig. 211

Figure 212. Subependymal hemorrhagic infarction with intraventricular hemorrhage (blood extending through the ventricular system into the subarachnoid space, as in Figure 211). Frontal section of the brain. Tan coloration of the blood deposits due to degeneration of the blood hemoglobin, characteristic of subacute process.

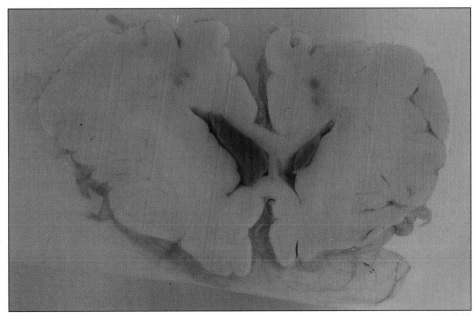

Fig. 212

A Case of **_Severe intrauterine growth retardation._**

This infant was premature and, according to the mother's history, was of 29 weeks' gestation. Weight was 900 grams (2 pounds). The average newborn weight at 29 weeks' gestation is 1,200 grams (2 pounds 11 ounces). This was a long, thin baby, with little subcutaneous tissue, a picture of severe intrauterine growth retardation (IUGR), severe dysmaturity (Figure 213). The emaciated appearance of the body made the head look very large.

Characteristic of severely dysmature infants, the face had the wizened appearance of an old man.

Was this infant, weighing 2 pounds, actually of 29 weeks' gestation? Though small and withered, he had physical features consistent with near-term gestational age — pronounced growth of head hair, well-developed ears — at autopsy the cerebrum showed a pattern of advanced development of the convolutions (Figure 214). The kidney, microscopically, showed a pattern of advanced cortical, glomerular, development.

Regarding causation of the intrauterine growth retardation, the maternal history provides distinct clues. The circumstances of this pregnancy were not optimal. The mother had a poor reproductive history (page 41); her two children born previously had been premature. In this pregnancy there had been recurrent vaginal bleeding. Although diabetes was not diagnosed in this mother, she had a strong history of familial diabetes. IUGR is known to occur at times in offspring of mothers with latent diabetes conditions.

Although there was no history of premature rupture of membranes, the placenta showed severe chorioamnionitis (Figure 215).

At birth, the infant appeared lifeless, limp, and cyanotic but responded to resuscitation. He seemed to improve during the first 3 days, despite difficulty in maintaining nutrition and hydration. On day 4 he became increasingly apneic, became unresponsive, and expired.

In summary, this was an example of severe intrauterine deprivation, and although one never knows all the things that happen during a pregnancy, in this case, the maternal factors noted, with the severe chorioamnionitis, manifestly impacted unfavorably on the fetus.

Figure 213. Dysmaturity of severe degree in a newborn. **(a).** A long thin baby with little subcutaneous tissue. Head hair present and large, well-developed ears, consistent with near-term gestation. **(b).** The face, with its wizened appearance, like an old man, is characteristic of dysmaturity.

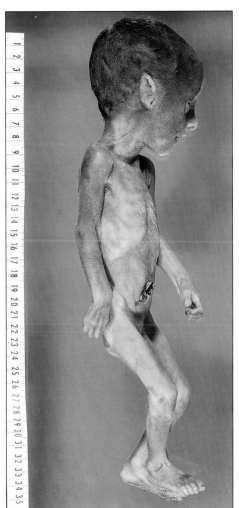

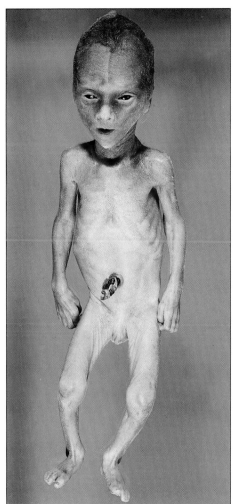

Fig. 213(a)

(b)

Figure 214. Brain showing pattern of cerebral convolutional development consistent with near-term gestation.

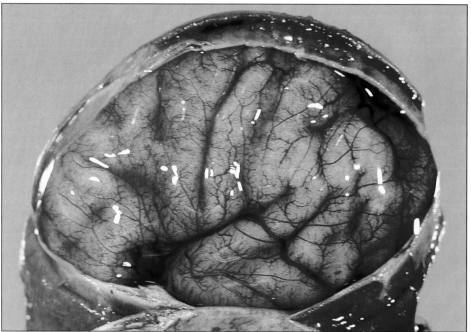

Fig. 214

Figure 215. Severe chorioamnionitis. The microscopic section of the membranes shows the amniotic surface above; below the amnion is a thick layer of deeply staining inflammatory tissue composed of an infiltration of acute and chronic inflammatory cells, the histopathologic picture of chorioamnionitis.

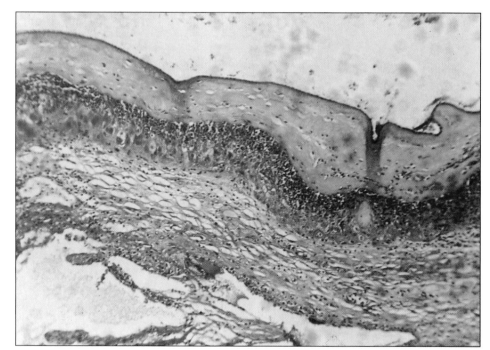

Fig. 215

A Case of   *Compound presentation, prolapse of the legs and one arm; premature labor.*

Premature rupture of the membranes occurred at 26 weeks of gestation, 2 days before delivery. Vaginal examination and x-rays revealed the head at the pelvic brim and the feet and an arm presenting in the vagina (Figures 216 and 217). A cesarean section was done. The newborn infant had an Apgar score of 1 at five minutes. The infant improved somewhat during the first hour, with gasping respiration, but later deteriorated, and died at 2 hours.

Findings at autopsy indicated that death was due to the inordinate stress of labor that this premature fetus encountered in this complicated presentation, with the newborn exhausted at birth, dying in congestive heart failure.

Figure 216. A graphic demonstration of the descending fetus during delivery, the white line representing the cervical ring, creating a caput succedaneum and edema and reddening of the prolapsed feet and right arm.

Figure 217. Edema and congestion of the feet and right arm, the consequence of prolapse of these extremities during delivery.

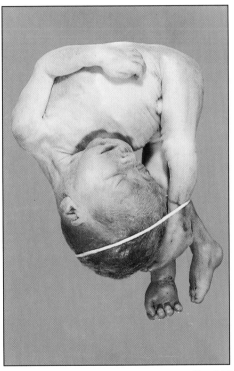

Fig. 216

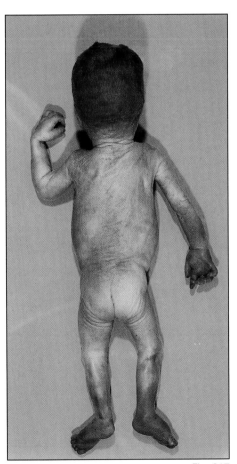

Fig. 217

A Case of *Cerebral venous thrombosis with periventricular infarction consequent to placental abruption.*

Premature labor occurred at 29 weeks' gestation, associated with premature detachment of the placenta. At birth, the umbilical cord was wrapped around the neck twice. The infant was in poor condition at birth and remained limp, with unstable vital function, with recurrent apnea. Death occurred at 30 hours.

In addition to the hypoxia-producing processes of the placental abruption and nuchal cord, the autopsy revealed hyaline membrane disease.

Pathologic studies of the brain revealed thromboses of the draining dural sinuses. The process of thrombosis extended retrograde to the large cerebral veins, to the Galen vein, and to small tributaries deep in the cerebrum. This led, consequently, to deep periventricular hemorrhagic infarction, to germinal matrix infarction (Figure 218).

This case demonstrates graphically basic mechanisms in the pathogenesis of fetal-neonatal hypoxic cerebral damage, linking hypoxia-producing complications and consequent circulatory failure, with the development of cerebral venous thrombosis and cerebral infarction (pages 11 and 14).

Figure 218. Cerebral thromboses with associated periventricular matrix infarction.
(a). Thrombosis of Galen vein. Frontal section of the whole brain (hematoxylin-eosin stain). The Galen vein, distended with fresh thrombosis, lies centrally between the cerebral hemispheres and above the midbrain.

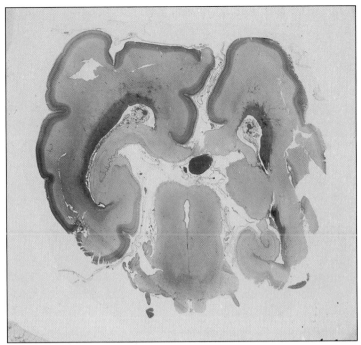

Fig. 218(a)

Figure 218(b). Hemorrhagic periventricular germinal matrix infarction. Premature brain; gestational age 29 weeks; clinical history of placental abruption, nuchal cord, and hyaline membrane disease.

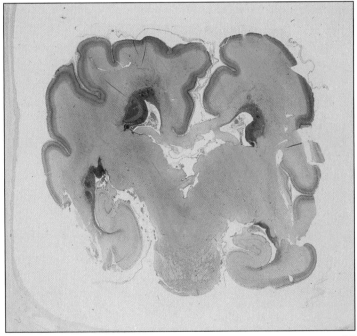

(b)

A Case of   *Hypoxic damage to the cerebral cortex during fetal life.*

The present case is a classic example of hypoxic cerebral cortical neuronal damage incurred during fetal life.

This was a term pregnancy. Vaginal bleeding had occurred during pregnancy. Loss of fetal activity, fetal death, was diagnosed prior to labor.

The placenta showed a retroplacental hematoma, partly old and yellow but composed mostly of fresh red blood clot.

The fetus was mature. Autopsy revealed severe venous congestion of the organs. The brain grossly was congested and edematous.

The cerebral cortex showed a patchy distribution of hypoxic damage in a pattern known pathologically as "laminar necrosis" (Figure 219), the pattern of damage that is commonly observed in adults who have suffered severe hypoxia and survived for a period of days (page 20).

With hypoxic laminar necrosis, the cortex is left with patchy necrotic pale areas depleted of nerve cells. This is the pattern of damage that occurred in this mature fetus. Hypoxia is the only pathologic process that can cause laminar neuronal necrosis.

This case is of special importance clinically. In cases that survive, cortical neuronal damage contributes to the development of clinical cortical manifestations of organic mental retardation, seizure disorder, psychopathy, and blindness, depending on what parts of the cerebral surface are devastated.

A question is at times raised critically as to the validity, the occurrence, of hypoxic cerebral neuronal damage during fetal life: Are neuronal alterations noted pathologically in the fetal brain attributable to antecedent intrauterine hypoxic exposure of the fetus — or are the microscopic neuronal changes artifacts, developing postmortem? The present case is a hallmark example, demonstrating that, yes, hypoxic neuronal damage does occur in the mature fetus.

Figure 219. Cortical hypoxic damage. Histologic section of cerebral convolutions; the cortex shows patchy pale areas with cellular elements wiped out; also, portions of preserved cortex with characteristic lamella pattern with six layers of nerve cells. Associated with the focal areas of patchy necrosis are neighboring veins occluded by thromboses.

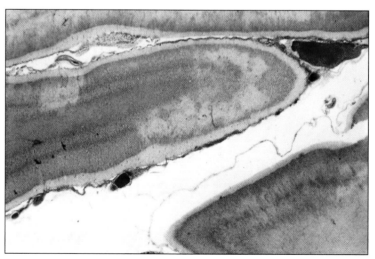

Fig. 219

A Case of   *Periventricular germinal matrix hemorrhagic infarction; massive intraventricular hemorrhage. Premature newborn, lived 2 days.*

The pregnancy was noted to have been uneventful until spontaneous contractions developed at 28 weeks, followed by spontaneous breech birth.

The Apgar score was 3 at 1 minute and 6 at 5 minutes. The infant was crying and breathing at 20 minutes and gradually improved. Intermittent apnea episodes increased, and at 47 hours respiration ceased.

At autopsy the brain showed cerebral intraventricular hemorrhage that originated in infarction of the germinal matrix (Figure 220). The hemorrhage extended through the third and fourth ventricles, out through the foramina in the fourth ventricle, into the subarachnoid space around the cerebellum and brain stem.

Figure 220. Massive intraventricular hemorrhage. Frontal section through the midlevel of the brain. On the lateral aspects of the distended cerebral ventricles, germinal matrix is evident as dark subependymal deposits.
On the right, the blood in the germinal matrix pad is in continuity with the blood cast in the third ventricle. A blood cast fills the lateral ventricles and the third ventricle.

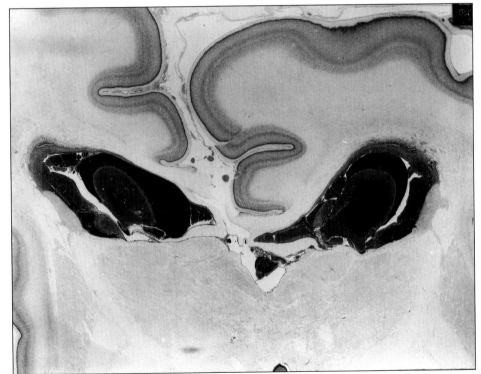

Fig. 220

A Case of ***Brain stem, cerebellar injury; difficult forceps delivery.***

Labor was prolonged, of poor quality. High forceps were applied, without success, then reapplied, achieving a difficult extraction (page 125).

At delivery, the infant was in poor condition, with an Apgar score of 3 at five minutes. The infant was cyanotic; fontanelles became bulging. Respirations were depressed during the 4 hours of survival.

At autopsy the brain showed diffuse subarachnoid hemorrhage. The cerebrum was congested and edematous, swollen, with the cerebral convolutions much flattened.

There were bodily changes of congestive heart failure, with cyanosis, cardiac dilatation, and congestion of viscera.

Detailed examination of the brain specimen revealed a heavy accumulation of hemorrhagic material, with tissue debris over the brain stem, over the basilar region, and over the ventral surface of the cerebellum. The spinal cord had prominent meningeal hemorrhages with adherent thick deposits of epidural blood clot. The thalamus showed focal hemorrhagic lesions. The cerebral ventricles were compressed.

The cerebellar hemispheres, as is evident in Figure 221, showed hemorrhagic discoloration and ragged surface erosion, particularly medially, in areas positionally related to the margin of the foramen magnum. Histologic section through the cerebellum, Figure 222, shows the nature of the damage — contusion and fragmentation — manifestly the effects of acute herniation injury incurred during the complicated forceps delivery. With excessive traction of the head during delivery, the cerebellum is drawn into the foramen magnum and becomes squeezed, torn, and abraded against the bony edge of the foramen (page 137).

Figure 221. Ventral aspect of the brain showing hemorrhagic discoloration and ragged surface erosion of the cerebellum in areas positionally related to the margins of the foramen magnum. Clinical history: high forceps applied; forceps slipped, reapplied. This is an example of mechanical injury; with excessive traction on the head, the brain stem and cerebellar area are drawn forcefully into the foramen magnum, compressed against the bony edge of the foramen.

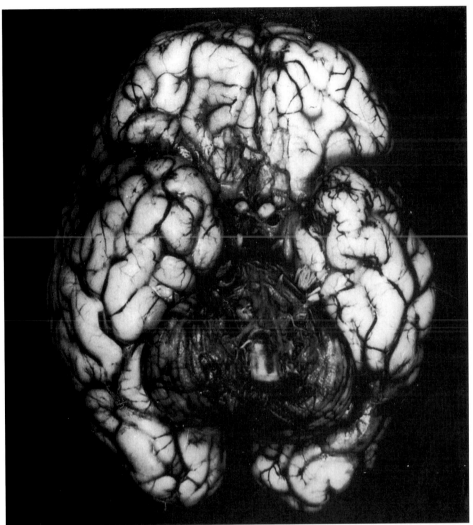

Fig. 221

Figure 222. Cerebellar damage incurred at birth; contusion with fragmentation, the effects of acute herniation incurred during complicated forceps delivery. This histologic section shows the surface damage, fragmentation and hemorrhage, corresponding to the ragged hemorrhagic erosion evident in Figure 221.

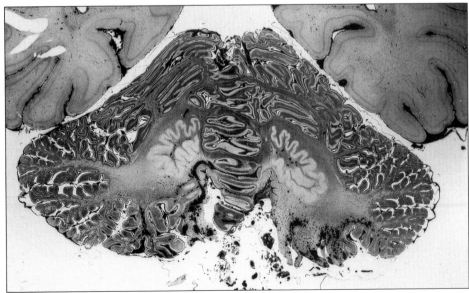

Fig. 222

A Case of **Maternal diabetic condition; dysmaturity and anemia of the newborn.**

This was a 19-year-old mother with a poor reproductive history, three previous miscarriages. The mother had a diabetic condition, with 3+ glucose and acetone in the urine. The mother had had an ongoing otitis media during the last five months of the pregnancy. Also, she had had cystitis. Pregnancy was at term.

Premature rupture of membranes occurred 2 days before delivery. The mother developed sepsis with fever of 104 degrees. Labor lasted 18 hours, with little progress. The fetal heart became irregular. A cesarean section was done. At delivery, the umbilical cord was entangled, wrapped twice around the neck and around the left arm. The infant was meconium-stained and very pale; she weighed 5 pounds 11 ounces (2,560 grams), a small-for-dates dysmature term infant (Figure 223).

At delivery a fresh retroplacental hemorrhage was present, with approximately one-third of the placenta prematurely detached. The placenta, examined in the pathology laboratory, with the fresh blood clot detached, showed patchy old retroplacental hematoma deposits on the maternal surface (Figure 224).

The anemic dysmature infant responded to care after delivery but remained in poor condition in the nursery. At 17 hours seizures developed; seizures were controlled with anticonvulsants. During the second day, respiratory difficulty developed and the weakened infant died.

At autopsy, the skin was very pale. Body changes of congestive heart failure were present, with the heart dilated, distended with blood (Figure 225), with congestion of the viscera, and edema and congestion of the brain (Figure 226). Microscopically, the cerebrum showed hypoxic damage in the nerve cells in the cortex (Figure 227); hypoxic damaged nerve cells appear shrunken, dark staining, with loss of cellular detail (page 21).

This case demonstrates the compound effects of chronic and acute compromise of the fetus, the chronic effects on the fetus due to adversive maternal factors, with resulting dysmaturity and anemia in the newborn. The fetus was additionally acutely compromised by the retroplacental hemorrhage and the neck and arm entanglement of the umbilical cord.

Figure 223. Pale, anemic, term newborn, of low birth weight (5 pounds 11 ounces).

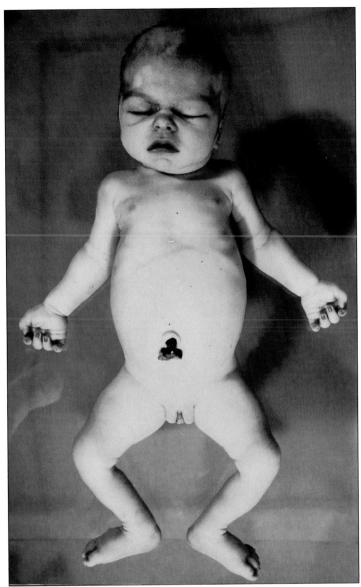

Fig. 223

Figure 224. Placenta with membranes. At delivery, premature detachment had occurred, with fresh blood clot covering about one-third of the placenta. The maternal surface, after the accumulation of fresh clot slipped away, showed marginal flat deposits of adherent old retroplacental hematoma.

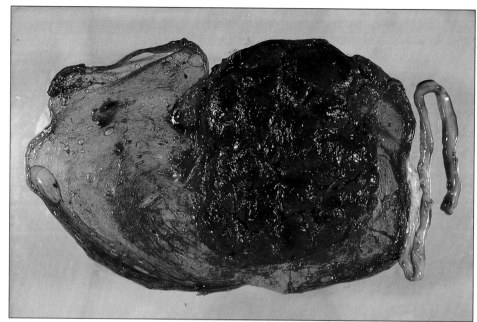

Fig. 224

Figure 225. The heart, distended with blood, in congestive heart failure.

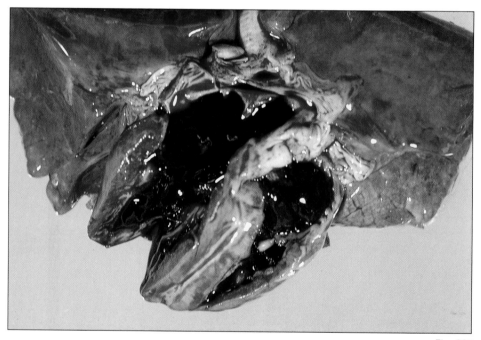

Fig. 225

Figure 226. Severe cerebral edema; convolutions flattened, the effect of hypoxic circulatory failure.

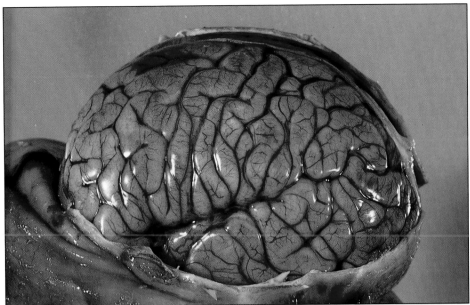

Fig. 226

Figure 227. Hypoxic damage to nerve cells in the cerebral cortex. The histologic section shows a group of dark, shrunken nerve cells, damaged by hypoxia, together with nerve cells relatively preserved, less affected by the hypoxic exposure.

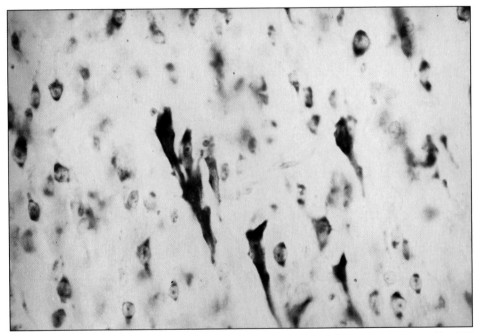

Fig. 227

A Case of **Brain stem and spinal cord injury; breech presentation with difficulty in delivery of the aftercoming head.**

This was a difficult breech birth, with prolonged labor and difficulty in delivering the trunk and aftercoming head.

The mother's previous pregnancy had terminated with a stillbirth after a prolonged labor.

In the present case, premature labor occurred at 35 weeks; labor lasted 8 hours. Breech extraction was carried out under spinal anesthesia. There was difficulty in rotating the trunk and delivering the arms. Considerable difficulty was encountered in delivering the aftercoming head, the cervix being tightly clamped about the neck. Extraction of the head was attempted unsuccessfully with forceps; ultimately the head was delivered by traction, with a finger placed in the infant's mouth (page 134).

The newborn infant was severely depressed, apneic. He remained cyanotic and hypotonic during the 2 1/2 hours of life.

Autopsy showed major spinal injury and brain stem damage.

The spine showed fracture of the third thoracic vertebra, laceration of the dura, and crushing transsection of the thoracic cord. Also there was paravertebral hemorrhage with extension of the hemorrhage into both pleural cavities.

The brain stem was encased in blood. Stretch injury of the brain stem had occurred, with tearing of the cerebellar peduncles and other structures about the fourth ventricle (Figure 228).

Spinal cord and brain stem damage result from exposure to excessive mechanical stress applied to the spinal axis in the form of hyperflexion, hyperextension, forceful traction, or forceful torsion (page 138).

In the present case spinal damage initially may have occurred internally, due to hyperflexion of the spinal column in the breech presentation. Plainly, the main damage occurred during the traction in delivering the trunk and in forceful manipulation in delivering the entrapped aftercoming head.

Figure 228. Brain stem injury incurred at delivery. Stretch injury with laceration and hemorrhage involving cerebellar peduncles and other structures about the fourth ventricle. Clinically, a complicated breech extraction with difficulty in delivering the aftercoming head. Postmortem examination revealed a major spinal injury as well as the stretch injury of the brain stem.

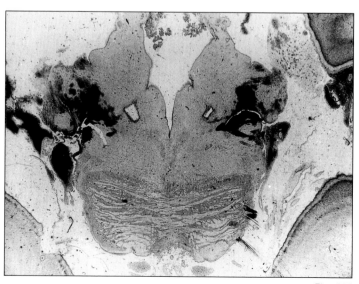

Fig. 228

A Case of   *Periventricular hemorrhagic infarction with intraventricular hemorrhage in a premature newborn of 24 weeks' gestation who lived 38 hours.*

The mother was admitted leaking foul-smelling amniotic fluid. The mother's temperature was 102 degrees.

The infant had an Apgar score of 4 at five minutes.

The infant remained depressed, with poor vital signs, failed to respond to care, and died at 38 hours.

The brain specimen showed massive periventricular infarction and intraventricular hemorrhage (Figure 229). The bleeding had extended through the ventricles, through the foramina in the fourth ventricle, with the consequent subarachnoid hemorrhage around the brain stem observed at autopsy (Figure 230).

Although molding of the head of a severe degree was present (Figure 231), it is pertinent to emphasize that the molding did not cause the brain hemorrhage that occurred (page 130); the intracranial hemorrhage was due to hypoxic cerebral damage.

The placenta showed acute chorioamnionitis with placentitis (Figure 232), accounting for the foul-smelling amniotic fluid and the mother's sepsis (page 88).

Figure 229. Massive periventricular and intraventricular hemorrhage; hemorrhage through the third ventricle and in the subarachnoid space around the base of the brain stem. Gross section (in celloidin) through the midportion of the cerebrum.

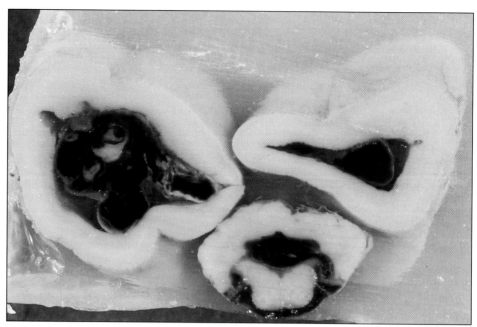

Fig. 229

Figure 230. Ventral view of the brain; subarachnoid hemorrhage about the brain stem. Extension of blood through the ventricular system resulting in blood in the subarachnoid space.

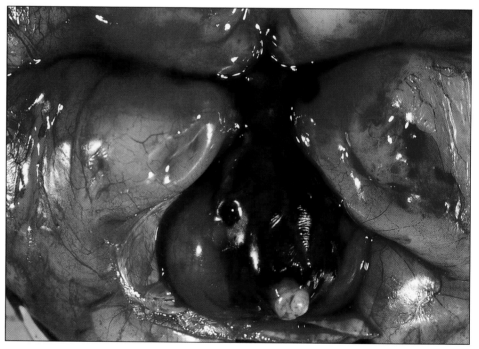

Fig. 230

Figure 231. Severe vertical molding of the head due to prolonged labor.

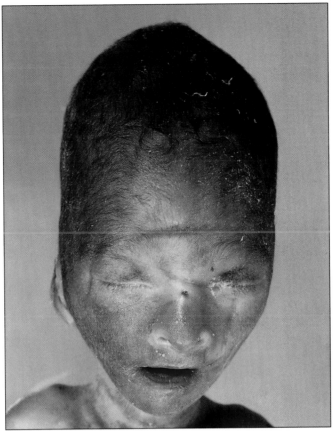

Fig. 231

Figure 232. Acute chorioamnionitis. Microscopic section of the membranes, the amniotic sac, showing diffuse infiltration of deeply staining acute inflammatory cells.

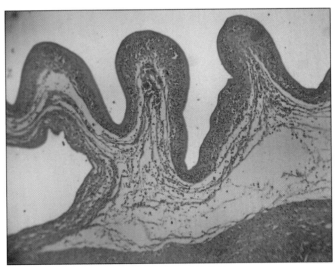

Fig. 232

A Case of   *Spinal injury in a premature newborn; death due to respiratory depression.*

This infant was prematurely delivered at 30 weeks of gestation. Birth was spontaneous, a vaginal delivery, cephalic presentation. Apgar score was 4 at five minutes. The newborn infant was limp and showed gradually deepening respiratory depression with apnea and expired after 16 hours (page 138).

The main findings at autopsy were in the spinal cord structures. Epidural hemorrhage was present through the length of the spinal canal. The spinal cord showed patchy thick deposits of blood adhering to the dura (Figure 233). Pathologic examination of the cord at serial levels revealed epidural hemorrhage and laceration of the dura; spinal roots were torn, surrounded by hemorrhage (Figure 234).

This case demonstrates an example of spontaneous intrinsic injury to spinal cord structures, developing during birth, in a fragile premature fetus compressed and forced through the birth canal at a time when the birth canal is still tight, unrelaxed physiologically, not prepared for passage of the fetus.

Figure 233. Spinal cord with dura; gross specimen. Epidural accumulations of blood. Premature delivery; cephalic presentation. Clinically, respiratory depression at birth; death after 16 hours.

Figure 234. Histologic section through the cervical portion of the spinal cord shown in Figure 233. Epidural hemorrhage; dural hemorrhage at the exit of spinal nerve root.

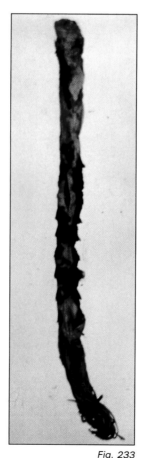

Fig. 233

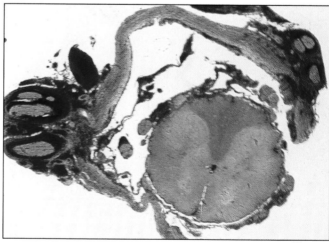

Fig. 234

A Case of **_Spinal cord injury; intranatal death during delivery of a large, macrosomic fetus; maternal diabetes._**

The mother was admitted to the hospital after being in labor over seven hours. The mother had borne three children previously. Apparently there had been little prenatal care. The pregnancy was thought to be post-term, at 43 weeks by dates.

At the time of admission, membranes had ruptured; there was leakage of meconium-stained amniotic fluid. Labor progressed very slowly. The head was delivered with difficulty. The fetus was alive at this time. Further difficulty developed in delivering the shoulders; a shoulder impaction developed. Effort was made to rotate the shoulders to overcome the shoulder dystocia. During the eight-minute period required to manipulate and deliver the shoulders, fetal death occurred (page 138).

At autopsy, the fetus was very large, weighed 5,120 grams (11 pounds 3 ounces) and was 55 centimeters (22 inches) long.

Maternal diabetes was suspected in this case because of the very large, macrosomic, fetus. Macrosomia often is the first sign of maternal diabetes. Further, at autopsy, in the pancreas there was hyperplasia of the islets, the tissue that produces insulin; this pathologic finding is common in offspring of diabetic mothers. With the diabetic mother producing inadequate insulin, the fetus tries to augment the insulin supply of the maternal-fetal system.

At autopsy extensive spinal injury was evident. The soft tissue around the neck, around the cervical spine, showed extravasation of blood. Hemorrhagic lesions were present in the meninges and spinal cord. The spinal cord grossly showed epidural hemorrhage from the fourth cervical to the midthoracic levels.

Microscopically, the spinal cord showed heavy epidural hemorrhage and laceration of the dura (Figure 235). Focal injury to the substance of the cord, focal and confluent hemorrhage, was present.

Spinal injury in this case was plainly due to fetal dystocia, to mechanical stress applied in rotation and traction on the spinal axis in dislodging the impacted shoulder and in delivering this large fetus.

Figure 235. Epidural spinal hemorrhage. Microscopic section of the cervical cord; a large epidural hemorrhage, a thick deposit of blood on the left side of the dura. At the upper right, there is laceration of the dura and escape of blood into the subdural space.

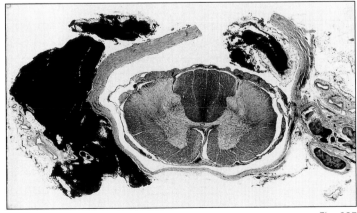

Fig. 235

A Case of   *Subacute cerebral damage present at birth in a term infant.*

Maternal hepatitis had occurred during the last weeks of gestation. The pregnancy was maintained to term. The infant was stillborn.

The brain at autopsy, disproportionately small, in the cranial vault was loosely suspended from the dura by strands of thick veins. The frontoparietal portion of the right cerebrum, with arachnoid removed, was smooth, of rubbery texture; posteriorly, superficial cerebral veins were dilated, filled with thromboses (Figure 236).

Figure 237, a section through the cerebrum, shows extreme destruction of the cerebral walls, creating a hydranencephalic structure (page 29).

The cerebral infarction, subacute pathologically, several weeks old, reflects the effects of an intrauterine hypoxia-producing process during the period of maternal illness prior to delivery (page 24).

Figure 236. Subacute cerebral damage subsequent to maternal hepatitis during the last trimester. Term gestation; infant stillborn. Cerebral surface showing far-advanced old, subacute, infarctional damage. Right frontoparietal region smooth, rubbery, leathery; posterior of the right cerebral surface covered with a network of large thrombosed veins. Posterior of the left hemisphere similarly affected, destroyed. The left hemisphere anteriorly, with surface convolutional pattern appearing preserved.

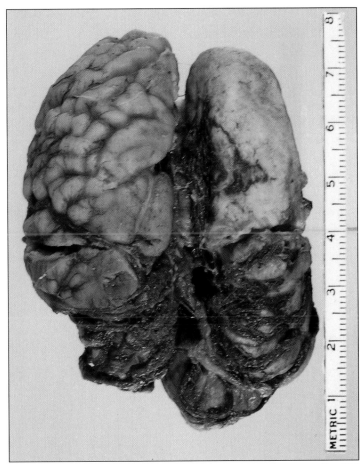

Fig. 236

Figure 237. A histologic section through the whole cerebrum reveals the cerebrum reduced to a hydranencephalic structure, with destruction, scarring, and thinning of the walls, with consequent great enlargement of the ventricles; the cerebrum that remains appears as two bladder-like hemispheres. The preserved convolutional pattern of the left cerebrum (Figure 236) turns out to be a facade, masking the extreme destruction of the underlying hemispheric wall. Of importance pathologically is the presence of the large surface veins distended with thrombus material.

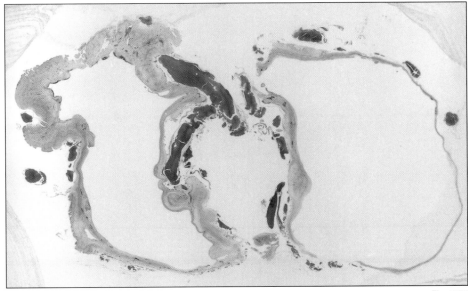

Fig. 237

A Case of   *Subacute cerebral damage in the fetus; twin transfusion syndrome.*

Premature labor ensued at 34 weeks of gestation. Labor lasted 5 hours. The first twin delivered was active and alert. The second twin, delivered eight minutes later, was stillborn. Fetal heart tones of both twins had been audible at the beginning of labor. However, after delivery of the first baby (liveborn), it was found that there was no fetal heart audible, that intranatal death of the other fetus had occurred, fetal death during labor.

The infants were of unequal size, characteristic of the twin transfusion syndrome. The liveborn infant, apparently the recipient in the fetus-to-fetus placental transfusion process, weighed 2,600 grams (5 pounds 2 ounces). The stillborn infant, apparently the transfusion donor, weighed 1,460 grams (3 pounds 4 ounces).

(It is of note that the liveborn infant, although appearing in good condition postnatally, later developed cerebral palsy.)

The stillborn infant at autopsy revealed congestion of the viscera. The skin and the organs of the thorax and abdomen were generally well preserved.

The brain showed far advanced *subacute cerebral hypoxic damage.* The brain was edematous and externally showed severe congestion of surface veins. The cerebral convolutional pattern was preserved; convolutions were flattened by edematous swelling of the cerebrum (Figure 238).

The cerebrum, the inner structures, showed deep portions of the white matter with far-advanced old, subacute infarction (Figure 239). The deep white matter of the parieto-occipital regions showed focal infarctional necrosis, periventricular leucomalacia (page 18). The cerebral cortex was relatively well preserved, even in the regions overlying the large areas of cerebral infarction.

The cerebral veins, both on the cerebral surface and in the deep tributaries, were dilated, engorged with blood.

In summary, this is a classic example of the accumulation of subacute cerebral damage during intrauterine life, old damage originating long before birth in a chronically compromised fetus.

Figure 238. Cerebrum showing edematous swelling, flattening of convolutions; external surface overall intact.

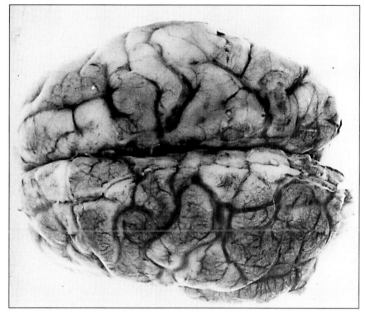

Fig. 238

Figure 239. Subacute cerebral damage in the (left) parieto-occipital region. Sagittal section of the cerebrum. Diffuse necrotic disintegration of the white matter. Overlying cortex relatively preserved.

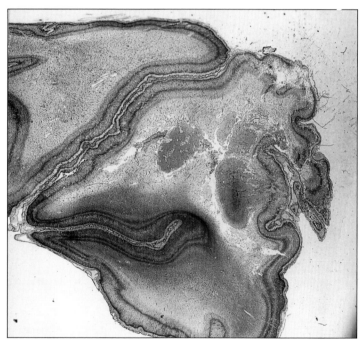

Fig. 239

A Case of   *Pneumothorax and pulmonary interstitial emphysema; trisomy 13.*

Severe respiratory distress developed rapidly; the infant presented multiple malformations.

This near-term infant was depressed at birth but responded to oxygen and positive pressure ventilation; subsequently the infant's respiration rapidly deteriorated, became increasingly labored, with depression of vital function, with death at 7 hours.

The infant showed multiple bodily abnormalities (Figure 240a). The eyes were small, microphthalmia. The forehead was long and slanting. The nose was broad and flat; cleft lip and palate were present. Polydactyly was present, with six toes on each foot (Figure 240b).

These stigmata were clinically suggestive of trisomy 13 (trisomy D) chromosome abnormality (page 147). The diagnosis was confirmed in the laboratory by chromosome analysis (Figure 241).

Clinically, of immediate concern was the rapid development of the severe respiratory distress that led to death. X-ray of the body at autopsy revealed pneumothorax, most evident in the left pleural cavity (Figure 242a). The intestinal tract showed ballooning distention with air (pneumo-intestinalis) as frequently occurs with positive pressure resuscitation.

At autopsy, corresponding to the x-ray findings, there was severe pneumothorax with compression atelectasis of the lungs (Figure 242b). The lung surfaces showed glistening air bubbles, characteristic of interstitial emphysema.

Visceral abnormalities characteristic of trisomy 13 were present at autopsy. The heart showed a malformation, a septal defect. The brain showed absence of the olfactory tracts, arhinencephaly.

Figure 240(a). Trisomy 13 (trisomy D). External bodily characteristics: long slanted forehead; microphthalmia; broad flat nose; cleft lip and palate; distortion of limbs.

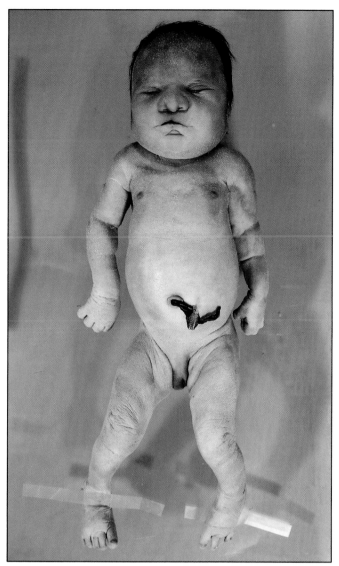

Fig. 240(a)

Figure 240(b). Polydactyly (six toes); trisomy 13.

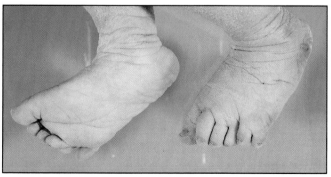

(b)

Figure 241. Trisomy 13 karyotype. The paired chromosomes in groups 13 to 15 are similar; an extra chromosome, a third, is present at the 13 location (arrow).

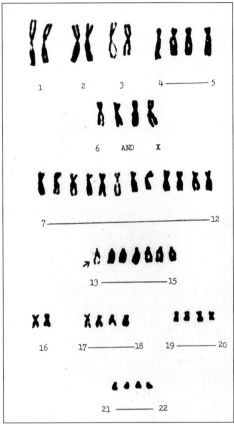

Fig. 241

Figure 242(a). Pneumothorax. Whole-body x-ray, postmortem. The left pleural space is filled with air, appears empty; severe pneumothorax. The lung is compressed, out of sight. The intestinal tract, distended with air, a complication of positive pressure resuscitation.

Figure 242(b). Pneumothorax; pneumo-intestinalis. Body viscera viewed at autopsy. Corresponding to the x-ray (a), the left pleural sac appears empty, with the lung compressed into the posterior of the thoracic cavity. Interstitial emphysema present, with many small shiny air bubbles on the lung surface. The loops of intestine are greatly distended with air, corresponding to the appearance in the x-ray.

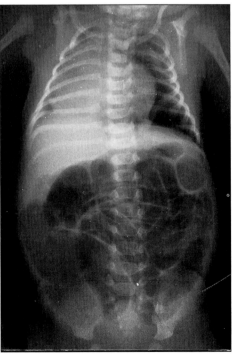

Fig. 242(a)

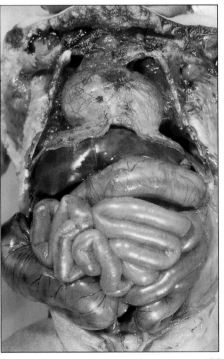

(b)

A Case of   *Premature detachment of the placenta, vaginal bleeding; maternal sudden exsanguinating intrauterine hemorrhage; shock.*

The mother, at 34 weeks of pregnancy, developed bright red vaginal bleeding at home. After admission to the hospital, vaginal bleed stopped. At 12 hours after admission, the mother complained of faintness; she went into shock, with the blood pressure dropping to 80/56. The uterus became enlarged and woody hard.

A stillborn infant was delivered by cesarean section. The placenta was found floating free in about 1,500 milliliters of blood in the uterine cavity.

The placenta, examined after delivery, had a large blood clot on the maternal surface, a retroplacental hematoma, weighing 170 grams (Figures 243a and b).

The stillborn infant was cyanotic and noticeably edematous overall (Figure 243a).

Intrauterine death was attributable to fetal hypoxic congestive heart failure. At autopsy, the heart was large, dilated, distended with blood; lungs were congested (Figure 244). Liver and spleen were enlarged, congestive hepatosplenomegaly (Figure 245); the brain was edematous, congested (Figure 246).

This case demonstrates the sequence of pathologic processes affecting the mother and fetus consequent to acute placental abruption (page 66).

Figure 243. Retroplacental
hematoma. **(a).** Cyanosis and
edema of the newborn infant.
(b). Placenta transected, with
adherent retroplacental
hematoma.

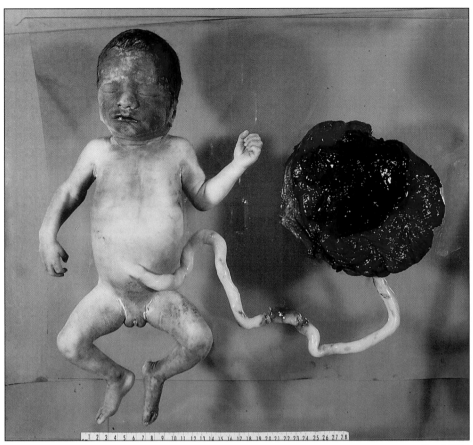

Fig. 243(a)

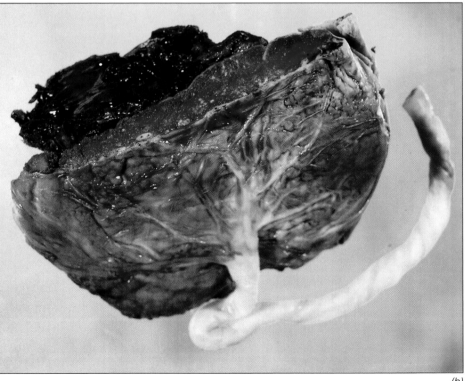

(b)

Figure 244. Congestive heart failure. Enlarged heart, dilated, distended with blood. Lungs congested.

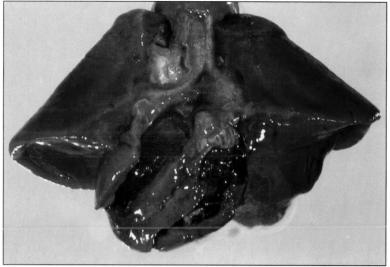

Fig. 244

Figure 245. Liver and spleen enlarged, congestive hepato-splenomegaly. Abdominal viscera viewed at autopsy.

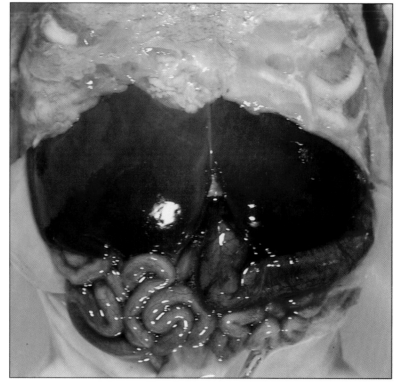

Fig. 245

Figure 246. Congestion of brain; edema and flattening of the cerebral convolutions.

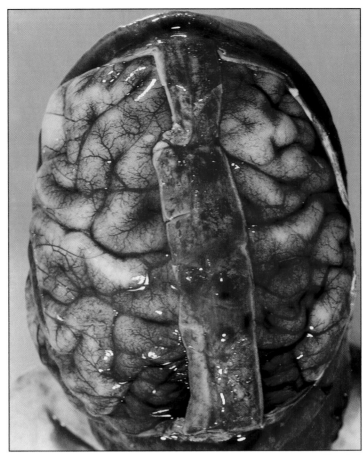

Fig. 246

A Case of *Nuchal cord; intrauterine meconium aspiration pneumonia.*

The mother apparently had had no prenatal care and was alone at the time of birth. Birth occurred at term.

According to the mother, the infant was stillborn, showed no signs of life, no respiration.

At autopsy, externally there was a strikingly noticeable pale ring on the skin of the neck (Figures 247a and b); this is characteristic of the encircling imprint made by a nuchal cord (page 83).

Meconium aspiration pneumonia was present (page 108). The lung, microscopically, showed many large meconium-stained cells and meconium-stained aspirated amniotic fluid (Figure 248).

Meconium is a chemical irritant in the fetal lung; when aspiration occurs, hours or days before birth, a chemical pneumonia develops in utero.

In the present case it is evident that the nuchal cord was tight and present for a long time. The consequent fetal hypoxia stimulated respiratory effort by the fetus, with resulting meconium aspiration. Intrauterine pneumonia developed (Figure 249).

Had this infant lived, the full-blown effects of the meconium aspiration syndrome would have ensued clinically.

Figure 247. Nuchal cord imprint; two views of the neck (**a** and **b**) showing a sharply demarcated pale ring, the impression in the skin caused by the umbilical cord being wrapped around the neck. Associated cyanosis of the body.

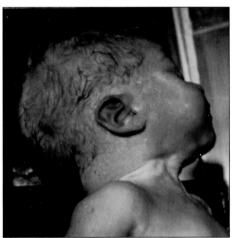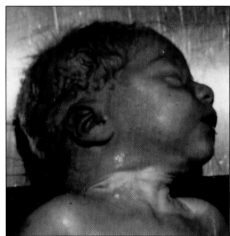

Fig. 247(a)   *(b)*

Figure 248. Meconium aspiration; microscopic section of the lung. At the upper right, brown-stained aspirated amniotic fluid material; alveoli with aspirated pigmented bubble-like elements.

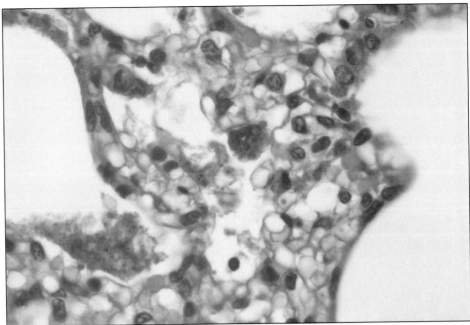

Fig. 248

Figure 249. Intrauterine meconium pneumonia. Microscopic section of lung showing a small bronchus surrounded by heavy infiltration of inflammatory cells, pathologically a form of bronchopneumonia.

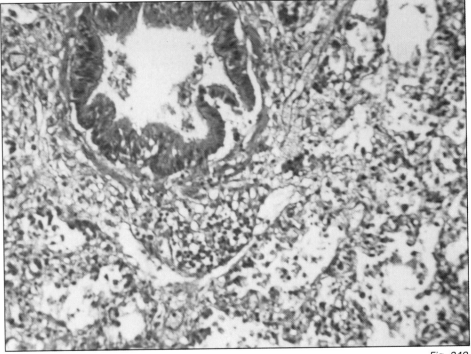

Fig. 249

A Case of ***Potter's syndrome with cystic kidneys; pneumothorax; posterior fossa subdural hemorrhage. Oligohydramnios.***

Persistent transverse presentation was present. Delivery was by cesarean section. Oligohydramnios was noted at delivery.

The infant, born at term, was small (5 pounds 6 ounces) and pale.

At delivery it was noted that the infant was dysmorphic; the ears were low placed, large, floppy (Figure 250). It was suspected that this infant was an example of Potter's syndrome (page 91), a genetic disorder characterized by a combination of ear deformities and kidney abnormalities. This impression was confirmed later at autopsy with the finding of hypoplastic cystic kidneys (Figure 251).

Relative to this, the oligohydramnios previously noted at delivery, is attributable to the failure of the kidneys to produce urine, the main constituent of amniotic fluid. Lack of amniotic fluid had caused compression distortion of the feet (Figure 250).

After the delivery the infant was depressed and required positive pressure resuscitation. The infant responded at first with improved respiration; however, he later developed severe respiratory distress. X-ray of the chest revealed bilateral tension pneumothorax with collapse of the lungs. Despite efforts to relieve the trapped air by inserting a tube into the thoracic cavity, the infant died at 5 hours. The pneumothorax was attributable to the positive pressure ventilation (page 111).

At autopsy, pneumothorax of a severe extent was demonstrated, with compression atelectasis of both lungs (Figure 252).

Molding distortion of the head had accrued during labor (page 130). Excessive compression of the head that had occurred due to the transverse presentation and to the oligohydramnios, caused irregular molding of the cranial bones, with depression displacement inward of the right parietal bone (Figure 253).

The molding distortion of the cranium led to a stretch-tear of the tentorium (page 131); bleeding from the tentorial tear caused posterior fossa subdural hemorrhage (Figures 254 and 255).

Figure 250. Potter's syndrome. Abnormality of the ears: large, low placed, floppy. Distortion of the feet, flexed and turned inward, due to intrauterine compression of the fetus resulting from lack of amniotic fluid, oligohydramnios, in this case. Infant, pale; intrauterine growth retardation; term infant weighed 5 pounds 6 ounces.

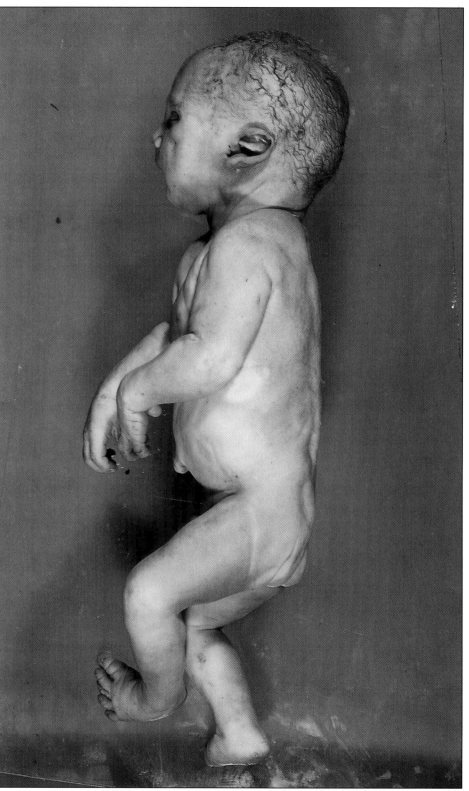

Fig. 250

Figure 251. Cystic hypoplastic kidney, related to Potter's syndrome. The kidney(s), less than one-half average size for a term newborn, with many small shiny bubble-like cysts on the surface.

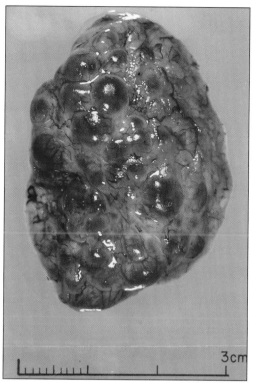

3cm

Fig. 251

Figure 252. Pneumothorax. At autopsy, the thoracic cavities with large vacant dark spaces devoid of lung structure. The lungs, compressed and small, with many minute shiny emphysematous blebs present on the surface and in the tissue around the pericardial sac.

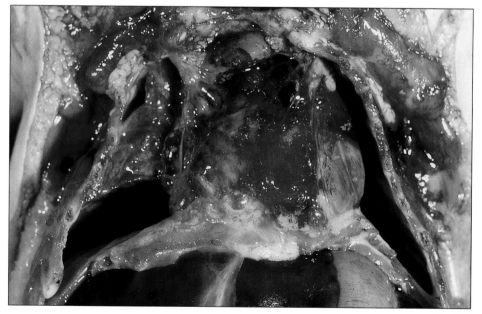

Fig. 252

Figure 253. Molding of the head, of irregular form, with depression of the right parietal bone; overlapping of the right frontal and left parietal onto the right parietal bone.

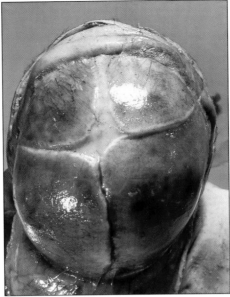

Fig. 253

Figure 254. Posterior fossa subdural hemorrhage. At autopsy, the cerebrum retracted posteriorly exposes the posterior cranial fossa, with blood in the subdural space around the brain stem.

Figure 255. Tentorial stretch-laceration. The temporal-occipital cerebral structures are retracted upward by gloved fingers, exposing the upper surface of the tentorium. An oval dehiscence, a tear, is present in the mid-upper portion of the tentorium. Posterior fossa hemorrhage due to bleeding from the tentorial laceration.

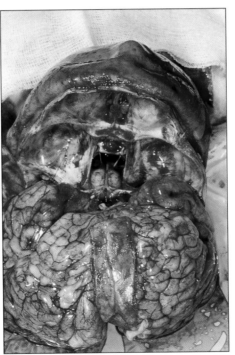

Fig. 254

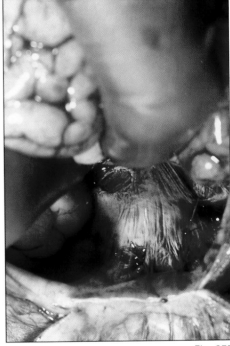

Fig. 255

A Case of   *Premature rupture of membranes; chorioamnionitis; dysmaturity; hyaline membrane disease.*

Premature rupture of membranes occurred at 28 weeks of pregnancy. At 37 hours after the rupture, with signs of fetal distress developing, a cesarean section was done. The amniotic fluid was cloudy and foul smelling. The newborn infant had spontaneous respiration with good heart action, with occasional spontaneous movements. The infant showed evidence of intrauterine growth retardation, weighing 765 grams (average weight at 28 weeks, 1,100 grams) (Figure 256).

Respiratory distress developed and the infant died at 5 hours.

The placenta microscopically showed severe chorioamnionitis with a heavy infiltration of acute inflammatory cells extending through the membranes (Figure 257).

At autopsy, congestive heart failure was evident, with congestion of the brain and other viscera, with congestive enlargement of the liver and spleen. Adrenal infarction was present (Figure 258), resulting from vein thrombosis.

The lungs showed hyaline membrane disease (Figure 259); this was consistent with prematurity of the infant (page 106).

Figure 256. Premature newborn; 28 weeks' gestational age. Intrauterine growth retardation; infant's weight, 765 grams (average for 28 weeks, 1,100 grams).

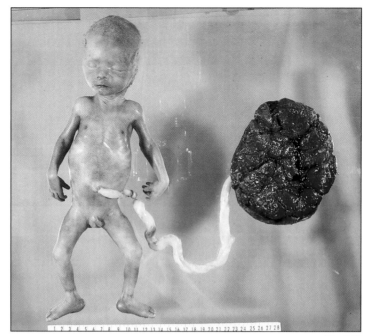

Fig. 256

Figure 257. Chorioamnionitis. Histologic section through the amniotic surface of the placenta. The amniotic surface, upper portion of the illustration, coated with a thick layer of inflammatory exudate.

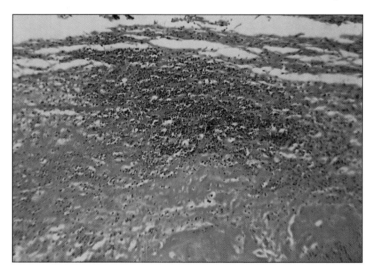

Fig. 257

Figure 258. Adrenal, cut surface, with circumscribed hemorrhagic infarction. Microscopic study showed thrombosis of adrenal veins.

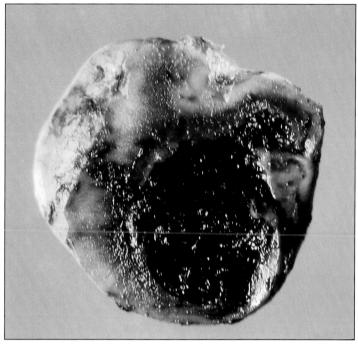

Fig. 258

Figure 259. Hyaline membrane disease; microscopic section of lung. Dilated alveolar sacs with some alveoli partly lined with thick pink glassy "hyaline" material.

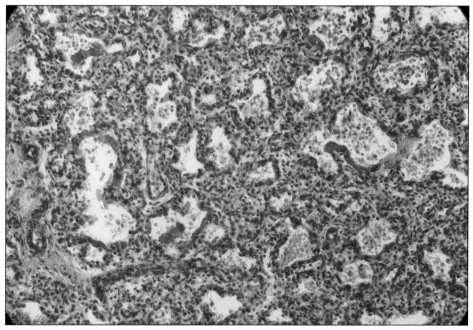

Fig. 259

A Case of **Premature rupture of membranes; chorioamnionitis. Newborn infant with congestive heart failure; intracerebral hemorrhagic infarcts.**

Rupture of membranes occurred 5 weeks before delivery. The newborn infant, of 26 weeks' gestational age, was severely depressed at birth and died at 4 hours.

The placenta showed far-advanced chorioamnionitis (Figure 260), attributable to the long existing premature rupture of the membranes (page 87).

Congestive heart failure was evident at autopsy, with engorgement of veins and dilated right heart (Figure 261). Viscera were congested. The brain at autopsy was edematous and congested.

The brain showed periventricular hemorrhagic infarction and intraventricular hemorrhage (Figure 262), consequent to hypoxic congestive heart failure.

Figure 260. Chorioamnionitis and placentitis. Histologic section through the amniotic surface of the placenta. The amnion appears in a convoluted pattern at the right and above. Acute inflammatory cells, deep-staining cells, extend from the amnion diffusely in the underlying placental tissue, forming an inflammatory exudate.

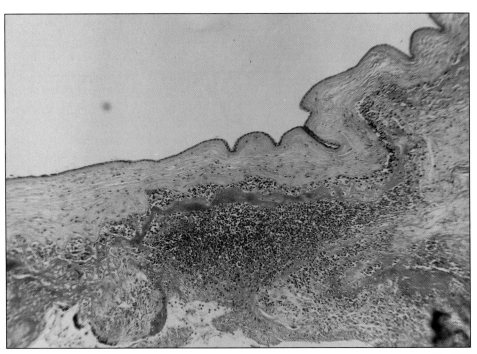

Fig. 260

Figure 261. Congestive heart failure. Venous stasis, engorged large veins draining into the distended right atrium, pattern characteristic of "backward" congestive failure.

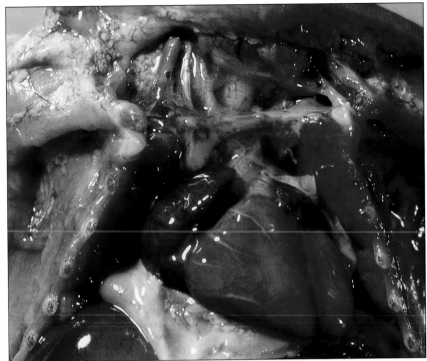

Fig. 261

Figure 262. Hemorrhagic periventricular germinal matrix infarction, consequence of congestive heart failure. Intraventricular hemorrhage from extension of bleeding from periventricular hemorrhagic infarcts. Accumulation of dark blood clot appears in the infarcted periventricular hemorrhage. Serial gross sections of the brain embedded in plastic.

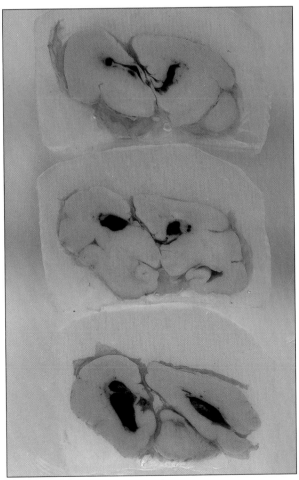

Fig. 262

A Case of **Subacute, old, cerebral hypoxic damage. Newborn polycythemia, the hyperviscosity syndrome.**

This pregnancy was complicated by a severe viral infection of the mother at 31 weeks of gestation. Pregnancy was maintained to term.

The newborn infant was severely depressed, with respiratory distress and cyanosis. Death occurred at 31 hours of age.

Of importance clinically was the finding of the newborn hematocrit of 73 percent indicating neonatal polycythemia. The average hematocrit at term is 61 percent. Hematocrit levels above 65 percent are indicative of polycythemia, the hyperviscosity syndrome (page 104).

The baby weighed 2,770 grams (6 pounds 1 ounce). At autopsy the heart was large; severe congestion of the viscera was present. Veins of the body were engorged; small vessels were described as "choked" with conglutinated blood.

The head size, 33 centimeters in circumference, was average. At autopsy the cranial cavity, surprisingly, was occupied by murky watery fluid and, at the base of the skull, was a shrunken small brain (Figure 263).

The brain weighed 130 grams (average brain weight at term is 358 grams). Externally, the convolutional pattern of the cerebrum was grossly distorted.

Figure 264 (the cerebrum in a whole-brain histologic section of the brain) shows far-advanced old, subacute, cerebral periventricular infarction (page 24). Significantly, the surface layer of the cerebrum was relatively preserved. This pattern of damage, predominantly deep periventricular infarction, indicates the causal hypoxic insult occurred when the cerebrum was premature, immature, corresponding to the time of the acute maternal viral illness two months before term.

The shrunken brain, its smallness, was due to the loss of deep cerebral substance.

As to the pathogenesis of the cerebral infarction: With polycythemia the vascular system is overloaded with viscous, thickened blood (the hyperviscosity syndrome), causing congestive heart failure, as in this case. With hyperviscosity, blood flow is slowed, leading to stasis-thrombosis. The cerebral infarcts in this case are attributable to the thrombosis of deep cerebral veins.

Figure 263. Small shrunken brain, about one third the average size of a term newborn brain. (Decreased size due to loss of deep cerebral substance; see Figure 264.)

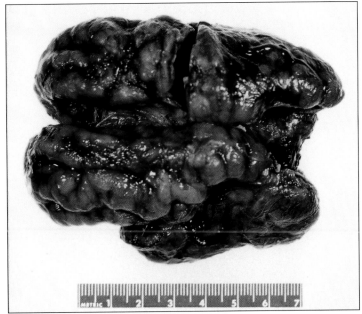

Fig. 263

Figure 264(a). Subacute, old, periventricular cerebral infarction. Whole-brain histologic section. The deep periventricular pink-staining areas are devitalized subacute infarctions.

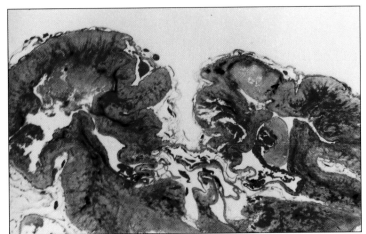

Fig. 264(a)

Figure 264(b). Higher magnification of a portion of the histologic section of (a). The surface layer of the cerebrum, relatively preserved, is separated from the deep infarcted tissue by an irregular hemorrhagic layer of tissue.

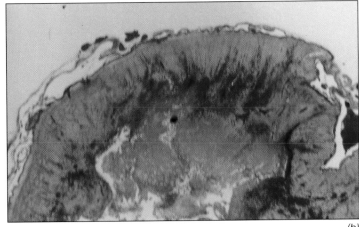

(b)

A Case of   ***Chorioamnionitis; maternal sepsis. Prematurity;
               footling breech delivery; fetus with posterior fossa
               subdural hemorrhage.***

The mother reported leaking of amniotic fluid, indicating premature rupture of membranes, at 23 weeks of gestation, a week before delivery. Culture of the leaking amniotic fluid revealed *Staphylococcus albus*. The amniotic fluid became purulent. The mother became septic, with fever of 104 degrees.

This was a footling breech presentation; the premature rupture of the membranes is attributable to protrusion of the fetus' foot through the amniotic sac, through the cervix into the vagina (page 88).

With footling presentation, the protruding leg is rendered edematous and reddened (Figure 265).

The infant died 5 hours after birth.

Examination of the placenta and membranes revealed purulent chorioamnionitis (Figure 266).

Autopsy revealed an intracranial, posterior fossa, subdural hemorrhage (Figure 267). In this breech birth, with delivery of the aftercoming head, apparent stretch-tearing of the dura occurred, resulting in the posterior fossa hemorrhage, the immediate cause of death (page 133).

Figure 265. Footling presentation; the left leg, protruding during delivery, became edematous and reddened.

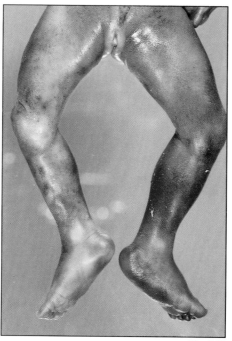

Fig. 265

Figure 266. Chorioamnionitis. Section through the amnion (above) and extending into the underlying placental tissue. Hematoxylin-eosin stain. The deep layer of the tissue section shows an irregular thick blue-staining deposit of acute inflammatory cells, purulent chorioamnionitis.

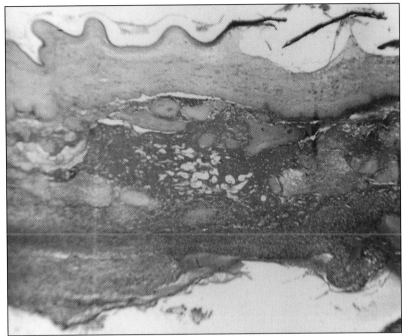

Fig. 266

Figure 267. Intracranial posterior fossa subdural hemorrhage. Autopsy view of the base of the skull, with the cerebrum raised and laid back, exposing the ventral structures of the brain. The midportion of the illustration shows the posterior fossa of the cranial cavity; the sides of the tentorium have been removed, exposing the pons lying in the posterior fossa. Surrounding the pons is a lake of fresh blood that filled the posterior fossa (some of the blood escaped during the dissection).

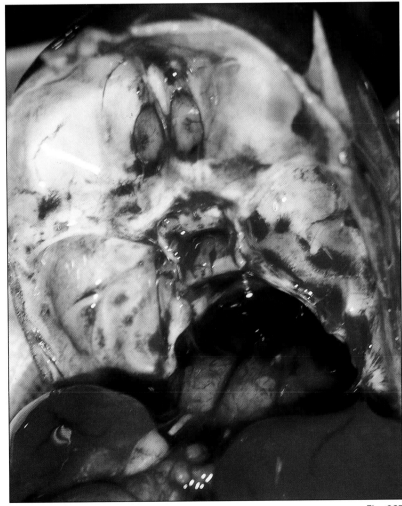

Fig. 267

A Case of   *Loss of fetal activity; placental infarction; retroplacental hemorrhage; intrauterine death with congestive heart failure.*

The mother, at term, reported decreased fetal activity during the 10 days before delivery. Examination 7 days before delivery revealed good cardiac function. At delivery, however, intrauterine death was evident.

This case demonstrates the hypoxia-producing effects of premature detachment of the placenta (page 66) and placental infarction (page 71).

The placenta showed a retroplacental hemorrhage, a circumscribed crater partly occupied by adherent blood clot. On section, the placenta showed extensive old and recent areas of infarction lying in the bed of the hematoma crater (Figures 268 and 269).

Autopsy revealed that the fetus had died in congestive heart failure with findings of cardiac dilatation and hydrothorax present (Figures 270 and 271).

The decreased fetal activity is attributable to mounting intrauterine hypoxia due to the compromise of placental function by the retroplacental hemorrhage and the extensive placental infarction, processes that resulted in congestive heart failure, ultimately to fetal death.

Figure 268. Retroplacental hematoma. In the upper part of the placenta the surface shows a crater, created by retroplacental hemorrhage; surrounding the crater is an irregular broad expanse of pale (infarcted) tissue.

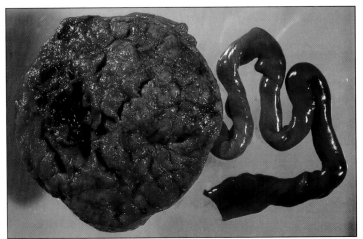

Fig. 268

Figure 269. Placental infarction. The placenta (after formalin fixation), sectioned through the area of retroplacental hematoma. Irregular broad mottled zone of recent (reddened) and old (yellowed) infarction extends outward from around the hematoma crater.

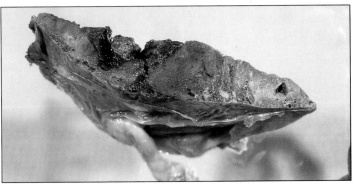

Fig. 269

Figure 270. Cardiac failure; heart dilated, distended with blood.

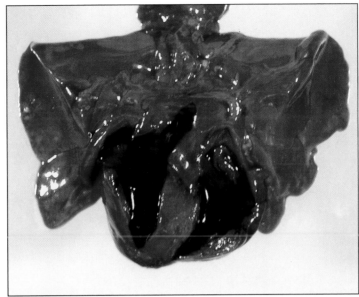

Fig. 270

Figure 271. Hydrothorax related to congestive heart failure. As depicted here, the right pleural cavity contained 7 milliliters of watery bloody fluid; the left, 15 milliliters. View of thoracic viscera at autopsy.

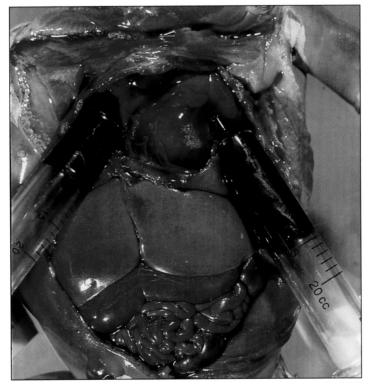

Fig. 271

*Maternal diabetes; maternal diabetic acidosis;
loss of fetal activity. Fetal death with congestive
heart failure; hydrothorax.*

This mother was an uncontrolled diabetic. She was admitted at 32 weeks of gestation with severe diabetic acidosis: glucosuria 4+, acetonuria 4+, blood sugar 490, electrolyte imbalance. The mother reported decreased fetal activity during the week before admission to the hospital.

Soon after admission there was loss of fetal heart tone, and a cesarean section was done. The infant was stillborn.

The infant appeared bloated, showing peripheral edema, puffiness of the face, the eyelids (Figure 272). There was focal denuding of the skin, maceration.

The placenta was large and edematous, characteristic of maternal diabetes.

Congestive heart failure was evident in the fetus, with the presence of hydrothorax (Figure 273) and ascites, in addition to the peripheral edema (page 9).

This case demonstrates the adverse effects on the fetus of uncontrolled maternal diabetes, diabetic acidosis, leading to decreased fetal activity, to fetal congestive heart failure, ultimately to fetal death.

Figure 272. Fetal death; mother with uncontrolled diabetes, with acute diabetic acidosis. Fetus with peripheral edema, puffiness of the face. Abdomen large and flabby (ascites); large edematous placenta.

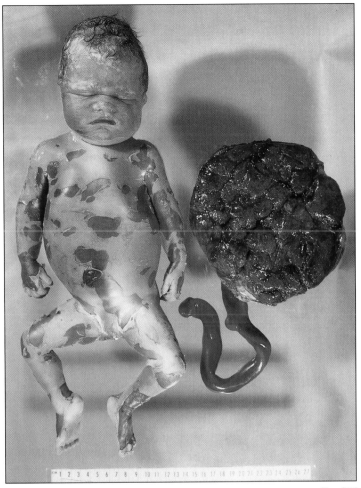

Fig. 272

Figure 273. Hydrothorax due to fetal hypoxic congestive heart failure.

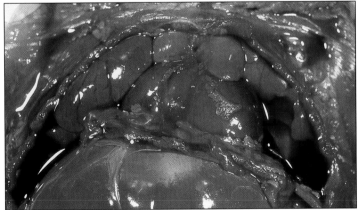

Fig. 273

A Case of   *Laceration of the cerebellum; premature delivery.*

This is an example of injury to the cerebellum due to herniation of the cerebellum into the foramen magnum during parturition (page 137). Birth occurred at 29 weeks of gestation.

At times, as in this case, the ventral surface of the cerebellum becomes compressed against the opposing sharp edges of the foramen, causing mangling hemorrhagic laceration of the folia (Figures 274 and 275).

Figure 274. Hemorrhagic physical injury of the right side of the cerebellum; ventral surface of the brain; 29 weeks' gestation. The right cerebellum, adjoining the brain stem, is fragmented and hemorrhagic, the result of cerebellar herniation into the foramen magnum.

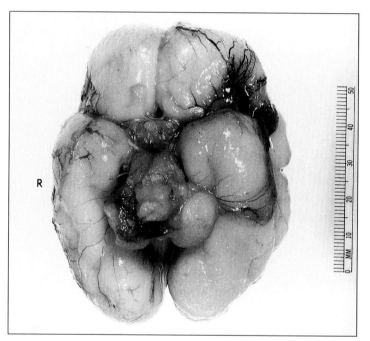

Fig. 274

Figure 275. Section through the brain stem and cerebellum showing hemorrhagic damage to the right cerebellar hemisphere, corresponding to that evident externally in Figure 274.

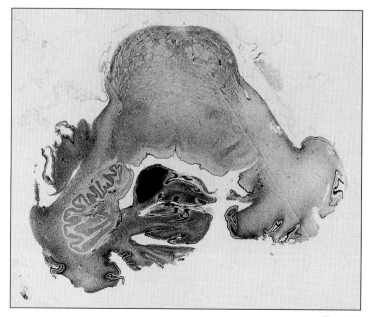

Fig. 275

A Case of   *Erythroblastosis fetalis with hydrops.*

The mother was Rh-negative. She had a history of three prior stillbirths. She was admitted at 28 weeks of gestation with premature rupture of membranes, with fever of 101.4 degrees.

The newborn infant showed characteristic changes of hydrops fetalis (page 98). The infant, stillborn, was of excessive weight, 1,580 grams (average for 28 weeks, 1,058 grams), due to the presence of hydrops; the infant had a bloated appearance, a puffiness about the face (Figure 276). The subcutaneous tissue was waterlogged, edematous (Figure 277). The abdomen was large, flabby, with a demonstrable fluid wave (ascites). Characteristic of erythroblastosis fetalis, the liver and spleen were enlarged (Figures 278a and b).

The brain was edematous. A subarachnoid collection of blood was present along the left side of the brain stem, lateral to the pons (Figure 279a). The subarachnoid hemorrhage had its origin from within the cerebrum, from a periventricular hemorrhagic infarct in the cerebral germinal matrix (Figure 279b).

Figure 276. Hydrops fetalis; Rh-negative mother. The infant edematous, with puffiness prominent about the face.

Figure 277. Subcutaneous edema, described at autopsy as "water runs freely from the sectioned surfaces."

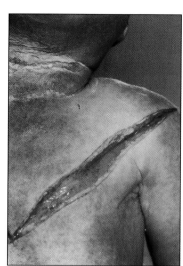

Fig. 277

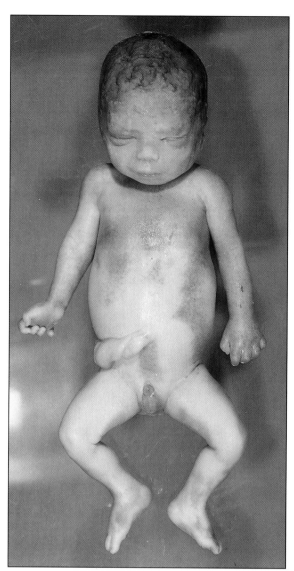

Fig. 276

Figure 278(a). Enlarged liver, characteristic of erythroblastosis. Body viscera exposed at autopsy.

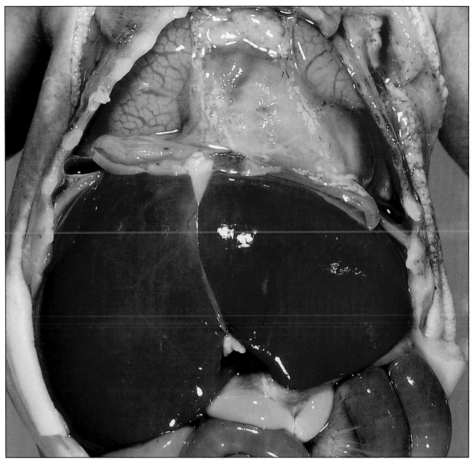

Fig. 278(a)

Figure 278(b). Spleen enlargement. (At autopsy, the abdominal viscera retracted to the right, exposing the large spleen.)

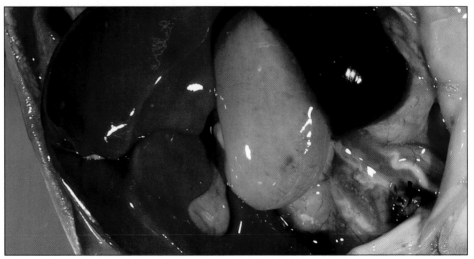

(b)

Figure 279(a). Edematous brain. Extravasation of subarachnoid blood along the left side of the brain stem.

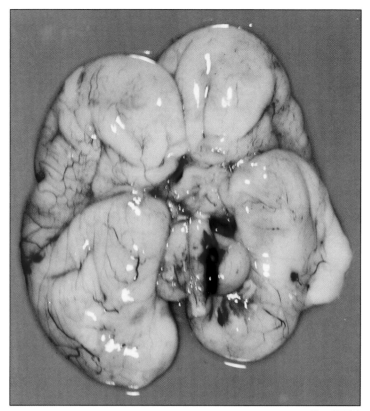

Fig. 279(a)

Figure 279(b). Cerebral periventricular matrix hemorrhagic infarction. (Brain specimen embedded in plastic, frontal section.) The origin of the subarachnoid hemorrhage, seen in (a), from the deep periventricular hemorrhage.

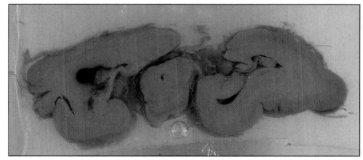

(b)

A Case of   ***Erythroblastosis fetalis; fetal hydrops;***
hepatosplenomegaly; jaundice.

The mother was a multipara, known to be Rh-negative, with a history of one stillbirth and one liveborn infant that required transfusion.

The pregnancy in this case was at term. During labor fetal distress became evident. The newborn infant was depressed, apneic, limp, failed to respond, and died 19 minutes after delivery.

The infant was large and hydropic, weighed 8 pounds 11 1/2 ounces. The infant showed obvious subcutaneous edema about the face, neck, and chest. The skin was pale, noticeably yellowed, jaundiced (Figure 280).

The placenta was boggy, large, and edematous, was 19 centimeters wide and up to 6 centimeters thick (Figure 281).

At autopsy, the abdomen was distended, contained 50 milliliters of clear amber watery ascitic fluid.

Hepatosplenomegaly was present. The greatly enlarged liver occupied over two-thirds of the abdominal cavity (Figure 282). The spleen likewise was about five times the normal size (Figure 283).

This case, the infant of an Rh-negative mother, presents the classic pathologic sequels of erythroblastosis fetalis: the newborn infant was pale (anemic), slightly jaundiced; had bodily edema, ascites; hepatosplenomegaly was present (page 145).

Figure 280. Erythroblastosis fetalis. Newborn infant bloated, edematous, pale and slightly jaundiced.

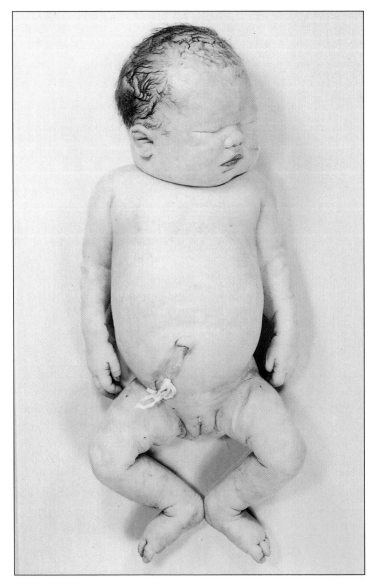

Fig. 280

Figure 281. Placenta, large, thick, and edematous, characteristic of erythroblastosis fetalis.

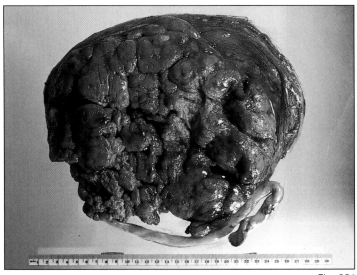

Fig. 281

Figure 282. Liver greatly enlarged. Abdominal viscera exposed at autopsy.

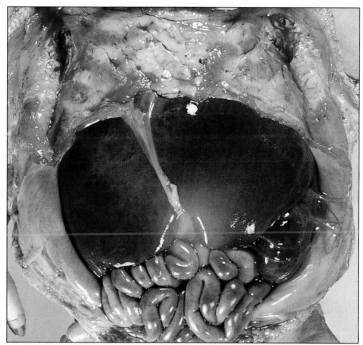

Fig. 282

Figure 283. Splenomegaly. Abdominal organs removed *en bloc* at autopsy.

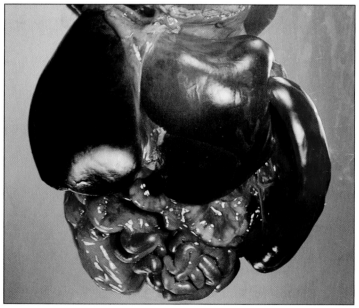

Fig. 283

A Case of   *Maternal influenzal infection; premature delivery, newborn with hyaline membrane disease; hypoxic cerebral damage.*

Premature labor developed at 30 weeks of pregnancy. The mother had had the flu during the previous week. There had been recurrent vaginal bleeding.

Delivery was precipitous. At birth the infant was depressed but improved, had an Apgar score of 7 at five minutes. Respirations were immediate, spontaneous; there was a weak cry.

The infant developed respiratory distress. Recurrent apnea began at 7 hours. Despite supportive efforts, the infant died at 15 hours.

Autopsy revealed a superficial liver injury, a subcapsular hemorrhage (Figure 284), referable to the precipitous delivery (page 102). More significant was the sequence of respiratory complications, with apnea and hyaline membrane disease (Figure 285) (page 106), leading to hypoxic cerebral damage, with cerebral periventricular hemorrhagic infarction, intraventricular hemorrhage, with subarachnoid hemorrhage (Figures 286 and 287).

Figure 284. Subcapsular hemorrhage of liver, related to the precipitous birth. View of abdominal viscera at autopsy.

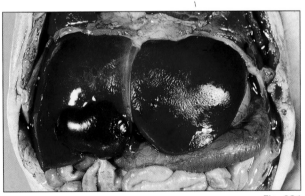

Fig. 284

Figure 285. Hyaline membrane disease. Histologic section of lung. In the midportion of the illustration are thick pink glassy deposits along the lining of the alveoli, the characteristic picture of hyaline membrane disease.

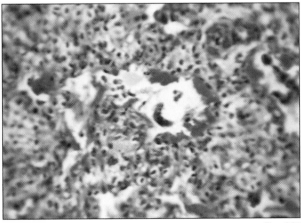

Fig. 285

Figure 286. Subarachnoid hemorrhage over the ventral aspect of the brain stem and cerebrum. The formalin, used to preserve the specimen, changes the color of the blood to dark brown.

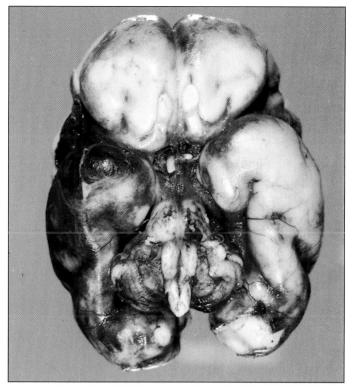

Fig. 286

Figure 287(a). The cerebrum, frontal section. On the left, a large hemorrhagic periventricular infarction and hemorrhage bulging into the ventricle.

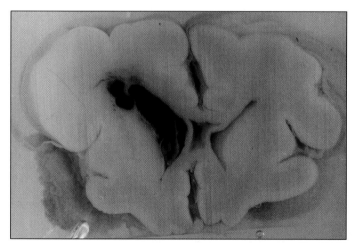

Fig. 287(a)

Figure 287(b). Extension of intracerebral hemorrhage into the fourth ventricle. A section through the posterior of the brain. Blood, escaping from the ventricular system and outward around the brain stem, giving rise to the subarachnoid hemorrhage seen in Figure 286.

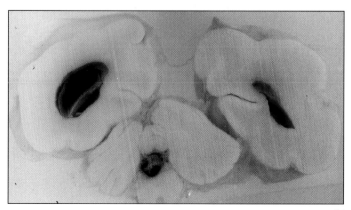

(b)

A Case of *Spinal injury in the newborn; respiratory distress syndrome (hyaline membrane disease).*

Labor developed at 37 weeks of pregnancy in this case. The mother had been sick with a sore throat prior to the onset of labor.

After prolonged labor, a cesarean section was done. The baby was in good condition at birth but soon developed respiratory distress. Respirations were grunting and labored. Chest x-rays revealed evidence of pneumonitis. The infant died after 2 1/2 days.

At autopsy there were significant pathologic findings in the spinal structures and in the lung. Examination of the spinal canal revealed a thick hemorrhagic deposit in the spinal epidural tissue, around the cord in the cervical and upper thoracic levels (Figures 288a and b). It is apparent that spinal damage contributed to early respiratory compromise that developed in this infant (page 138).

The lungs were large and heavy, mottled dark red, and of a firm consolidated consistency (Figure 289). The lung tissue, on section, was soggy and bloody.

Microscopically, the lung showed alveolar spaces crowded with inflammatory cells blotting out the normal lung architecture, a picture of far-advanced lung consolidation, pneumonitis (Figure 290a). Figure 290b shows alveoli with remnants of hyaline membrane deposits.

As a consequence of the postnatal pulmonary complication, the infant developed hypoxic congestive heart failure; this resulted in ascites and hydrothorax, together with edema and congestion of the brain and other body organs.

Figure 288(a). Spinal epidural hemorrhage. Autopsy view of the spinal canal, with the spinal cord removed. A thick extravasation of blood in the epidural tissues of the lower cervical and upper thoracic level.

Figure 288(b). Spinal cord, with dura in place around the cord. Blood clots, adherent to the dura, corresponding to the epidural hemorrhage in (a).

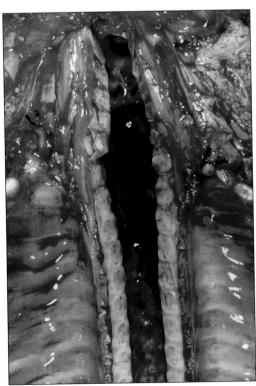
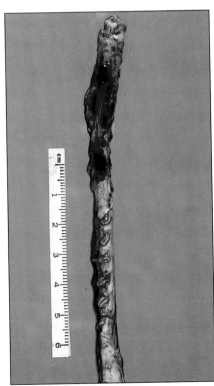

Fig. 288(a)   *(b)*

Figure 289. Hyaline membrane disease. The lungs at autopsy, large, dark red, of doughy consistency.

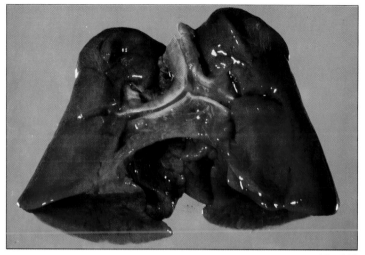

Fig. 289

Figure 290(a). Hyaline membrane disease. Histologic section of lung; an overall heavy consolidating infiltration of inflammatory cells.

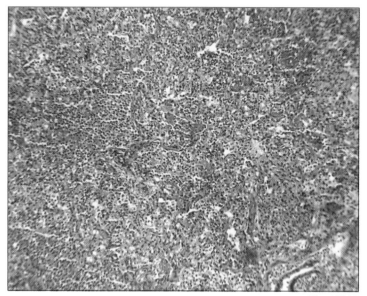

Fig. 290(a)

Figure 290(b). Hyaline membrane disease. Alveoli with hyaline membrane deposits, together with surrounding heavy inflammatory reaction.

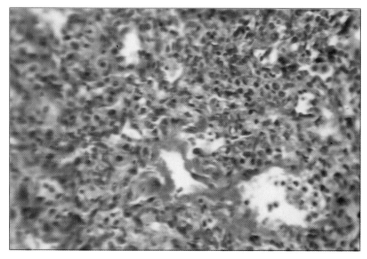

(b)

A Case of   *Hyaline membrane disease; neonatal hypoxic congestive heart failure.*

This infant, born at 36 weeks of gestation, was in good condition at birth but soon deteriorated, developing respiratory distress, with grunting respirations and cyanosis. The infant became lethargic, floppy, and appeared septic, with fever of 103.4 degrees. He developed increasing respiratory distress with grunting respiration.

X-ray of the chest soon after birth showed a noticeable amount of pneumothorax bilaterally, with changes of lung atelectasis. A second x-ray of the lung showed opacification of the lung fields and residual pneumothorax (Figure 291).

Death occurred at 16 hours.

At autopsy, there was pronounced cyanosis and slight jaundice of the skin. Most prominent was the appearance of the lungs — large, mottled dark red and purple, consolidated (Figure 292). The tissue on section was firm, rubbery. The lung microscopically showed alveolar walls thickened and infiltrated with acute inflammatory cells; alveoli and small bronchioles were lined with waxy glassy pink hyaline material (Figures 293a and b).

Hypoxia, imposed by the fulminating hyaline membrane disease, resulted in acute congestive heart failure (page 8). The heart was large, dilated, especially the right chambers (Figures 294a and b). The cardiac failure caused visceral congestion, with ascites and hydrothorax present, with the brain showing vascular engorgement and edematous swelling (Figure 295).

Figure 291. X-ray of the chest prior to death showing evidence of lung consolidation and a degree of pneumothorax. Lung fields showing opacification, evidence of diffuse consolidating pathologic process in the lungs due to hyaline membrane disease. Clear areas laterally, pneumothorax.

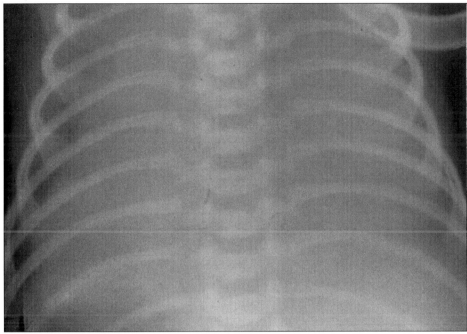

Fig. 291

Figure 292. The lungs, with hyaline membrane disease; appearance at autopsy. External surfaces dark red, mottled. The lungs firm, rubbery, in consistency.

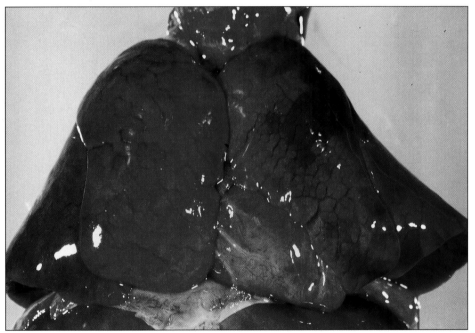

Fig. 292

Figure 293(a). Hyaline membrane disease. Histologic section of the lung; alveolar walls thick, infiltrated with acute inflammatory cells.

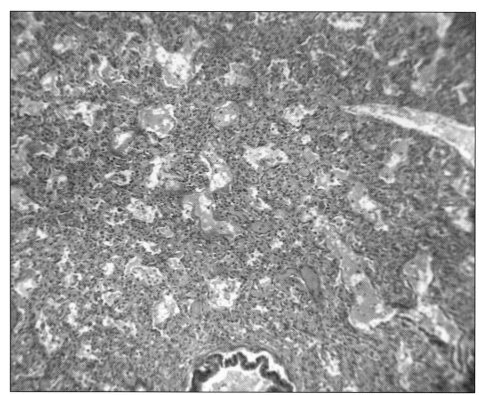

Fig. 293(a)

Figure 293(b). Higher magnification of the lung showing shreds of pink glassy hyaline material lining alveolar spaces.

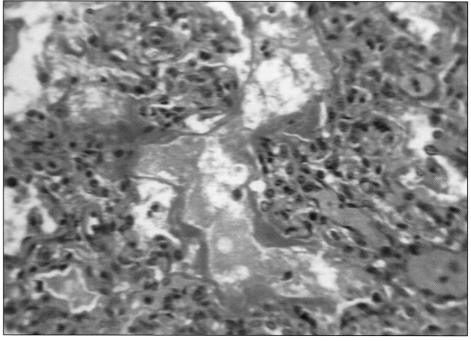

(b)

Figure 294(a). Cardiac failure due to hypoxia; the heart, much increased in size, especially the right side.

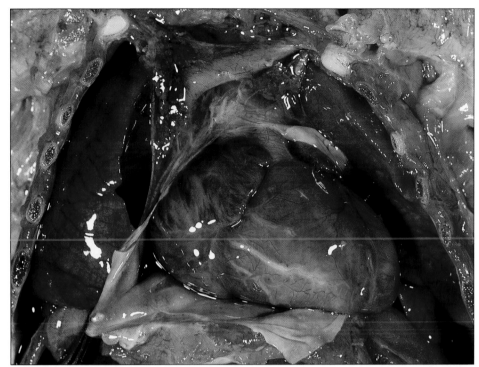

Fig. 294(a)

Figure 294(b). Heart, dilated, decompensated; chambers distended with blood.

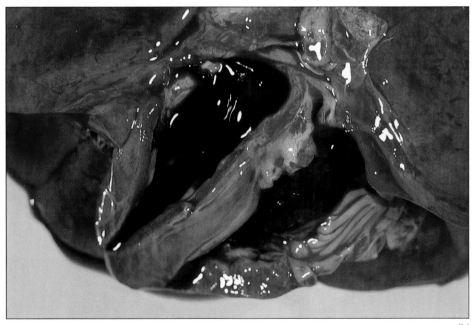

(b)

Figure 295. Brain, edematous and congested; flattening of cerebral convolutions; the effects of congestive heart failure.

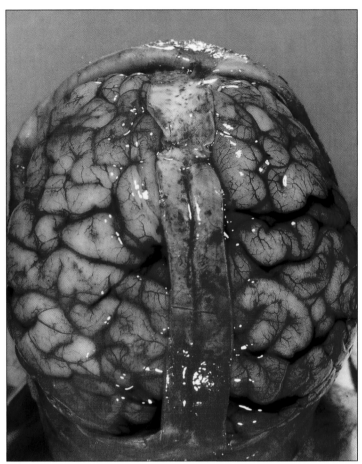

Fig. 295

A Case of   *Placental abruption, premature newborn with hyaline membrane disease; heart with subepicardial venous infarct; cerebral intraventricular and subarachnoid hemorrhage.*

Premature labor, with vaginal bleeding, developed at 29 weeks of gestation. At delivery the placenta showed retroplacental and retromembranous hemorrhage (Figure 296).

The infant was in good condition at birth, then developed labored respiration with periods of apnea, became pale and cyanotic (Figure 297). Death occurred at 21 hours.

Prior to death, x-ray of the chest showed evidence of hyaline membrane disease (page 106). This was confirmed at autopsy (Figures 298a and b). Congestive heart failure was present, with cardiac dilatation and diffuse venous engorgement of the body viscera. The surface of the heart showed an area of venous infarction in the subepicardial myocardium (Figures 299a and b).

The brain at autopsy showed a deposit of blood in the subarachnoid space around the cerebellum (Figure 300). Subsequent examination of the brain specimen revealed that the source of the blood was from within the cerebrum, from periventricular hemorrhagic infarction (Figure 301).

In summary, this is an example of the two distinctive complications that affect prematurely born infants: hyaline membrane disease and intraventricular hemorrhage (page 15). This infant succumbed to the prenatal intrauterine hypoxic effects of premature placental detachment and postnatal hyaline membrane disease; consequent congestive heart failure with systemic venous congestion resulted in visceral infarctional damage, in the heart. and in the brain; damage in the cerebrum led to intraventricular hemorrhage.

Figure 296. Retroplacental (retromembranous) hemorrhage. On the left, the membranes at the edge of the placenta with an adherent fresh hematoma.

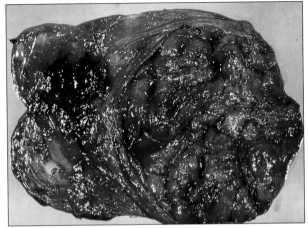

Fig. 296

Figure 297. Infant at death, pale, cyanotic. Gestational age, 29 weeks; lived 21 hours. Increasing respiratory distress due to hyaline membrane disease.

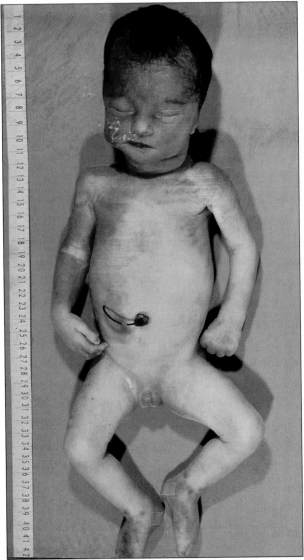

Fig. 297

Figure 298(a). Hyaline membrane
disease; lung histologic section;
in the middle of the lung section,
a bronchiole lined with a waxy,
pink layer of hyaline material.
Tissue is congested.

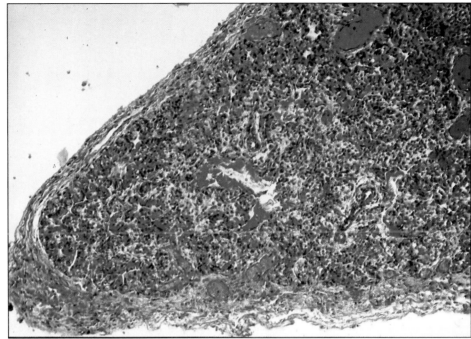

Fig. 298(a)

Figure 298(b). Higher magnification
of the area showing bronchiole
lined with hyaline membrane.

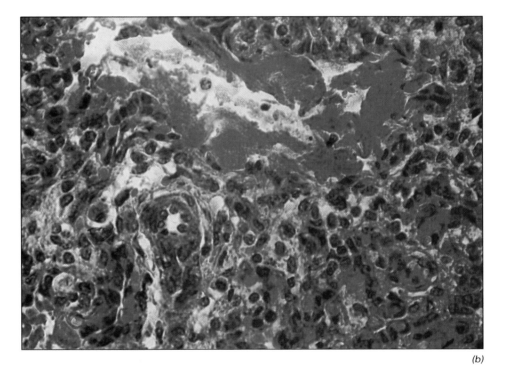

(b)

Figure 299(a). Myocardial infarction in a premature newborn. Left ventricle wall; histologic section. Near the upper left margin, an area of venous infarction, marked by prominent venous congestion.

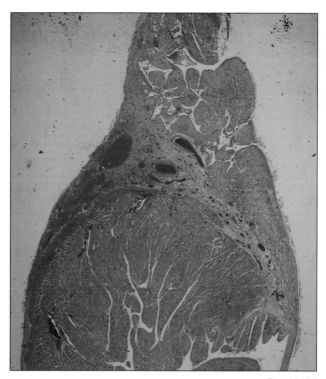

Fig. 299(a)

Figure 299(b). Myocardial infarction in a premature newborn. Devitalized infarcted tissue suffused with blood.

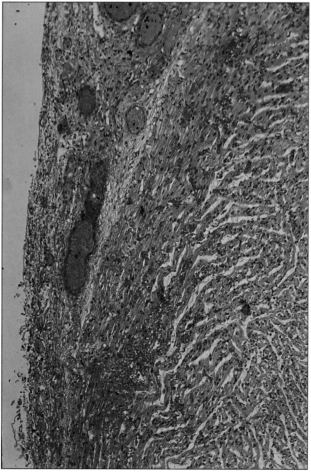

(b)

Figure 300. Ventral aspect of brain; a deposit of subarachnoid blood around the cerebellum.

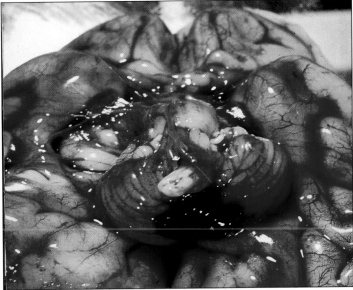

Fig. 300

Figure 301. Subependymal hemorrhagic matrix infarct, on the right forming a hematoma bulging into the ventricle. Blood oozing from the hematoma, extending through the ventricular system, out into the subarachnoid space, giving rise to the subarachnoid hemorrhage as in Figure 300. Frontal section of the brain; specimen embedded in plastic.

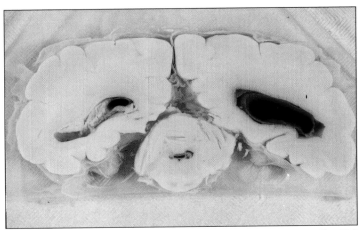

Fig. 301

A Case of   *Intrauterine growth retardation, fetal death; chorioamnionitis; circumvallate placenta; short umbilical cord malformation.*

This case is a good example of intrauterine growth retardation (IUGR). The newborn, near term, weighed 2 pounds 9 ounces, grossly underweight, reflecting adversive gestational conditions. Physical features of maturity, long black hair, well-developed ears, were evidence of near term gestation, despite the low birth weight (Figure 302).

The infant was stillborn.

It is evident that the adversive gestational process that caused intrauterine deprivation ultimately led to lethal compromise, fetal death.

Autopsy revealed that the fetal death was associated with congestive heart failure, evidenced by the presence of massive hydrothorax (Figure 303).

The placenta showed chorioamnionitis, placentitis, of severe degree (Figure 304), contributing to the fetal demise.

Of interest too, the placenta showed a circumvallate malformation (page 77). Also present was a short-cord malformation (page 79). The significance of these malformations in this case is unclear.

Figure 302. Intrauterine growth retardation; stillborn fetus near term, 2 pounds 9 ounces. Circumvallate placenta, a raised thickening around the placental margin. Umbilical cord malformation, short cord, 25 centimeters long (average at term, 50 centimeters).

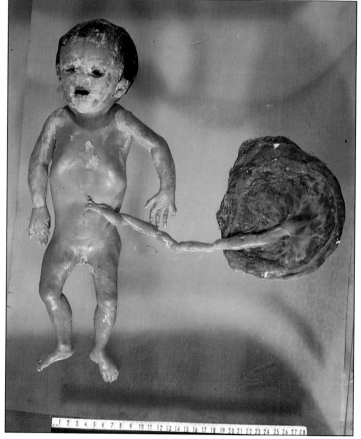

Fig. 302

Figure 303. Hydrothorax, evidencing congestive heart failure. The right pleural cavity with 12 milliliters of fluid, the left, 8 milliliters. Autopsy view of thoracic structures.

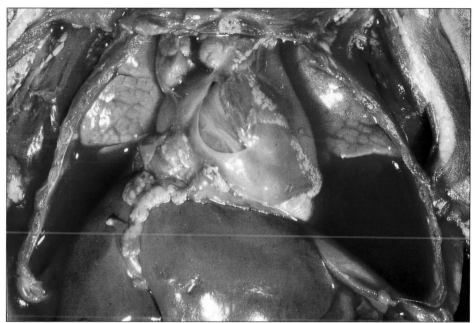

Fig. 303

Figure 304. Chorioamnionitis with placentitis. Histologic section of the amnion (upper left corner) with subjacent placental tissue heavily infiltrated with acute inflammatory cells.

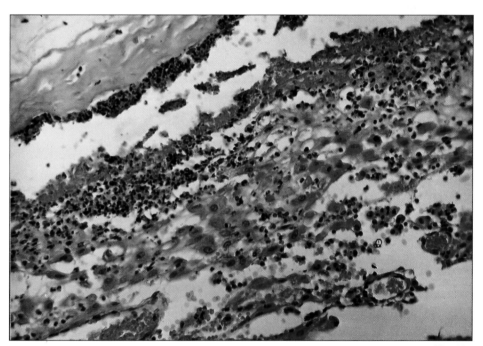

Fig. 304

A Case of ***Precipitous premature delivery; spinal injury with respiratory depression; hypoxic cerebral damage.***

This premature infant (28 weeks' gestation) was delivered precipitously. The infant lived 4 hours and had respiratory depression throughout life.

At autopsy, extensive spinal injury was evident, spinal epidural hemorrhage (Figure 305), together with perivertebral and perioccipital hemorrhage. That the fetus was subjected to forceful labor was evidenced by the presence of a prominent caput succedaneum.

The brain at autopsy presented a thick layer of subarachnoid blood around the ventral surface of the cerebellum (Figure 306). The subarachnoid hemorrhage was the result of intraventricular hemorrhage; the intraventricular hemorrhage was the consequence of hypoxic hemorrhagic periventricular matrix infarction (Figure 307), with bleeding into the ventricles and out into the subarachnoid space around the cerebellum (page 15).

This is a good example of the sequence of spinal injury causing respiratory depression, with resulting hypoxic (cerebral) damage (page 138).

Figure 305. Spinal epidural hemorrhage. Premature newborn with spinal injury due to forceful precipitous delivery.

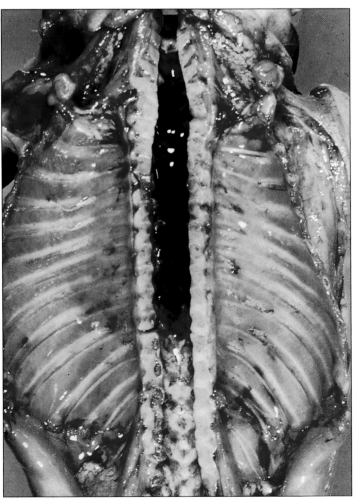

Fig. 305

Figure 306. Subarachnoid hemorrhage around the base of the brain, over the ventral aspect of the cerebellum. (Brain specimen after preservation in formalin.)

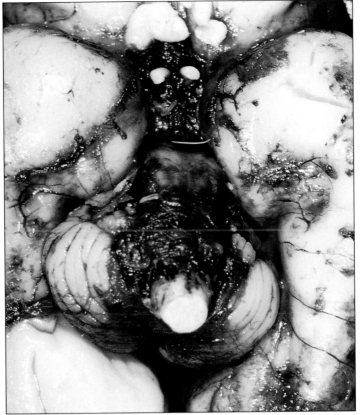

Fig. 306

Figure 307. Hemorrhagic periventricular infarction, giving rise to intraventricular hemorrhage and subsequently to subarachnoid hemorrhage (Figure 306). Frontal section of brain, embedded in plastic.

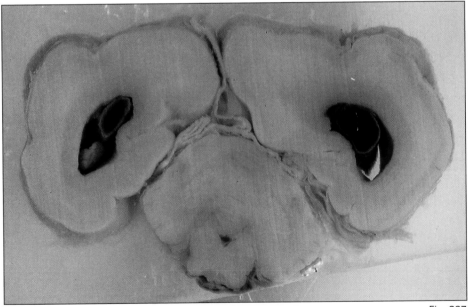

Fig. 307

A Case of **Shoulder presentation, vaginal delivery; crush laceration of liver, hemoperitoneum.**

This was a small premature, of 19 weeks' gestation, a shoulder presentation, delivered vaginally, stillborn.

With shoulder presentation, the fetus descends through the birth canal with the upper part of the body flexed, with the head pushed against the abdomen (Figure 308), compressing the abdominal viscera. The liver, squeezed by the external pressure, is subjected to crush injury, to laceration. Bleeding occurs into the abdominal cavity, hemoperitoneum. This sequence of pathologic processes occurred in the present case.

At autopsy, on opening the abdomen, a large amount of blood escaped. Figure 309, the abdomen opened at autopsy, shows residual hemoperitoneum, with blood around and between the viscera.

On further dissection, with removal of the rib cage, the right lobe of the liver presented a large blood-bleb, a subcapsular hematoma; the adjoining liver surface was ragged, torn (Figure 310a). Further study revealed extensive crush laceration of the liver (Figure 310b).

This case is an extreme example of crush injury of the liver, with exsanguination into the abdomen. Relevantly, in cases with less severe liver laceration, with less bleeding, the fetus, the newborn, is gradually rendered anemic. Anemia leads to mounting hypoxia, with the infant, surviving, incurring hypoxic brain damage postnatally (page 102).

Figure 308. Shoulder presentation, with the fetus flexed, the head compressing the abdomen.

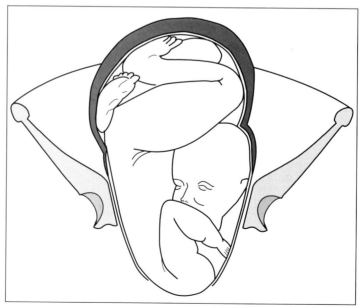

Fig. 308

Figure 309. Hemoperitoneum. (At autopsy, on opening the abdomen, a large amount of blood escaped.) Residual blood present around and between the organs.

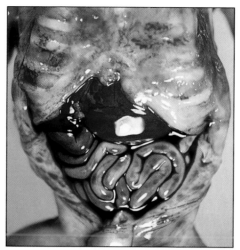

Fig. 309

Figure 310(a). Liver with subcapsular bleb, hematoma, and ragged laceration of the right lobe. **(b).** Severe laceration of the liver, crush injury. (The body viscera removed together, *en bloc,* and preserved in formalin.) The block of organs, rotated to expose the liver, shows massive liver laceration.

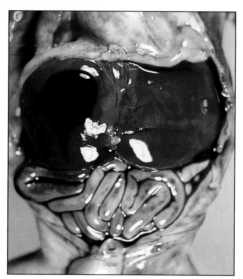

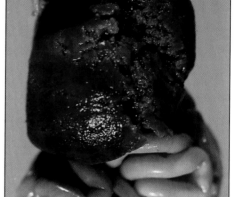

Fig. 310(a)   *(b)*

A Case of *Placental abruption. Postnatally, infant developed hypoxic congestive heart failure; infarcts of lungs; hypoxic cerebral damage.*

Premature labor developed at 34 weeks of gestation. The placenta showed an adherent marginal retroplacental hematoma (Figure 311).

The infant was in good condition at birth, with a five-minute Apgar score of 9. Subsequently the infant developed increasing respiratory distress. X-ray of the chest showed densities in the lung fields. Neurologic depression appeared on day 3; seizure activity developed. The infant died on day 4. The clinical impression was that a major intracranial complication had occurred terminally.

At autopsy, congestive heart failure was evident, with cardiac dilatation, visceral congestion, and collection of free fluid in the pleural sacs and in other body cavities.

The lungs showed large areas of consolidation and red discoloration, areas of hemorrhagic infarction (Figure 312a). Histologic studies confirmed that these areas in the lung were venous infarcts (Figure 312b); areas of infarction corresponded to the lung densities seen in the chest x-rays prior to death.

The brain showed diffuse subarachnoid hemorrhage over the cerebrum (Figure 313a) and around the brain stem and cerebellum (Figure 313b). Further study of the brain revealed that periventricular hemorrhagic infarction had occurred, with resulting intraventricular hemorrhage (Figure 314a); extension of the intraventricular hemorrhage outward led to subarachnoid hemorrhage around the brain stem (Figures 313b and 314b) and around the cerebrum (Figure 313a).

This case demonstrates that while hypoxic congestive heart failure commonly causes infarctions in the brain, the same pathologic sequence at times affects other body viscera, as in this case, causing lung infarction.

Figure 311. Marginal retroplacental hematoma; premature labor at 34 weeks of pregnancy. The hematoma was adherent and had depressed the underlying surface of the placenta, indicating the accumulation of blood was of some age.

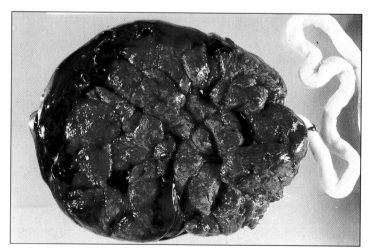

Fig. 311

Figure 312(a). Lungs, with hemorrhagic infarcts, dark red consolidated areas.

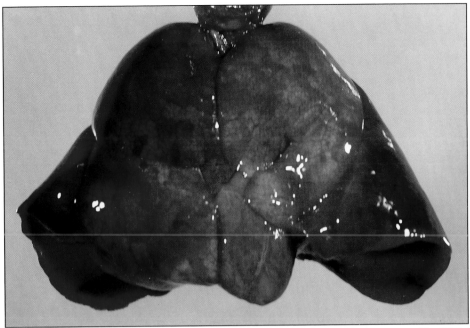

Fig. 312(a)

Figure 312(b). Lung, venous infarction; histologic section. The area of infarction, dense, congested. Extending through the infarcted area is a large vein, occluded by a thrombus.

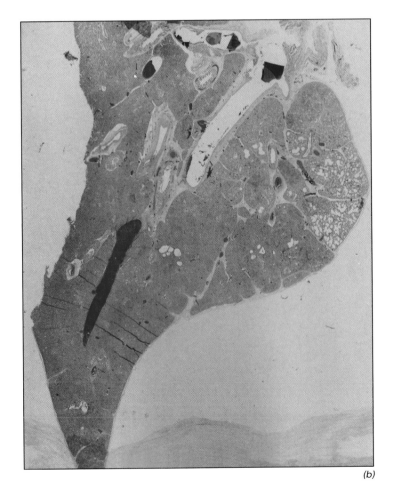

(b)

Figure 313(a). Subarachnoid hemorrhage extending over the cerebrum.

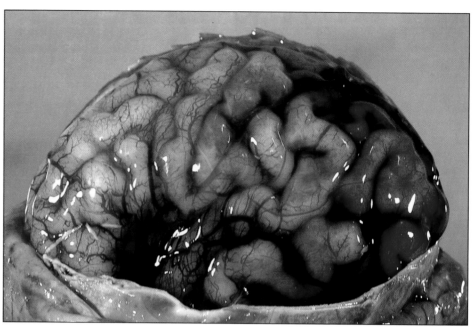

Fig. 313(a)

Figure 313(b). Subarachnoid hemorrhage over the brain stem and ventral aspect of the cerebrum. Subarachnoid hemorrhage due to extension of intraventricular bleeding (Figure 314).

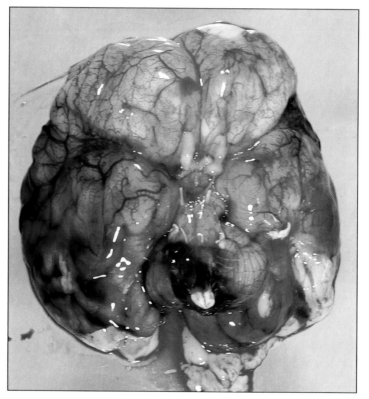

(b)

Figure 314(a). Intraventricular hemorrhage leading to subarachnoid hemorrhage. Intraventricular hemorrhage in the right lateral ventricle with extension into the third ventricle.

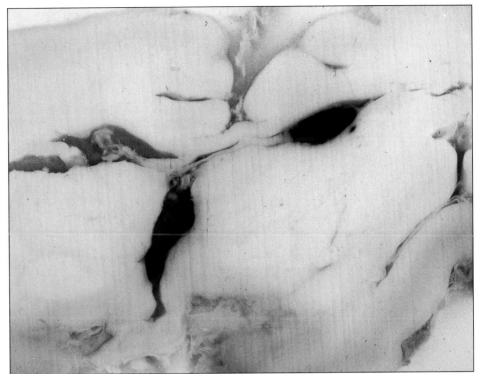

Fig. 314(a)

Figure 314(b). Subarachnoid hemorrhage around the brain stem, the extension of hemorrhage from within the ventricles.

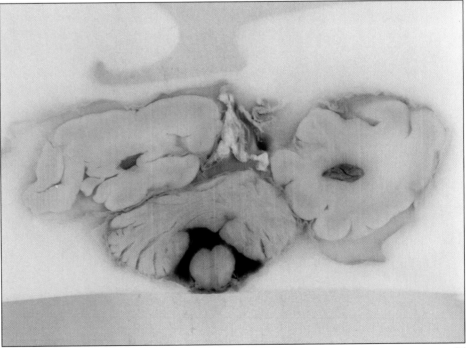

(b)

A Case of   *Fetal distress; nuchal cord; midforceps delivery; spinal injury; posterior fossa hemorrhage.*

Pregnancy had been uncomplicated, was at term. The mother reported normal fetal activity.

After six hours of labor, with a cephalic presentation, with the cervix fully dilated, with the head engaged, rupture of membranes occurred releasing "pea soup" meconium-stained amniotic fluid. The fetal heart became irregular, with bradycardia of 80 per minute. With these signs of fetal distress, midforceps delivery was performed, with rapid extraction of the fetus. The infant, stillborn, was cyanotic (Figure 315).

The umbilical cord was tightly wound around the neck four times. When the cord was uncoiled, a pale indented groove around the neck remained, evidence that the tight cord had been present for a considerable period (Figure 316).

Of relevant significance, too, was the fact that the umbilical cord was short, only 25 centimeters long (average at term, 50 centimeters).

At autopsy the viscera were congested, the effect of hypoxic circulatory failure.

Two important injuries were present, spinal injury and posterior fossa subdural hemorrhage.

Spinal injury was evident as spinal epidural hemorrhage (Figure 317).

In the cranial cavity, the posterior fossa contained a large fresh blood clot, a subdural hemorrhage (Figure 318). The hemorrhage arose from a stretch-tear of the tentorium. Blood accumulating in the posterior fossa compresses the brain stem, compromising vital function (page 133).

In summary, the clinical and autopsy data indicate that the sequence of pathologic events was as follows: The loops of cord around the neck were manifestly innocent until the fetus started to descend in the birth canal; with the short cord present, there was no slack in the cord and, with the descent, the loops around the neck tightened; the fetus was rendered hypoxic, with bradycardia, and meconium amniotic fluid developing, evidencing fetal distress. Rapid midforceps extraction was done, with resulting spinal injury and tentorial laceration with posterior fossa hemorrhage.

Was the fetal death due to (1) intranatal hypoxia imposed by the nuchal cord, or (2) physical injury, spinal injury, and the posterior fossa hemorrhage? Probably both.

Figure 315. Cyanotic fetus; term gestation; intranatal death.

Figure 316. Nuchal cord; neck showing pale groove, imprint of nuchal cord.

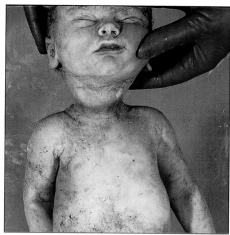

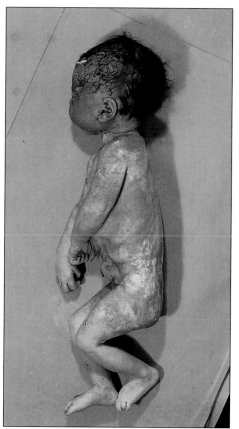

Fig. 316

Fig. 315

Figure 317. Spinal injury; epidural hemorrhage. Autopsy view of spinal canal. The cord has been elevated and retracted to the side, revealing a thick gelatinous deposit of blood in the spinal epidural tissue, extending through the cervical and upper thoracic segments.

Figure 318. Posterior fossa subdural hemorrhage. A tentorial stretch tear was present. (At autopsy, the tentorium incised, the cerebellum retracted upward revealing subdural accumulation of fresh blood around the brain stem.)

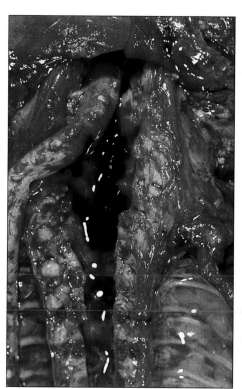

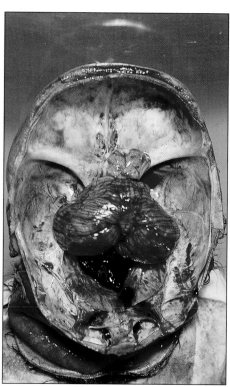

Fig. 317

Fig. 318

A Case of   *Cerebral laceration; precipitous birth.*

This was a precipitous vaginal delivery of a large baby, with a large head (pages 41 and 124).

The infant was moribund at birth; increasing rigidity with opisthotonos developed. Death occurred on the second day.

Excessive distortion of the head had occurred during the descent of the fetus. Compression of the head in the fronto-occipital diameter resulted in an increased biparietal diameter. As a consequence, the corpus callosum was stretched and torn. Neighboring cerebral convolutions were lacerated, creating large hematomas and intraventricular hemorrhage (Figure 319).

Figure 319. Cerebral laceration and hemorrhage due to physical injury, precipitous delivery. Frontal section of the brain. Corpus callosum and adjoining cerebral structures torn, with formation of large cerebral hematomas and intraventricular hemorrhage.

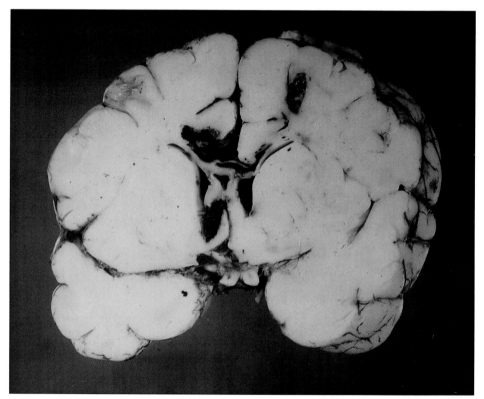

Fig. 319

A Case of   *Excessive molding of the head; intraventricular hemorrhage; premature newborn.*

The infant, born at 30 weeks of gestation, was depressed at birth but responded to care and improved. On the second day the infant developed respiratory distress, became increasingly hypoxic, cyanotic, with collapse of vital function. Death occurred at 31 hours of life.

At autopsy the head was elongated, due to persisting caput succedaneum and severe molding of the head (Figure 320a and b).

The bulging caput, over the posterior of the head, examined at autopsy, consisted of an edematous hemorrhagic thickening of the scalp.

The molding of the head, due to lateral compression of the head during descent of the fetus, resulted in extensive overriding of the parietal bones over the frontal and occipital bones (Figure 321a and b) (page 130).

The lungs were firm and dark, and microscopically showed hyaline membrane disease (accounting for the respiratory distress terminally). Hypoxic congestive heart failure was evident, with ascites and congestion of viscera.

The brain showed subarachnoid hemorrhage, with a large deposit of subarachnoid blood around the cerebellum, compressing the brain stem (Figure 322). Study of the brain specimen revealed periventricular hemorrhagic infarction (related to the terminal congestive heart failure) with intraventricular hemorrhagic blood from the ventricles extending out into the subarachnoid space around the cerebellum (Figure 323).

What is the significance, what are the effects, of the severe molding of the head in this case? Although molding is at times linked to intracranial injury, to tentorial tear, with subdural hemorrhage, in the present case this did not happen. Death was due to hypoxic brain damage, with intraventricular and subarachnoid hemorrhage.

Figure 320(a). Severe molding of the head together with a caput succedaneum. Elongation molding of the head due to lateral compression on the head during descent. Elongated appearance of the head exaggerated by the presence of the caput succedaneum. Anterior view of molded head.

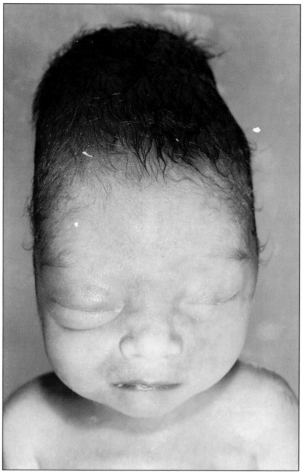

Fig. 320(a)

Figure 320(b). Side view of molded head.

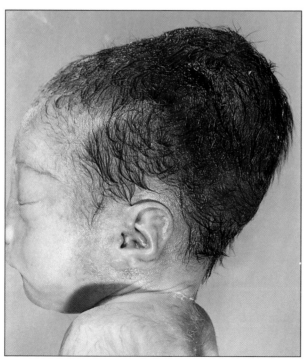

(b)

Figure 321(a). Molding of the head. Autopsy view of the skull bones after reflection of the scalp. Viewed posteriorly, with the occipital bone tucked under the overriding parietal bones.

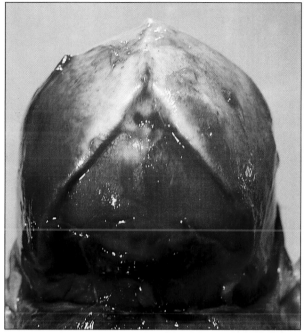

Fig. 321(a)

Figure 321(b). Molding of the head (viewed from above); overriding of the frontal bones by the parietal bone.

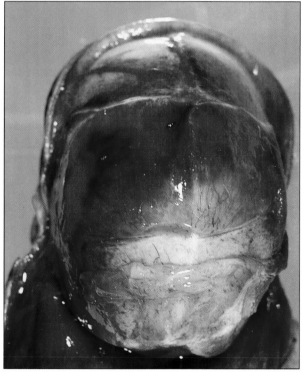

(b)

394

Figure 322. Subarachnoid blood around the cerebellum compromising the brain stem. Autopsy view of ventral surface of brain.

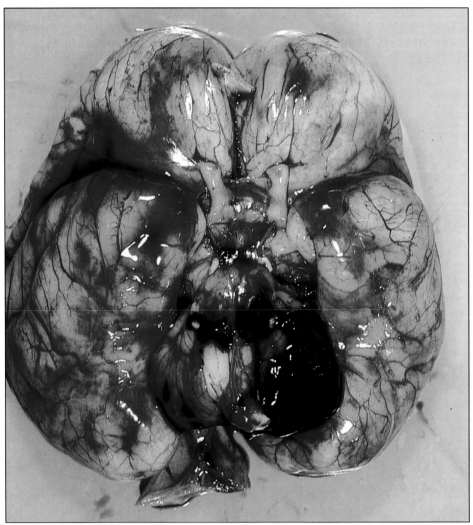

Fig. 322

Figure 323. Intraventricular hemorrhage with extension out into the subarachnoid space around the brain stem, as seen in Figure 322. (Brain specimen preserved in formalin; frontal section through the posterior of the brain.)

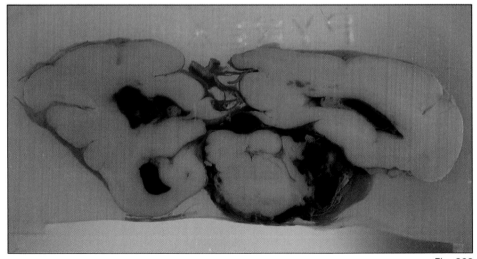

Fig. 323

A Case of   *Massive intraventricular hemorrhage in a premature newborn.*

Severe vaginal bleeding occurred at 18 weeks of pregnancy; bleeding recurred at 24 weeks and labor ensued. Placental infarcts and retroplacental hemorrhages were present at delivery.

The newborn infant was depressed, was apneic and flaccid. He responded to resuscitation. Subsequently the infant deteriorated neurologically. Death occurred on the second day.

At autopsy the brain was swollen and congested. The deep structures of the cerebrum showed infarctional destruction of the germinal matrix, giving rise to massive intraventricular hemorrhage (Figure 324) (page 15).

This is a clear example linking hypoxia-producing placental disease (placental infarction and retroplacental hemorrhage) with consequent fetal-neonatal hypoxic cerebral damage.

Figure 324. Massive intraventricular hemorrhage; premature newborn infant. Parasagittal section of the cerebrum (a lengthwise section of the cerebrum, taken in a plane halfway between the midline of the brain and the outer lateral edge of the cerebrum). Whole brain histology section stained cresyl violet.

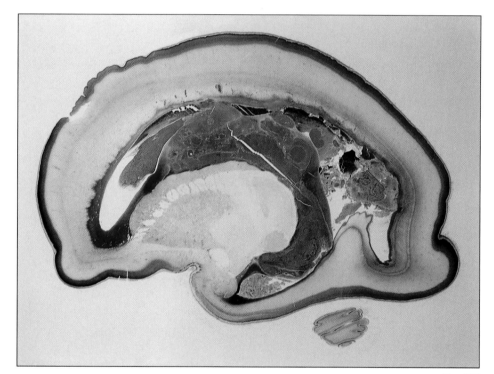

Fig. 324

A Case of **Cerebellar and spinal injury; precipitous breech birth.**

An episode of severe vaginal bleeding occurred at 12 weeks of gestation. The mother was in poor condition, having lost weight during the pregnancy. Labor developed at 26 weeks. The fetus was delivered from a footling breech presentation; birth was precipitous.

The infant remained severely depressed, limp, but survived for 14 hours.

At autopsy, the body externally showed the effects of the footling breech presentation, with edematous red discoloration of the back and right leg (Figure 325).

The placenta, on the maternal surface and on the adjoining membrane, had retroplacental, retromembranous hemorrhages, old and recent deposits of blood clot, the cause of the vaginal bleeding that had occurred (page 44).

At autopsy, examination of the cranial cavity revealed the posterior fossa with a large amount of fluid blood (Figure 326). The cerebellum was coated with a thick cake of blood that obliterated the external features of the cerebellum (Figure 327a). Also there was subarachnoid blood around the base of the brain.

The question was — Where did the blood encasing the cerebellum and around the cerebrum come from? From within the cerebrum, from intraventricular hemorrhage? Transection through the cerebrum showed there was no blood in the ventricles. Transection of the cerebellum showed the cerebellar hemispheres were largely destroyed, permeated deeply with blood clot (Figure 327b). It was conclusive that this was a case of physical injury, damage to the brain stem, cerebellum, due to foramen magna herniation (page 137). In cases of breech presentation, with the head extracted at the end of the delivery, with traction exerted on the fetus' body in order to deliver the aftercoming head, at times the brain stem, cerebellum, is drawn into the foramen magnum at the upper end of the spinal canal, and in this process the cerebellum is ground against the edge of the foramen magnum.

Spinal injury in the form of spinal epidural hemorrhage was evident at autopsy, attributable to traction in the delivery of the aftercoming head (page 138).

Figure 325. Edema and red discoloration of right buttocks and leg, the effects of delivery from footling breech presentation. The edema and redness here is analogous to caput succedaneum in cephalic presentation.

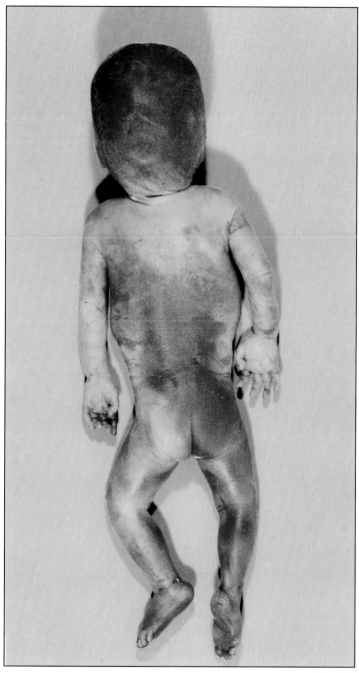

Fig. 325

Figure 326. Posterior fossa hemorrhage. (Autopsy view of base of the skull, the posterior fossa, with the brain retracted forward.)

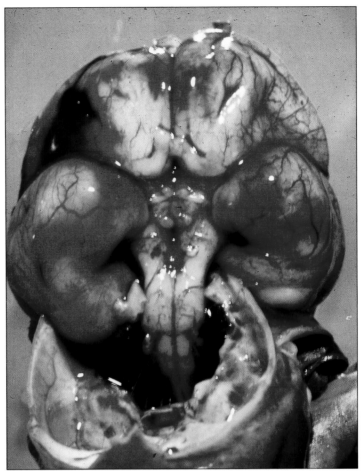

Fig. 326

Figure 327(a). Cerebellum encased in adherent blood clot in the subarachnoid space. Ventral view of brain at autopsy.

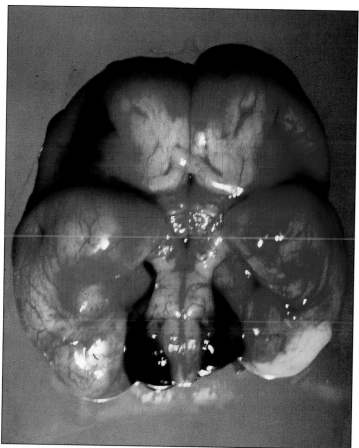

Fig. 327(a)

Figure 327(b). (Section of the brain preserved in formalin, embedded in plastic.) Hemorrhagic destruction of cerebellar hemispheres attributable to cerebellar herniation at delivery.

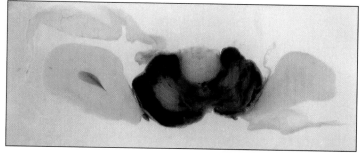

(b)

A Case of *Nuchal cord; long umbilical cord; placental infarcts; intrauterine growth retardation; fetal hypoxic congestive heart failure; intrauterine death.*

This gestation was complicated by two intrauterine hypoxia-producing pathologic processes: (1) nuchal cord and (2) placenta with multiple infarcts.

This was the second pregnancy for this mother, the first having ended with a miscarriage at 3 months. With the present pregnancy the mother was admitted to the hospital two times for vaginal bleeding during the early part of the pregnancy.

Fetal heart was heard during the week before delivery.

The mother was admitted in active labor at 34 weeks of gestation.

The infant was stillborn.

At birth, the umbilical cord was coiled around the neck; the cord was noted to be excessively long (Figure 328). This is a classic example of the occurrence of nuchal cord linked to the presence of a long umbilical cord (pages 80 and 83).

The infant was small, weighed 1 pound 15 ounces (872 grams; average weight at 34 weeks' gestation, 1,800 grams), reflecting chronic intrauterine deprivation, intrauterine growth retardation.

The placenta was small, weighed 136 grams, about half the normal weight for 34 weeks' gestation. The maternal surface, over about one-third of the placenta, showed depressed, irregular, furrowed, tan, indurated tissue, old infarction, and areas of red discoloration, recent infarction (page 71). The massive infarction resulted in placental insufficiency (page 76), contributing to fetal deprivation, to IUGR (Figure 329)

An adherent retroplacental hematoma, present over the infarct, accounted for the recurrent vaginal bleeding (page 102).

The hypoxia-producing effects of the nuchal cord and the placental infarct resulted in fetal hypoxic congestive heart failure, evidenced at autopsy by the presence of hydrothorax (Figure 330) and severe congestion of the brain (Figure 331) and other organs.

While the placental pathologic processes caused chronic fetal deprivation, IUGR, it is likely that the nuchal cord was the ultimate lethal factor.

Figure 328. Nuchal cord; the umbilical cord, excessively long, wound tightly around the neck at delivery. Infant, at 34 weeks' gestation, small for dates, IUGR.

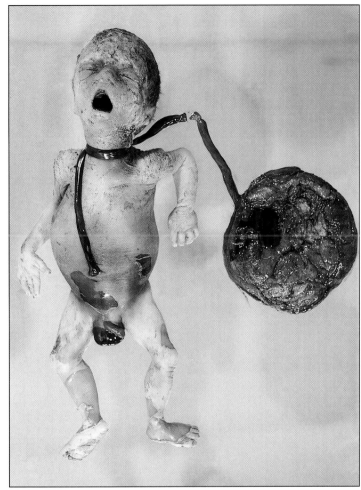

Fig. 328

Figure 329(a). Placental infarcts. The maternal surface in the lower third of the placenta depressed, tan, indurated; old infarction. A small adherent retroplacental hemorrhage over part of the infarcted surface.

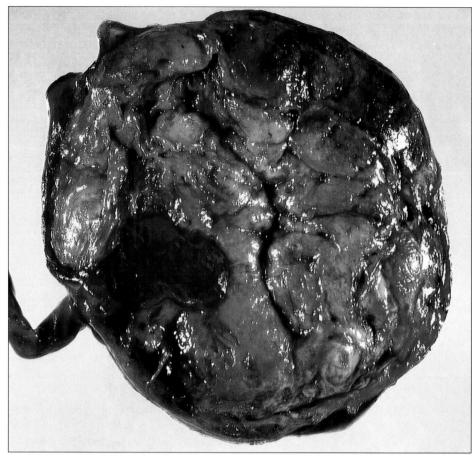

Fig. 329(a)

Figure 329(b). Placenta, cut surface. Areas thinned and scarred; pale areas, old infarction; mottled red areas of recent infarction. (Placenta specimen preserved in formalin, transected.)

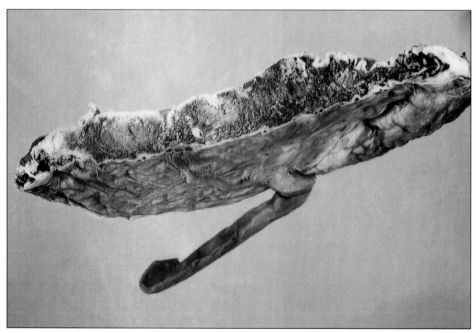

(b)

Figure 330. Hydrothorax due to hypoxic congestive heart failure. View of thoracic viscera at autopsy.

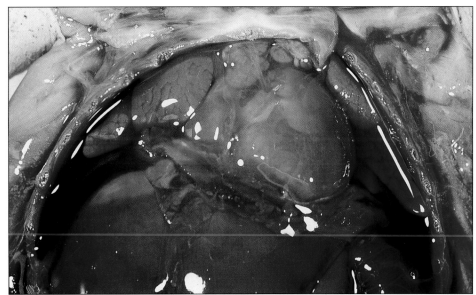

Fig. 330

Figure 331. Cerebral edema and congestion. Convolutions flattened due to cerebral swelling. Prominent venous congestion.

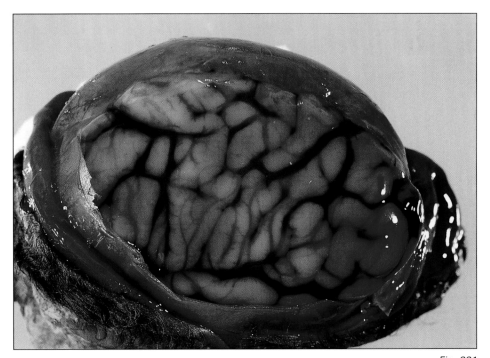

Fig. 331

A Case of **Tight nuchal cord; long umbilical cord; fetal death with congestive heart failure.**

The mother was admitted in labor at 39 weeks of gestation. There were no fetal heart tones. The infant was stillborn. The umbilical cord was tightly wrapped around the neck two times (Figure 332a). At autopsy, after the umbilical cord was uncoiled, the neck was left with a deep pale groove, the imprint of the nuchal cord. The pale imprint, persisting after death, indicated that the tight nuchal cord had been present for a period of time before death.

The umbilical cord was not only wrapped around the neck but also extended posteriorly, entangled around the left shoulder (Figure 332b).

Tight nuchal cord causes death, not due to choking, of course, but death results from compression of the loops of tight cord, with consequent blocking of fetal circulation, with death of the fetus due to hypoxic congestive heart failure. This occurred in the present case. At autopsy, congestive heart failure was manifested as cardiac dilatation, hydrothorax, congestion of the lungs and other bodily viscera, especially the brain (Figures 333 and 334).

Contributing to the occurrence of the nuchal cord was the presence of a long umbilical cord malformation; the umbilical cord was 107 centimeters long (average length is 50 centimeters at term).

Figure 332(a). Nuchal cord. Umbilical cord wrapped tightly around the neck two times. **(b).** Nuchal cord extending backward, entangled about the left shoulder.

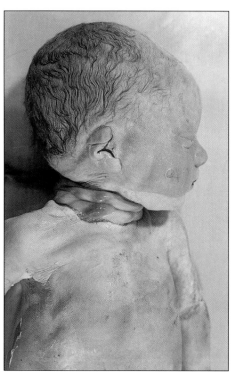

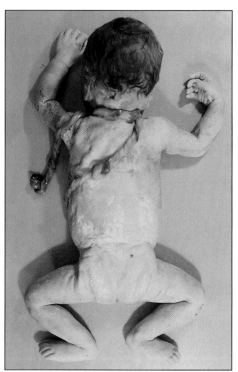

Fig. 332(a)

(b)

Figure 333. Congestive heart failure due to compression of the umbilical cord circulation. Cardiac dilatation; hydrothorax; lungs congested with petechiae present. Thoracic viscera viewed at autopsy.

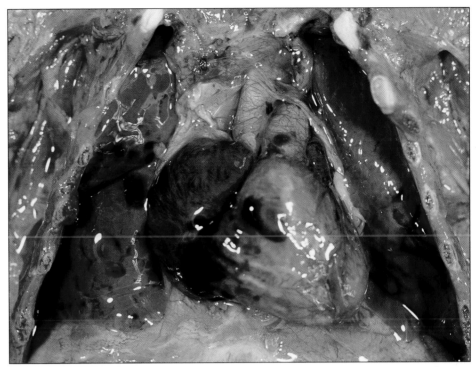

Fig. 333

Figure 334. Brain congested, edematous; flattening of cerebral convolutions.

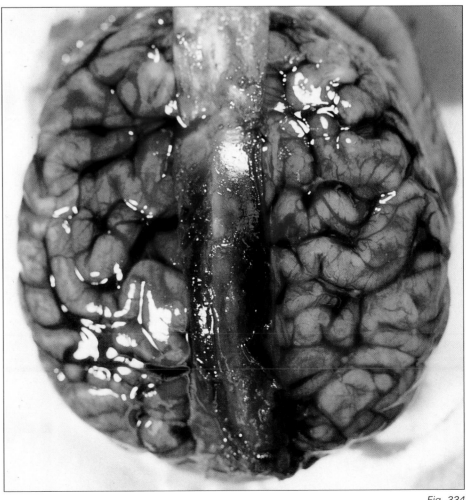

Fig. 334

A Case of   *Intrapartum death of a large postmature fetus;
placental insufficiency (infarcts); meconium aspiration.*

In this 43-week gestation, fetal death occurred during labor. The stillborn infant was large, 22 1/2 inches long and weighing 9 pounds 12 ounces. The infant was cyanotic (Figure 335).

The placenta, the fetal surface, and the umbilical cord were dark olive-green, heavily meconium-stained (Figure 335). The presence of heavy meconium staining in this case is reflective of severe intranatal fetal hypoxia.

Meconium aspiration had occurred (page 108). Meconium material oozed from the nose. The oral cavity contained tan meconium; likewise the trachea and bronchi contained tan meconium-stained mucus (Figure 336).

The placenta, in addition to being meconium-stained, showed a thinned scarred indurated central area of tan discoloration, with focal points of calcification; this scarred area occupied about one-half of the placenta (Figure 337a). Microscopically this proved to be an area of old placental infarction (Figure 337b).

The autopsy revealed the effects of hypoxia-producing placental insufficiency; congestive heart failure was evident, with cardiac dilatation and engorgement of large veins (Figure 338); body organs showed severe congestion.

The brain presented cerebral venous congestion of severe degree, with consequent edematous swelling of the brain (Figure 339a). Dural sinuses contained adherent thrombi (Figure 339b), reflecting circulatory failure, venous stasis thrombosis.

Regarding the causes of death, the conclusion emerges that this was an example of placental insufficiency, placental infarction, with the placenta inadequate to sustain fetal life, with the stress of labor proving to be the final lethal factor.

Figure 335. Macrosomic stillborn postmature infant. Cyanotic infant. Placenta and umbilical cord with heavy dark-green meconium staining.

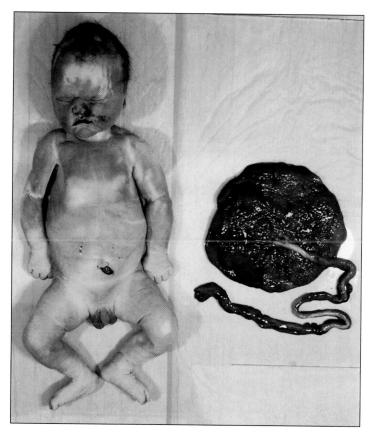

Fig. 335

Figure 336. Meconium aspiration. Trachea coated with thick tan meconium-stained mucus. Autopsy examination of thoracic viscera.

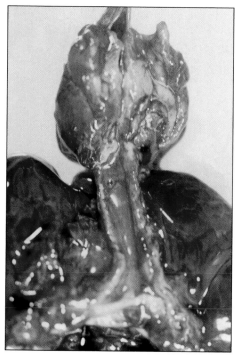

Fig. 336

Figure 337(a). Placental infarction. Maternal surface of placenta. Central area of placenta thinned, tan, indurated, due to old infarction.

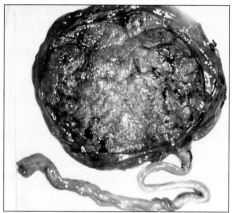

Fig. 337(a)

Figure 337(b). Microscopic structure of the placental infarction; section taken through the tan area in (a). On the left, the placental chorionic villi are effaced, replaced by scar tissue. On the right, residual chorionic villi.

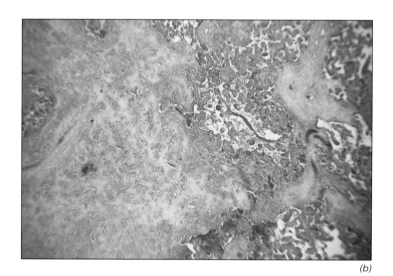

(b)

Figure 338. Congestive heart failure. Autopsy view of thoracic viscera. The heart enlarged, dilated, especially the right atrium. Lung dark red, severely congested.

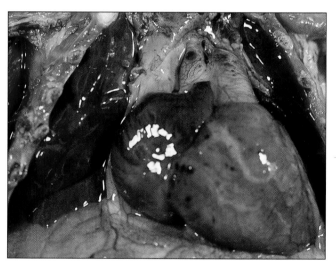

Fig. 338

Figure 339(a). Cerebral edematous swelling (brain weight, 520 grams; average term brain weight, 350 to 400 grams); flattening of convolutions due to cerebral swelling. Engorged superficial cerebral veins. Dissection at autopsy, cerebrum with a midline strip of dura (containing the superior longitudinal dural venous sinus).

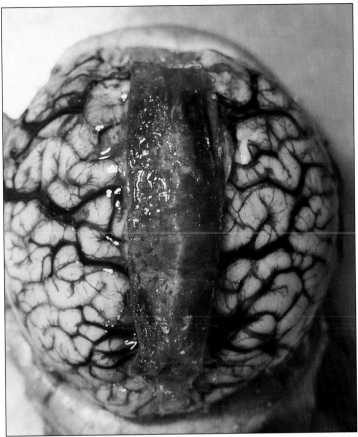

Fig. 339(a)

Figure 339(b). Thrombosis of superior longitudinal dural venous sinus. The dural strip, in Figure 339(a), transected, viewed on end. In the illustration, the longitudinal dural sinus, lying in the triangle at the junction of the horizontal piece of dura with the vertical piece of falx cerebri, contains an adherent thrombus. The engorgement of the superficial cerebral veins in Figure 339(a) due to thrombotic occlusion of the superior longitudinal sinus.

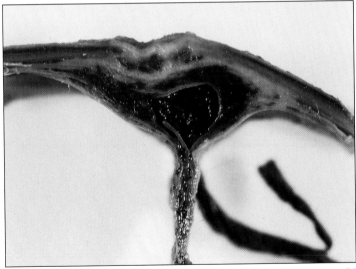

(b)

A Case of   *Germinal matrix infarction. Premature newborn with hyaline membrane disease and congestive heart failure.*

This was a complicated pregnancy. The mother gained excess weight with associated increasing peripheral edema. During the third month the mother was sick with the "flu" and was febrile for 3 days.

Labor developed at 30 weeks of gestation. The infant was in poor condition at birth and remained depressed postnatally. Terminally, with the development of mounting respiratory distress, the infant became increasingly cyanotic, hypoxic. Death occurred at 24 hours.

Autopsy revealed hyaline membrane disease. Changes of hypoxic congestive heart failure were present, with hydrothorax and congestion of viscera.

The brain showed subarachnoid hemorrhage, mainly around the brain stem and cerebellum.

The cerebrum presented a large hemorrhagic infarction of the periventricular germinal matrix (page 14). This was located abutting the caudothalamic groove, overlying the deeply located *vena terminalis* (Figure 340). The matrix infarction is attributable to circulatory stasis in the tributaries of the *vena terminalis*.

Blood oozing from the periventricular infarction into the ventricular system and out into the subarachnoid space accounted for the subarachnoid hemorrhage around the brain stem, observed at autopsy.

This case is a good example of the sequence of postnatal pulmonary complication leading to hypoxic congestive heart failure, with consequent visceral venous congestion, with deep cerebral venous stasis, ultimately leading to germinal matrix infarction.

Figure 340. Germinal matrix hemorrhagic infarction; intraventricular hemorrhage. Infarcted germinal matrix, located in the groove between the caudate nucleus and the thalamus. Germinal matrix cells destroyed, with the residual tissue suffused with blood. (Parasagittal histologic section of the cerebrum in a longitudinal plane, halfway between the midline and the lateral surface of the cerebrum.)

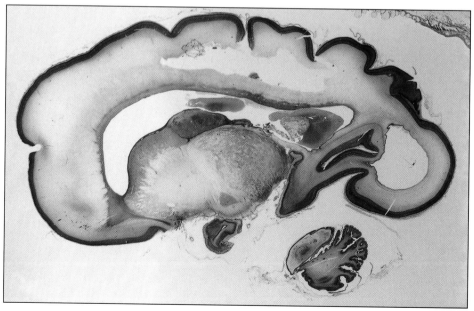

Fig. 340

A Case of   ***Placental insufficiency due to large placental infarcts; intrauterine growth retardation (IUGR); intrauterine death.***

The mother was examined a week before delivery; a good fetal heart tone was present. According to the mother, during the day before delivery there was decreased fetal activity. At delivery the infant was cyanotic, stillborn.

Gestation was 38 weeks, term.

The infant was small, weighed 4 pounds 1 ounce, evidencing intrauterine deprivation, IUGR (Figure 341a).

The placenta was small, weighed 210 grams, about half the average weight for a term placenta, an example of placental insufficiency (page 76).

The maternal surface was of irregular pattern, with about half of the placental plate occupied by bulky indurated tan cotyledons. The cut surface of the placenta (Figure 341b) revealed large confluent pale portions of indurated tissue, histologically old infarcts (Figure 341c).

The autopsy revealed bodily evidence of death due to congestive heart failure, with visceral congestion, ascites, and hydrothorax (Figure 342).

In summary, this is an example of placental insufficiency due to multiple old placental infarcts; the compromised placenta, causing chronic fetal deprivation (IUGR), was ultimately unable to support fetal life.

Figure 341(a). Small cyanotic term stillborn infant (4 pounds 1 ounce), IUGR. Placenta small with large islands of infarction.

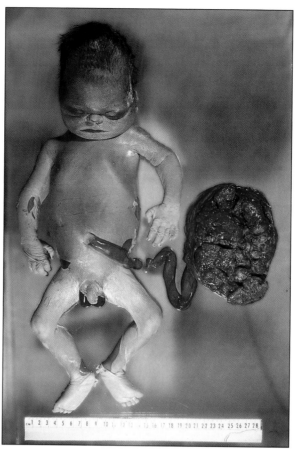

Fig. 341(a)

Figure 341(b). Placenta transected; large pale infarctions. (Placenta after preservation in formalin.)

Figure 341(c). Placental infarction, old. Histologic section through the thickness of the placental plate, through pale portion in Figure 341(b). Microscopically, most of the placental architecture effaced, replaced by scar tissue.

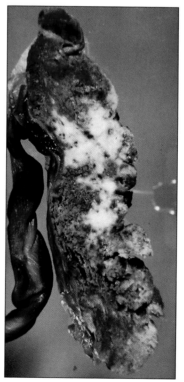

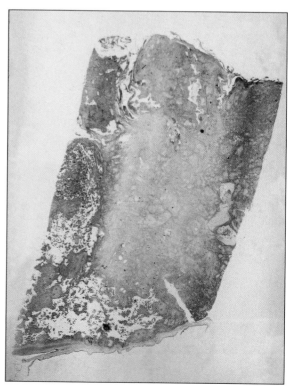

(b)

(c)

Figure 342. Hydrothorax, consequent to hypoxic congestive heart failure; placental insufficiency. View of thoracic organs at autopsy.

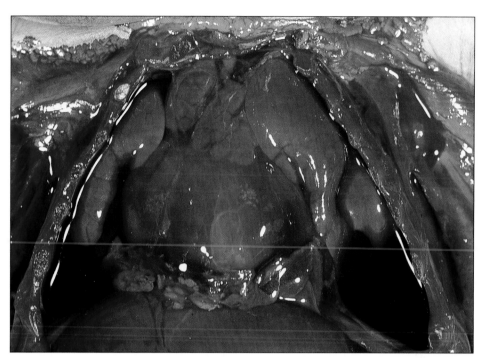

Fig. 342

A Case of **_Massive placental infarction; intrauterine growth retardation; intrauterine death with fetal congestive heart failure._**

The mother experienced an abrupt onset of explosive labor, expelling the infant and placenta, precipitously, at home (page 41). The infant was apparently stillborn.

This was the mother's third pregnancy; the first baby was delivered at term; the second pregnancy terminated in a miscarriage.

In the present case, the third gestation, vaginal bleeding had occurred repeatedly during the second and the third trimester; however, the pregnancy was maintained to near term, to 37 weeks.

Office examination of the mother the day before the delivery revealed a vertex presentation, fetal heartbeat 140 per minute; no abnormalities were evident.

The baby was small for dates (IUGR), very cyanotic (Figure 343).

The placenta was small. The surface of the placenta was of irregular pattern, with confluent firm mottled areas of yellow occupying about half of the surface (Figure 343), and underneath the mottled tan areas were broad portions of old infarction (Figure 344). This is a good example of placenta insufficiency due to infarction.

Retroplacental blood clots — some red, soft, fresh and some tan, old — were adherent to the maternal surface of the placenta and to the attached membranes (Figure 343).

The fetus died in congestive heart failure, evidenced by the severe cyanosis and, at autopsy, showing enlargement of the heart, engorgement of the great veins in the neck, and congestive hepatosplenomegaly (Figure 345).

In summarizing the clinical and pathologic processes in this case, this is an example of maternal poor reproductive function (previous spontaneous abortion; vaginal bleeding in this pregnancy), with vaginal bleeding linked to placental infarction, with retroplacental hemorrhage, with placental insufficiency causing intrauterine growth retardation and, ultimately, fetal death.

Figure 343. Cyanotic stillborn infant, weight 4 pounds 9 ounces, small for gestational age (37 weeks), intrauterine deprivation, IUGR.

Placenta attached, small (weight 250 grams; average weight at 37 weeks gestation, 400 to 450 grams). Maternal surface of placenta with yellow indurated areas in contrast to the adjoining soft gray-red intact placental tissue.

Retroplacental hemorrhage and retromembranous hemorrhage present, with some adherent clots red, fresh, and some tan, old.

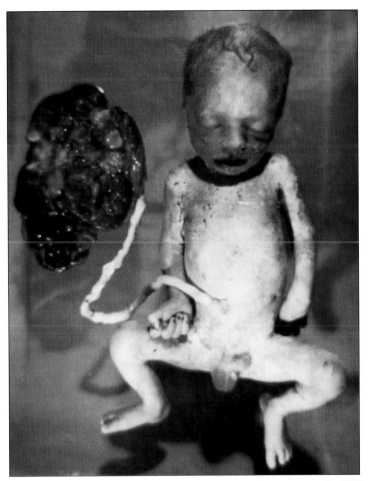

Fig. 343

Figure 344. Placental infarcts (the placenta after preservation in formalin, transected). Tan indurated tissue (corresponding to tan areas in Figure 343), occupying most of the placental plate; pathologically, confluent old scarred infarcts.

Figure 345. Fetal congestive heart failure. Heart large, dilated; engorged large veins in the mediastinum and neck. Liver and spleen enlarged due to congestion.

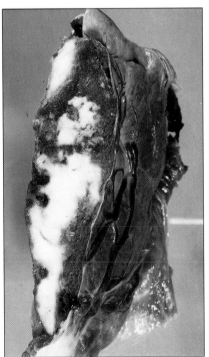

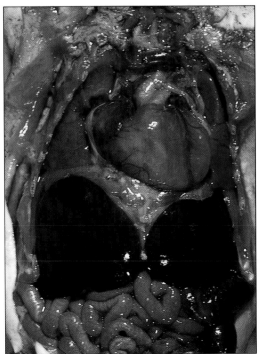

Fig. 344

Fig. 345

A Case of **_Placental infarction; intrauterine growth retardation; intranatal death; fetal congestive heart failure with hydrothorax and lung infarction._**

The mother was admitted at term in active labor. This was her second pregnancy; the first had terminated in an incomplete abortion at 9 weeks.

Fetal heart tones were absent during labor. The infant was stillborn.

Amniotic fluid was dark brown. The fetal surface of the placenta was meconium stained.

The infant was severely cyanotic. She appeared undernourished, with spindly extremities and little subcutaneous adipose tissue; although of term gestation, she only weighed 3 pounds 13 ounces, reflecting intrauterine deprivation (IUGR) (Figure 346).

The placenta had multiple indurated yellow areas, infarcts pathologically (Figure 347).

Autopsy revealed evidence of fetal death due to hypoxic congestive heart failure. In addition to deep cyanosis, severe congestion of viscera was present, together with ascites and hydrothorax (Figure 348). The lungs (Figure 349) presented thrombotic occlusion of large veins with hemorrhagic infarctions (page 158).

The brain was congested and edematous (Figure 350).

This case demonstrates the clinical-pathologic sequence encountered commonly in cases of placental insufficiency due to placental infarction: placental infarction causing intrauterine hypoxia, nutritional deprivation (IUGR), with the marginally surviving fetus unable to tolerate the superimposed stress of labor, intranatal death.

Figure 346. Intrauterine growth retardation, term infant, 3 pounds 13 ounces. Severe cyanosis at delivery reflecting hypoxic intrauterine death.

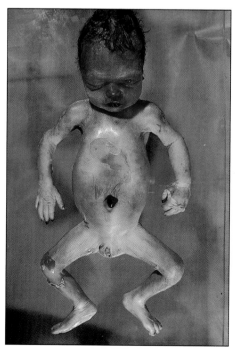

Fig. 346

Figure 347(a). Placenta, maternal surface with multiple confluent indurated yellow areas of infarction.

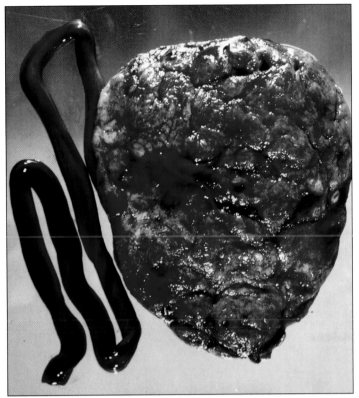

Fig. 347(a)

Figure 347(b). Transection of placenta; area of indurated yellow discoloration on the right (old infarction); on the left, a circumscribed area of red and yellow, a more recent infarction. (Placenta after preservation in formalin.)

Figure 347(c). Old placental infarction. Histologic section of the yellow indurated portion of placenta in Figure 347(b), showing placental structure destroyed, replaced by scar tissue.

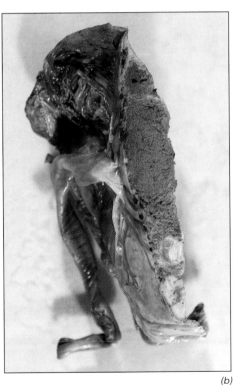

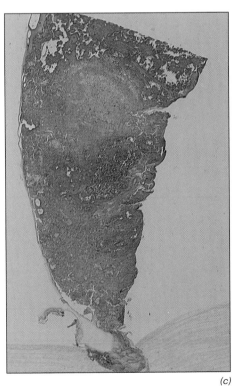

(b)

(c)

Figure 348. Hydrothorax consequent to hypoxic congestive heart failure. (View of thoracic cavity at autopsy.)

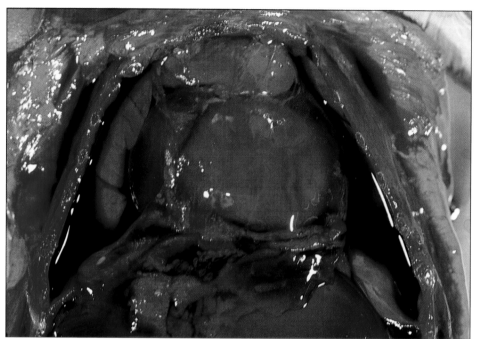

Fig. 348

Figure 349. Lung with large veins distended with thrombi. Lower lobe with confluent areas of hemorrhagic infarction.

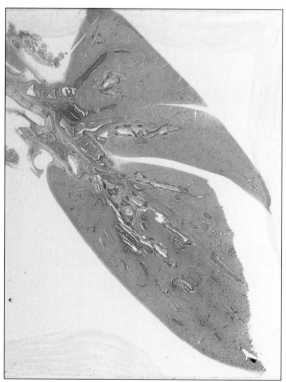

Fig. 349

Figure 350. Brain,
congested, edematous.

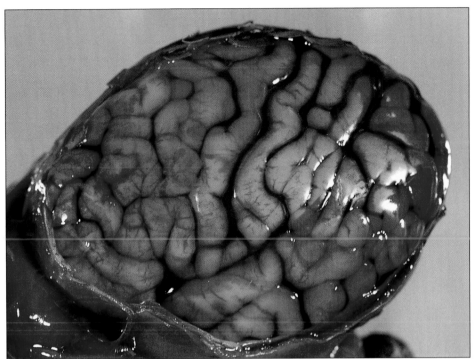

Fig. 350

A Case of *Placental insufficiency; placental infarction; intrauterine growth retardation; intrauterine death; fetal hypoxic congestive heart failure.*

This mother presented a record of poor reproductive function. The mother's first pregnancy produced a large 9-pound baby. A second pregnancy ended with a spontaneous abortion. The present case was her third pregnancy. She previously had had pelvic inflammatory disease and nephritis. At the time of admission, the mother stated there had been decreased fetal activity during the previous 2 weeks. The mother was admitted with blood pressure of 150/110; she was treated for toxemia. Fetal bradycardia developed. A stillborn infant was delivered. Gestation was at 32 weeks.

The infant weighed 2 pounds 3 ounces (992 grams) (average weight at 32 weeks is 1,600 grams) reflecting chronic intrauterine deprivation, IUGR.

The placenta showed multiple old and recent infarcts (Figure 351), creating placental insufficiency.

At autopsy, reflecting chronic hypoxia, there were pathologic findings of congestive heart failure, with hydrothorax (Figure 352) and ascites. Related to the circulatory failure was the presence of acute intestinal infarction (Figure 353).

This case portrays the adverse impact of placental disease on the well-being of the fetus: intrauterine growth retardation; compromise of vital function leading to decreased fetal activity terminally; death due to hypoxic congestive heart failure.

Figure 351(a). Placental infarcts. Placenta transected; a large red subacute infarct occupying the middle third; on the left, a small pale old infarct.

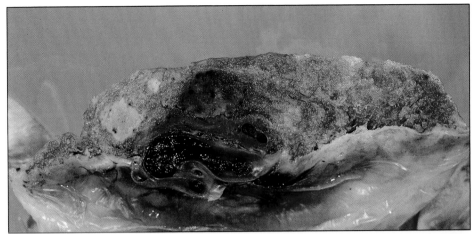

Fig. 351(a)

Figure 351(b). Histologic section; on the left, placental architecture destroyed, replaced by scar tissue; on the right, remnants of placental villi.

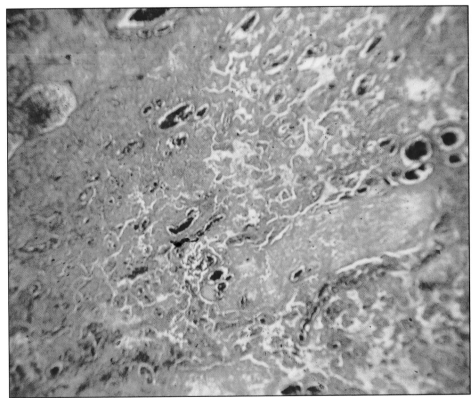

(b)

Figure 352. Hydrothorax; both pleural cavities containing large fluid collections. View of thoracic cavity at autopsy.

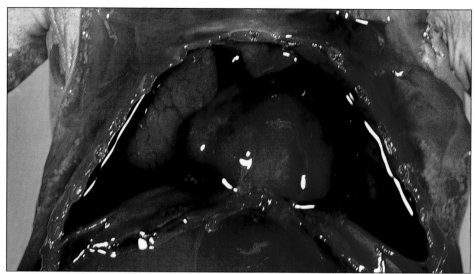

Fig. 352

Figure 353. Intestinal infarction. Intestinal loops distended, with angry red discoloration.

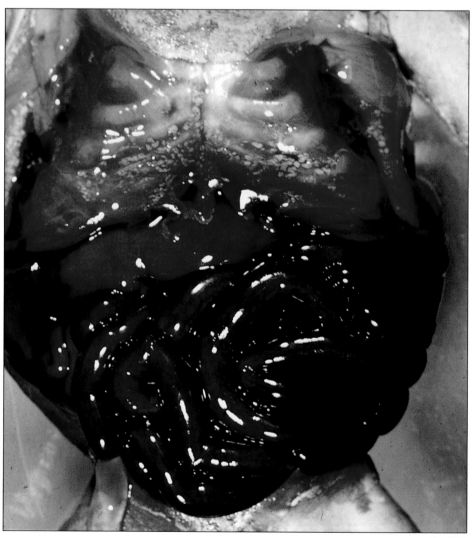

Fig. 353

A Case of   **Placental insufficiency (placental infarcts); intranatal death; fetal hypoxic congestive heart failure; fetal hydrops; IUGR.**

The mother was admitted in active labor. During the first stage of labor, at 11 1/2 hours, fetal heart rate was normal, with tones of good quality. The second stage was short; fetal heart tones were lost during this period of delivery. The infant was stillborn.

The gestational age was open to question. According to dates given by the mother, the pregnancy was of 32 weeks' duration. However, although the baby was small, it was evident that the gestation was term or near term. This conclusion was based on the physical characteristics of the baby, the hair growth, the well-developed ears and, on subsequent anatomic studies, the mature appearance of the cerebral convolutional pattern, together with the far-advanced development of the kidney structures microscopically.

Plainly, this was a case of intrauterine growth retardation (IUGR).

The placenta was large, edematous, and showed multiple areas of infarction, causing placental insufficiency. Some infarcts were dark red, fresh; others were tan, indurated, old (Figure 354).

At autopsy, the infant appeared plump; the body was edematous, characteristic of hydrops fetalis (Figure 355a). The subcutaneous tissue was extremely edematous (Figure 355b). The hydrops was attributable to congestive heart failure that preceded the fetal death (page 9).

Autopsy revealed the changes of congestive heart failure with the heart greatly enlarged, distended with blood (Figure 356). Ascites and hydrothorax were present. The lungs and other organs were congested; congestive hepatosplenomegaly was present (Figure 357). The brain was swollen, edematous, with pronounced flattening of the cerebral convolutions (Figure 358).

It is of interest to note that the thymus and adrenals were small, atrophied, characteristic of cases of intrauterine growth retardation, indicative of prolonged intrauterine compromise, fetal deprivation.

In this case, with function of the placenta insufficient, compromised by multiple infarcts, the fetus, surviving marginally during intrauterine life, was unable to tolerate the superimposed stress of vaginal birth.

Figure 354. Placenta showing multiple confluent tan (rubbery) areas of old infarction.

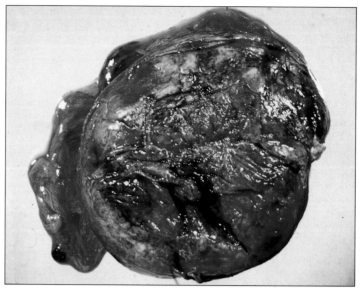

Fig. 354

Figure 355(a). Hydrops fetalis. The baby appears pudgy, due to bodily edema.

Figure 355(b). Hydrops fetalis (initial autopsy incision through the skin); subcutaneous tissue edematous, waterlogged; watery fluid oozing from the tissue, at the upper end of the incision.

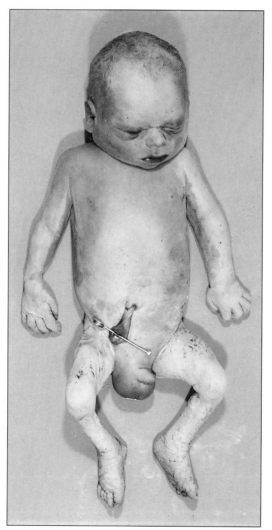

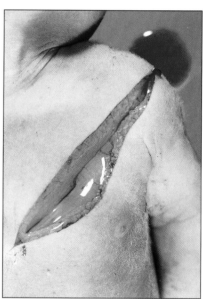

(b)

Fig. 355(a)

Figure 356. Congestive heart failure (autopsy view of thoracic viscera). Heart enlarged, dilated, distended with blood.

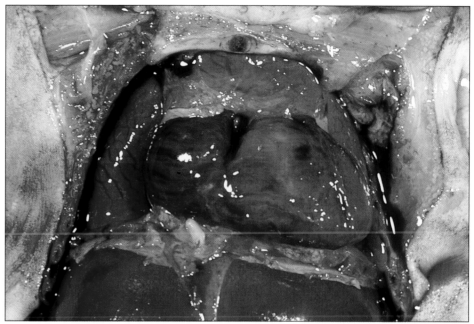

Fig. 356

Figure 357. Congestive hepatosplenomegaly due to prolonged congestive heart failure.

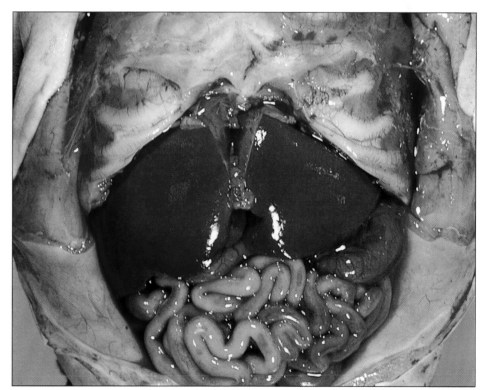

Fig. 357

Figure 358. Cerebral edema, severe swelling with flattening of cerebral convolutions.

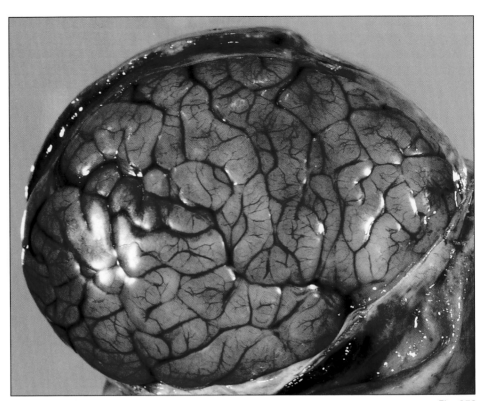

Fig. 358

A Case of   *Pneumothorax in a 2-day-old premature; intraventricular hemorrhage and subarachnoid hemorrhage.*

This is an example of neonatal pneumothorax leading to hypoxic cerebral damage.

Labor developed at 32 weeks of gestation. The infant at birth was in good condition with an Apgar score of 10 at one minute and 10 at five minutes. Subsequently the infant developed respiratory distress, with periods of apnea. The infant was treated with positive pressure ventilation. The infant's condition deteriorated; death occurred at 30 hours of age. It was thought the infant had developed hyaline membrane disease.

At autopsy the infant was cyanotic. Abdomen was tensely distended, tympanitic (Figure 359).

Postmortem x-ray of the body showed pneumothorax together with pneumo-intestinalis (Figure 360).

This was confirmed at autopsy. Bilateral pneumothorax was present (Figure 361a). The intestines were distended with air, pneumo-intestinalis.

In addition to pneumothorax, interstitial emphysema was present. The lungs were diminished in size; the pneumothorax had compressed the lungs, leaving empty space around the lungs (page 111).

Pulmonary interstitial emphysema was of a pronounced degree, with clusters of air-containing blisters appearing on the lung surfaces (Figure 361a), with the process of interstitial emphysema extending through the substance of the lungs (Figure 361b).

The autopsy also revealed visceral changes of congestive heart failure; the heart was enlarged, distended with blood; the body organs showed severe congestion microscopically.

The brain presented a thick deposit of subarachnoid blood over the brain stem (Figure 362a). The subarachnoid blood proved to originate from intraventricular hemorrhage, from periventricular hemorrhagic matrix infarcts (Figure 362b).

In summary, the sequence of clinical and pathologic events after birth: Positive pressure ventilation contributed to the development of interstitial emphysema and pneumothorax; pulmonary failure led to hypoxic congestive heart failure, with systemic congestion, cerebral venous infarction, intraventricular hemorrhage, and subarachnoid hemorrhage.

Figure 359. Cyanotic premature
infant; abdomen tensely distended.
Infant of 34 weeks' gestation;
death at 30 hours.

Figure 360. Pneumothorax.
X-ray of the body postmortem.
The right pleural cavity shows
the lung decreased, atelectatic;
around the lung there is a broad
space with increased translucency,
an extensive pneumothorax.
The left chest shows prominent
pneumothorax.

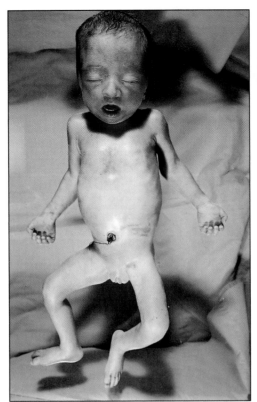

Fig. 359

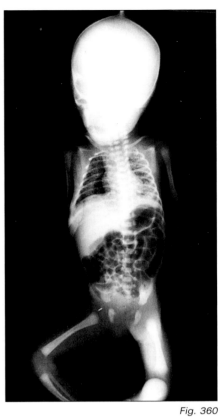

Fig. 360

Figure 361(a). Bilateral
pneumothorax; view of the
thoracic cavities at autopsy. As
evident in the x-ray in Figure 360,
the lungs are compressed by the
pneumothorax, with open spaces,
free air, occupying much of the
thoracic space around the lung.

   Pulmonary interstitial emphysema
present, evident as blister-like
bubbles of air about the surfaces
of the lungs.

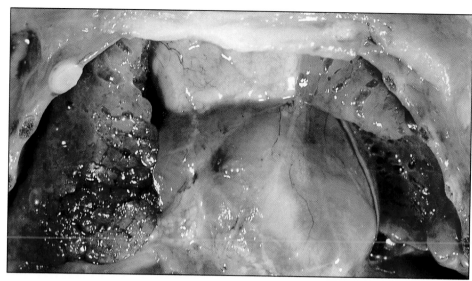

Fig. 361(a)

Figure 361(b). Interstitial
emphysema extending into
the deep structures of the lungs,
creating air cysts in the lungs.
(Histologic section of the lung)

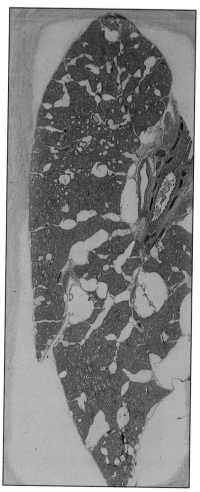

(b)

Figure 362(a). Subarachnoid hemorrhage over the ventral aspect of the brain stem.

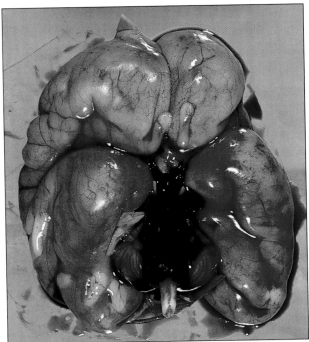

Fig. 362(a)

Figure 362(b). Intraventricular hemorrhage, arising from periventricular matrix infarction, giving rise to subarachnoid hemorrhage. (Sections of brain embedded in plastic) In the section of brain at the top, there are focal hemorrhagic infarcts in the germinal matrix, appearing as dark brown deposits protruding into the lateral ventricles.
The lower two sections of brain show blood extending through the ventricles.

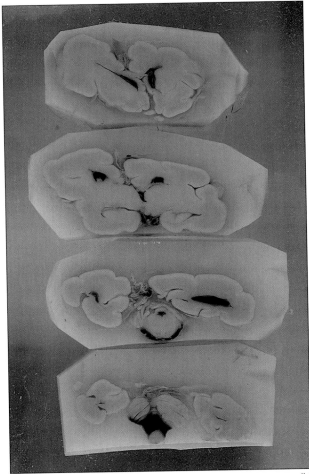

(b)

A Case of   *Precipitous delivery; subdural hemorrhage; resuscitation with positive pressure ventilation; pneumothorax, Potter's syndrome.*

This was a precipitous breech delivery. The aftercoming head was rapidly expelled, unmolded. Gestation was at term.

The infant, depressed at birth, was resuscitated with positive pressure ventilation. The infant failed to respond and died 1 1/2 hours after delivery.

Postmortem x-ray revealed pneumothorax, with most of the thoracic space of increased translucency, with the lungs small, compressed medially (Figure 363).

Correspondingly, the autopsy revealed the lungs compressed, leaving most of the thoracic space empty, an example of far-advanced pneumothorax (Figure 364). The lung surfaces presented clusters of air-containing blebs, interstitial pneumothorax. Related to this, microscopic sections of the lung tissue showed numerous clear cysts (Figure 365). Rupture of emphysematous blebs on the lung surface leads to escape of air into the pleural sacs, creating pneumothorax (page 111).

Examination of the cranial cavity revealed posterior fossa hemorrhage (Figure 366). This was due to a stretch-tear of the tentorium (Figure 367).

Of incidental interest, the autopsy revealed elements characteristic of Potter's syndrome, with ear malformation, kidneys hypoplastic, and uterus bicornuate.

In summary, this infant was subjected to a precipitous breech birth. The aftercoming head, unmolded, rapidly expelled, incurred intracranial damage, tentorial laceration with posterior fossa hemorrhage (page 133). Compression of the brain stem by the posterior fossa hemorrhage resulted in compromise of vital function, to central respiratory depression. This, together with the unrelieved pneumothorax, led to death.

Figure 363. Pneumothorax. Postmortem x-ray of the chest. Increased translucency of most of the thoracic space, indicating absence of lung structure due to pneumothorax with compression of the lungs medially.

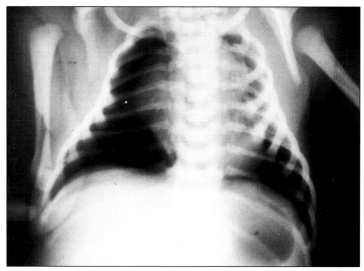

Fig. 363

Figure 364. Pneumothorax; thoracic structures at autopsy. The pleural cavities are empty. The lungs, much reduced, with only small tags of lung structure visible. Lung surfaces present clusters of shiny air-containing blisters, interstitial pneumothorax.

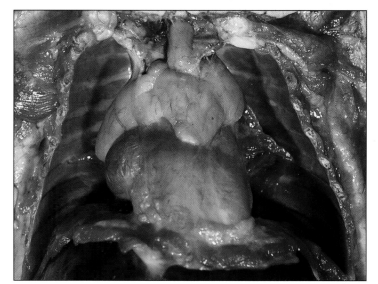

Fig. 364

Figure 365. Pulmonary interstitial emphysema. Histologic section showing thin-walled cysts formed by the dissection of air into connective tissue.

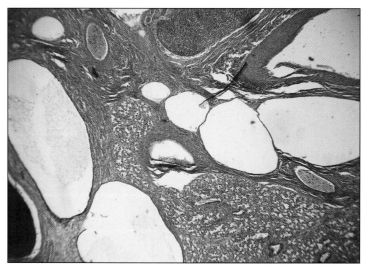

Fig. 365

Figure 366. Posterior fossa hemorrhage, arising from tear in the tentorium (Fig. 367). (Most of the blood that had accumulated in the posterior fossa was lost during autopsy dissection.)

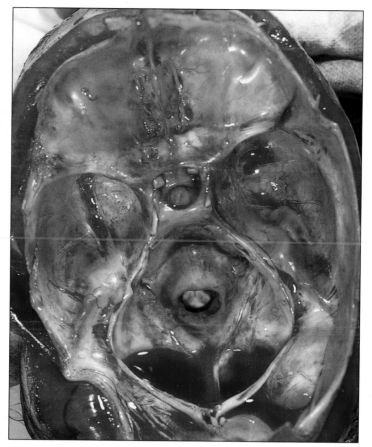

Fig. 366

Figure 367. Stretch-tear of the tentorium. This view at autopsy, with the cerebrum retracted upward, shows the upper surface of the tentorium in the lower part of the illustration; in the middle of the tentorium, the smooth surface is disrupted, pulled apart, a stretch-tear. The tear, penetrating the thickness of the tentorial sheet, led to posterior fossa hemorrhage.

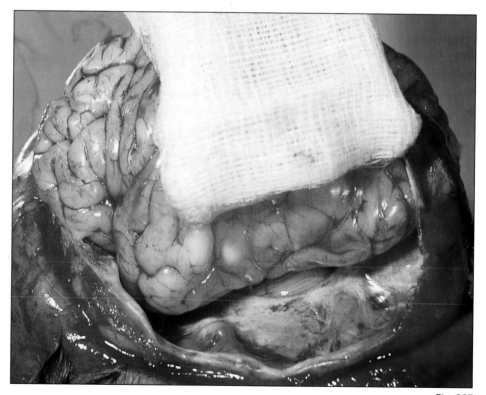

Fig. 367

A Case of *Intrauterine pneumonia following premature rupture of membranes.*

Premature rupture of membranes was reported by the mother the day before the onset of labor. Gestation was 34 weeks. This was a vaginal delivery with forceps extraction of the fetus.

The infant, cyanotic, in poor condition at birth, developed increasing respiratory difficulty and died on the second day.

The lungs at autopsy were large, dark red, of boggy texture. The pleural surfaces presented speckled gray-yellow patches, 2 to 4 millimeters wide (Figure 368). The tissue beneath these patches was yellowed and indurated. Microscopically these focal areas proved to be abscesses (Figure 369).

Of interest, at autopsy the cerebellum showed a surface hemorrhagic lesion, laceration, of the right hemisphere (Figure 370), apparently incurred during delivery, the consequence of forceps traction, with herniation of the cerebellum into the foramen magnum (page 137).

Regarding the cause of the pneumonia, was the lung infection incurred in utero, prior to birth? Or was it a postnatal process? It is conclusive, based on the far-advanced pattern of the pneumonia, with abscess formation, that the pathologic process in the lung was of a duration longer than 2 days, longer than the period the infant survived. It is evident that the infection originated during intrauterine life, and is attributable to the premature rupture of membranes (page 112).

Figure 368. Lung abscesses. Posterior view of the lungs (after preservation in formalin). The pleural surfaces, of mottled appearance, with circumscribed gray-yellow patches that proved to be abscesses (Figure 369a).

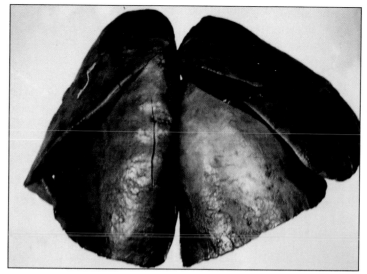

Fig. 368

Figure 369(a). Lung abscess. Histologic section through a yellow patch seen in Figure 368. On the left, lung tissue with architecture obliterated, consolidated, forming an abscess; on the right, at the margin of the abscess, an area of pneumonia, with persisting lung tissue, with alveoli containing inflammatory cells.

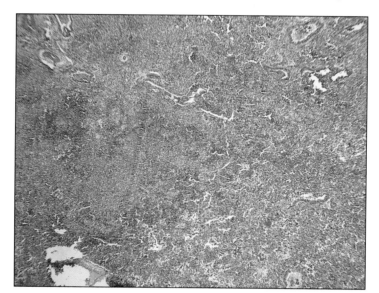

Fig. 369(a)

Figure 369(b). Pneumonia; higher magnification of area of pneumonia in Figure 369(a), showing details of the acute inflammatory process, with polymorphonuclear leukocytes, pus cells, in the alveolar spaces.

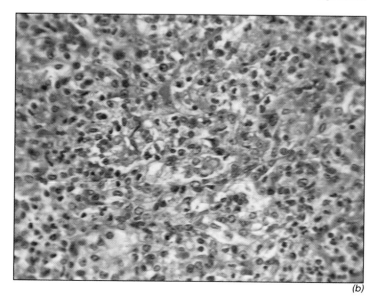

(b)

Figure 370. Cerebellum with surface laceration of the right hemisphere.

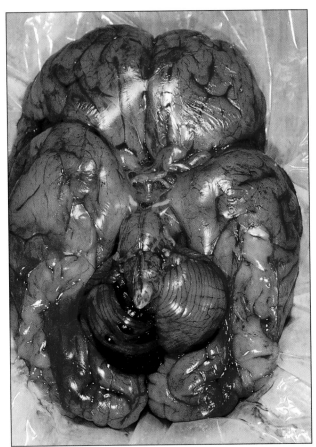

Fig. 370

A Case of   *Intrauterine pneumonia; premature rupture of membranes.*

Premature rupture of membranes occurred 2 months before delivery (page 87); intermittent leakage of amniotic fluid occurred. The mother was treated with antibiotics. Labor developed prematurely, at 26 weeks, according to the mother's history. Fetal heart tones were good during delivery. There were no signs of maternal sepsis. This was a breech birth.

The newborn infant on physical examination appeared of approximately 28 to 30 weeks' gestation.

The infant was in poor condition, cyanotic, with gasping respiration. He was intubated; there was difficulty in attempting to expand the lungs. Death occurred at 2 hours.

At autopsy, bronchopneumonia was the main pathologic finding (page 112). The lungs were rubbery, mottled gray-pink and red. Microscopically, bronchopneumonia, far advanced, was present (Figure 371). For the most part, the lung architecture was obliterated by heavy deposits of acute inflammatory cells, most pronounced around the small bronchi.

Also, at autopsy, congestive heart failure was evident; the subcutaneous tissue was edematous; the abdomen contained 20 milliliters of clear ascitic fluid; viscera were congested; the brain was firm, congested.

Of added interest was the presence of spinal epidural hemorrhage (Figure 372). This was apparently the consequence of excessive flexion of the spinal column during breech birth (pages 134 and 135).

Figure 371(a). Bronchopneumonia. Lung section, near the hilum, microscopically showing acute inflammatory cell infiltration in alveoli walls and within alveoli. On the left, abscess formation with focal concentration of pus cells. Adjoining bronchi with inflammatory debris.

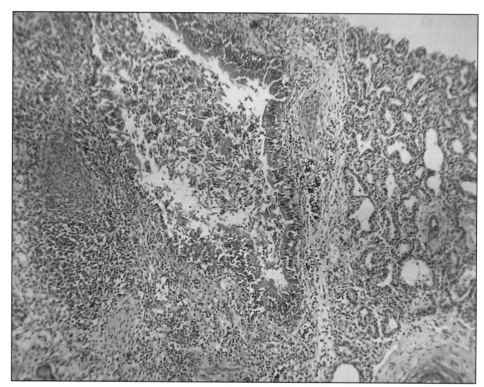

Fig. 371(a)

Figure 371(b). Bronchopneumonia. Lung section from periphery of lung; heavy inflammatory cell infiltration through the consolidated lung tissue.

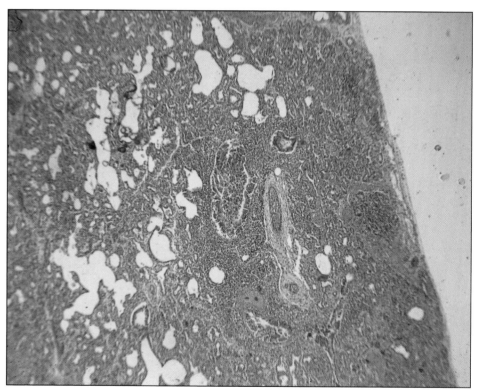

(b)

Figure 372. Spinal injury; spinal epidural hemorrhage. Breech delivery; premature infant, 28 to 30 weeks' gestation.

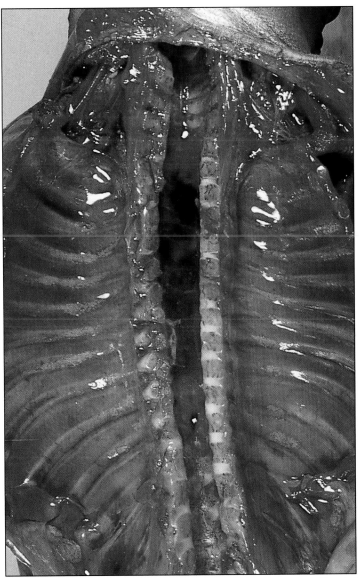

Fig. 372

A Case of   *Intrauterine pneumonia following premature rupture of membranes; chorioamnionitis.*

The mother had received no prenatal care until a week before delivery.

Premature rupture of membranes had occurred 2 days before the onset of labor. The mother indicated there were no fetal movements in the 3 hours before labor onset.

The infant was stillborn. Gestation, based on the mother's dates, was thought to be at 35 weeks; however, at birth, the physical features of the infant indicated a term gestation. The infant was severely cyanotic (Figure 373).

The amniotic fluid "had a fetid odor." (Culture of the fluid yielded a mixed growth of bacteria.)

Chorioamnionitis was present, with the inflammatory process extending into the placental tissue (Figure 374).

At autopsy, the lungs were firm, mottled red and purple. Microscopically, sections showed a pattern of far-advanced pneumonia, with alveolar walls thickened, infiltrated with acute inflammatory cells (Figure 375).

Alveolar spaces contained inflammatory cells together with aspirated squames and yellow-stained clumps, apparently meconium. Although no mention was made in the delivery record of meconium staining of the amniotic fluid, it is evident that meconium had been present, contaminating the amniotic fluid, and had been aspirated by the fetus. This process contributed to the inflammation in the lung.

In summary, this is a case of intrauterine pneumonia of dual causation: (1) bacterial infection (premature rupture of membranes; bacterial infection of placenta; chorioamnionitis), and (2) meconium aspiration pneumonia.

Figure 373. Severe cyanosis; stillborn infant with intrauterine pneumonia; term gestation.

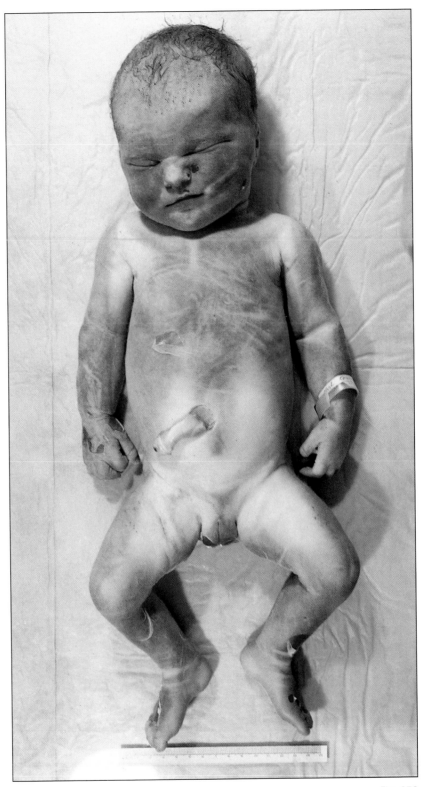

Fig. 373

Figure 374. Chorioamnionitis. Histologic section; amniotic membrane over the upper surface of the placenta. Heavy concentration of acute inflammatory cells forming thick, dark blue-staining deposits, extending into the placental tissue. Maternal history of premature rupture of membranes 2 days before delivery. Culture of placenta yielded mixed growth of bacteria.

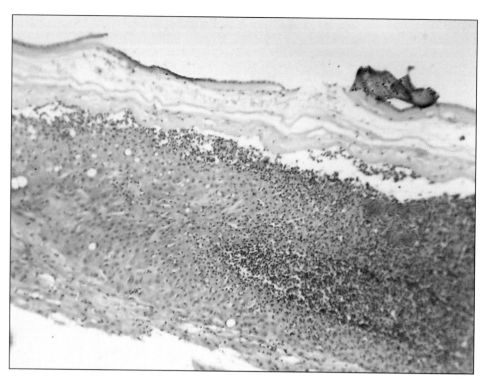

Fig. 374

Figure 375. Intrauterine pneumonia. Histologic section of lung; alveolar walls thickened, infiltrated with inflammatory cells. Alveolar spaces contain inflammatory cells and brown pigment, clumps of meconium.

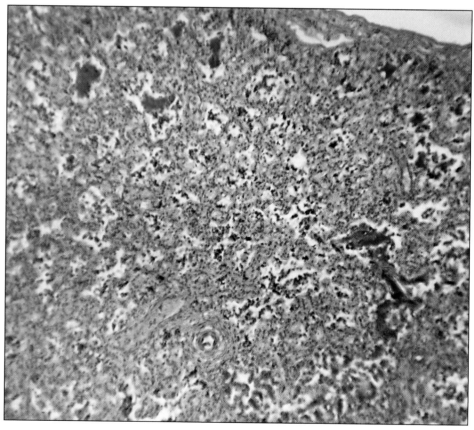

Fig. 375

A Case of *Premature placental detachment; massive retroplacental hemorrhage; cerebral periventricular, intraventricular, and subarachnoid hemorrhage.*

The mother was admitted in premature labor, at 24 weeks of pregnancy. At delivery, the newborn infant appeared lifeless, with only a faint heartbeat, and was pronounced dead at eight minutes.

The infant was intensely cyanotic (Figure 376).

Premature separation of the placenta had occurred. The placenta at delivery had a large dark-red adherent retroplacental hemorrhage of recent origin, occupying over half of the maternal surface. Also, at the edge of the placenta there was a deposit of gray-yellow old blood clot (page 66).

At autopsy there were findings of hypoxic congestive heart failure, with a large dilated heart distended with blood (Figure 377).

The brain was edematous. Blood was present in the subarachnoid space around the brain stem (Figure 378). The blood oozing from the foramina in the brain stem indicated the presence of cerebral intraventricular hemorrhage. This origin of the blood was confirmed in subsequent studies of the brain, studies demonstrating cerebral periventricular hemorrhagic infarction with intraventricular hemorrhage (Figure 379).

This case demonstrates the sequence of placental compromise, premature placental detachment, with consequent fetal hypoxic congestive heart failure, with resulting hypoxic cerebral damage.

Figure 376. Premature detachment of placenta; retroplacental hemorrhage, recent (dark red), and old (tan-brown). Premature newborn; 24 weeks' gestation, lived briefly, severe cyanosis.

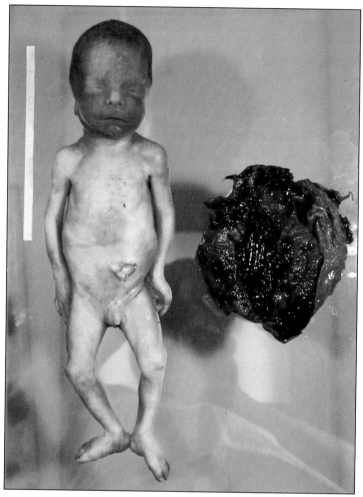

Fig. 376

Figure 377. Hypoxic congestive heart failure. Right atrium distended with blood. View of thoracic viscera at autopsy.

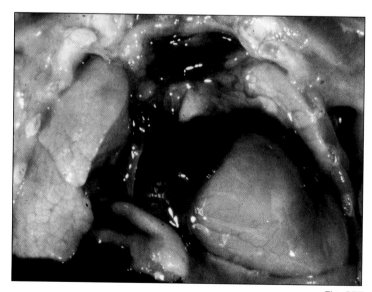

Fig. 377

Figure 378. Subarachnoid hemorrhage; extravasation of blood into the subarachnoid space around the brain stem. Blood from within the ventricles escaping through the foramina in the brain stem into the subarachnoid space.

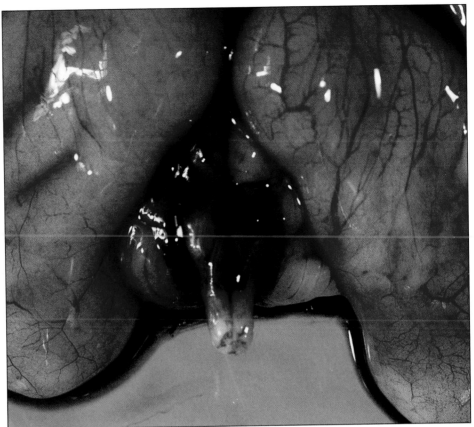

Fig. 378

Figure 379. Periventricular hemorrhagic infarction; intraventricular hemorrhage. Extension of the hemorrhage through the ventricular system into the subarachnoid space (Figure 378).

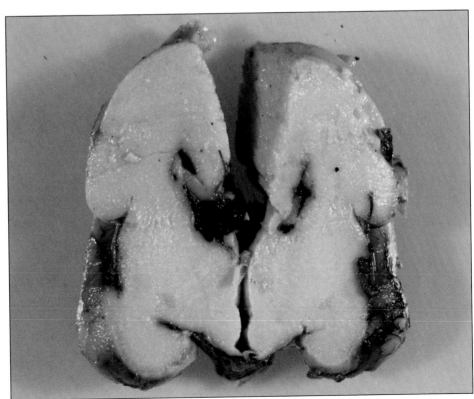

Fig. 379

A Case of *Retroplacental hematoma; vaginal bleeding; intrauterine growth retardation (IUGR).*

Recurrent vaginal bleeding had occurred at 8 weeks and 16 weeks of pregnancy. Premature labor developed at 30 weeks. Presentation was breech. The newborn infant, in very poor condition at birth, lived 1 hour.

The weight of this infant was 790 grams (average weight at 30 weeks, 1,200 grams), evidencing fetal deprivation, intrauterine growth retardation.

The placenta presented an old red-brown retroplacental hematoma firmly attached to the maternal surface (Figure 380).

In summary, the link, pathologically, between the presence of an old retroplacental hematoma and the occurrence clinically of recurrent vaginal bleeding is clearly demonstrated in this case (pages 67, 68).

The case also demonstrates the chronic compromising influence of placental disease on the fetus, the effect of an old retroplacental hematoma, causing intrauterine growth retardation.

Figure 380. Old retroplacental hematoma. The maternal surface of the placenta in the lower portion covered by a smooth pad of retroplacental blood clot; the red-brown color indicates the clot is old.

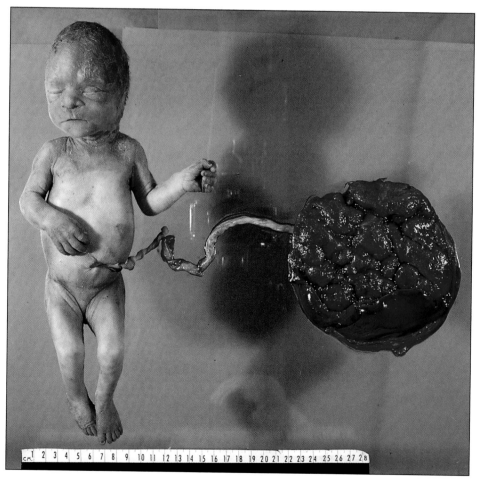

Fig. 380

A Case of   *Placental abruption; underlying placental infarction.*
Premature newborn; intrauterine growth retardation.

The mother was admitted in active labor at 33 weeks of pregnancy (prenatal information was not available) and delivered a stillborn infant. Intrauterine death apparently had occurred a period of time prior to delivery, evidenced by early maceration, slipping of the skin, with denuded areas about the legs. The infant was cyanotic (Figure 381).

The placenta presented an adherent large retroplacental hemorrhage, the cause of the intrauterine death.

Placental infarction was present, in addition to the retroplacental hemorrhage. Transection of the placenta revealed an extensive indurated pale portion of the placenta, an old infarction, under the retroplacental hemorrhage (Figure 382).

Autopsy indicated the fetus had died with hypoxic congestive heart failure, with the heart greatly enlarged, distended with blood (Figure 383), with viscera congested. The brain was swollen, edematous, with severe venous congestion (Figure 384).

This case is of special interest with regard to the pathogenesis of placental abruption: With placental infarction, the necrotic area of placental tissue at times becomes detached from the inner aspect of the uterine wall; bleeding from torn vessels in the uterine wall leads to the formation of a retroplacental hemorrhage, to placental abruption. With the fetus rendered hypoxic, fetal congestive heart failure, fetal death, follows. This pathologic sequence apparently occurred in the present case (pages 66 and 71).

Figure 381. Cyanotic premature infant, 33 weeks' gestation, stillborn. Early maceration, denuding of skin about the legs, indicating intrauterine death had occurred a period of time prior to birth. Placenta with large fresh adherent retroplacental hemorrhage.

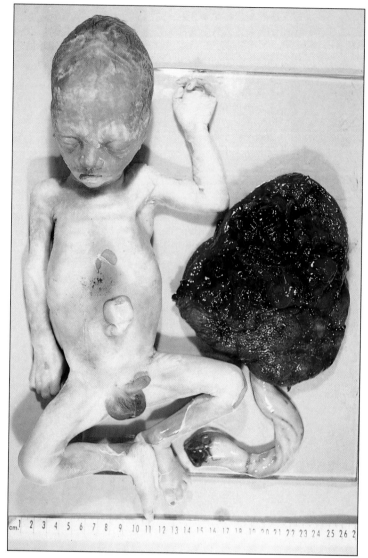

Fig. 381

Figure 382. Retroplacental hematoma with underlying extensive old placental infarction. Transection of the placenta (after preservation in formalin). Retroplacental hematoma over the pale tan infarcted area; compression, indentation, of part of the infarcted area.

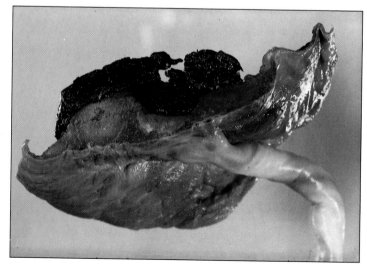

Fig. 382

Figure 383. Congestive heart failure. Heart, at autopsy, enlarged, distended with blood.

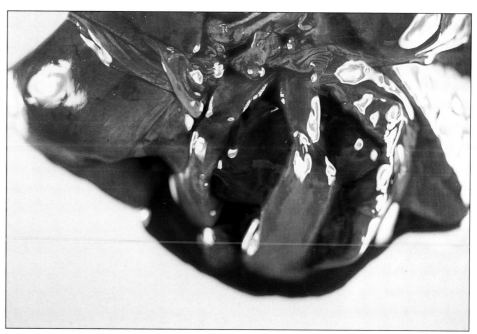

Fig. 383

Figure 384. Edematous swollen brain; surface veins engorged, consequence of congestive heart failure.

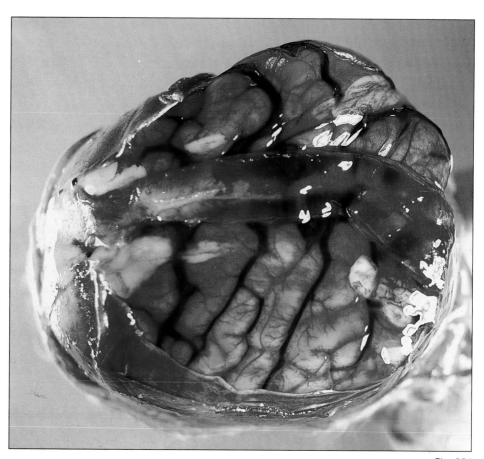

Fig. 384

A Case of

Toxemia; placental infarction; retroplacental hemorrhage; prolapse of cord; intranatal death.

The mother was obese; weight was 240 pounds. She was admitted near term with signs of preeclampsia, with hypertension, edema, excessive weight gain (page 51). She improved and was discharged.

Ten days later she was readmitted in labor. The mother indicated she had not felt fetal movement for some time. No fetal heart tones were audible. Further examination revealed prolapse of the umbilical cord (page 81).

At delivery the fetus, full term, was cyanotic (Figure 385). There was early maceration of the skin, denuded areas, evidencing that fetal death had occurred a period of time prior to delivery; this was consistent with the mother's report of loss of fetal activity prior to labor.

The placenta at delivery showed "50% premature detachment, with a mass of blood, approximately 300 ml., lightly adherent to the maternal surface."

At autopsy, the infant presented physical features of term maturity, with thick growth of head hair, well-developed ears. The weight was 2,510 grams (5 pounds 9 ounces, low birth weight for term), indicating intrauterine deprivation, IUGR. The skin, as noted at delivery, showed focal denuded areas.

The segment of umbilical cord attached to the fetus was thick, edematous and congested. The middle portion of the cord, apparently the prolapsed part, was thinned, flattened, pale.

The placenta, examined in the pathology laboratory, showed broad areas of the maternal surface covered with adherent blood clot (Figure 385), together with focal indurated areas of yellow discoloration that, on transection of the placenta, proved to be areas of infarction (Figures 386a and 386b).

The effect of the accumulated pathologic processes, causing intrauterine hypoxia, was evidenced at autopsy. Internal examination indicated that the fetus had died with hypoxic congestive heart failure, with enlargement, dilatation, of the heart, congestive hepatomegaly (Figure 387), congestion of the other body organs. The brain was swollen, edematous, congested (Figure 388).

In retrospect, did the preeclampsia affect the well-being of the fetus? The literature indicates there is an increased incidence of placental infarction in cases of eclampsia.

Low birth weight, IUGR, present in this case is attributable to the adverse effects of the old and recent placental infarctions compromising nutrition of the fetus.

As in other cases here presented, as in Case 83, page 447, this is an example demonstrating the link, pathologically, between the occurrence of placental infarction and placental abruption, retroplacental hemorrhage (page 66).

Regarding the cause of death, this fetus had three strikes against it, three major hypoxia-producing gestational complications — placental infarction and placental abruption, culminating in the third strike, the cord prolapse.

Figure 385. Cyanotic term infant; intrauterine death; early maceration, with patchy denuded areas of skin. Placenta with retroplacental hemorrhage; focal tan areas of infarction. The umbilical cord segment attached to the fetus is thick, edematous, congested. The middle portion of the cord is notably thin, pale; this is apparently the segment of cord that had been prolapsed.

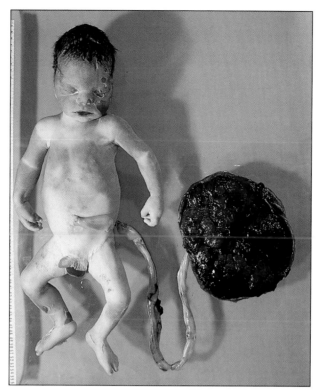

Fig. 385

Figure 386(a). Placenta, transected, revealing recent infarcts (dark red) and old yellow infarcts. (The placenta preserved in formalin, then transected.)

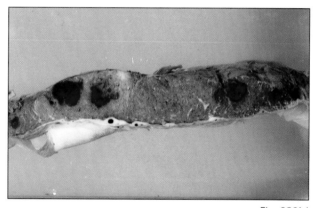

Fig. 386(a)

Figure 386(b). Placental infarcts (histologic section). Infarcts appear as large dense dark-staining areas.

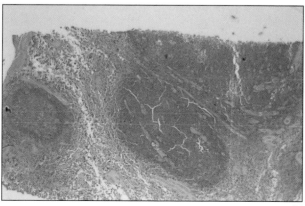

(b)

Figure 387. Congestive hepatomegaly; enlarged congested liver extending far below the rib margins. (View of abdominal organs at autopsy.)

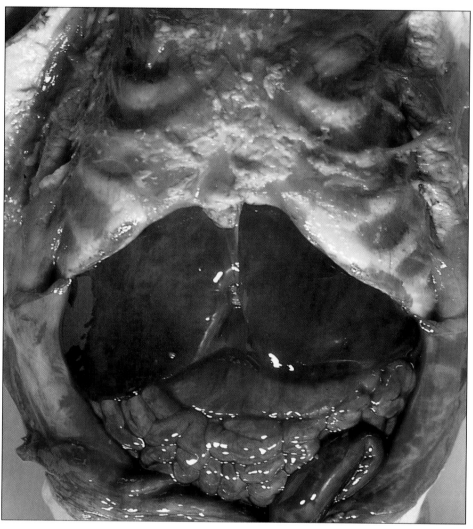

Fig. 387

Figure 388. Cerebral swelling, edema, congestion consequent to hypoxic congestive heart failure.

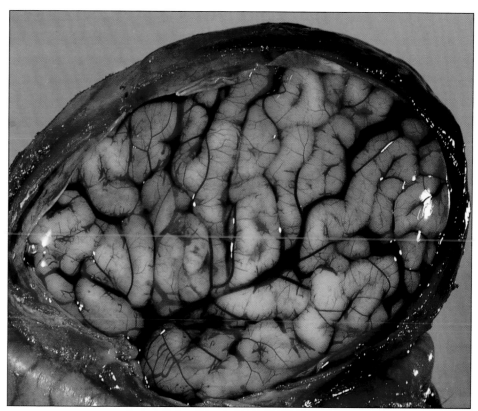

Fig. 388

A Case of   *IUD present during pregnancy; recurrent vaginal bleeding; placental abruption; premature birth at 32 weeks.*

Episodes of vaginal bleeding, increasing in frequency, occurred in the last months of this pregnancy. Premature labor developed at 32 weeks, with delivery of a liveborn infant, in poor condition; death occurred at 3 hours after birth.

An IUD was delivered with the placenta. The maternal surface of the placenta was coated with a thick layer of adherent dark red fresh hematoma together with a deposit of old tan blood clot (Figures 389 and 390).

The presence of an IUD during pregnancy is adversive to the mother and the fetus, frequently resulting in spontaneous abortion and sepsis. Vaginal bleeding and premature labor at times occur, as in the present case (page 88).

Figure 389. IUD delivered with placenta; extensive recent dark red retroplacental hemorrhage; focal deposits of old tan blood clot.

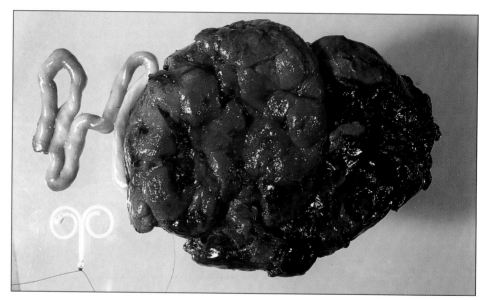

Fig. 389

Figure 390. Retroplacental hematoma, adherent to the maternal surface of the placenta. Histologic section through the edge of the retroplacental hemorrhage in Figure 389.

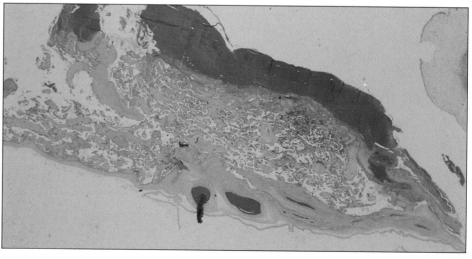

Fig. 390

A Case of **Old retroplacental hemorrhage; premature birth. IUGR newborn with congestive heart failure.**

The mother was admitted at 28 weeks of pregnancy in active labor; footling breech presentation was followed by the live birth of an infant in poor condition, limp, with weak respiratory effort. The infant's legs were edematous, cyanotic (Figure 391), reflecting the effects of the footling presentation (analogous to edema of the scalp, caput succedaneum, with cephalic delivery).

Apgar score was 2 at one minute and never improved. The infant remained flaccid and unresponsive.

The infant, weighing 850 grams (1 pound 14 ounces; average weight at 28 weeks, 1,100 grams), was underweight, and was long and thin, evidencing intrauterine nutritional deprivation, IUGR.

Death occurred at 3 hours.

The placenta had a large tan and red retroplacental hematoma that depressed the maternal surface and was tightly adherent (Figure 392). It was apparent that the retroplacental hematoma had compromised placental function, contributing to the development of IUGR (page 68).

The autopsy revealed pathologic changes of congestive heart failure. Ascites and hydropericardium were present. The heart was large, dilated, distended with blood, especially the right atrium and neck vein tributaries (Figure 393). The viscera were severely congested. The brain was edematous (Figure 394).

Figure 391. IUGR; premature infant of 28 weeks' gestation; 3-hour survival. Lower extremities cyanotic, edematous, due to footling breech birth.

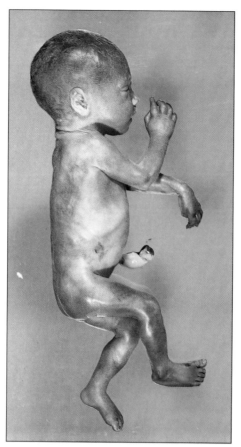

Fig. 391

Figure 392. Old retroplacental hematoma, mottled tan and red, depressing the placental surface, indicating the blood clot is of some age.

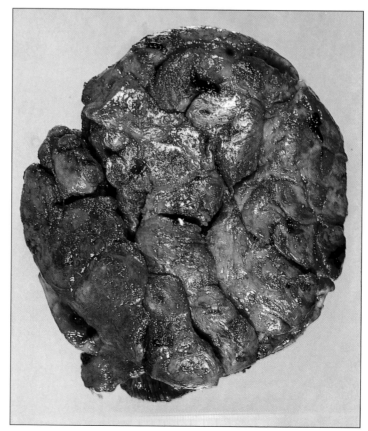

Fig. 392

Figure 393. Cardiac dilatation; right atrium and neck tributaries engorged with blood, effects of congestive heart failure. (View of thoracic viscera at autopsy.)

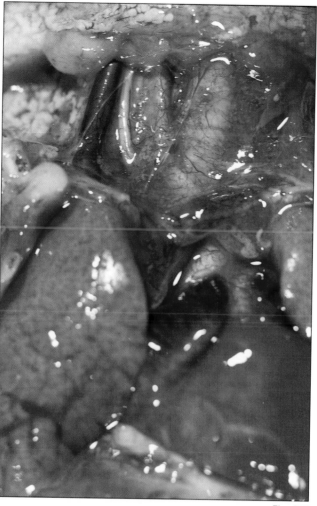

Fig. 393

Figure 394. Cerebrum, edematous; the primitive surface veins are congested.

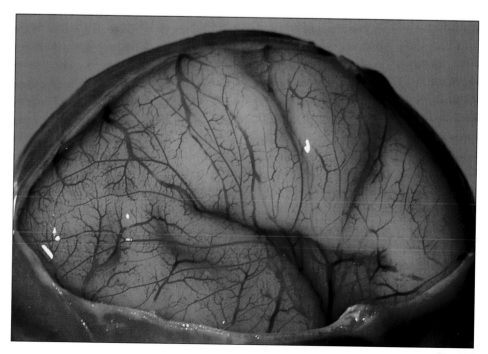

Fig. 394

A Case of   *A mother with poor reproductive history; multiple miscarriages. Placental abruption; premature newborn.*

Some mothers manifestly have faulty reproductive function, commonly with an obstetric history punctuated by repeated miscarriages, pregnancies terminated prematurely by placental abruption, retroplacental hemorrhage. The present case is an example of this (page 41).

This 30-year-old mother had been pregnant nine times. There were six miscarriages in early pregnancy, one stillbirth at term (Down syndrome), one stillbirth at 7 months.

With the ninth pregnancy, the present case, she delivered prematurely at 29 weeks; this was the first infant that survived. The Apgar score at one minute was 6 and at nine minutes was 8.

At delivery, placental abruption was present, massive retroplacental hemorrhage (Figure 395). Premature detachment had occurred in a pattern that commonly terminates pregnancy in mothers with poor reproductive function (page 66).

Figure 395(a). Placental abruption; massive retroplacental hemorrhage present at delivery. Premature delivery at 29 weeks; surviving newborn with good Apgar score.

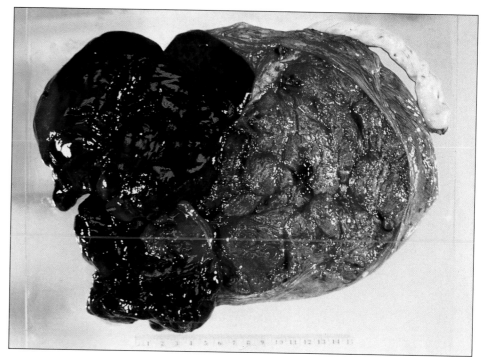

Fig. 395(a)

Figure 395(b). Placenta transected. Thick layer of adherent retroplacental blood over half of the placenta; underlying portion of placenta compressed, thinned, by the clot, indicating the clot was present for a long time.

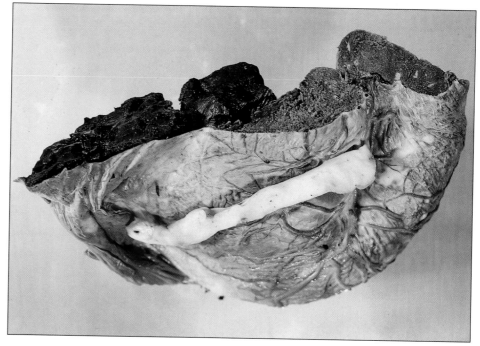

(b)

A Case of   *Respiratory depression at birth related to spinal injury.*

This premature infant was delivered spontaneously, vaginally, at 32 weeks of gestation. Delivery was recorded as "easily accomplished." Respiratory depression was present directly after birth. The infant was pale and cyanotic. Respiratory depression continued with periods of apnea. The infant died at 36 hours.

The main finding at autopsy was extensive spinal epidural hemorrhage (Figure 396). A thick extravasation of blood was present on the posterior aspect of the spinal canal, extending from the cervical through the upper thoracic segments. No other significant pathologic findings were evident at autopsy.

This is a good example of central respiratory depression due to spinal injury, due to compromise of respiratory centers in the spinal cord and brain stem (page 138). It is of interest to note that, as in this case, spinal injury at times occurs in cases in which the delivery is spontaneous, easily accomplished.

Figure 396. Spinal epidural hemorrhage; extravasation of blood in the cervical and thoracic regions. View of the spinal canal at autopsy; spinal cord removed, revealing spinal epidural hemorrhage. Premature infant of 32 weeks' gestation. Respiratory depression present at delivery and continued unrelieved, with death at 36 hours.

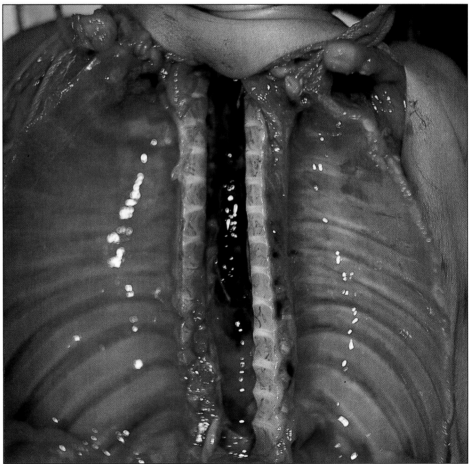

Fig. 396

A Case of   *Subacute hypoxic cerebral damage in a very premature newborn.*

Spontaneous labor developed at 25 weeks of gestation. This very premature infant responded to care initially, survived for 5 weeks.

At autopsy the cerebrum showed irregular disintegration of the tissue in the region of the periventricular germinal matrix — old subacute hypoxic infarctional damage (Figure 397a). Posteriorly the cerebral damage, penetrating deeply into the white matter, created extensive hemorrhagic cavitation (Figure 397b).

While the cerebral infarction may have originated in fetal life, it is probable that the hypoxic damage continued postnatally, accruing during the 5 weeks of survival, becoming subacute pathologically (page 24).

Figure 397(a). Subacute hypoxic cerebral damage. The area of the periventricular germinal matrix shows fragmentation and discoloration of the tissue. Section through the cerebrum in the frontal region.

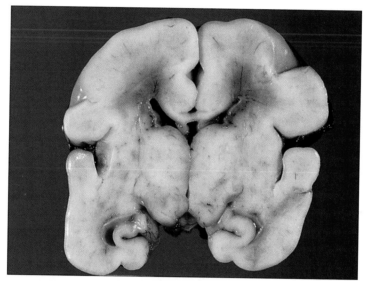

Fig. 397(a)

Figure 397(b). Subacute hypoxic cerebral infarctional damage in the periventricular white matter, appearing hemorrhagic, with cavitation. Section through the posterior of the cerebrum.

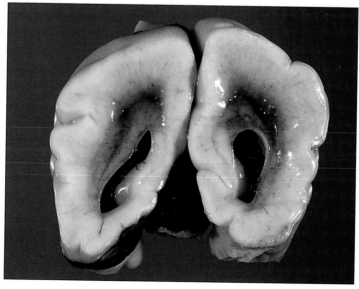

(b)

A Case of **_Complicated breech delivery; rupture of liver; fracture dislocation of spine._**

Labor developed spontaneously at 18 weeks of pregnancy, with frank breech presentation. The trunk of the flexed fetus was rapidly delivered, expressed through the rigid, only partly dilated, cervix. The cervix clamped down on the aftercoming head; manual extraction of the trapped head was necessary.

Death occurred during the process of the traumatic delivery.

Autopsy revealed major damage to the spine and to the liver. The trunk and buttocks showed hemorrhagic discoloration, the consequence of breech birth (Figure 398) (page 128).

The skin over the back of the head was avulsed, torn loose, during the difficult delivery, during the manual extraction of the aftercoming head.

X-ray of the body postmortem revealed spinal injury, cervical vertebral fracture dislocation (Figure 399) (page 135).

At autopsy, the internal examination revealed massive hemoperitoneum due to rupture of the liver (Figure 400). The liver injury is attributable to the breech delivery, with the trunk flexed, with the head pressed against the abdomen, compressing the liver, causing rupture of the liver (page 102).

It is apparent that this traumatic process, occurring early in the descent through the birth canal, leading to laceration and exsanguinating hemoperitoneum, was the cause of fetal death.

Figure 398. Traumatic delivery of small premature. Breech birth resulting in edema and hemorrhagic discoloration of the buttocks, back, and legs. (Overall tan appearance of the skin due to formalin preservative.) Avulsion of the skin over the occipital area due to difficulty in delivering the aftercoming head.

Figure 399. Spinal injury. Postmortem x-ray. In the neck the vertebral bodies are out of alignment, with irregular, increased, spacing between dislocated vertebrae.

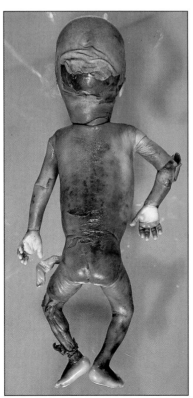

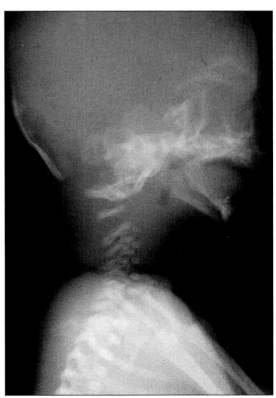

Fig. 398   *Fig. 399*

Figure 400. Rupture of the liver with resulting massive hemoperitoneum. The right lobe of the liver shows an irregular crush laceration, the source of the hemorrhage.

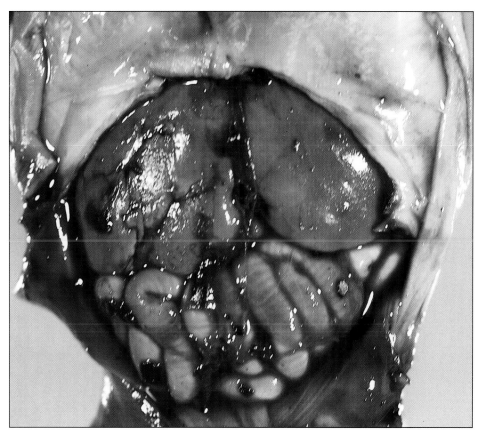

Fig. 400

A Case of   ***Sudden unexpected death of a large term newborn
due to tentorial tear with posterior fossa hemorrhage.***

The mother was 28 years old, para 1, gravida 2. This pregnancy was uncomplicated according to the record. The mother was admitted at term, in active labor. Presentation was cephalic, left occipito-anterior (LOA). The length of labor was 4 hours, 20 minutes. Delivery proceeded without difficulty. There was no dystocia.

The infant at birth was in good condition, with good vital function, good cry. She was large, weighed 9 pounds, and measured 21 inches in length.

At 9 hours after birth, the infant was examined and appeared in good condition. Observed one-half hour later, at 9 1/2 hours, the infant appeared quiet. One-half hour after this, at 10 hours, the nurse found the infant pale and mottled, not breathing, lifeless.

At autopsy, the main findings were intracranial, a posterior fossa hemorrhage due to a tear in the tentorium (see Figure 85, page 132).

On exposing the upper surface of the tentorium, a jagged laceration, a stretch tear, was present at the junction of the tentorium and the falx cerebri. The tear in the tentorium was 10 millimeters long, with the edges of the tear separated 3 to 6 millimeters.

When the tentorium was reflected, a large posterior fossa subdural hemorrhage was exposed (Figure 401).

It is of interest to note that the infant at death had become pale; this is attributable to the infant having bled out, with the occurrence of the intracranial hemorrhage (page 102).

The newborn infant, weighing 9 pounds, had a large head. It is apparent that during descent of the fetus, with molding of the large head, the tentorium was subjected to intolerable stretch strain and was torn.

This case is an example of injury incurred during birth, with the injury at first latent, silent, with the effects delayed, coming on catastrophically, unexpectedly, in the postnatal period. The reason for the delay is not entirely clear. It is apparent that the bleeding from the torn tentorium, at first oozing gradually, builds up; ultimately, the hemorrhage into the posterior fossa, mounting, causes compression of vital centers in the brain stem and results in death (page 133).

Figure 401. Posterior fossa subdural hemorrhage. (View of base of skull at autopsy.) Posterior fossa with about 30 milliliters of fluid blood.

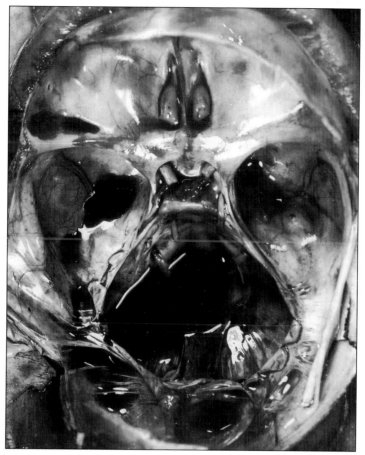

Fig. 401

A Case of   *Posterior fossa subdural hemorrhage;*
              traumatic delivery of the aftercoming head.

This infant was delivered at 37 weeks of gestation from a footling breech presentation. Respiratory difficulty and cyanosis were present at birth. The infant lived briefly.

At autopsy the infant appeared pale. The intracranial examination revealed a 1-centimeter tear in the tentorium. A large posterior fossa subdural hemorrhage was present (Figure 402).

With breech delivery, with the aftercoming head unmolded, intracranial injury, stretch-tear of the tentorium, with posterior fossa hemorrhage, is relatively common (page 133).

Figure 402. Posterior fossa subdural hemorrhage consequent to laceration of the tentorium. Autopsy view of base of the skull.

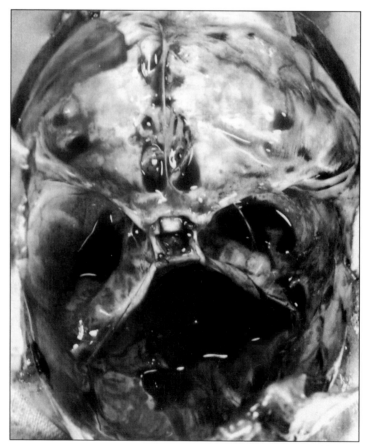

Fig. 402

A Case of   ***Twin transfusion syndrome; intrauterine death of one (hydropic) twin.***

The mother, a 21-year-old primipara with known twin pregnancy, was admitted in labor at term. Peripheral edema had developed; blood pressure rose to 170/120. The mother was treated for toxemia. Labor was desultory. Fetal heart tones became faint. Cesarean section was performed.

Twin A was stillborn; weight was 8 pounds 2 1/2 ounces. Twin B, somewhat smaller, weighing 7 pounds 9 ounces, was in good condition at birth and continued well clinically.

Twin A, at autopsy, was extremely edematous, the picture of hydrops fetalis (Figure 403). The face appeared bloated, the abdomen was distended. The body showed early maceration, with denuding of skin over the abdomen and extremities; this indicated that fetal death had occurred a period of time before delivery (page 9).

The placenta was large, weighed 1,400 grams. The fetal surface was separated by a thin midline septum. Microscopically, the septum, near its attachment to the placenta, showed remnants of chorionic villi, indicating these were apparently dichorionic (dizygotic) fraternal twins.

The fetal surface had prominently congested vessels. Although this was manifestly a case of twin transfusion syndrome, anastomotic connections between the vascular systems of the two twins were not demonstrated

The two sides of the maternal surface of the placenta were strikingly different (Figure 403). The part of the placenta belonging to the stillborn infant, twin A, was larger, mottled pale tan, and, like this twin, was edematous, boggy. The portion of umbilical cord attached to this side, like the segment attached to this fetus, was edematous and reddened.

The part of the placenta belonging to twin B, the survivor, was soft, dark red; the umbilical cord on this side was of ordinary appearance, tan and relatively thin.

Microscopically, portions of tissue from the two sides of the placenta were different, reflecting the dissimilarity grossly. The tissue from the portion of the placenta related to the stillborn twin, the pale side of the placenta, microscopically showed chorionic villi that were shrunken and without visible blood vessels (Figure 404a). In contrast, in the tissue from the part of the placenta that served the liveborn twin, the dark-red side, the chorionic villi were well preserved, plump, well vascularized (Figure 404b).

The autopsy indicated that the hydropic condition of twin A was due to fetal congestive heart failure (page 8). The subcutaneous tissue, the muscles, were edematous. Hydrothorax and hydropericardium were present (Figure 405). The heart was dilated, engorged with blood (Figure 406). Body viscera were congested. The brain was edematous, swollen, with flattened cerebral convolutions and venous congestion (Figure 407).

In cases of twin transfusion syndrome, one twin becomes the donor, the other, the recipient. Commonly, it is the donor that proves more vulnerable, becoming bled out and hypoxic and, if surviving, is born with hypoxic cerebral damage, or the infant is stillborn (page 97).

Less often it is the recipient that is worse off; becoming overloaded with blood, the fetus becomes plethoric, hydropic, due to congestive heart failure. Intrauterine hypoxia develops leading to intrauterine cerebral hypoxic damage; the hypoxic congestive heart failure at times results in fetal death, as occurred in the present case.

Figure 403. Twin transfusion syndrome; hydrops fetalis (recipient fetus). Bodily edema due to fetal congestive heart failure; stillborn (other twin liveborn). Early maceration, areas of denuded skin, indicating intrauterine death occurred a period of time before delivery. Placenta large, weighing 1,400 grams. Maternal surface; the portion of the placenta related to the stillborn infant pale, mottled gray-tan. The other side of the placenta (the liveborn twin) dark red.

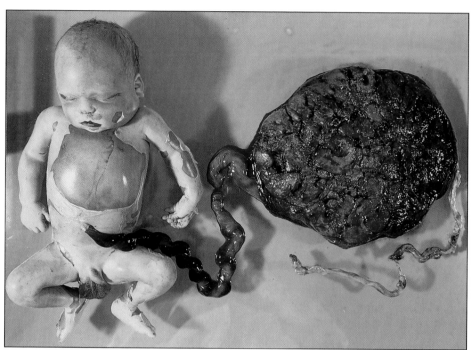

Fig. 403

Figure 404(a). Placental tissue from the pale part of the placenta (Figure 403), the part belonging to the stillborn twin; histologic section showing chorionic villi devitalized, shrunken, avascular. **(b).** Placental tissue from dark-red side of the placenta, the part belonging to the liveborn twin, showing well-preserved structures, with chorionic villi plump and well vascularized.

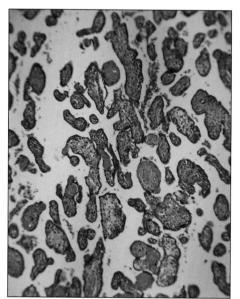 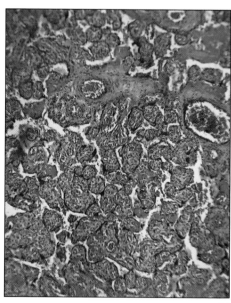

Fig. 404(a) (b)

Figure 405. Hydrothorax. Hydropic fetus manifesting congestive heart failure. Right pleural cavity containing 15 milliliters of clear watery fluid; the left, 14 milliliters. Hydropericardium; the heart visible within the enlarged pericardial sac; sac distended with 9 milliliters watery fluid. View of thoracic viscera at autopsy.

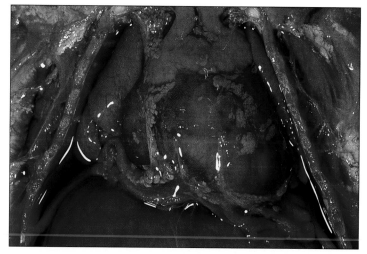

Fig. 405

Figure 406. Cardiac failure. Heart enlarged, dilated, distended with blood.

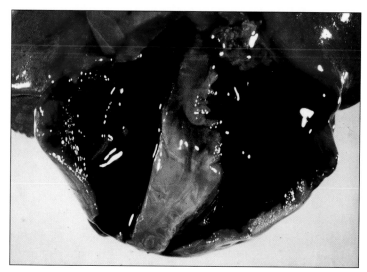

Fig. 406

Figure 407. Cerebral edema, swelling, with convolutions flattened. Veins congested.

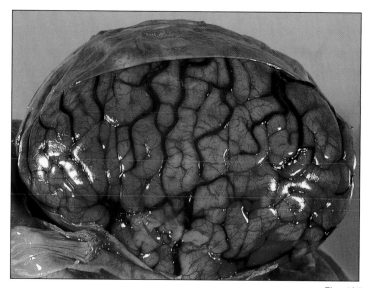

Fig. 407

A Case of   *Tight umbilical cord knot; newborn infant in good condition.*

This pregnancy was regarded as uneventful clinically. Spontaneous rupture of membranes occurred 12 hours before admission. Amniotic fluid was clear. Vertex presentation. Labor was induced with oxytocin. There was no sign of fetal distress during labor. The newborn infant was in good condition at birth with an Apgar score of 6 at one minute, 10 at five minutes.

The umbilical cord had a tight knot (Figure 408). Also there were several "false" knots.

This case is of clinical importance, demonstrating that, in a delivery, with no fetal distress evidenced, with the newborn in good condition at birth, the presence of an umbilical cord knot, even a tight knot, is not reason to conclude that hypoxic damage had occurred (page 85).

Figure 408. Tight knot in the umbilical cord; the newborn infant in good condition at delivery. It is of note that the cord, near the cut end, has two "false" knots, varicosities in the vein, appearing as red protrusions on the cord surface.

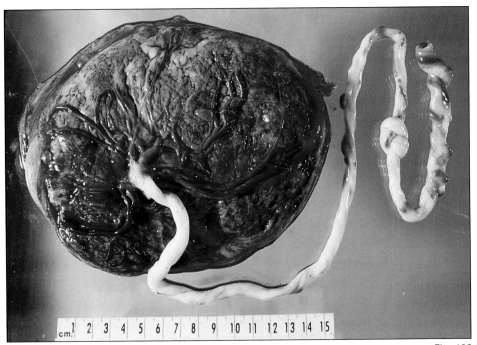

Fig. 408

A Case of   *Long umbilical cord; cord entanglement with nuchal cord and two tight cord knots.*

Decreased fetal activity was noted by the mother 2 days before admission (page 169). Pregnancy was near term. There were four previous pregnancies, with infants at term, liveborn.

At delivery, fetal heart was not audible. Amniotic fluid was dark brown.

The infant, stillborn, showed far-advanced maceration, in a degree commensurate with the history of loss of fetal activity during the 2 days before delivery.

The umbilical cord was tightly wound around the neck, a tight nuchal cord, and was entangled around the left shoulder, under the armpit, and just beyond this, the cord had two tight knots (Figures 409a and b).

The umbilical cord, unentangled from the fetus, was abnormally long, 120 centimeters, 4 feet, more than twice as long as is normal at term (average, 50 centimeters, about 2 feet long).

This case demonstrates the hazard to the fetus posed by an abnormally long cord. With the fetus afloat in the amniotic sac, even the ordinary 2-foot-long umbilical cord invites entanglement. When the cord is twice that long, the hazard is much increased (pages 80, 83 and 84).

Figure 409(a). Umbilical cord entanglement, with nuchal cord, cord around the left shoulder, under the armpit; two tight knots. Long cord malformation, 120 centimeters in length. Fetus with advanced maceration, indicating intrauterine death long before delivery. **(b).** Close-up of the tight knots in the umbilical cord.

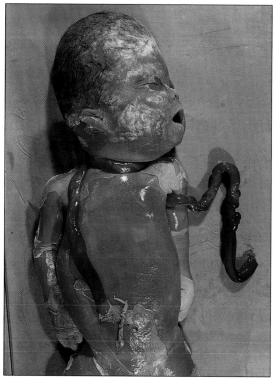

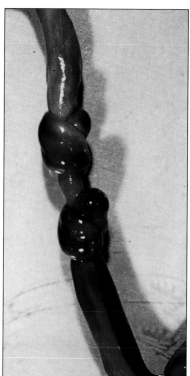

Fig. 409(a)   *(b)*

A Case of   *Intrauterine death due to umbilical cord tight knot.*

Intrauterine death had occurred a few days prior to birth. Gestation was estimated to be 35 weeks.

At delivery there was diffuse maceration of skin, reflecting intrauterine death a period prior to birth. The main finding was the presence of a tight knot in the umbilical cord, the cause of the fetal death (Figure 410) (page 84).

Figure 410(a). Tight umbilical cord knot; stillborn infant; diffuse maceration, areas of denuded skin, indicating fetal death a period prior to birth. **(b).** Tight knot in umbilical cord; enlarged view of knot shown in (a).

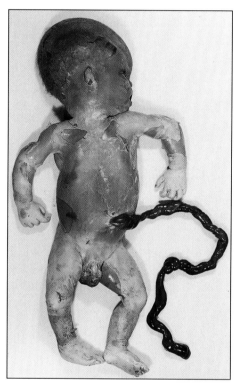

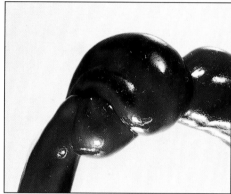

Fig. 410(a)

(b)

A Case of   *Maternal low weight gain during pregnancy; intrauterine growth retardation; pneumothorax; umbilical cord with multiple loose knots.*

Adversive gestational processes, of acute to chronic nature, occurred in this case, processes adversive to the well-being of the fetus, to the newborn infant.

This was a term pregnancy of 41 weeks. The mother was gravida 5, para 4. In this pregnancy manifestly she had a nutritional problem; she gained only 8 pounds. Maternal low weight gain is adversive to the fetus and often is associated with fetal nutritional deprivation, intrauterine growth retardation (page 94). The mother reported decreased fetal activity during the last week before delivery. During labor, meconium staining of the amniotic fluid appeared.

At birth, the infant was in poor condition, cyanotic, almost lifeless. He was resuscitated with oxygen and positive pressure ventilation. Death occurred at 3 hours.

At autopsy, severe cyanosis was present (Figure 411). The infant was small, with spindly extremities and little subcutaneous adipose tissue. Although of 41 weeks' gestation, the infant weighed only 4 pounds, 5 ounces (1,954 grams), reflecting the nutritional deprivation, IUGR, that had occurred.

The thorax at autopsy revealed large bilateral pneumothorax with compression atelectasis of the lungs (Figure 412). In addition to the pneumothorax, mediastinal interstitial emphysema had developed (page 111).

The pneumothorax, attributable to the positive pressure resuscitation efforts, causing unremitting bodily hypoxia, was the immediate cause of death.

The heart was large, dilated, distended with blood, the effects of congestive heart failure. Likewise, the bodily viscera were congested.

The cerebrum showed periventricular damage appearing as focal red-brown lesions at the caudothalamic angle on each side (Figure 413). These lesions, of subacute nature pathologically, were the residue of germinal matrix infarction, reflecting hypoxic insult during early intrauterine life. The damage in the cerebrum extended outward into the deep white matter (page 17).

Of interest were the presence in the umbilical cord of several loose knots (Figure 414). The question arises as to whether these knots were tightened at times during intrauterine life, contributing to fetal hypoxia.

In summary, in this complex case, the cause of death can be related to chronic factors, IUGR occurring in a gestation with maternal low weight gain, and to acute neonatal factors, a newborn infant who developed pneumothorax, leading to hypoxic congestive heart failure and death.

Figure 411. Cyanotic pale newborn, of 41 weeks' gestation; small for gestational age, IUGR.

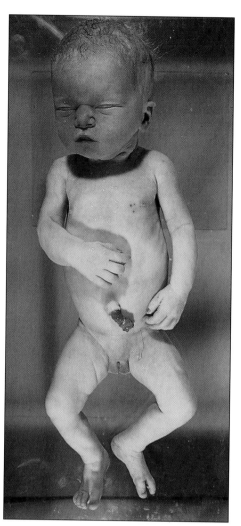

Fig. 411

Figure 412. Pneumothorax; compression atelectasis of lungs. More severe on the right, with over half of the pleural cavity appearing empty; vacant space created by the pressure pneumothorax displacing, compressing, the lung.

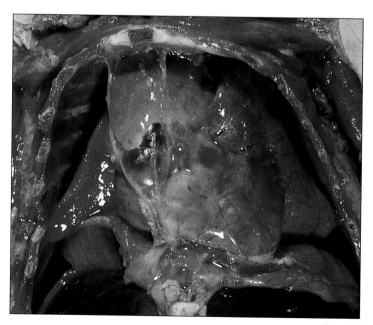

Fig. 412

Figure 413. Subacute cerebral infarctional damage, focal red-brown lesions at the caudothalamic angles on each side, the residues of hypoxic damage incurred during early fetal life. Damage extending into the cerebral white matter, in areas of gray discoloration. Frontal section of brain, embedded in plastic.

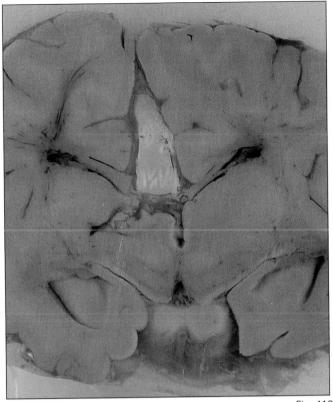

Fig. 413

Figure 414. Loose knots in the umbilical cord.

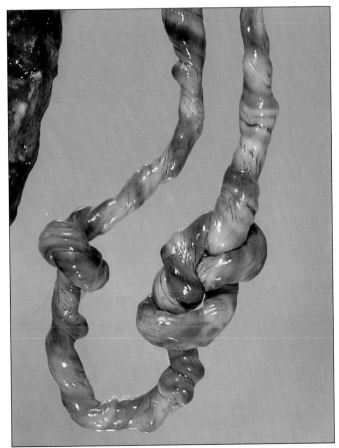

Fig. 414

A Case of   *Umbilical cord knot; newborn with no hypoxic manifestation.*

The infant was delivered by cesarean section. The mother was a primipara, with prolonged labor and failure of parturition to progress.

At delivery there was a firm knot in the umbilical cord (Figure 415a and b). It merits note that the part of the umbilical cord to the left of the knot, the segment going to the fetus, is thickened, edematous, evidencing that circulation through the cord was impeded. Manifestly this degree of circulatory compromise did not impact on the fetus; the newborn infant had an Apgar score of 10/10 (page 84).

Figure 415(a). Umbilical cord with firm knot. The segment of umbilical cord on the left (the part toward the fetus), thickened, edematous, reflecting some degree of obstruction of circulation. **(b).** Close-up view of knot.

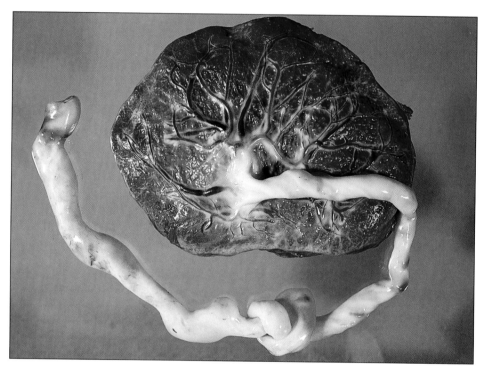

Fig. 415(a)

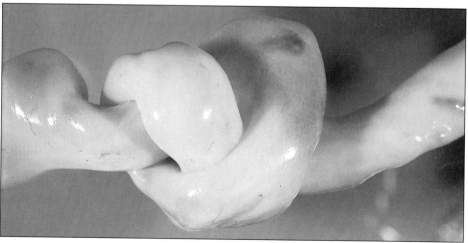

(b)

A Case of   *Long umbilical cord; nuchal cord wound round the neck six times; newborn infant with good Apgar score.*

Labor developed at term; presentation was full breech. During the second stage of labor, after the trunk was delivered and the neck exposed, a nuchal cord was evident. The nuchal cord, as it was removed, proved to be wound around the neck six times.

The infant at birth was in good condition, with an Apgar score of 8 and 10.

When the placenta was delivered, most notable was the unusually long umbilical cord (Figure 416). The length of the cord was 105 centimeters (4 feet 5 inches), twice as long as the average cord length at term (50 to 60 centimeters).

A long cord is a hazard to the fetus, prone to become entangled, prone to lead to nuchal cord (pages 80 and 83). If the cord around the neck becomes tightened, circulation through the cord is compromised, rendering the fetus hypoxic.

Manifestly, in the present case, as in most cases of nuchal cord, the cord remained loose around the neck and the fetus was not jeopardized.

Figure 416. Long umbilical cord; fetus with nuchal cord wound six times around the neck. Umbilical cord length, 105 centimeters. As evident in the illustration, the cord length is approximately seven times the width of the placenta (15 centimeters wide).

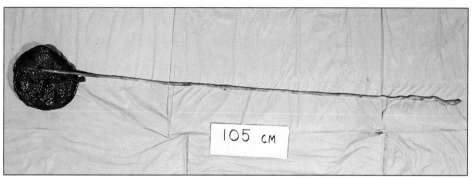

Fig. 416

A Case of   *Hypoxia-producing sickle cell disease and the development of congestive heart failure with visceral venous infarcts in the fetus.*

Manifestations of sickle cell disorder were evident pathologically in both the mother and the fetus in this case. Premature stillbirth occurred at 33 weeks of gestation. Prior to this pregnancy, the mother had given birth to two children with sickle cell disorder, one of whom had severe manifestations.

Sickle cell disorder causes anemia with resulting hypoxia in the mother and in the fetus. Fetal mortality is of increased incidence in mothers with sickle cell disorder.

There is evidence pathologically that red cell sickling was present in this case, in both the mother and the fetus. Red blood cells normally have the shape of a round biconcave plate. In persons with sickle cell disorder, when the red cells are subjected to decreased oxygen, some of the red cells assume a half-moon shape, a sickle shape (Figure 417).

Sickle cells manifestly are "sticky," so that when blood flow slows down, the distorted sticky cells become conglutinated, clumped together — stasis thrombosis. Stasis thrombosis of veins leads to hemorrhagic infarction of the tissue related to the thrombosed, occluded, vessel.

Pathologically, this syndromic sequence — red cell sickling, stasis-thrombosis, infarction — is evident in this case, affecting significantly the placenta, the fetal lung, and other organs.

The placenta in a case with maternal sickle cell disorder is characterized by the presence of multiple infarcts. Pathologic examination of the placenta in the present case showed a pattern of infarction. The infarcts were multiple. The presence of infarcts compromised the function of the placenta, creating placental insufficiency. With placental insufficiency, blood supply to the fetus, oxygenation of the fetus, was decreased. Circulation from the fetus to the placenta was slowed, reduced.

Placental insufficiency due to whatever cause renders the fetus hypoxic. While some fetuses may survive this hypoxic process, in some instances, as in the present case, placental insufficiency led to lethal fetal hypoxia.

When the fetus is subjected to increasing hypoxia, the first organ affected, evident clinically, is the heart. The muscle of the heart, the myocardium, lacking oxygen support, gradually becomes exhausted, weakened, and the heart slows down, bradycardia.

When the hypoxia is prolonged, cardiac weakening develops gradually and commonly the dominant effect is "backward failure," blood flow in the venous system slows down; stasis-thrombosis occurs in organs of the body. Stasis-thrombosis leads to congestion and infarction in the viscera. Viscera are congested and edematous; often watery edema fluid oozes out into the thoracic cavities and into the abdominal cavity (page 9).

The autopsy examination revealed the typical findings of hypoxic congestive heart failure: free fluid in the chest and abdomen; venous congestion of all the organs; stasis-thrombosis (conglutination of blood) in visceral veins; infarctional damage in the lungs, adrenals, and other organs.

The autopsy revealed bodily structures relatively well preserved but with some early degenerative postmortem-type changes indicating that fetal death had occurred a period of time before delivery.

Premature rupture of membranes had occurred a period of time prior to delivery; chorioamnionitis, far advanced, was evident pathologically (Figure 418).

It was thought by some that death had occurred during the process of birth. The pathologic findings at autopsy indicate that the lethal process developed long before birth, an hypoxic pathologic process related to the presence of sickle cell disorder, placental infarction with insufficiency, leading to a compromise of fetal oxygenation with consequent lethal hypoxic congestive heart failure, with visceral infarcts in the body.

Figure 417. Sickle cell abnormality of red cells. A chorionic villus, in cross section; histologic preparation. Many of the red cells are half-moon, sickle-shaped (normally red cells are round, biconcave).

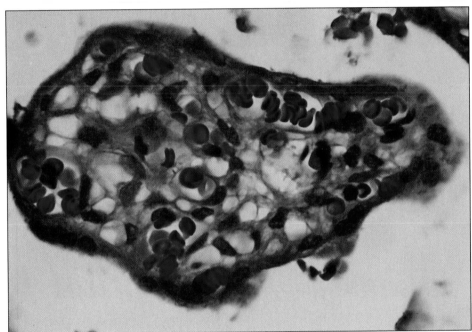

Fig. 417

Figure 418. Chorioamnionitis; histologic section. A strip of membranes, folded over; the deep strata with heavy infiltration of blue-staining inflammatory cells.

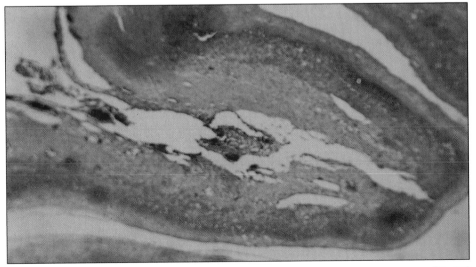

Fig. 418

A Case of   *Myocarditis in a newborn; antecedent maternal viral infection, anemia; maternal drug abuse; fetus with nuchal cord; fetal-neonatal anemia; hemorrhagic subacute cerebral lesion; basal ganglia calcification. Cerebral palsy, mental retardation, seizure disorder, microcephaly, hydrocephaly, and porencephaly developed later in infancy.*

Myocarditis in this newborn was diagnosed early in the postnatal period and was considered related to maternal viral infection during pregnancy.

Clinically this was manifest as a sudden onset of cardiac symptoms with bradycardia and shock in a previously stable newborn — a clinical picture characteristic of neonatal myocarditis.

The newborn in this case presented evidence of intrauterine deprivation. The infant, of 42 weeks gestation, was malnourished, long and thin, characterized as being scrawny. Additionally, the newborn was anemic. At birth there was a tight nuchal cord compromising the infant. Meconium staining was present; however, the infant did not aspirate and did not develop meconium pneumonia. The newborn, although with a good Apgar, 9 at five minutes, in the course of the first day developed cardiac complications and became neurologically depressed.

Maternal causal factors contributing to the compromise of fetal well-being included drug abuse during early pregnancy, maternal anemia, acute viral infection, and borderline diabetes.

With regard to the CT studies, this is a key case in that the sequence of CT scans demonstrates the transition of a large cerebral lesion, present at birth, undergoing changes gradually over a period of time, ultimately, at 1 year, present as porencephalic cavitations in the cerebrum; hemorrhagic lesions in the basal ganglia seen postnatally subsequently became calcified.

CT scans taken neonatally showed an apparent hemorrhagic lesion in the left temporoparietal region, consistent with a bleeding subacute cerebral infarction having origin early on, during intrauterine life (Figure 419). Subarachnoid blood was present, indenting the lesion in the left temporoparietal region and extending posteriorly over the cerebrum. At other levels of the scan, intraventricular blood was evident, apparently due to bleeding from the hemorrhagic lesion in the temporoparietal region, with blood passing through the ventricular system into the subarachnoid spaces.

In this scan it is significant that the ventricles are large, indicating an absence of cerebral edema, absence of ventricular compression, indicating that the cerebral damage is subacute; if this were acute cerebral damage, the brain would be edematous, swollen, with compressed, obliterated ventricles.

The CT scan taken 4 days later shows the lesion in the left temporoparietal area with a pale center, a deposit of blood, surrounded by a rarefied translucent border extending to the surface, a border of necrotic tissue indicating slow disintegration of tissue (Figure 420).

The CT scan taken at 9 days shows the lesion in the left temporoparietal area with less evidence of blood but a broadened area of rarefaction, indicating progression of necrosis (Figure 421)

The CT scan of the brain taken at 6 weeks (Figure 422) shows ventricles much enlarged due to increased intracerebral pressure resulting from blood clot obstructing the outflow of cerebral spinal fluid from the cerebrum, the blood apparently originating from the hemorrhagic infarct (page 157).

In the CT scan of the brain taken at 3 months, subsequent to the insertion of a ventricular shunt (Figures 423a and b), placed to establish drainage and relieve intraventricular pressure, the ventricles are smaller than in the scan 2 months previous.

In Figure 423(a), in the region of the right basal ganglia, there is a density, an apparent focus of hemorrhage or calcification. The left temporoparietal area shows a patchy translucency, a honeycombed lesion, the residue of the lesion seen originally in Figures 419 and 420.

Figure 423(b), a scan through an upper level of the cerebrum, shows large porencephalic cysts in both frontal lobes.

The CT scan of the brain taken at 1 year (Figure 424) shows an area of density (calcification) in the right basal ganglia, in the caudate nucleus, corresponding to the large hemorrhagic lesion in this area seen previously. The left temporoparietal lesion persists.

Neurologic sequels that developed in this infant included spastic cerebral palsy, mental retardation, seizure disorder, transient hydrocephaly, and microcephaly. The calcified lesion in the basal ganglia is of particular interest with regard to the development of cerebral palsy in this case.

Figure 419. CT scan of the brain taken at 2 days. In the deep strata of the left temporoparietal region there is a large pale area indicating the presence of a hemorrhagic infarcted lesion of subacute nature having origin during intrauterine life. This portion of the cerebrum is indented due to the presence of an accumulation of subarachnoid blood. Subarachnoid blood is also apparent (pale area) over the left posterior part of the cerebrum. Significantly ventricles are widely patent.

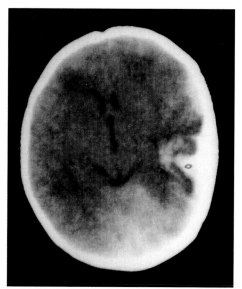

Fig. 419

Figure 420. CT scan taken at 6 days shows the lesion in the left temporoparietal region with a pale center, a deposit of blood surrounded by a rarefied translucent border extending to the surface.

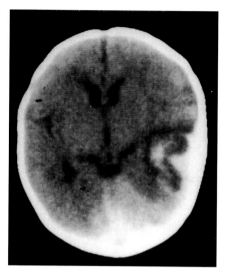

Fig. 420

Figure 421. CT scan taken at 9 days shows the left temporoparietal lesion seen previously, now with less intracerebral blood and with an enlarged area of rarefaction from the ventricle outward through the cerebral wall. The subarachnoid collection of blood indenting the left temporoparietal region persists.

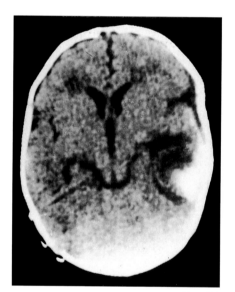

Fig. 421

Figure 422. CT scan of the brain taken at 6 weeks shows the ventricles much enlarged.

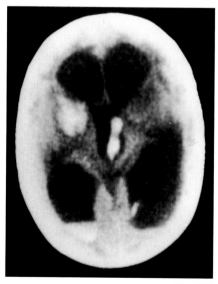

Fig. 422

Figure 423. CT scan of the brain taken at 3 months after insertion of ventricular shunt. The ventricles are reduced in size. **(a).** In the region of the right basal ganglia, a persisting hemorrhagic lesion corresponding to the lesion seen in Figure 422. The left temporoparietal area shows a translucency, a honeycombed lesion, the residue of the lesion seen originally in Figures 419 and 420.
(b). A scan through an upper level of the cerebrum shows large porencephalic cysts in both frontal lobes.

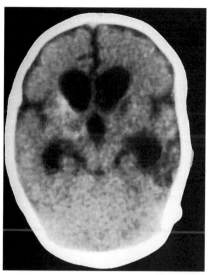 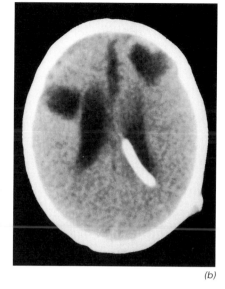

Fig. 423(a)

(b)

Figure 424. CT scan of the brain taken at 1 year shows an area of density (calcification) in the right basal ganglia, in the caudate nucleus, corresponding to the large hemorrhagic lesion in this area seen previously. The left temporoparietal lesion persists.

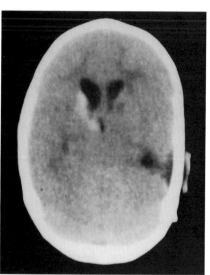

Fig. 424

A Case of   *Microcephaly vera; severe mental retardation.*

The history indicated that this child was the product of a normal term gestation with uneventful labor and delivery. The parents noted that the baby was quiet, inactive, and almost never cried.

Examination at 2 1/2 months noted that the child was microcephalic. She was listless and thought to be developmentally retarded.

Two older siblings in the family had developed normally, physically and mentally.

At 10 months her head was noticeably small, microcephalic (head circumference, 40.3 centimeters; normal at 10 months, 45 centimeters).

On examination at 25 months her head circumference was 41.5 centimeters (normal at 25 months, 48 centimeters). Motor movements were of a gross undifferentiated form.

Psychological testing at 3 years indicated a social quotient of 9, equivalent to a social age of 3 months, reflecting a severe degree of mental retardation.

There was little increase in size of the head in subsequent years.

The infant had frequent respiratory infections with high fever. She died at 6 years of age.

At autopsy, the head was small, with a circumference of 43 centimeters. The brain was small and weighed 690 grams (average weight at 6 years, about 900 grams). The convolutional pattern of the cerebrum appeared simplified with a paucity of tertiary sulci. The cortex showed no evidence of damage (Figure 425).

Considering the clinical and pathologic aspects of the case, this is an example of the relatively rare group of cases of microcephaly vera, cases with severe mental retardation due to an intrinsic failure in development and growth of the cerebrum. Although the occurrence of microcephaly vera commonly has a familial lineage, at times cases make their appearance without an apparent underlying genetic basis.

Figure 425. Microcephaly vera. Clinically the infant had a small head, was microcephalic. Little increase in size of the head during childhood. Death at 6 years. At autopsy the brain weighed 690 grams, approximately a third less than average.

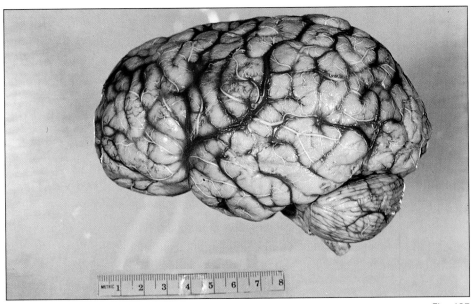

Fig. 425

A Case of   *Maternal gestational illness with severe psychiatric stress, with chronic colitis; abruptio placentae. Offspring with hemiplegic cerebral palsy, partial blindness and seizure disorder.*

Hypoxic cerebral damage in the premature immature fetus often affects the cerebrum asymmetrically, one hemisphere being more damaged than the other. The sequelant manifestations usually reflect this, affecting one side of the body more than the other (page 182). The present case is an example of this.

The mother had a history of chronic medical and emotional stress illnesses, beginning at the age of 16 years and extending through this pregnancy at age 25 years. The mother's emotional stress processes had serious visceral pathologic effects, resulted in psychosomatic inflammatory disease of the intestine, manifestations of functional colitis resembling Crohn's disease. Psychosomatic processes, compromising visceral function of the mother, pose a hazard to the well-being of the fetus. During the pregnancy, the mother had headache, dizziness, "nerves" — recorded through months of this pregnancy (page 53).

The pattern in the present case is reflective of an infant with chronic intrauterine compromise, bearing latent subacute cerebral damage that originated long before labor, latent damage that became manifest in later infancy as cerebral palsy and other cerebral disabilities.

At term the mother had a sudden onset of vaginal bleeding. Abruptio placentae was diagnosed. Figure 426 is a histologic section of the placenta showing retroplacental hemorrhage.

The newborn infant was in good condition, with an Apgar of 6 and 7.

The newborn did well on the first day. On the second day an episode of apnea (seizure apnea?) occurred. After that, the infant did well and was discharged on the seventh day.

For the next 11 months the infant did well, with no apparent neurologic manifestations. At 11 months the infant experienced a seizure, beginning in the right extremities and extending over the body. CT studies of the brain at this time showed a decrease in size of the left cerebral hemisphere, with damage affecting mainly the posterior of the left cerebrum. The left lateral ventricle was enlarged (Figure 427).

This CT study and subsequent imaging studies demonstrate the pattern of late chronic cerebral damage related clinically to the development of cerebral palsy (page 188).

A CT scan taken at 2 years 9 months again showed the left side of the cerebrum much decreased, with progressive enlargement of the lateral ventricle (Figure 428).

At 6 years of age an MRI scan showed much decrease of the deep strata of white matter, particularly in the posterior portion of the left cerebrum (Figure 429). In contrast, overall, most of the cerebral cortex remained.

At age 7 years, clinically the child showed minimal manifestations of hemiplegic cerebral palsy, with involvement of the right side of the body, reflecting damage to the left cerebrum and partial blindness (right homonymous hemianopsia) affecting the right visual field, reflecting damage to the left posterior (occipital) portion of the cerebrum. There was a decrease in fine motor skills. The child developed seizure disorder and was mildly retarded.

This case demonstrates the progressive loss of left cerebral substance over a period of years, resulting in asymmetrical cerebral palsy, hemiplegia.

It merits emphasis that the primary damage is deep, periventricular, evidenced by the left enlarged lateral ventricle at 11 months; this loss of deep white matter is particularly evident in the left posterior parietal lobe. In contrast to the loss of deep white matter strata, most of the cortex is still present.

Figure 426. Retroplacental hemorrhage. The histologic section of the placenta in this case shows an accumulation of blood behind the placental tissue, apparent in the lower right portion of the illustration; the fetal surface of the placenta is present, convoluted, extending diagonally through the illustration.

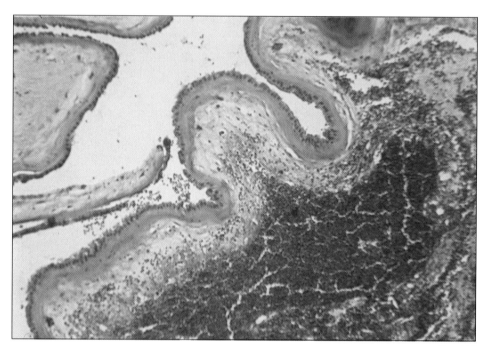

Fig. 426

Figure 427. Asymmetrical cerebral damage in this case; CT scan taken at 11 months. The left cerebral hemisphere is smaller than the right and shows an enlarged lateral ventricle (the black oval); these changes reflect damage to the deep periventricular white matter and consequent growth attenuation of the left cerebrum.

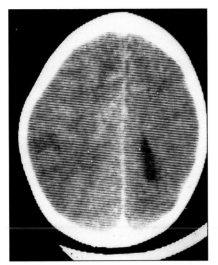

Fig. 427

Figure 428. CT scan of cerebrum in this case taken at 2 years 9 months, some 2 years after that shown in Figure 427. Progression of pathologic changes, the left hemisphere proportionately much smaller than the right.

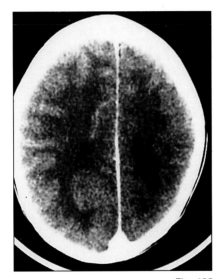

Fig. 428

Figure 429. MRI scan at 6 years shows the chronic, "end-stage," pattern of damage. The left parieto-occipital region (in the illustration the lower half of the left cerebrum) shows much decrease of the deep strata of white matter, compared with that on the right. In contrast, most of the cerebral cortex is still present.

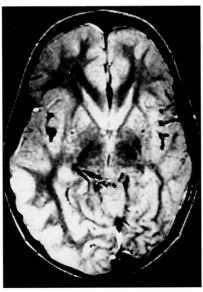

Fig. 429

A Case of ● ***Xanthochromic spinal fluid at birth indicating presence of old brain damage. Infant ultimately developed cerebral palsy, mental retardation, seizure disorder, and microcephaly.***

When a "spinal tap" is done, one of the most important details is the color of the fluid. Xanthochromic spinal fluid means the fluid, instead of being water-clear, colorless, has a yellow tinge (*xantho-,* yellow; *-chromia,* color) (page 173).

The fluid that is removed at the time of the spinal tap is a sample of cerebrospinal fluid that is produced in the cerebral ventricles and then circulates out into the subarachnoid space. The subarachnoid space lies beneath the arachnoid membrane surrounding the brain and spinal cord.

The finding of xanthochromic subarachnoid spinal fluid is of major importance in defining the time of incurrence of the cerebral damage.

The presence of xanthochromic spinal fluid in a newborn is substantial evidence of old, subacute, cerebral hemorrhagic damage that originated long before birth.

In the present case, a lumbar spinal tap was done 1 hour and 15 minutes after birth. The spinal fluid was bloody. (In the laboratory, a tube of the spinal fluid is centrifuged so that the blood cells become packed at the bottom of the tube. The fluid above the packed cells, the supernatant, is examined.) The supernatant fluid in the present case was slightly xanthochromic, yellowed.

Xanthochromia, yellow coloration of the spinal fluid, is due to the presence of old hemorrhagic damage in the brain.

With hemorrhage in the brain, with blood escaping into the ventricles, into the spinal fluid, red cells become lysed, broken down; the hemoglobin from the red cells first gives the spinal fluid a pink color. The hemoglobin gradually degenerates to a yellow pigment, giving the spinal fluid a yellow color — xanthochromia. (Just like a hemorrhagic black and blue bruise in the skin gradually becomes yellow-green after a period of time.)

This change in color takes many days, and continues to be present for weeks and months when there is an old hemorrhagic lesion in the brain.

Xanthochromia does not develop in a few hours, or even in a day or two. This is my experience as a laboratory pathologist in observing spinal fluid specimens in cases of head injury, cases in which the time of damage is known.

The finding of xanthochromia in the present case is firm evidence that the brain damage in the fetus, the infant, occurred a long time before labor and delivery.

Relevant to this, this term gestation was complicated by substantial clinical-pathologic processes. Vaginal bleeding occurred in the middle trimester, reflecting a placental disorder. The placenta at delivery was pathologic, fibrotic. Adding to this was the presence of a nuchal cord. These factors, the occurrence of placental and umbilical cord disorders, manifestly compromised the fetus, causing chronic fetal hypoxia.

How did the xanthochromia of the spinal fluid come about? The presence of xanthochromic spinal fluid means that there had been extravasation of blood into the subarachnoid fluid at a point previous to the time of birth.

The first CT scans, on day 1, were reported as showing intraventricular hemorrhage with blood extending out into the subarachnoid space. Considering that the subarachnoid fluid was xanthochromic, it is conclusive that the bleeding seen in the CT scan originated at a time prior to birth.

With blood present in the ventricles, the origin of the blood in this term infant was no doubt from a deep periventricular source, from (subacute) damage originating during premature fetal life. Like a chronic duodenal ulcer, these cerebral lesions have areas of hemorrhagic necrosis, and bleed. Deep periventricular damage is incurred specifically in the premature cerebrum; it does not originate in the mature cerebrum.

The later CT scan at 13 weeks showed extreme wasting away of the cerebral walls, especially in the frontal lobes, with extensive loss of deep white matter, ex vacuo hydrocephalus. Pertinently, the surface strata, the cortical and subcortical strata, were relatively preserved (Figure 430). Pathologically, this pattern of damage, with loss of deep periventricular tissue, reflects damage incurred during the premature period of intrauterine fetal life.

The loss of periventricular tissue involving white matter, as well as neighboring basal ganglia, evident in the CT scans (ex vacuo hydrocephalus), accounts for spastic cerebral palsy in this case and accounts for the retardation of brain growth, microcephaly, present. The manifest extension of damage to the surface, to the cortex, accounts for the mental retardation and seizure disorder.

Figure 430. Cerebral damage evident in the CT scan taken at 13 weeks of age in this case. Clinical evidence of brain damage originating during early fetal life, with spinal fluid found to be xanthochromic at birth. Lateral ventricles are enlarged due to loss of deep periventricular white matter. Cerebral convolutions anteriorly are shrunken, atrophied, due to loss of white matter; surface cortical strata relatively preserved.

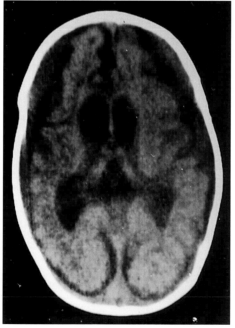

Fig. 430

A Case of   *Intrauterine growth retardation with associated cerebral damage and sequelant mental retardation and psychopathy.*

This infant, born at term, weighed 3 pounds, reflecting intrauterine growth retardation (IUGR). In infancy she was a weakling, developmentally retarded. At age 13 chronologically, her mental age was about 7 years; IQ was 52. The child became increasingly psychotic (page 212), difficult to manage. She developed diabetes and at age 46 she died of pneumonia.

The brain at autopsy was small, weighed 950 grams (average for the age, about 1,150 grams). The cerebral convolutional pattern was simplified, underdeveloped, lacking tertiary sulci, as compared with the normal adult brain. The frontal and occipital poles of the cerebrum were blunted, characteristic of maldeveloped brains (Figure 431).

The left side of the cerebrum showed a distorted convolutional pattern; the convolutions around the sylvian fissure were irregular, some enlarged, some shrunken (Figure 432). This view also demonstrates a structural disproportion between the main parts of the brain, with the relatively undersize cerebrum and the large (normal) cerebellum.

The internal structure of the cerebrum was abnormal, with a paucity of white matter, particularly posteriorly where there were areas of gray discoloration, old brain damage (Figure 433). On the left side of the cerebrum the temporal convolutions were narrowed, shrivelled, corresponding to the convolutional abnormalities evident in Figure 432.

This is a case that demonstrates the link between intrauterine fetal deprivation, with IUGR, and manifest cerebral compromise, cerebral damage, with the surviving infant, and later the adult, developing sequelant cerebral disabilities of organic mental retardation and psychopathy.

What is the genesis of the brain damage?

Special studies in this case indicated that the damage was of venous infarctional nature having its origin in fetal life (page 11). In the fresh brain specimen the deep venous system was injected with radiopaque substance; the brain was then x-rayed. The x-rays showed a striking difference in the deep venous system on the two sides; the venous structures of the left were much reduced compared with the right (Figure 434). The reduced pattern of veins on the left is attributable to remote thrombotic occlusion. Pathologically, the reduced venous function on the left can be correlated with the abnormal, damaged, convolutions on the left as seen in Figure 433.

Figure 431. The brain in this case, on the left, is small compared with the normal-size brain on the right. The convolutions appear large, underdeveloped, lacking tertiary sulcation. Frontal and occipital poles are blunted.

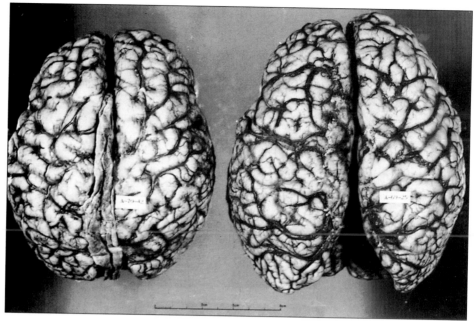

Fig. 431

Figure 432. The left side of the cerebrum showing abnormal convolutional pattern around the sylvian fissure, some convolutions being large and some, in the temporal lobe, appearing compromised, shrunken. The sylvian fissure anteriorly is open, undeveloped, resembling the fetal brain of 35 weeks' gestation.

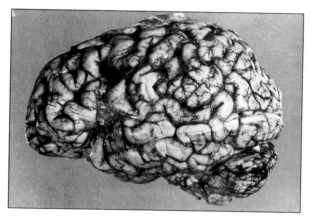

Fig. 432

Figure 433. Cerebrum showing abnormal architecture (horizontal section through the cerebrum); decreased white matter. Posteriorly, on the left, broad areas of gray discoloration, areas of old damage. On the left, temporal convolutions are irregular, shrivelled, corresponding to the abnormal convolutional pattern evident on the left side of the cerebrum externally (Figure 432).

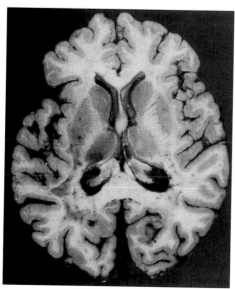

Fig. 433

Figure 434. X-ray of the brain specimen in this case. **(a).** The deep venous system has been injected with radiopaque substance. On the right, the deep venous tributaries are richly distributed through the cerebral white matter. In contrast, the venous distribution on the left is less prominent. In the x-ray, the structures of the left cerebral hemisphere are noticeably distorted, diminished. This can be correlated with the pattern of less venous branches on the left.

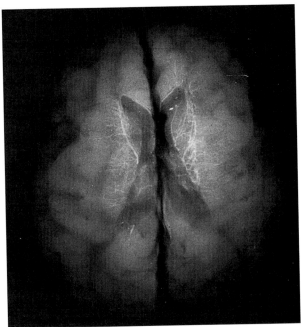

Fig. 434(a)

Figure 434(b). A close-up view of the injected cerebrum showing the difference between the relatively intact venous system on the right compared with the diminished venous pattern on the left.

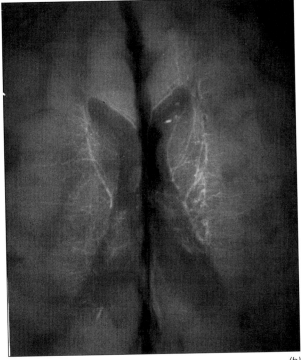

(b)

A Case of   *Intrauterine growth retardation; basal ganglia damage. Infant developed cerebral palsy, mental retardation, seizure disorder, and microcephaly.*

This term newborn weighed 4 pounds 8 ounces (2,000 grams), an example of intrauterine growth retardation (IUGR) (page 94). The pregnancy was reported to have been uncomplicated; the cause of the IUGR was unclear.

During early infancy microcephaly was apparent, and at 5 months spastic cerebral palsy was diagnosed. The child developed seizure disorder and was severely mentally retarded.

The infant failed to thrive. The size of her head remained small, severe microcephaly. At age 10, her head circumference was 43 centimeters (average at 10 years is 52 centimeters). There were frequent respiratory infections. She expired at age 10 years.

At autopsy the severe microcephaly evident externally (Figure 435) was associated with a correspondingly small brain (Figure 436). The weight of the brain, 530 grams, was about one-half the average weight for the age (average weight at 10 years, about 1,000 grams). The frontal and parietal portions of the cerebrum were much reduced structurally compared with the temporal and occipital regions.

The internal structures of the cerebrum (Figure 437) showed old chronic damage to periventricular structures, with scarring and loss of tissue, resulting in ex vacuo hydrocephalus (page 29). As illustrated, the white matter around the ventricles was decreased, with scarring and distortion of the caudate nuclei (basal ganglia) (page 185). The temporal lobe structures were less affected.

The clinical manifestations of microcephaly and cerebral palsy are directly attributable to the damage to the deep structures, the scarring of the caudate nuclei and loss of periventricular substance. Likewise the mental retardation and seizure disorder in this case were the consequence of diffuse cerebral damage.

Figure 435. Severe microcephaly due to brain damage incurred during fetal life. The side view of the head shows the outline of the face of ordinary proportions; the upper part of the head is flattened, lacking ordinary roundness, fullness.

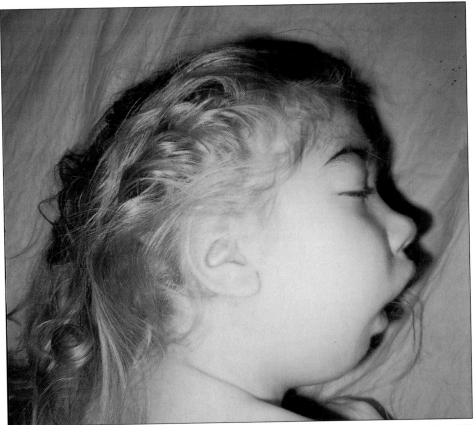

Fig. 435

Figure 436. Brain, right lateral view, corresponding to the right side of the head in Figure 435. The brain is about one-half average size for the age. The temporal and occipital lobes are of ordinary proportions, while the frontal and parietal regions are much reduced.

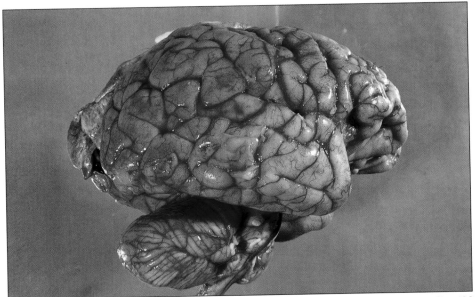

Fig. 436

Figure 437. Cerebral damage in a case of cerebral palsy, mental retardation, seizure disorder, and microcephaly. Enlargement of the lateral ventricles due to periventricular damage, loss of periventricular white matter; caudate nuclei (basal ganglia) scarred and distorted, more evident on the right.

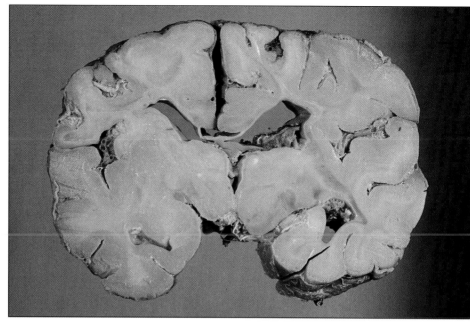

Fig. 437

A Case of   ***Microcephaly present at birth. Cerebral palsy
(basal ganglia damage present), mental retardation
and seizure disorder in childhood.***

This was a term newborn described as being spastic the day after birth. Little relevant prenatal information was available. The newborn infant weighed 6 pounds. Soon after birth, the fontanelles were tense; the infant became lethargic. Postnatally there was increasing spasticity. The infant developed seizure activity on the fifth day.

Examination at 1 year showed an underdeveloped infant with a small head; head circumference was 41 centimeters (average for 1 year is 47 centimeters).

The infant failed to thrive, remained severely underdeveloped physically. At age 3, the child was functioning at the level of 2 months. At 5 years, physical examination indicated moderate quadriplegia, severe mental retardation, and seizure disorder, in addition to microcephaly. The child was still functioning at the level of 2 months. The head size remained small, with virtually no increase in size between the first and fifth year. The child developed pneumonia and died at the age of 5 years.

At autopsy, externally the outstanding feature was the severe microcephaly (Figure 438a and b); head circumference was 41.5 centimeters (average at 5 years is 50 cm.). Viewing the microcephalic head anteriorly, the face appeared of proportionate size, with a pronounced narrowing and smallness of the upper part of the head.

The brain was small (Figure 439a), weighed 500 grams (average at age 5, about 850 grams). Viewed from the side, the brain showed a striking smallness of the cerebrum in contrast to the large, normal-size cerebellum (Figure 439b). The convolutional pattern of the cerebrum was much distorted; the cerebral convolutions in the frontal region, and especially in the occipital region, were shrunken and irregular.

Study of the deep structures of the cerebrum showed distortion, scarring, and cavitation of the caudate nuclei (Figure 440).

In summary, this is a good example of a case of cerebral palsy attributable to deep cerebral damage, to caudate nuclei damage, with encephaloclastic microcephaly. The mental retardation and seizure disorder in this case can be related to the convolutional cortical damage (pages 195, 205).

Figure 438. Microcephaly due to encephaloclastic brain damage. Child, 5 years old, with a head circumference equivalent to the head size of an infant 4 months old.

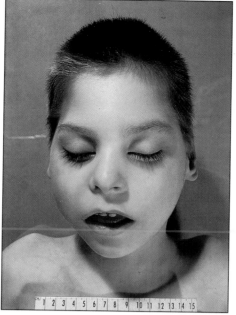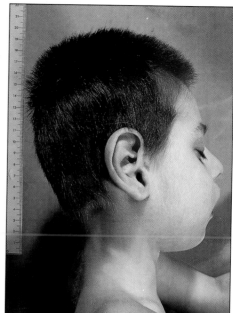

Fig. 438(a)   (b)

Figure 439(a). Cerebrum, upper surface; convolutions in the anterior and posterior regions irregular, shrunken.
(b). Cerebral convolutional damage; microcephaly. Side view of the brain; cerebrum small in contrast to the normal proportions of the intact cerebellum.

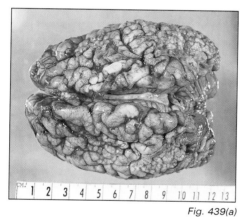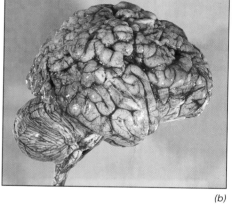

Fig. 439(a)   (b)

Figure 440. Brain specimen showing deep damage. Section through the anterior portion of the cerebrum. (Section of brain after preservation in formalin) The caudate nuclei (basal ganglia) located below the lateral ventricles, with notched scarred distortion and with focal deposit of old, tan hemorrhage.

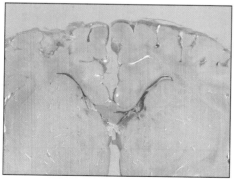

Fig. 440

A Case of

Twin pregnancy. Maternal illness with acute enteritis, gestational weight loss, anemia; prediabetes. Newborn with macrosomia. Infant later developed cerebral palsy, mental retardation, seizure disorder.

This mother had previously produced macrosomic, oversize, babies. Macrosomic offspring are evidence of underlying disturbed metabolism in the mother, commonly the first sign of latent prediabetes (page 48). Her first three babies were macrosomic (one, over 10 pounds); the twins, likewise (applying standard table of weights for twins), were in the eightieth to ninetieth percentile by weight. The offspring of mothers with diabetic metabolic abnormalities have an increased incidence of cerebral palsy (page 49).

This was not a robust pregnancy. During the pregnancy the mother was sick, had diarrhea with weight loss; she became anemic.

Labor was induced at term.

The first twin was delivered vaginally, with no apparent problem (the postnatal and follow-up information on this infant is not available).

Delivery of the second twin was impeded by a compound presentation with prolapse of an arm. The infant, subsequently delivered by cesarean section, was initially depressed.

The question arose as to whether there was acute hypoxic damage present in the brain of this newborn. Plainly, the presence or absence of acute brain damage is validly determined not by monitor tracing, or by meconium staining, etc., but is validly determined clinically and pathologically by the performance of the newborn in the immediate post delivery hours, the first day (page 164).

At delivery, although depressed, this infant, still affected by the labor stress, responded quickly to the attention given in the delivery room and, within half an hour, was improved, active, breathing on her own, with good cry, good color, and, in the succeeding hours, in the nursery, was alert and out to her mother to nurse.

Clearly, this is not the picture of a newborn with severe acute cerebral damage incurred during birth or in the delivery room.

Infants with acute cerebral damage present at birth have a specific clinical pattern: They are depressed at birth and stay that way for hours, comatose, with depressed vital function.

The newborn in this case was not that way. The pattern in the present case is reflective of an infant with chronic intrauterine compromise, bearing latent subacute cerebral damage that became manifest in later infancy as cerebral palsy and mental retardation.

The occurrence of subacute cerebral damage in the newborn is well known to pathologists who study brain damage. It is not well known to clinicians, who tend to attribute cerebral palsy and related cerebral disabilities, automatically, to events that occur during labor and delivery or postnatally.

The improved condition of this newborn on the first day was compromised by the early onset of seizure activity requiring phenobarbital sedation that depressed the newborn infant neurologically. Early onset of seizures in the newborn is increasingly recognized to be due to causes other than acute brain damage; the early onset reflects damage, an epileptogenic focus, imprinted antenatally, a period of time before birth.

This child developed the dyskinesias of cerebral palsy. Cerebral palsy is known to be due to deep cerebral (basal ganglia) damage incurred at a time during premature immature fetal life prior to 34 or 35 weeks. It does not occur related to events of labor and delivery in mature birth (page 190).

A Case of   *Maternal illness, with chronic heart disorder, celiac disease, psychiatric disorder; acute viral infection. Newborn IUGR infant later developed cerebral palsy and seizure disorder.*

The circumstances underlying this gestation were not favorable to the well-being of the fetus. This was a mother with many chronic and acute medical problems, with problems of emotional stress.

Just prior to this pregnancy, this mother had a long hospitalization with thrombophlebitis. She had lost 10 pounds.

Any kind of maternal illness during pregnancy, physical or emotional, directly affects the maternal-placental-uterine-fetal complex, compromising the fetus. Pathologically, the causal process exercises its effects through the common denominator of intrauterine hypoxia.

Rheumatic heart disease as manifested in this mother is due to remote damage involving the valves and the muscle of the heart (page 51).

The acute stage of rheumatic fever usually appears in children with symptoms of fever, toxicity, joint pain and swelling, heart murmurs, and congestive heart failure. This is the pattern as it occurs in its classic form. Very often, clinical manifestations are much subdued and the illness is commonly passed off as flu, viral infection.

During the acute stage, the heart valves, most commonly the mitral, develop inflammatory deposits on the surface of the valve leaflets, and the heart muscle develops focal acute inflammation. After the acute stage quiets down, the focal lesions in the heart become scarred, and affected valves "heal" with scarring, causing thickening of the valve leaflets and adhesions of the leaflets to one another, so that the valve becomes rigid and narrowed, stenotic, forming a bottleneck to the flow of blood through the heart.

Very often, all this goes on quietly and the effects of the heart damage remain muted. Cardiac symptoms usually are delayed for many years.

Then, unexpectedly, many years later, cardiac symptoms appear, usually in the adult during a period of physical stress, during an unrelated illness, or during pregnancy, as in this case.

Congestive heart failure develops with peripheral edema, with shortness of breath. When this happens during pregnancy, with the function of the heart compromised, oxygenation of the mother (and the fetus) at best is marginal. (In the present case, the seriousness of the mitral stenosis condition is evident by the fact that the mother needed a valve replacement after this pregnancy.)

Viral-type upper respiratory infection (URI) occurred in this mother a few weeks before labor, at about 27 weeks of gestation. This infection, with fever, occurred during a very critical period, at a time when the fetal brain is highly vulnerable to (hypoxic) damage (page 118). With acute illness, with fever, the metabolic oxygen requirements of the mother are sharply increased, leaving the fetus oxygen-deprived, hypoxic.

Celiac disease, nontropical sprue, was diagnosed prior to the pregnancy; the mother was troubled with recurrent diarrhea; she reported having tarry stool during this gestation. Visceral disorders, such as celiac disease, are commonly precipitated by emotional stress.

Psychiatric problems of long standing were indicated in the mother's record, (page 53). She had a history of manifest emotional problems with associated visceral disorders. Prior to this pregnancy, when she was hospitalized for abdominal pain, a psychiatric evaluation indicated that her symptoms were exaggerated by emotional stress.

Emotional stress is known to cause visceral disorders, ulcers (as had occurred with this mother), and occurring during pregnancy, it affects the fetus.

Just prior to this pregnancy, the mother had gone through a divorce, and in addition to her physical problems, she found herself unmarried and pregnant, and not certain who the father was.

Maternal illness, physical, emotional, is at times a factor in precipitating premature labor. This circumstance appeared in the present case.

Labor developed at 31 weeks and 3 days, following a prolonged URI. Effort to halt the labor with ritodrine failed. Congestive hear failure developed due to the mother's chronic rheumatic heart disease. Cesarean section was done, with delivery at 32 weeks.

The condition of the newborn at birth was good. The Apgar score of 4 and 7, for a very small preemie, is very good (comparable to 9, 10 for a term infant). As with all very premature babies, this was not a sturdy infant, and like other very small prematures, she needed respiratory assistance. None of this reflects the presence of acute brain damage. The baby developed moderate hyaline membrane disease; this is a predictable constant for very young prematures. The baby was maintained pink, well oxygenated.

During the first day the baby was described as resting quietly, color was pink; at the time of the initial exam in the nursery, her eyes were open, muscle tone good. During day one her vital signs were stable; and the baby was crying lustily, very active. Fontanelles were soft and flat.

This was not the clinical picture of a baby with acute fresh brain damage. This newborn infant, on neurologic examination, did not have manifestations of acute brain damage. Newborn infants that have acute brain damage show it: with low Apgar score; at delivery they are limp, comatose, with depressed vital signs, in congestive heart failure — and they stay that way for hours and days. This baby wasn't like that.

That the adverse gestational conditions had impacted on the fetus is evidenced by the outcome, by the fact that the newborn showed intrauterine growth retardation (IUGR). This premature newborn infant was inordinately small, weighed 1,219 grams. At 32 weeks, the average newborn weight is 1,600 grams, putting this baby at the 10th percentile, a pound underweight.

IUGR varies in severity and is due to periods of fetal deprivation resulting from maternal disorders, uterine, placental abnormalities, or any process that compromises the integrity of the maternal-uterine-placental-fetal complex. Taking this into consideration, the IUGR affecting this newborn is attributable to the chronic and acute illnesses of the mother.

IUGR is associated with inadequate fetal nutrition and inadequate oxygenation, so that the fetus is subject to the accruing of varying severity of silent subacute hypoxic cerebral damage. Pathologically, this kind of latent subacute damage has been confirmed in the past in autopsy studies, observed in IUGR infants that die during delivery or soon after birth. In infants surviving, the latent cerebral damage ultimately is manifested as cerebral palsy and other cerebral disability. A high incidence of cerebral palsy develops in IUGR infants.

This infant developed cerebral palsy. Cerebral palsy is due to damage to the deep cerebral structures, to the basal ganglia, during early intrauterine life. With acute cerebral damage incurred by the early immature fetus, if the fetus survives, the damage "quiets down" and the fetus (newborn) is delivered bearing latent old subacute damage, not manifested neonatally. After an interval, months, manifestations of the cerebral damage, latent at birth, surface, with the development clinically of cerebral palsy and other cerebral disabilities.

This is the clinical-pathologic sequence in the present case.

A Case of **Maternal psychiatric stress. Newborn with xanthochromic spinal fluid indicating subacute cerebral damage; development of cerebral palsy, mental retardation, and seizure disorder in infancy.**

The effect of maternal stress as a factor compromising the well-being of the fetus has attracted increasing clinical attention. The present case presents an example in which there was no significant medical illness during pregnancy reported. The main clinical factor in the pregnancy was severe maternal psychiatric stress (page 53).

The mother, early in pregnancy, was abandoned by her husband and required ongoing care in the local mental health clinic. The mother, Catholic, filed for divorce in midpregnancy.

The infant, born at term, was depressed but responded to care. However, he developed seizure activity at 17 hours. Spinal tap at 30 hours revealed xanthochromic spinal fluid.

The clinical pattern is consistent with incurrence of brain damage during early fetal life, the damage becoming subacute in the infant born at term. That the damage anteceded the birth process, that the damage present at birth was old, not fresh, is evidenced by the presence of xanthochromic spinal fluid in the newborn (page 173). Xanthochromia is due to the presence of degenerated hemoglobin, a process that takes a long period of time to develop, more than 30 hours.

The infant's postnatal performance—the fact that he improved, became active, stable with good muscle tones in the hours after birth — is further evidence that the newborn infant did not have acute cerebral damage.

Consistent with the presence of old brain damage at term, this infant subsequently developed cerebral palsy, mental retardation, and seizure disorder.

A Case of   *Low weight gain during pregnancy, maternal hypotension, maternal anemia. Newborn anemia; newborn subacute cerebral damage. Infant developed cerebral palsy, mental retardation, and seizure disorder.*

In addition to the severe anemia that was present in this infant, at birth there were also other factors, maternal gestational problems, adversive to the fetus. The mother had failed to gain an appropriate amount of weight during the pregnancy; she had symptomatic hypotension; she was anemic. These problems compromise the nutrition and oxygenation of the fetus.

Anemia in this newborn was evident at delivery (page 95). The infant was noted to be pale. The suspected anemia was confirmed in the hematology examination: hemoglobin level was 14 grams (normal for the newborn is 19 grams); the hematocrit was 45 percent (normal is 61 percent) (page 95).

Anemia, in the fetus as in the adult, causes hypoxia. The red cell is the oxygen-carrying vehicle in the blood. The decrease in the hematocrit by one-third means this fetus existed with much less than the average amount of oxygen.

Intrauterine hypoxia leads to fetal hypoxic visceral damage. The brain is the most sensitive target tissue in the body; with chronic intrauterine hypoxia, the fetus accrues subacute and acute cerebral damage.

What caused the chronic anemia? The question is of more than academic interest.

Essentially, there are four possible causes of the fetal-neonatal anemia: (1) infections, as with cytomegalic virus, (2) hemolytic disease, as with Rh incompatibility, (3) an acute hemorrhage in the newborn, (4) fetal-maternal transfusion syndrome.

Regarding the first two, there are no bases for implicating these mechanisms in the present case. There was no substantial evidence of sepsis, infection. There was no hyperbilirubinemia to go with an hemolytic causation.

Regarding the third possibility, hemorrhage within the infant, there was no clinical or radiologic evidence of this.

Regarding the fourth, the fetal-maternal transfusion syndrome, the transfer of blood from fetal to maternal circulation occurs regularly in some degree in most if not all gestations (page 97). The degree, the amount of transfusion varies, is severe in some instances.

In most cases of serious fetal-maternal transfusion the exact cause is not clear. Some cases are attributable to pathologic processes in the placenta.

As noted, the mother in this pregnancy failed to gain a healthy amount of weight. Women gain most of their weight during the last two trimesters, averaging an increase of 0.8 pound per week. In the present case, from the beginning of the second trimester and in the following 20 weeks, this mother gained 7.5 pounds. She should have gained 16 pounds. Low maternal weight gain is adversive to the needs of the fetus (page 46).

Hypotension in this mother, with diastolic pressure ranging from 50 to 60, was symptomatic, with episodes of fainting. In pregnancy, hypotension is associated with deficient profusion of blood flow through the mother's body to the uterus and placenta, with consequent oxygen deprivation of the fetus (page 53).

Maternal anemia during gestation, as occurred in this case, is an hypoxia-producing mechanism, affecting both mother and fetus.

Despite the fetal-neonatal anemia and despite maternal adversive gestational factors, the infant at birth had a good Apgar score and did well during the first 4 hours — indicating that the newborn infant did not have fresh cerebral damage.

Fontanelles remained flat, indicating an absence of cerebral edema, absence of acute cerebral damage (page 167).

CT scan of the brain a day after birth (Figure 441) likewise showed lateral ventricles patent, absence of cerebral edema. Significantly, the brain scan showed evidence of far-advanced subacute cerebral damage (page 33).

This infant later developed manifestations of cerebral palsy. CT scans showed evidence of deep periventricular cerebral damage. Cerebral palsy is known to be due to deep cerebral basal ganglia damage incurred during premature immature fetal life prior to 34 or 35 weeks. The deep cerebral damage present in this newborn is of a subacute form, attributable to anemia in the fetus and to hypoxia-producing maternal problems during this gestation.

Figure 441. CT scan of brain taken a day after birth. The frontal lobes show wide areas of decreased density, loss of substance, in an area of deep white matter adjoining the lateral ventricles. The lateral ventricles are open. Taking into account the facts that the lateral ventricles are not compressed and that, clinically, fontanelles were flat, it is conclusive that the frontal damage is not acute, but is old, subacute.

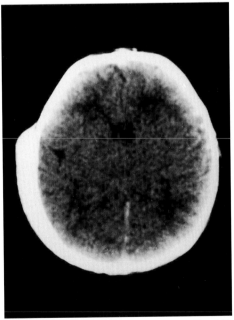

Fig. 441

A Case of   ***Twin gestation, complicated presentation, dysmature newborn with subacute deep cerebral damage; basal ganglia damage. Maternal low weight gain; vaginal bleeding. Infant developed cerebral palsy, mental retardation, seizure disorder, and microcephaly.***

The infant in this case was delivered as the second of twins. At delivery, vertex presentation with prolapse of an arm occurred, requiring cesarean section. The first twin, delivered vaginally, without complications, developed no neurologic problems.

The question arises as to why, in twin births, as in this case, one baby comes out without injury, and the other infant is born with brain damage.

Experience, clinical and pathologic, demonstrates that, as occurred in this case, in twin gestations, adverse conditions during intrauterine life at times have a damaging effect on one fetus, leaving the other fetus unscathed.

Did the complications at delivery that occurred with this (second) twin cause brain damage? There is substantial evidence, clinical and pathological, indicating there was no acute brain damage in this newborn infant. The intrauterine lives of twin embryos, twin fetuses, are not the same, particularly when considering fraternal twins, a female and a male in the present case, with two placentas.

It is a common lay and medical misconception that twin fetuses, because they are twins, react in the same way to intrauterine pathologic conditions. The two fetuses in this gestation are biologically different, each with different organ constitution, reacting individually to noxious processes. While both fetuses are subject to the same adverse gestational complications of the mother, the fetuses do not react the same way pathologically.

This was a term pregnancy. The mother had had hypotension, low weight gain, and vaginal bleeding with cramps during this pregnancy. At midpregnancy she was sick with a viral infection, with a sore throat.

Hypotension during pregnancy compromises body circulation, oxygenation of the mother and fetus. Low weight gain during pregnancy indicates a disordered maternal metabolism, adverse to the fetus. Bleeding with cramps is an ominous sign, reflecting placental disorder, a hazard to the fetus.

The pregnancy problems of the mother manifestly exercised an adverse effect on the fetuses in this case. Although the first-delivered twin was a "good baby," the second twin was not. This newborn infant was long and thin, dysmature, reflective of intrauterine deprivation. The enfeebled newborn was depressed at birth; however, he responded to the attention given in the delivery room: his vital functions, respirations, soon improved. He soon became active and alert, with good respirations. Fontanelles were soft.

The clinical picture of this newborn is not consistent with the presence of acute fresh cerebral damage. Infants with acute, fresh, diffuse cerebral damage remain comatose, limp, and unstable continuously, from delivery on, for hours and days. This newborn was not that way.

The CT scan taken at 2 days showed evidence of far-advanced pathologic change in the cerebrum (Figure 442). The white matter deep in the cerebrum showed decreased density, an extensive loss of tissue substance. Considering that this infant after delivery was soon active and alert, with soft fontanelles, it is conclusive that this white matter damage was not of an acute nature, but was of a subacute form, damage incurred remotely during intrauterine life (pages 24, 33).

Pathologic processes affecting the fetus during early intrauterine life are by nature latent, silent clinically. The common denominator of these adversive processes is hypoxia — the fetus is subjected to varying degrees of oxygen deprivation, which leads to an accruing of subacute cerebral damage in the fetuses that survive to term or near term. Newborn infants, so affected, are born harboring old, subacute cerebral damage — damage not manifested at birth. The occurrence of subacute cerebral damage in infants at birth is well known to pathologists who study brain damage. It is not well known to clinicians, who tend to attribute cerebral palsy and related cerebral disabilities, automatically, to events that occur during labor and delivery or postnatally.

The present case graphically demonstrates the relationship of deep cerebral damage, damage to basal ganglia, and the consequent development of cerebral palsy.

The CT scan taken at 3 weeks, in addition to depletion of cerebral white matter, shows focal cavitations in the basal ganglia (putamen) on each side (Figure 443), the residue of early fetal damage (pages 13, 28, 185). Correlating this with clinical sequels, this child developed cerebral palsy with mental retardation, seizure disorder. Microcephaly was present.

Microcephaly with cerebral palsy, as in the present case, is due to failure of the brain to grow consequent to the damage to the deep cerebral strata.

Figure 442. CT scan of brain at 2 days; decreased density of white matter in the frontal and posterior regions. The white matter damage is far advanced, of subacute nature. Ventricles and cavum septi pellucidi are visible.

Figure 443. CT scan at 3 weeks. Basal ganglia (putamen) on both sides show focal areas of low density, cavitations. The white matter, especially frontally, shows a depletion of tissue substance.

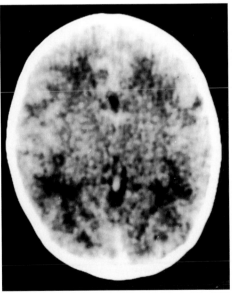 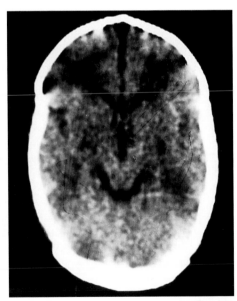

Fig. 442   Fig. 443

A Case of   *Maternal viral infections; teenage pregnancy.*
              Dysmature newborn; basal ganglia lesions.
              Cerebral palsy and other neurological disabilities
              in infancy; microcephaly.

This was a teenage pregnancy. The mother had protracted recurrent upper respiratory infections during pregnancy. With acute viral illness, with fever, the metabolic oxygen requirements of the mother are sharply increased, leaving the fetus oxygen-deprived, contributing to hypoxic brain damage.

The mother gained 40 pounds during pregnancy; however. the infant, born at 41 weeks, was relatively underweight at 6 pounds 4 ounces, was long and thin, dysmature.

The infant was depressed at birth but improved. Seizures developed at 3 hours.

The CT scans at 4 months showed enlarged ventricles and lesions in the basal ganglia, structural changes typical of the pathologic pattern that evolves in the brain in cases of cerebral palsy.

In addition to cerebral palsy, the infant, at 3 years, had mental retardation, seizure disorder, and microcephaly.

A Case of   *Genetic optic hypoplasia with hypothalamic dysfunction; mental retardation, seizure disorder, motor dysfunctions with clinical misdiagnosis of cerebral palsy.*

This was a case of genetic optic hypoplasia. There was a sibling with the same optic hypoplasia.

The infant had an Apgar score of 9 and 10 at birth. A nuchal cord was present. The infant had a temperature of 100.4 degrees on day 3, with seizure activity; these symptoms soon receded. The infant was discharged home on the fifth day in satisfactory condition. During infancy a diagnosis of hypothalamic dysfunction was made. The condition is known to occur syndromically in cases of optic hypoplasia.

At the age of 9 years the child showed a degree of mental retardation, had a seizure disorder, and had defective motor function.

Initially the motor defects were called cerebral palsy. Later the neurologic assessment of the child indicated that the motor defects "do not fit the common pattern of cerebral palsy."

This case illustrates an example of motor disability due to a formative defect of the central nervous system.

Pathologically and clinically, this type of case should not be categorized as cerebral palsy. Clinically, cerebral palsy has three distinctive patterns, with spasticity or hypotonia or athetosis. Pathologically, it is due to damage to the premature immature cerebrum. It is not due to genetic malformation of the brain.

A Case of

Severe maternal illness during pregnancy; retroplacental hematoma. Newborn anemia; basal ganglia damage. Infant developed cerebral palsy, mental retardation, seizure disorder, and microcephaly.

The mother during this pregnancy was sick with a viral-type illness, flu and diarrhea, a period during which she lost weight. Viral illness during pregnancy is a hazard to both mother and fetus, associated with increased morbidity and mortality (page 118).

At delivery a large retroplacental hematoma was present, occupying about one-half of the diameter of the maternal surface of the placenta. This was an "occult" type of retroplacental hematoma formation; this hemorrhage had been silent clinically, with no vaginal bleeding or other clinical manifestations prior to delivery (page 68).

Anatomically, the placenta is tightly adherent to the inner aspect of the uterine wall. At times a part of the adherent placenta becomes loosened, separated from the uterine wall. The cause of such detachment is not precisely known.

With detachment of a part of the placenta, a pocket forms between the placenta and the uterine wall, a pocket filled with blood clot, a retroplacental hematoma. At times, the hematoma remains walled off, forming an "occult" retroplacental hematoma.

In this case — with no prepartum vaginal bleeding, no bleeding into the amniotic sac and no inordinate amount of bleeding at delivery — the blood present was mainly in the formed retroplacental clot, the hematoma. It was evident that this detachment, the retroplacental hematoma, had formed a period of time, days or more, before birth.

The importance of this pathologic pattern is that it indicates that, with the hematoma behind the placenta present for a long time before birth, oxygenation of the fetus was consequently compromised for a long time during intrauterine life.

Placental abruption, retroplacental hemorrhage, is associated with a high incidence of cerebral palsy in offspring.

The gestational problems — the mother's illness, the retroplacental hematoma — manifestly affected the fetus adversely. The newborn infant was enfeebled, pale, anemic, and required transfusion soon after birth.

This newborn, although depressed at birth, responded to treatment and improved, and at 4 hours was pink, vigorous, with good color, good respiration, lungs clear, crying lustily. This was not the picture of a newborn with severe acute cerebral damage. Infants with acute cerebral damage at birth have a specific clinical pattern. They are depressed at birth and stay that way for hours, days. The newborn in this case was not that way.

Although in the hours after birth this infant improved, this clinical progress was compromised by the early onset of seizures on the first day, a complication requiring heavy sedation with phenobarbital rendering the infant neurologically depressed.

The CT scan taken on day 2 showed changes of cerebral edema, swelling; however this was not severe; clinically fontanelles remained soft and flat.

CT studies of this brain at 3 months showed evidence of severe pathologic changes, broad areas of loss of substance. Pertinently, there were large areas of decreased density, cavitations in the basal ganglia (Figure 444).

Although the CT scan taken neonatally failed to reveal it, it is evident that the newborn cerebrum harbored pathologic changes of severe nature, of subacute origin, damage originating in fetal life, resulting from the adverse processes present during this gestation.

The severe cerebral damage revealed in the CT scan at 3 months is reflected in the infant's subsequent clinical course. The damage in the basal ganglia and white matter relates to the development of cerebral palsy in this child (page 185). With the severe damage in the cerebral white matter, the cerebrum failed to grow, microcephaly. With the damage reaching the cerebral cortex, severe mental retardation and seizure disorder were present in the child.

Figure 444. CT scan of brain at 3 months. **(a).** Scan at the level of the basal ganglia showing large areas of decreased density in the putamen and caudate nucleus on both sides. Loss of substance in the frontal and temporal region, with narrowing, atrophy, of convolutions.

Figure 444(b). Scan through the lower level of the cerebrum. Evidence of large cavitations in the basal ganglia (putamen) as well as defects in the thalamus on both sides.

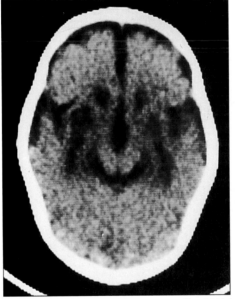 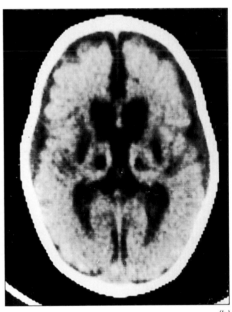

Fig. 444(a)   (b)

A Case of   *Vascular malformation (encephalofacial hemangio-endothelioma), present at birth. Hemiparesis, seizure disorder, mental retardation; Sturge-Weber syndrome.*

The newborn infant had a "port-wine stain," a capillary hemangioma, over the right side of the forehead and extending about the nose and upper lip. In the weeks postnatally the infant developed increasing seizure activity, clonic seizures, involving the left side of the body. Craniotomy revealed a diffuse angiomatous malformation (hemangioendothelioma) extending over the surface of most of the right cerebral hemisphere.

Seizures were controlled with anticonvulsant medication. The child was severely mentally retarded. There was moderate left hemiparesis. Death occurred at age 26.

At autopsy the right side of the cerebrum was much reduced in size; the right cerebral hemisphere was occupied by a massive invasive bulbous hard tumor (a hemangioendothelioma) up to 6 centimeters in diameter (Figure 445).

Figure 445. Tumorous mass, hemangioendothelioma; present in the right cerebrum. The presence of this neoplasm, originating as a vascular malformation, was identified at operation soon after birth. The tumor gradually increased. Death occurred at 26 years. Section of brain specimen shows the tumor occupying one half of the right cerebrum.

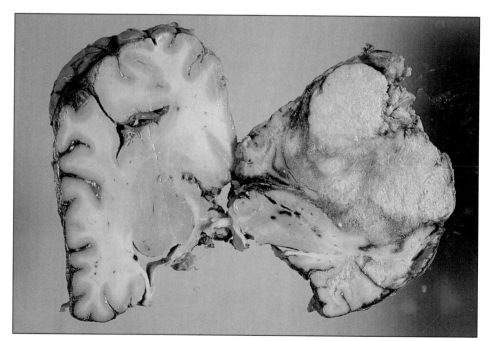

Fig. 445

A Case of

Dysmaturity and postmaturity. Maternal excessive weight gain and anemia. Newborn infant with CT evidence of subacute cerebral damage. Cerebral palsy and other neurologic disabilities later in infancy.

This case demonstrates the effects of gestational compromise, causing intrauterine deprivation, dysmaturity, with the newborn infant harboring latent, old brain damage at birth, with the effects of latent cerebral damage becoming manifest later in infancy.

The infant was post-term at 43 weeks' gestation, and had typical physical characteristics of postmaturity, with peeling skin and a plantar pattern of complex creases extending into the heel.

This is an example of an infant with a complex intrauterine development, a combination of dysmaturity as well as postmaturity.

In some cases, if the postmature fetus has been exposed to prolonged adversive gestational processes with deprivation of nutrition and oxygenation, the newborn infant, although showing physical and neurologic evidence of postmaturity, is small and underweight, the pattern of postmaturity-dysmaturity.

This postmature infant was underweight, dysmature (IUGR) (page 94). He weighed 2,977 grams (6 pounds 10 ounces), in the twentieth percentile. The average weight at term is 3,300 grams; the infant was about 1 pound underweight.

The length of this newborn was 53 centimeters, in the ninetieth percentile. This was a long lean baby. The newborn was described as "thin." Likewise, in the initial examination, it was noted that the infant had "very little subcutaneous fat." This is typical of malnourished dysmature newborn infants.

The **Ponderal Index** (page 94), a measure of fetal nutrition, was 1.99, far below the tenth percentile, indicating that this fetus was chronically deprived, malnourished, dysmature.

In the postmature, pathologically, the causes of intrauterine compromise that lead to dysmaturity, to hypoxic cerebral damage, are essentially the same adversive processes that may occur in other gestations. Regarding causation in the present case, this mother gained weight excessively. The recorded prepregnancy weight was 130 pounds. This mother by the thirty-fifth week weighed 180 pounds, a weight gain of 50 pounds. The overall optimal weight gain in pregnancy is about 25 pounds. This mother gained twice that amount.

Weight gain may in part be due to retention of fluid, with excessive swelling of the limbs. This was not a factor apparent in the present case.

Excessive maternal weight gain, of the degree in the present case, is usually of metabolic origin, reflecting endocrine dysfunction, metabolic disorders, such as diabetes or thyroid disorder, and it exercises an adversive effect on the fetus (page 47).

The mother was marginally anemic, with the hematocrit 35 percent early in pregnancy. Maternal anemia is associated with fetal deprivation.

This dysmature enfeebled fetus was unable to tolerate the stress of parturition; the newborn was transiently depressed. After the delivery he responded quickly, with an Apgar score of 8 at five minutes, and was soon pink and crying. The newborn infant was described at the initial physical examination as being "in no acute distress." Blood pH was normal; lung fields were clear.

Clinically and pathologically, this is not the picture of a newborn with acute cerebral damage. Infants with acute cerebral damage at birth have a specific clinical pattern: They are depressed at birth and continue that way, comatose, with depressed vital function. This infant at delivery was not like that.

However the clinical improvement of this newborn was compromised by the early onset of seizures. Seizure activity in this newborn required heavy sedation with phenobarbital, rendering the infant neurologically depressed. It is increasingly realized clinically that the early onset of seizures in the newborn is not due to acute brain damage, that such seizures are attributable to antecedent early fetal cerebral damage (page 208).

The CT scan studies show in sequence a transition of the subacute cerebral damage present at birth, to a later pattern at 7 days, and to the chronic form of damage present at 9 months.

The CT scan done on day 2 (Figure 446) shows evidence of old brain damage, subacute damage far advanced, indicating an origin long before birth; the scan shows patent ventricles, indicating absence of acute cerebral swelling (page 33).

That the changes are old, not acute, is substantiated by the facts that (1) the ventricles are open, indicating an absence of edema, an absence of acute pathologic process, and (2) clinically, at the time, on day 2, the fontanelles were flat and soft, reflecting an absence of acute brain damage. If the CT scan changes were indicative of acute cerebral damage, this infant would show it clinically, and after delivery would have remained comatose and limp — which was not the case with this newborn.

The CT scan taken later, on day 7, again shows patent ventricles reflecting a lack of edema, consistent with old brain damage (Figure 447). There is evidence of hemorrhagic damage in the occipital regions. Pathologically, hypoxic damage in the newborn is due to the process of venous infarction. In venous infarction, of old, subacute form, recurrent bleeding occurs, producing the pattern evident in the CT scans taken on day 7.

The CT scan taken at 9 months (Figure 448) shows the late effects of the hypoxic damage observed neonatally (page 34). The ventricles are enlarged, due to loss of deep periventricular white matter: ex vacuo hydrocephalus.

In the occipital regions there are areas of rarefaction, cavitations, in the areas of hemorrhagic infarction noted neonatally. The devitalized infarcted tissue is gradually absorbed, leaving cavitations.

The child, examined at the age of 5 years, had the dyskinesias of cerebral palsy, was severely mentally retarded, had a seizure disorder, was a behavior problem, and was microcephalic. Taking into account the maternal medical problems, the dysmaturity of the newborn evidencing intrauterine deprivation, and the evidence in the newborn CT scan of old brain damage, it is conclusive that the cerebral damage, responsible for the child's disabilities, was due not to acute cerebral damage at birth but was attributable to subacute damage originating during premature immature fetal life.

Figure 446. CT scan of the head taken on day 2 showing evidence of old subacute brain damage and lack of evidence of acute damage. **(a).** Decreased density in the temporal, parietal, and occipital lobes, areas of old subacute brain damage. The lateral ventricles are visible, indicating absence of edema. **(b).** CT scan at an upper level through the cerebrum; decreased density over the posterior cerebral region, consistent with old brain damage.

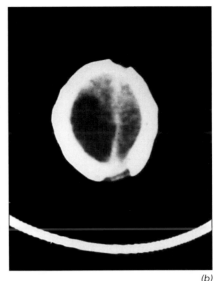

Fig. 446(a)

(b)

Figure 447. CT scan of the head taken on day 7. **(a).** Patchy areas of density in the occipital and posterior parietal regions; areas of damage corresponding to that seen in Figure 446(a). Ventricles are slightly enlarged. **(b).** CT scan at an upper level through the cerebrum corresponding to Figure 446(b); broad areas of increased density consistent with deep hemorrhagic infarction.

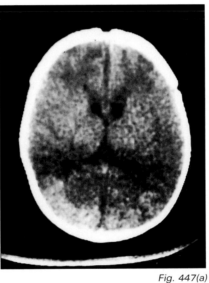
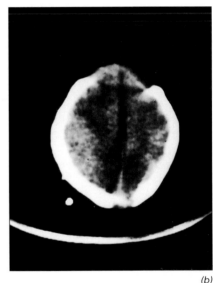

Fig. 447(a)

(b)

Figure 448. CT scan taken at 9 months. **(a).** Section through the cerebrum; enlarged lateral ventricles; posteriorly, large areas of decreased density, cavitations, corresponding in location to damage evident in Figure 447(a). **(b).** CT scan at an upper level through the cerebrum corresponding to Figure 447(b); large irregular areas of decreased density, confluent cystic lesions in the posterior cerebrum.

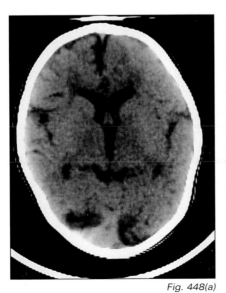
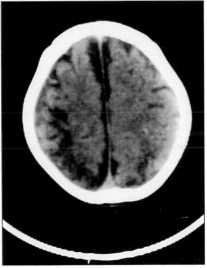

Fig. 448(a)

(b)

A Case of   *Maternal poor reproductive record; pregnancy vaginal bleeding, anemia. Newborn with intrauterine growth retardation, fetal-neonatal anemia, spinal fluid xanthochromia; spasticity in early infancy; death at 21 months; autopsy findings of hydrocephaly and cystic lesions in basal ganglia.*

This mother had a poor reproductive record, with two spontaneous abortions prior to this pregnancy (page 41). The pregnancy in this case was punctuated by episodes of vaginal bleeding, the portent of a threatened abortion; the mother became anemic.

With a clinical history of poor reproductive performance of the mother in past pregnancies, with miscarriages, vaginal bleeding as in the present case, there is an increased incidence of cerebral palsy in the offspring.

Although the previous pregnancies had ended in spontaneous abortion, paradoxically this pregnancy was carried to 42 weeks. The newborn infant was small for gestational age (IUGR), weighed 2,900 grams, in the fifteenth percentile.

At delivery the infant was depressed but had an Apgar score of 6 at five minutes. Clinically the infant was considered postmature. He improved in the hours after delivery, was pink, crying, alert, and had good reflexes. Seizure activity appeared at 17 hours. Seizures responded to treatment.

The newborn infant was anemic.

The spinal fluid had a yellow discoloration, was xanthochromic. The finding of xanthochromic (*xantho-*, yellow; *-chromia*, color) spinal fluid is of major importance in defining the time of incurrence of the cerebral damage (page 173).

Xanthochromia of spinal fluid was present in the spinal tap specimen at 14 1/2 hours after delivery. Xanthochromia, yellow discoloration of the spinal fluid, is due to the presence of old hemorrhagic damage in the brain. With hemorrhage in the brain, with blood escaping into the ventricles, into the spinal fluid, red cells become lysed, broken down; the hemoglobin from the red cells first gives the spinal fluid a pink color. The hemoglobin gradually degenerates to a yellow pigment and gives the spinal fluid a yellow color — xanthochromia. (Like a hemorrhagic black-and-blue bruise in the skin that gradually becomes yellow-green after a time.) This change in color takes many days, and continues to be present for weeks and months when there is an old hemorrhagic lesion in the brain. Xanthochromia does not develop in a few hours, or even in a day or two. The finding of xanthochromia is firm evidence that the brain damage in this fetus, this infant, occurred a long time before labor and delivery.

The head failed to grow, and by the tenth month microcephaly was evident. The CAT scan at 1 month showed enlarged ventricles with scattered lucencies, thought to be infarcts.

At 5 months there was increasing spasticity. The infant developed a seizure disorder.

He expired at 21 months, after a respiratory disorder.

At autopsy, the brain showed greatly enlarged ventricles. There were bilateral cystic lesions in the basal ganglia. The cystic lesions were old, with scarring.

A Case of **Twin gestation, one stillborn, both small for gestational age. Surviving newborn twin with fetal-neonatal anemia; spinal fluid xanthochromia; cerebrum with subacute damage. Cerebral palsy and other neurologic disabilities developed later in infancy.**

Prenatal clinical information was scanty. Mother had symptomatic hypotension with periods of faintness.

One twin was liveborn, the other was stillborn. Both twins were undersize, showed intrauterine growth retardation, reflecting adversive gestational processes. The stillborn twin showed slight maceration, indicating intrauterine death occurred a period of time, hours or days, before labor (no autopsy performed).

The placenta examination indicated a monochorionic, diamniotic gestation. The placental portions were joined. The portion of placenta belonging to the stillborn twin showed a pattern consistent with degeneration, devitalization, beginning a long time before delivery.

The surviving twin was severely anemic, with the hematocrit at birth 26 percent; average for a term newborn is 61 percent. Decreased hematocrit means decreased oxygenation of the body.

Anemia occurring in one newborn twin, as occurred in this case, is indicative of the syndrome of fetus-to-fetus placental transfusion (page 97). However, at times, in single or twin gestation, there is a defect in the placenta that leads to substantial fetal-maternal transfer of blood (page 97). In the present case, it is possible that the anemia in the surviving twin was due to a fetal-maternal transfusion, a process that led to the anemia in one and death of the other twin.

The newborn infant, pale and depressed at birth, with low Apgar, responded to treatment, with transfusions, and was soon stable, with improved vital functions, lung fields clear. Fontanelles were soft, not bulging, indicating there was no acute edematous swelling, no acute brain damage.

The CT scan of the brain taken on day 2 (Figure 449) showed a diffuse low-density appearance of both left and right hemispheres; ventricles were open, average size. The presence of open ventricles indicates an absence of cerebral edema and indicates that the loss of substance in the cerebral hemispheres was of *subacute* nature, of remote origin (pages 24, 33).

Improvement in the newborn was compromised by the early onset of seizure activity during the first day, reflecting damage incurred during early fetal life and triggered by the stress of the birth process (page 207).

The finding of xanthochromic (*xantho-*, yellow; *-chromia*, color) spinal fluid is of major importance in defining the time of incurrence of the cerebral damage. Xanthochromia of spinal fluid was present in the spinal fluid specimen taken 9 hours after delivery. Xanthochromia is due to the presence of old hemorrhagic damage in the brain (page 173).

With hemorrhage in the brain, the hemoglobin from the red cells gradually degenerates to a yellow pigment and gives the spinal fluid a yellow color —

xanthochromia. This change in color takes many days, and continues to be present for weeks and months, when there is an old hemorrhagic lesion in the brain.

The follow-up CT scan taken on day 12 (Figure 450) confirmed the severe loss of cerebral white matter, subacute damage, evident in the previous scans. The disintegration of the white matter led to corresponding enlargement of the lateral ventricles.

The surviving infant later manifested cerebral palsy, mental retardation, seizure disorder, and was microcephalic.

The CT scan taken at 3 years (Figure 451) showed pathologic changes corresponding to those present in the neonatal scans, with diffuse loss of cerebral substance creating a honeycomb appearance in the white matter, cystic porencephaly. Ventricles were much enlarged due to loss of periventricular white matter, ex vacuo hydrocephalus (page 29).

In this case the question arose as to whether there was acute brain damage present at birth, incurred during delivery. Infants with acute, fresh, brain damage remain unresponsive, with unstable vital signs, for prolonged periods and commonly show clinical and CT evidence of edematous swelling at birth.

The newborn infant in this case was not like that. He responded to treatment and was soon stable in the hours after birth. The CT scan of the brain and the xanthochromic spinal fluid are evidence that the damage was old, subacute, incurred long before birth.

The sequence of brain CT scans presented in this case offers a classic example of consecutive pathologic changes beginning with subacute cerebral damage present in the newborn and going on over a period of years to the end stage of cystic porencephalic disintegration of the cerebrum, resulting clinically in cerebral palsy, mental retardation, seizure disorder, and microcephaly (page 189).

Figure 449. CT scans of the brain on day 2. **(a)** shows evidence of decreased cerebral white matter (appearing as darkened zones through the intermediate strata). The ventricles appearing in **(b)**, located centrally, black, triangular, are of average size, reflecting an absence of acute edema.

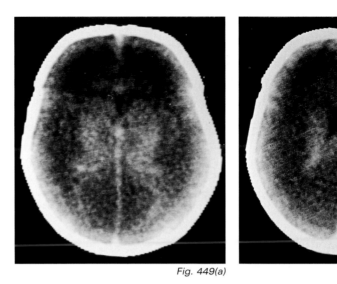

Fig. 449(a)   *(b)*

Figure 450. CT scans taken on day 12 show a progression of pathologic changes compared to day 2; diffuse darkened areas in the intermediate zones, indicating severe subacute loss of white matter; corresponding enlargement of ventricles. **(a).** Scan of cerebrum at the level of the basal ganglia. **(b).** Scan of cerebrum at an upper level.

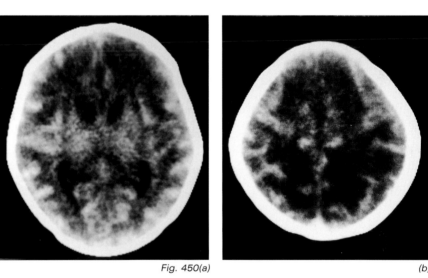

Fig. 450(a)   *(b)*

Figures 451(a) and **(b).** CT scan of cerebrum at 3 years showing evidence of diffuse loss of white matter (areas of black) particularly affecting the posterior of the cerebrum. Ventricles much enlarged due to loss of surrounding cerebral substance.

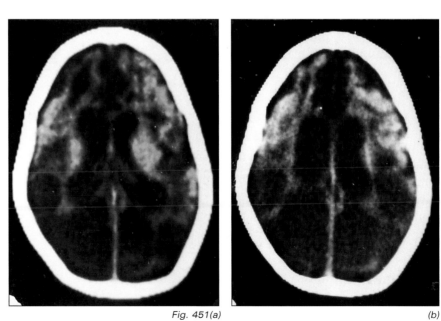

Fig. 451(a)   *(b)*

A Case of **_Prolonged vaginal bleeding during pregnancy; premature birth; placental abruption. Manifestations of cerebral palsy and learning disorder developed in childhood._**

This mother's vaginal bleeding began in midpregnancy and gradually rendered her anemic. Maternal anemia is an hypoxia-producing process for both the mother and the fetus.

Labor developed at 35 weeks of gestation associated with abruption, premature detachment of the placenta. Present at delivery was a large retroplacental hematoma, partly fresh, partly old blood clot. The latter accounted for the prolonged bleeding during the pregnancy (pages 66 and 68).

With the gradual development of premature detachment of the placenta, with the placenta increasingly separated from the uterus by a hematoma, function of the placenta was compromised, rendering the fetus chronically hypoxic.

Intrauterine hypoxia was additionally caused by the mother's anemia.

The fetus, exposed to hypoxia during midpregnancy, prior to 35 weeks, when the fetal brain is immature, incurs deep cerebral damage, affecting periventricular structures, the basal ganglia. Basal ganglia damage causes cerebral palsy.

At the time of birth the question arose as to whether there was acute hypoxic brain damage present in this infant. The presence or absence of acute brain damage is validly determined clinically and pathologically by the performance of the newborn in the immediate postdelivery hours and in the first day (page 164).

Infants born with extensive cerebral damage, fresh _acute_ intranatal cerebral damage, have a characteristic clinical pattern. These infants remain limp, in shock, for hours after delivery, with congestive heart failure, with depressed vital signs.

This newborn was not like that. This newborn soon had stable vital function, was responsive and was noted to be in good condition during the hours after delivery.

Fetuses that survive after being subjected to chronic intrauterine hypoxia accrue subacute cerebral damage. Newborn infants, previously affected during early fetal life, are born harboring old, subacute cerebral damage — damage surfacing months later with manifestations of cerebral palsy and other cerebral disabilities.

A Case of   *Retroplacental hematoma, vaginal bleeding; premature labor. Newborn with polycythemia. Infant developed cerebral palsy, mental retardation, and microcephaly.*

This case illustrates the relationship between the occurrence of placental disorders and the development of fetal cerebral damage. This is sometimes referred to as the placenta-cerebral syndrome (page 64).

The placenta showed an old retroplacental organizing clot, an old retroplacental hematoma.

Anatomically, the placenta is tightly adherent to the inner aspect of the uterine wall. At times a part of the adherent placenta becomes loosened, separated from the uterine wall. (The cause of this detachment is not precisely known; sometimes it begins with a small infarct of the placental surface at its attachment to the uterus.)

With detachment of a part of the placenta, a pocket forms between the placenta and the uterine wall, a pocket filled with blood clot, a retroplacental hematoma.

At times, as in the present case, the hematoma remains walled off, for a long time clinically silent, forming a chronic, occult, retroplacental hematoma.

The retroplacental hematoma ultimately may penetrate beyond the edge of the placenta causing vaginal bleeding; this occurred in the present case.

The chronic occult retroplacental hematoma is of importance pathologically for two reasons: (1) The part of the placenta separated, walled off by the clot, is put out of function, leading to placental insufficiency, to interference with fetal oxygenation and nutrition. (2) The clot, lying against the uterine wall, represents an irritant to the uterine musculature, at times triggering contractions, premature labor. This happened in the present case, with premature contractions occurring at 33 weeks of gestation.

The infant, although premature at 33 weeks, at delivery was in good condition with an Apgar score of 7 and 9. The newborn infant was polycythemic (excessive red blood cells), indicative of chronic intrauterine hypoxia (page 104). Neurologically he was active, responsive, had good reflexes. His postnatal course was complicated by a brief period of RDS (respiratory distress syndrome), jaundice (jaundice per se is not a hazard), and the development of a feeding problem.

Although no neurologic abnormalities were present neonatally, the infant subsequently developed evidence of brain damage, the manifestations of cerebral palsy.

When was the brain damage incurred?

The clinical pattern in this case is consistent with the syndromic pattern of latent subacute cerebral damage present at birth, damage incurred a period of time prior to birth, damage related to adverse pathologic processes to which this fetus was exposed. Relevant to this, in the present case there was the old retroplacental hematoma, a pathologic condition that compromises the function of the placenta, leading to fetal hypoxia, fetal damage.

A Case of **_Premature newborn with xanthochromic spinal fluid; medication error. Maternal illness during pregnancy. Cerebral palsy and other neurologic disabilities developed later in infancy._**

This mother was sick during pregnancy with gastroenteritis and flu; she developed toxemia of pregnancy. Birth occurred prematurely at 34 weeks of gestation. This small premature was in good condition at birth, with an Apgar score of 8 and 9, with spontaneous respiration, crying, and vigorous activity. Fontanelles were flat. These clinical findings indicate there was no *acute* brain damage at the time of birth.

Later in the first day respiratory distress and other problems developed. Spinal fluid at 6 hours was xanthochromic; xanthochromia, yellow coloration of the spinal fluid, indicates the presence of old hemorrhagic damage in the brain (page 173).

With hemorrhage in the brain, with blood escaping into the ventricles, into the spinal fluid, red cells become lysed, broken down; the hemoglobin from the red cells first gives the spinal fluid a pink color. The hemoglobin gradually degenerates to a yellow pigment and gives the spinal fluid a yellow color — xanthochromia. (Like a hemorrhagic black-and-blue bruise in the skin that gradually becomes yellow-green after a time.)

This change in color takes many days, and the process continues for weeks and months when there is an old hemorrhagic lesion in the brain.

At one week after birth a medication error occurred: an overdose of potassium was administered. Subsequently the infant had a seizure and became unresponsive; he promptly responded to treatment and was soon stable.

Taking into account that this mother had medical problems during pregnancy, problems adversive to the fetus, and considering the fact that the spinal fluid was xanthochromic, reflecting old brain damage present at birth, it is conclusive that the cerebral palsy and other neurologic disabilities were due not to the medication error but to intrauterine pathologic processes during early fetal life, with the infant born with old brain damage.

A Case of

Maternal viral infection, emotional stress, pregnancy low weight gain, vaginal bleeding; birth premature. Newborn small for gestational age; neonatal CT scan evidence of periventricular damage. Infant developed cerebral palsy, mental retardation, seizure disorder, and microcephaly.

This case illustrates the relationship of early pregnancy complications associated with premature birth and the consequent development of cerebral palsy in the offspring.

This mother had substantial medical and emotional problems during this pregnancy. She had pelvic inflammatory disease, vaginal bleeding, viral infection, colds, bronchitis.

She had serious psychiatric problems. Reflective of this mother's poor condition is the fact that she failed to gain weight during the early part of this pregnancy.

This mother, at 4 weeks of pregnancy, was treated for symptoms of a viral syndrome. Again, at 8 weeks of this pregnancy, she was treated for a cold, URI, viral syndrome. That her illness was serious is evident in the fact that at this time, in a period of 3 weeks, she lost 6 pounds.

Three weeks later she developed a sore throat, bronchitis, and was treated with antibiotics.

Viral infection during pregnancy is a hazard to both the mother and the fetus. Pregnant women clinically have increased susceptibility to viral infections, to influenza, upper respiratory infections, viral sore throat, as well as the specific viral infections of rubella, chicken pox, and measles. Flu epidemics in times past resulted in maternal mortality rates of up to 50 percent in pregnant women. Miscarriage occurred in 35 to 60 percent of the flu epidemic cases. With acute illness, with fever, the metabolic oxygen requirements of the mother are sharply increased, leaving the fetus oxygen-deprived, hypoxic.

Low maternal weight gain compromises fetal well-being and is associated with impaired neonatal outcome. The present case is an example of this. Mothers with inadequate weight gain during pregnancy have increased rates of low birth weight infants.

During this pregnancy the mother was emotionally unstable, under manifest psychiatric stress. She received medication in treatment for this stress. Mental stress of the degree evident in this mother affects the physiologic functions of the body — cardiovascular (chest pain), respiratory (asthma symptoms), and metabolic (weight loss).

It is difficult to determine the role of emotional stress in causing perinatal fetal brain damage; however, there is no reason to think it is a minor one (page 53).

This mother had a poor obstetric track record. This was her fourth pregnancy. In the first delivery, the infant was severely depressed. The second pregnancy was terminated by abortion because of a pelvic problem. The third pregnancy was complicated by pyelonephritis, vaginal bleeding, threatened abortion, false labor. The pregnancy described here was superimposed on the presence of pelvic inflammatory disease. The presence of inflammatory disease is not a healthy environment for an embryo-fetus. The pregnancy in this case was complicated by vaginal bleeding. This mother, in a subsequent pregnancy, at four months of gestation, reported vaginal bleeding again.

Ultrasound study in the present case indicated a low-lying placenta, meaning the placental margin extended to, or near to, the cervical opening, creating a degree of placenta previa. This predisposed to episodic vaginal bleeding that occurred in this case (page 69). Recurrent bleeding during pregnancy, due to pathologic processes affecting the placenta, compromises the fetus, causing hypoxia.

A low-lying placenta, as in this case, not only is associated with vaginal bleeding but also is known to be conducive pathologically to premature detachment and premature labor.

This newborn infant, at 29 weeks of gestation, weighing 660 grams, was below the second percentile for weight, small for gestational age (SGA), (IUGR). The intrauterine growth retardation reflected the adverse conditions present for the fetus during intrauterine life (page 94).

Regarding the neurologic condition of the infant at birth, this newborn directly after delivery was in relatively good clinical condition (despite the fact that he was extremely premature and undersized, small for gestational age). The next day he was noted to be relatively stable.

On day 2 he suddenly deteriorated, became anemic, and developed ultrasound evidence of intracerebral periventricular infarction and intraventricular hemorrhage.

Ultrasound studies repeated during the next month showed cerebral periventricular necrosis with increasing ventricular dilatation. Obstructive hydrocephalus was evident, apparently resulting from impaction of the aqueduct by blood clot and necrotic tissue debris (page 157). The CT scan of the head at 3 months showed great dilatation of the ventricles, with thinning of the cerebral walls (Figure 452). The infant survived; the hydrocephalus required a ventriculo-peritoneal shunt.

The child at 5 years had cerebral palsy, mental retardation, seizure disorder, blindness, and microcephaly.

With the development of pressure hydrocephalus, initially the head size increased excessively. This was controlled by the shunt, and ultimately the opposite pattern occurred: the head failed to enlarge with age, microcephaly. With the deep cerebral strata damaged, the brain fails to grow, with resulting microcephaly.

Figure 452. CT scan of the brain at three months, showing wide dilatation of the cerebral lateral ventricles with thinning of the cerebral walls, hydrocephalus. **(a).** Scan at a lower level of the brain. **(b).** Scan at an intermediate level. **(c).** Scan at an upper level.

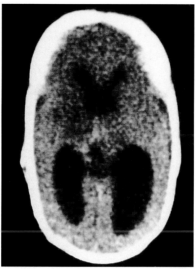

Fig. 452(a)

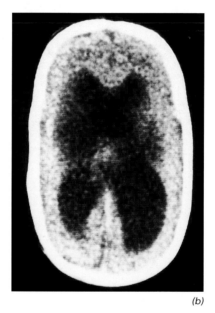

(b)

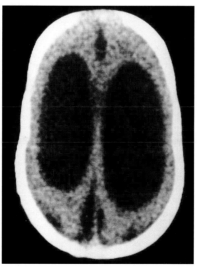

(c)

A Case of **Maternal psychiatric stress, antecedent multiple abortions, maternal viral infection, pregnancy low weight gain, familial diabetes. Newborn with macrosomia. Infant developed cerebral palsy and seizure disorder in the months after birth.**

This mother, gravida 7, with six previous elective abortions, was single and unemployed, under much emotional stress, reluctant to have a seventh abortion. There is increasing clinical and experimental evidence that psychiatric stress, in the same way as physical illness, has adversive effects on the fetus (pages 41, 53).

This was not a robust pregnancy. The mother had a viral upper respiratory infection; with maternal viral infection, with fever, the maternal oxygen demand increases, with resulting fetal oxygen deprivation.

This mother had had a problem with nutrition, with a low pregnancy weight gain. She had substantial factors indicating a metabolic disorder (latent prediabetes?). She had a family background of diabetes; the baby in this gestation was macrosomic; macrosomia is commonly the first manifestation of the disordered metabolism of latent diabetes (page 48).

This mother had had an abortion some months prior to the beginning of this pregnancy. This baby was born with an infiltrate in the lungs, a pneumonia originating during intrauterine life. With reasonable medical probability, the pneumonia, the lung infection, stemmed from a chronically postabortion infected uterus.

At delivery, the infant, still affected by the labor stress, was depressed. It is most important to recognize that the infant responded to the attention given in the delivery room; his vital functions, respiration, soon improved.

Regarding the concern that there was acute hypoxic brain damage present in this newborn — the presence or absence of acute brain damage is validly determined, not by a monitor tracing, or by meconium staining, etc., but is validly determined clinically and pathologically by the performance of the newborn in the immediate postdelivery hours and in the first day (page 164).

Infants born with extensive cerebral damage, with fresh *acute* intranatal cerebral damage, have a characteristic clinical pattern. These infants remain limp, in shock, for hours after delivery, with congestive heart failure, respiratory failure, depressed vital signs, often lasting for many days.

This newborn was not like that. This newborn soon had stable vital function, was alert, active, within the first hour, and had good color, good respiration, good muscle tone and reflexes during the first day.

However, the improved clinical course of this newborn was compromised by the early onset of seizure manifestations at the end of the first day, a complication requiring heavy sedation with phenobarbital, rendering the infant neurologically depressed for days.

Clinically the early onset of seizures in the newborn is increasingly recognized to be due to causes other than acute brain damage.

As noted, during pregnancy, gestational problems exercise an adversive effect on the fetus. These underlying pathologic processes often are latent, silent clinically. The common denominator of these adversive processes is *hypoxia* — the fetus is subjected to varying degrees of oxygen deprivation that leads to an accruing of subacute cerebral damage in the fetuses that survive to term. Newborn infants, so affected, are born harboring old, subacute cerebral damage, damage that later becomes manifest as cerebral palsy and other neurologic disorders.

This child developed the dyskinesias of cerebral palsy. Cerebral palsy is known to be due to deep cerebral (basal ganglia) damage incurred at a time during premature immature fetal life prior to 34 or 35 weeks. It does not occur related to events of labor and delivery in mature birth.

A Case of   *Vaginal bleeding during pregnancy; progressive placental detachment; premature labor. Newborn with intrauterine growth retardation and anemia. Infant developed spastic cerebral palsy.*

The mother had recurrent vaginal bleeding during this pregnancy and, in the last weeks, was sick with a viral-type infection.

Premature labor occurred at 34 weeks of gestation due to premature detachment of the placenta.

The vaginal bleeding in this case was caused by a long-existing ongoing premature placental detachment, as evidenced at the cesarean section and in the pathology studies of the placenta. With the detachment, a retroplacental hematoma was formed. Pathologically, this was diagnosed as a "partially organized progressive retroplacental hemorrhage" (Figure 453). The term "organized" means the hematoma clot was being attached to the placenta by connective tissue cells, scar cells, meaning that the process had been going on for a long time, weeks, months (page 67).

Anatomically, the placenta is tightly adherent to the inner aspect of the uterine wall. At times a part of the adherent placenta becomes loosened, separated from the uterine wall. The cause of such detachment is not precisely known. Sometimes it begins with an infarct of the placental surface at its attachment to the uterus; a placental infarction was diagnosed pathologically in this case.

With detachment of a part of the placenta, a pocket forms between the placenta and the uterine wall, a pocket filled with blood clot, a retroplacental hematoma. At times, the hematoma remains walled off forming a chronic "occult" retroplacental hematoma. Often, as in this case, the retroplacental hemorrhage penetrates beyond the edge of the placenta, forming a track down to the cervix, causing vaginal bleeding (Figure 42, page 66) (pages 44, 68).

The chronic occult retroplacental hematoma is of importance pathologically: (1) That part of the placenta that is separated, walled off by the clot, is put out of function, leading to placental insufficiency, to interference with fetal oxygenation and nutrition. (2) The clot, lying against the uterine wall, represents an irritant to the uterine musculature, triggering contractions, premature labor.

This fetus was chronically deprived, malnourished, had IUGR (page 94). Intrauterine growth retardation varies in severity and is due to periods of fetal deprivation resulting from maternal disorders, uterine, placental abnormalities, or any process that compromises the integrity of the maternal-uterine-placental-fetal complex. Fetal IUGR is associated with inadequate fetal nutrition and inadequate oxygenation, so that the fetus is born with varying silent subacute cerebral damage.

This newborn infant was noted to be pale. Pale means anemia. Anemia was confirmed in the newborn hematology reports. The anemia was substantial, and the newborn was transfused soon after birth to bring the blood level up.

In the context of the present case it is likely that the fetal-neonatal anemia was due to fetal-maternal transfusion syndrome (page 97).

The transfer of blood from fetal to maternal circulation occurs regularly, in some degree in most if not all gestations. The degree, the amount of transfusion, varies, but is severe in some instances. The cause, the pathogenesis, of the fetal-maternal transfusion process is thought to be associated with pathologic processes that damage elements of the placenta, as occurs with placental infarction. In the present case there was infarction of the placenta.

The main question neurologically was, When was the infant's brain damage incurred? There was concern that this infant, at birth, had *acute* hypoxic brain damage. However, in this case, there is substantial clinical-pathologic evidence that this newborn infant did not have *acute* cerebral damage.

Newborn infants with *acute* brain damage are depressed at delivery and stay depressed for hours and days. They remain comatose, limp, with unstable vital function, with bulging fontanelles reflecting edematous swelling of the brain, acute brain damage.

The newborn infant in this case was not like that. Although depressed at delivery, she soon responded the morning after delivery and was active, vigorous, pink. Vital functions were stable. During the first day clinically there was marked improvement. Fontanelles were flat. Neurologic assessment on day two indicated that the infant was neurologically intact, with no clinical evidence of brain damage. Plainly, this is not the picture of a newborn infant with *acute* diffuse cerebral damage.

The clinical course of the newborn infant in the present case is consistent with the syndromic pattern of infants who incur hypoxic cerebral damage in early premature fetal life, with the surviving fetus harboring old subacute deep cerebral damage, with the effects of the damage surfacing later during infantile life as cerebral palsy.

Infants born with old *subacute* cerebral damage, resulting from adversive gestational processes, are typically depressed at birth, but unlike newborn infants with acute cerebral damage, infants with subacute damage soon respond and are stable, have spontaneous activity, improved tone, and no evidence of cerebral edema, no bulging fontanelles. This was the clinical pattern in the present case (pages 24 and 166).

Figure 453. Placenta showing old and recent retroplacental hemorrhage; microscopic section. Above, a pale-staining layer of decidual tissue from the uterus; below, vascular placental tissue undergoing infarction. Between the decidual layer and the placental tissue is an irregular dark-staining layer, an extravasation of blood, apparently organized old and recent retroplacental hemorrhage.

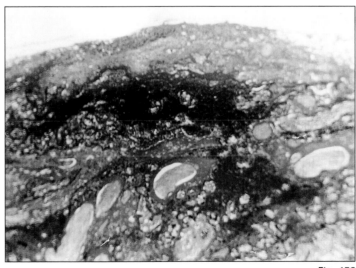

Fig. 453

A Case of   *Triplets; premature labor at 31 weeks; one triplet with postnatal hypoxia due to apnea, subsequent development of cerebral palsy.*

Premature labor occurred at 31 weeks of gestation with delivery of triplets by cesarean section. The infants responded well and left the delivery room in good condition. All were anemic and two were transfused. The second of the triplets developed severe recurrent apnea, much more than did the other two (page 105). Subsequently this infant developed motor symptoms at 5 months, was diagnosed as having spastic quadriplegia.

CT scan at 5 months showed enlarged lateral ventricles. The other two of the triplets had no manifest neurologic abnormalities.

On a clinical pathologic basis it is conclusive that the cerebral damage in the middle triplet had its origin postnatally, due to neonatal apnea, severe hypoxia, with associated acute deep cerebral damage and subsequent development of spastic cerebral palsy.

A Case of *Maternal recurrent viral infections, maternal anemia, decreased fetal activity, intrauterine growth retardation. Infant subsequently developed cerebral palsy, mental retardation, epilepsy, and microcephaly.*

The mother had periods of sickness with fever during this pregnancy, recurrent flu episodes, gastroenteritis. She was anemic. Low maternal weight gain was recorded. The mother was admitted to the hospital at 39 weeks with gastroenteritis and dehydration. The fetus was affected by this maternal illness, at one point showed decreased fetal activity during the hospitalization.

The fetus, though compromised, survived. The infant had a very low Apgar score, but she responded to treatment in the delivery room. The newborn infant showed chronic effects of gestational deprivation, showed intrauterine growth retardation.

What was the underlying cause of the initial depression in this newborn? Was it due to acute cerebral damage incurred during labor and delivery? Or was this a feeble newborn, previously compromised during early fetal life?

In newborn infants who do have *acute* cerebral damage, the clinical manifestations are characteristic: *Prolonged* depression of vital function occurs; the infant remains comatose, flaccid, for days.

In the present case, this newborn infant did not show this clinical pattern. Although this newborn infant had a low Apgar score, she was described as active with good color a few hours after birth.

This infant later was diagnosed as having mild cerebral palsy. These mildly affected children are characterized as being awkward, with a dyskinetic loss of fine motor function. Often there are gross motor defects (gait) and difficulty in articulation. Often associated with this are mental retardation, behavior problems (head banging), and seizure disorder, as in this case (page 218).

Pathologically, brain damage that leads to manifestations of cerebral palsy is due to hypoxic deep cerebral damage that takes place specifically in the premature period of fetal life (or in premature newborn) months before term. The newborn infant in this case was estimated to be of 41 weeks' gestation. At that time in gestation, damage to the deep structures, damage that leads to cerebral palsy, does not occur.

In fetuses that survive intrauterine deprivation, hypoxia, during early fetal life, incurring cerebral damage affecting the deep periventricular strata, the cerebral damage, initially pathologically acute, becomes subacute. Newborn infants, so affected, are born harboring subacute, old, cerebral damage.

This infant was observed to be microcephalic. In fact, microcephaly was apparent at birth, as well as in subsequent years. Microcephaly, common in cases of cerebral palsy, is the result of deep cerebral damage originating during premature immature fetal life, with consequent growth of the cerebrum compromised, reduced.

A Case of **Maternal emotional stress, malnutrition, anemia. Premature delivery, nuchal cord, intrauterine growth retardation, fetal-neonatal anemia, fetal-neonatal microcephaly. The infant developed spastic cerebral palsy, mental retardation, seizure disorder.**

This gestation presents a constellation of adversive conditions affecting the maternal-fetal complex. This mother had many health problems, stress problems, during pregnancy, problems that are known to exercise adverse effects on the fetus, effects that create fetal deprivation, fetal hypoxia. This mother was very young, pregnant at 17 years, an unfavorable factor for pregnancy. She had obvious emotional stress during this pregnancy; at 29 weeks she suffered a physical assault; she was destitute, living in a "rescue mission" with a husband who had a record of alcohol abuse and behavior problems. She was sick; she had bronchitis and asthma. She was malnourished and anemic.

The premature rupture of the membranes, the premature birth, that occurred at 36 weeks, did not of itself cause related fetal distress. However, the fetus, already compromised, weakened in utero by maternal factors, was further endangered by a nuchal cord, a complication that often originates at an early fetal age, subjecting the fetus to hypoxia. Added to this, this fetus (newborn) was anemic; anemia in the fetus causes hypoxia.

Despite this poor intrauterine environment, the fetus, although chronically compromised, blighted, survived and at birth the newborn had a good Apgar score.

This newborn infant did not show a clinical pattern of *acute* brain damage postnatally. On the contrary, this infant, with an Apgar score of 6 and 8, was described as "active and crying" after birth.

In newborn infants who do have *acute* cerebral damage, whether the damage is incurred during birth or postnatally, the clinical manifestations are characteristic: *Prolonged* depression of vital function occurs. The infant remains comatose, flaccid, for days, often in congestive heart failure. If the newborn survives, improvement is slow over the following days and weeks.

The good condition of this infant after delivery is incongruous with the diffuse cerebral damage manifested later by the infant. This provides support for the clinical-pathologic interpretation that the cerebral damage in this infant was incurred at a time other than the perinatal period, that this manifest diffuse cerebral damage is attributable to pathologic processes in the premature immature fetal period.

In fetuses that survive intrauterine deprivation, hypoxia — incurring cerebral damage affecting the deep periventricular strata — the cerebral damage, initially pathologically acute, becomes subacute. Newborn infants, so affected, are born harboring subacute, old, cerebral damage.

This newborn infant was observed to have a small head, even too small for a premature (head circumference at birth, 29.5 centimeters; average for 36 weeks' gestation is 32 centimeters). This is evidence that cerebral damage was incurred long before birth, with consequent failure of the damaged brain to enlarge appropriately — fetal-neonatal microcephaly.

Microcephaly became even more evident as the infant grew older, together with cerebral palsy, mental retardation, and seizure disorder.

The only CT scan taken in infancy, at 10 months, reflected the clinical disabilities in the infant (Figure 454). All the ventricles were dilated, the result of deep periventricular loss of substance. A massive defect appeared in the right posterior cerebral wall. Although most of the white matter in this part of the cerebrum was lost, there remained, persisting, a thin layer of cortical and subcortical tissue.

Figure 454. CT scan at 10 months. Ventricles are dilated, reflecting loss of periventricular tissue. The right posterior cerebral wall is decreased in thickness, reflecting loss of deep cerebral strata, leaving a thin cortical and subcortical layer.

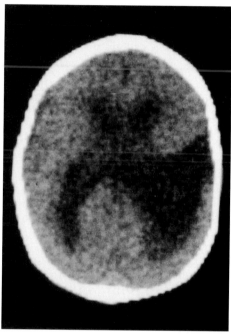

Fig. 454

A Case of   *Twin gestation; one stillborn, with old brain damage present at autopsy. Surviving twin developed cerebral palsy, mental retardation, seizure disorder, and microcephaly.*

Toxemia, preeclampsia, and gestational problems that developed during the last trimester led to the death of one fetus; the surviving twin later developed cerebral palsy and other severe cerebral disabilities. Regarding the time of origin of the brain damage, autopsy study of the brain in the stillborn infant revealed that, although the fetus was alive immediately prior to delivery, encephalomalacia, old brain damage, was present, indicating that the causal mechanism responsible for the brain damage had origin long before birth.

This was the mother's second pregnancy. The first pregnancy had also been complicated by preeclampsia and was terminated at 37 weeks by cesarean section.

In the present case, with the onset of labor at 37 weeks, with mounting signs of toxemia, and with abnormal fetal monitor signs appearing, the pregnancy was terminated by a repeat cesarean section.

In this case the mother was sick, with prelusive signs of toxemia beginning months before delivery. Although the maternal factors of toxemia clinically were essentially brought under control at the time, the fetuses manifestly incurred damaging effects.

This mother had an episode of premature labor at 32 weeks of gestation. Premature labor indicates that something pathologic has occurred in the gestation. The pathologic process that triggers the onset of premature labor is likewise hostile to the fetus.

This mother had become anemic. Anemia causes chronic bodily hypoxia, both maternal and fetal hypoxia.

Twin gestation has a high incidence of fetal-neonatal morbidity and mortality and a high incidence of cerebral palsy in twin survivors.

In this twin gestation, the chronic intrauterine pathologic environment was such that one twin did not survive, showing at autopsy evidence of old brain destruction, encephalomalacia. Not only was the brain damage pathologically old, but additionally the brain weight, at 210 grams, was 100 grams less than average for this gestational age, further indication of longstanding intrauterine encephaloclastic processes.

The other twin, likewise exposed and damaged by the adverse gestation processes, managed to survive. Sequelant cerebral disability of cerebral palsy reflects intrauterine fetal cerebral damage incurred long before birth.

The enfeebled surviving fetus did not tolerate the stress of labor and delivery and the newborn was depressed at birth, but in the nursery he improved and was awake and active, with stable vital signs soon after birth.

The progress of the newborn infant was compromised by the onset of seizures. It was necessary to sedate the infant with phenobarbital, rendering the infant clinically lethargic.

The newborn surviving infant showed evidence of intrauterine malnutrition, was long and thin.

Toxemia of pregnancy broadly affects the maternal-placental-fetal complex (page 57). The visceral changes in this disease compromise maternal kidney, liver, cardiovascular, and other visceral functions, beginning in a prelusive period, at a time before signs and symptoms appear in the mother. The adverse effects on the mother and fetus begin before albuminuria and hypertension appear. The mother in this case complained of headache and dizziness, had peripheral edema early in the last trimester. The signs of toxemia were increased at 32 weeks, with albuminuria and hypertension.

This surviving child, examined at 9 years of age, had spastic cerebral palsy. Pathologically, brain damage that leads to manifestations of cerebral palsy is due to hypoxic damage of the deep cerebral structures, damage that takes place specifically in the *premature* period of fetal life (page 190).

CT scan studies of the surviving child showed extensive, old deep cerebral damage with calcification (Figures 455 and 456).

The child showed microcephaly. With deep brain damage occurring during fetal life, with destruction of periventricular tissue, the brain is decreased in size, fails to grow normally, leading to microcephaly—evident in this case.

Figure 455. CT scan taken at 1 year 9 months shows in the cerebrum areas of decreased density in the frontal and temporal regions. The cerebral white matter is decreased and there is corresponding lateral ventricle enlargement.

Figure 456. Areas of decreased density similar to those in Figure 455; additionally, areas of increased density, apparently foci of calcification in the parieto-occipital regions bilaterally.

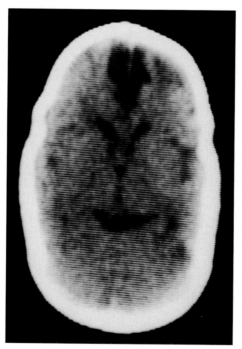

Fig. 455

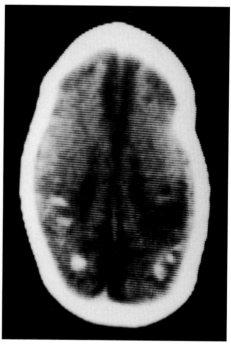

Fig. 456

A Case of

A macrosomic anemic newborn; maternal signs of prediabetes; morbid obesity; anemia. Infant later developed spastic cerebral palsy, mental retardation, seizure disorder, and microcephaly.

This mother was morbidly obese, 5 feet 5 inches in height and weighed 270 pounds. Obesity is a hazard to the pregnant mother and her fetus. Morbid obesity is reflective of a disturbed metabolism. Metabolic disorders in the mother exercise an adversive effect on the fetus. Obesity per se predisposes to hypertension and diabetes, both of which may be unveiled during pregnancy (page 47).

This mother produced a macrosomic baby, weighing 4,050 grams (9 pounds), over the ninetieth percentile in weight and more than a pound overweight for the gestational age (average at 40 to 42 weeks is 3,300 to 3,500 grams).

Macrosomia in offspring, as in this case, is commonly the first sign of latent prediabetes in the mother. In this direction, maternal obesity and macrosomic offspring are two important indicators of maternal latent prediabetes (page 48).

In people who become diabetic, the bodily dysfunctions have origin many years before the diabetes becomes overt. Maternal prediabetes (or diabetes) effects an unfavorable uterine environment, exercises a damaging effect on the fetus, extending over the entire length of the gestational period. In these circumstances there is a high incidence of stillbirths.

This mother became anemic at midpregnancy.

Anemia compromises oxygenation of the mother, with resulting decreased oxygen supply to the placenta and the fetus.

At the beginning of this gestation the mother had severe prolonged tonsillitis with fever up to 104 degrees. With fever, the metabolic oxygen demands of the mother are much increased, leaving the embryo, fetus, oxygen deprived, susceptible to hypoxic damage.

This newborn was anemic, a condition present in the fetus for a prolonged period.

At birth, the hematocrit was reported at 45.8. Average for a newborn is 61. The hematocrit measures the quantity of red cells in the blood. In the present case, correspondingly, the hemoglobin level was decreased, 15.5 (average for newborn is 19).

Chronic anemia, in the fetus as in the adult human, causes chronic hypoxia. The red cell is the oxygen-carrying vehicle in the blood. The decrease in hematocrit means this fetus existed with less than the average amount of oxygen supply, chronic severe fetal hypoxia.

This infant, months after birth, presented manifestations of cerebral palsy, mental retardation, seizure disorder.

It is of importance to recognize that this infant, although depressed at delivery, responded to care given in the delivery room, with her Apgar score at five minutes rising to 5. Her vital function, respiration, improved. At the initial examination in the nursery, she was still depressed but was active, crying; her lung fields were clear.

The fontanelles remained soft and flat—meaning there was no brain swelling, no acute edema. This was confirmed by the CT scan, which showed patent ventricles, no evidence of cerebral swelling or acute damage to the brain (pages 167, 168).

Considered retrospectively, this was a weak, anemic, macrosomic fetus — weakened, *not* by inordinate acute intranatal hypoxia, but was chronically enfeebled by maternal adversive gestational processes, a fetus unable to tolerate the stress of labor. This gestational background is compatible with the presence of latent subacute cerebral damage, damage accrued in a chronically unfavorable intrauterine environment, damage that ultimately led to the manifest disabilities.

A Case of   *Decreased fetal activity. Anemic dysmature infant born with old subacute cerebral damage. Infant developed cerebral palsy, mental retardation, seizure disorder, and microcephaly.*

During the last weeks of this gestation, fetal activity had decreased, reflecting gradual weakening of a chronically enfeebled, anemic fetus, compromised by adverse gestational processes (page 169).

During this pregnancy there were maternal factors adverse to the well-being of the fetus. This mother had a family history of diabetes and she gained weight excessively, up to 41 pounds at term, factors suggesting she had a disturbed metabolism, possibly reflecting a latent prediabetic condition.

The newborn infant was long and thin, dysmature (IUGR), anemic (pages 94, 95). He was depressed at birth but soon responded, with stable vital function after delivery, indicating that the infant did not have *acute* brain damage. Infants with acute brain damage do not respond, remaining depressed for hours, days. This newborn was not like that.

The neonatal CT scans indicated old, subacute, cerebral damage, decreased density of the white matter, damage reflecting onset a long time, weeks, before birth (Figure 457). Ventricles were patent; there was no evidence of cerebral edema (pages 24, 33).

Scans taken subsequently at 12 days and at 3 years show a progression of loss of cerebral substance (Figures 458 and 459).

This infant developed cerebral palsy, mental retardation, seizure disorder, and microcephaly.

The sequence of changes in the series of imaging studies, extending over a period of years, presents an example of the transition of fetal-neonatal hypoxic cerebral damage to the ultimate pattern of chronic residual cerebral damage in cases of cerebral palsy and related cerebral disabilities (page 189).

In view of the evidence in the newborn CT scans of old cerebral damage and the absence of acute cerebral edema and considering the good performance of the newborn during the hours after birth, considering the absence of prolonged coma, the absence of unstable vital function and the absence of other clinical signs of acute brain damage, the conclusion emerges that this brain damage was incurred, not at birth, but had origin long before birth.

Figure 457. CT scan of the brain at 4 days. **(a).** Far-advanced disintegration of deep white matter in the frontal and temporal regions of a form, a severity, indicating an origin beginning in utero a long time, days, weeks, before birth; subacute damage. **(b).** CT scan showing patent lateral ventricles indicating absence of acute cerebral edema.

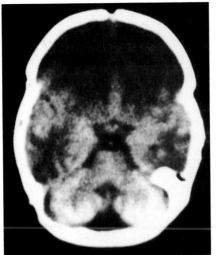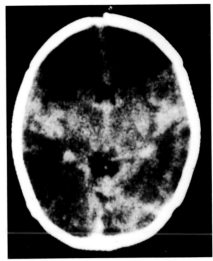

Fig. 457(a)   (b)

Figure 458. CT scan of the brain at 3 months. In the frontal region there is a loss of periventricular white matter. This loss of tissue generally corresponds to the white matter damage evident in the neonatal scan in Figure 457.

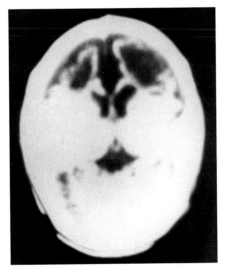

Fig. 458

Figure 459. CT scan of the brain at 3 years shows evolution of the cerebral damage observed in the neonatal (Figure 457) and 3-month (Figure 458) scans. The frontal lobes are diminished, appear contracted, almost obliterating the rarefied damaged areas evident in previous scans, leaving increased subarachnoid space around the atrophied lobes. The scan shows enlarged ventricles, reflecting loss of periventricular tissue.

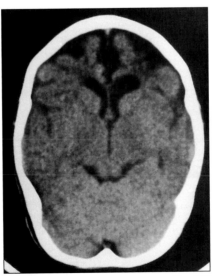

Fig. 459

A Case of *A mother with history of habitual abortion, morbid obesity, recurrent vaginal bleeding. Newborn, postmature, with intrauterine growth retardation. Infant later developed hemiplegic cerebral palsy, mental retardation, seizures, and microcephaly.*

This mother was an "habitual aborter" with a poor record of pregnancy performance, with three or four prior miscarriages, a record unpromising for the fetus (page 41). Relevantly, the mother had "spotting" vaginal bleeding in this and in other pregnancies. Vaginal bleeding during pregnancy is a clinical complication that reflects an intrauterine pathologic process, and often is prelusive to spontaneous abortion. The pathologic processes that four times caused fetal death previously for this mother proved sublethal for this fetus.

The mother was obese, with obesity of a degree characterized clinically as morbid obesity, a pregnancy problem adversive to the well-being of the fetus (page 47). There was no clinical record, no prenatal care, during the first 18 weeks of this pregnancy.

This newborn showed the effects of intrauterine compromise, was underweight, malnourished, showing intrauterine growth retardation. The enfeebled sick fetus did not tolerate the ordinary stress of labor and the newborn was depressed at birth. The newborn infant responded to resuscitation; lung fields were clear, muscle tone improved. Fontanelles remained normal, not bulging. This was not the picture of a newborn with acute brain damage. Newborn infants with acute brain damage are comatose for prolonged periods, with bulging fontanelles indicative of cerebral swelling, with congestive heart failure. This newborn was not like that.

The head size, average at birth, failed to grow, and at 1 month was in the tenth percentile, microcephalic. Beginning at 16 months the infant developed recurrent seizures. At 2 years there was delay in mental and motor function.

Diagnosis of right hemiplegic cerebral palsy was made.

The CT scan at 2 years showed enlargement of the left lateral ventricle; this correlated with the clinical pattern of asymmetrical cerebral palsy (page 182).

MRI studies at 5 years showed extensive damage in the left cerebral hemisphere (Figure 460). The left cerebral hemisphere was much smaller than the right. There was much enlargement of the left lateral ventricle, particularly posteriorly. There was decreased density in the deep strata of the left cerebral wall, especially periventricularly, in the frontoparietal region and in the parieto-occipital region, forming porencephalic cystic lesions.

This pattern of cerebral damage, affecting the deep periventricular strata, has its origin in premature immature fetal life, weeks or months before term.

Figure 460. MRI study of the brain at 5 years in a case of hemiplegic cerebral palsy.
(a). A coronal image through the fronto-parieto region shows dilated left lateral ventricle and indicates broad areas of porencephalic loss of tissue in the cerebral wall in the deep periventricular white matter.

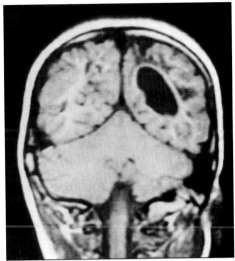

Fig. 460(a)

Figure 460(b). The left hemisphere is reduced; the lateral ventricle is much increased, especially posteriorly, due to loss of periventricular tissue. (Horizontal plane.)

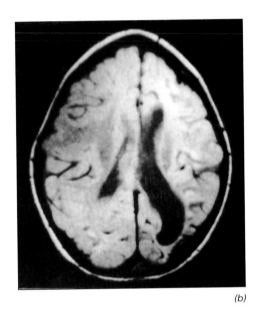

(b)

Figure 460(c). An image through the left cerebrum in a parasagittal plane showing dilated lateral ventricle and decreased densities, porencephalic lesions in the frontoparietal and occipital regions.

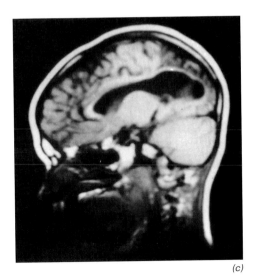

(c)

A Case of   *Maternal morbid obesity, maternal hypertension.*
            Newborn with intrauterine growth retardation
            and polycythemia. Infant developed hemiplegic
            cerebral palsy, mental retardation, seizure disorder,
            and microcephaly.

This mother was big, morbidly obese, 286 pounds at term. She was hypertensive. These are conditions adverse to the well-being of the fetus.

Marked obesity is a hazard to the pregnant mother and her fetus (page 47). Morbid obesity is reflective of a disturbed metabolism. Metabolic disorders in the mother exercise an adverse effect on the fetus.

Obesity per se predisposes to hypertension and to diabetes, both of which may be unveiled during pregnancy. This obese mother was a certain candidate for future diabetes (her father had diabetes).

This newborn showed the effects of chronic intrauterine deprivation, intrauterine malnutrition, and intrauterine hypoxia. The gestational age of this newborn was 39 1/2 weeks. This newborn weighed 6 pounds (2,720 grams). This is in the fifteenth percentile for 39 1/2 weeks; the average weight for 39 1/2 weeks is 3,100 grams. This newborn should have weighed at least 7 pounds.

Furthermore, big mothers make big babies ordinarily — so that at 6 pounds this baby was underweight.

This newborn infant had polycythemia. Polycythemia (*poly-,* many; *-cythemia,* cells in the blood) means there are excessive red cells in the blood.

The condition polycythemia is also known as the "hyperviscosity syndrome." In polycythemia, the increase in the number of red cells in the blood is associated with increased hematocrit (the percentage of blood volume made up of red cells), and corresponding increased hemoglobin concentration in the blood. This causes an increase in the viscosity of the blood and leads to stasis of blood flow (page 104).

Hemoglobin concentration in excess of 22.0 grams or a hematocrit of more than 65 percent anytime during the first week of life is considered evidence of polycythemia. This infant's hematology records showed: hematocrit 71 percent, hemoglobin 21 grams at 35 hours of life. Hemoglobin was 21.3 grams on day 3; the hematocrit was 68 percent on day 5.

Red cells are formed in the bone marrow. In the *primary* form of polycythemia, excessive red cells are formed pathologically, with the cause not known (this does not apply in this case).

In the *secondary* form, as in this case, excessive red cell formation is triggered by the presence of hypoxia (the Indians in the Andes have secondary polycythemia).

During gestation, if the fetus is subjected to ongoing hypoxia due to hypoxia-producing maternal factors, placental disorders, a degree of polycythemia results. The red cells carry oxygen to the fetus; the increase in red cells in polycythemia is an effort to increase oxygenation for the fetus.

In this case, maternal conditions of obesity and hypertension were adverse to the well-being of the fetus, contributing to intrauterine hypoxia.

A sonogram on day 4 showed hemorrhage in the right lateral ventricle and into the third ventricle; origin of the blood was attributable to a hemorrhagic lesion in the caudate nucleus.

The presence of blood in the brain is not necessarily due to acute brain damage. Subacute lesions, as well as fresh acute damage, are hemorrhagic. Relevantly, the CT on day 6 (Figure 461) and the sonograms on day 7 and day 10 revealed evidence of infarction associated with hemorrhage.

In a CT scan on day 20 (Figure 462), the necrotic tissue in the infarcted areas had begun to be absorbed, leaving porencephalic cavitations, greater on the left. Likewise, with the loss of deep cerebral tissue, the ventricles were enlarged.

With the cerebral damage greater on the left, the resulting disability was more pronounced on the right side of the body, right hemiplegic cerebral palsy.

Although the size of the head (and brain) were normal at birth, the head failed to increase in size with age, and by the tenth month, with a head circumference of 40 centimeters (below the second percentile), the infant was plainly microcephalic.

Figure 461. CT scan taken on day 6 shows large areas of decreased density in the left parietal region, indicating loss of deep cerebral white matter, suggesting far-advanced (subacute) infarction; similar smaller areas of low density appear in the right frontal and right occipital regions. Large areas of high density posteriorly in the cerebrum are consistent with areas of subacute periventricular hemorrhagic infarction.

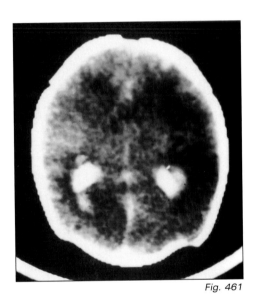

Fig. 461

Figure 462. CT scan taken on day 20 shows progression of the process of infarction. Large areas of low density in the deep periventricular white matter of the left parieto-occipital region and about the occipital horn of the right lateral ventricle are consistent with areas of porencephaly.

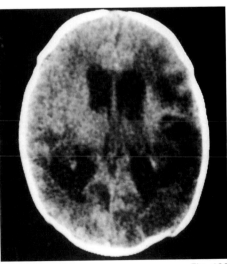

Fig. 462

A Case of   ***Periventricular and intraventricular hemorrhage present at birth and persisting during early infancy; intrauterine growth retardation. Child developed cerebral palsy, mental retardation, epilepsy; microcephaly.***

The present case deals with an infant born at 41 to 42 weeks of gestation. The newborn was underweight for his gestational age, weighing 6 pounds 2 ounces.

Relative to this fetal deprivation, although there was no account of maternal pregnancy illness, the record showed that in a 5 week period during midpregnancy, the mother failed to gain weight, suggesting that she was sick.

During the first hours after birth the newborn was stable, active, crying lustily.

The fact that this infant was responsive, active, and stable during the first hours after delivery is substantial evidence that there was not an *acute* process of brain damage present at birth.

The infant deteriorated on the second day and had seizure activity.

Ultrasound on day 2 showed an intraventricular hemorrhage. CT scans at 2 weeks showed, in addition to intraventricular hemorrhage, evidence of damage in the periventricular white matter in the frontal lobes (Figure 463). It is likely that the intraventricular hemorrhage had its origin from this periventricular damage. Repeated ultrasound studies during the first 2 months postnatally showed persisting subependymal and intraventricular hemorrhage.

The clinical pathologic pattern here is consistent with the presence at birth of a latent subacute subependymal periventricular hemorrhagic lesion (page 24). The location of the cerebral damage, periventricular, is characteristic of damage having origin in early premature fetal life. These lesions are hemorrhagic infarcts and, in fetuses that survive, the lesions become subacute, latent. In some cases the lesions continue to bleed into the ventricles, as appeared in this case.

The child at 4 years showed spastic cerebral palsy, mental retardation, seizure disorder, and microcephaly.

Figure 463. CT scan of brain at 2 weeks showing decreased density in frontal areas, indicating loss of white matter substance.

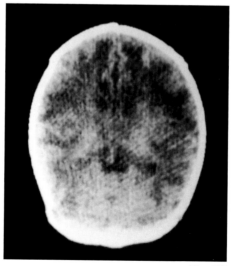

Fig. 463

A Case of **_Maternal obesity; pregnancy emotional stress; vaginal bleeding during pregnancy, preeclampsia. Intrauterine growth retardation. Infant developed cerebral palsy, mental retardation, seizure disorder._**

This mother, 5 feet 7 inches in height, weighing 261 pounds, was characterized as morbidly obese. Obesity is a hazard to both mother and fetus (page 47).

In the mother's background, in addition to obesity, was a family history of diabetes. The mother's obesity reflects a disturbed metabolism.

This mother had episodes of vaginal bleeding during this gestation. In many instances, vaginal bleeding reflects a pathologic condition in the placenta. There is a high incidence of cerebral palsy in offspring of mothers with a history of vaginal bleeding during pregnancy.

Another contributing factor, this mother was under substantial emotional stress, with personal problems. While it is difficult to assess the effect of maternal psychiatric stress on pregnancy outcome, there is increasing clinical opinion that such stress compromises the well-being of the fetus.

Near term the mother developed signs of toxemia.

The effect of adversive conditions on the fetus, the newborn, in this term pregnancy, is evidenced by the fact that this infant was underweight, weighing 6 pounds 1 ounce. However, the length was 20 1/2 inches (52 centimeters), at the ninethieth percentile. This was a long thin newborn, a dysmature newborn. Obese women usually produce heavy babies.

The head circumference of this newborn was small, 31.75 centimeters, in the fifteenth percentile.

In the CT scan on day 1, the ventricles appeared small but were visible; no edema or acute damage was evident.

The infant's head remained small, obviously microcephalic.

Functionally, at 6 years the child had cerebral palsy, mental retardation, and seizure disorder. The MRI at this time showed a pattern of late chronic cerebral damage, widespread loss of cerebral substance, the consequence of fetal-neonatal hypoxic cerebral damage (Figure 464).

Figure 464. MRI of brain at 6 years. In this scan and at other levels, there is much loss of cerebral white matter, leaving many regions with cystic spaces, reaching from the deep white strata to the subcortical layer. Diffuse loss of white matter, leaving ventricles enlarged.

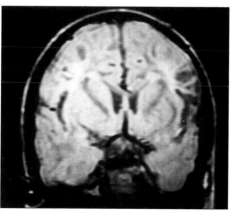

Fig. 464

A Case of　　*A premature newborn with hypoxic brain damage due to postnatal apnea; subsequent development of cerebral palsy and mental retardation.*

This mother was hospitalized and treated for acute pelvic inflammatory disease immediately prior to the time of conception. PID is a chronic disorder not readily cleared up.

Premature birth occurred at 34 weeks of gestation.

Pathologically, with pelvic inflammatory disease, even after symptoms are gone, the pathologic process remains embedded in the pelvic tissues, chronically "smoldering." With PID, as in this mother, the infectious process can become subacute and chronic, affecting the ovaries, tubes, and spreading through the lining of the uterus and into the cervix — and persisting.

PID is one of the common causes of miscarriage. There is substantial literature that links pelvic infectious disease to premature labor. The occurrence of the premature delivery was a major factor in this case, setting the stage for the development of hypoxic brain damage in the newborn infant postnatally and the consequent development of cerebral palsy.

Prematurity, per se, by itself, does not cause cerebral palsy. Prematurity *is a factor,* however, in that prematurity (in the fetus or newborn) *plus hypoxia* causes specific damage to the cerebrum that results in cerebral palsy.

It was thought by some of the clinicians in this case that the newborn infant had incurred acute hypoxic brain damage during labor and delivery.

The newborn was recorded as being in good condition in the delivery room, with spontaneous onset of respiration, with a good Apgar score, 7 and 8, which is excellent for a premature. In the nursery, he was described as active, crying lustily, and with good skin color.

An infant who has suffered severe hypoxic acute brain damage during labor and delivery does not perform that way.

The valid assessment of the presence or absence of acute brain damage is based, not on what may or may not have occurred during the events of labor and delivery, but is indicated by the performance of the newborn (page 164).

Infants that are born with massive *acute* cerebral damage are comatose at birth and remain comatose for prolonged periods, days, with depression of vital function and congestive heart failure. This was not the pattern in the present case. He did not perform as if he had acute, stroke-like brain damage.

This premature newborn infant developed recurring episodes of apnea (page 105). Apnea is an arrest of breathing for 20 seconds or more. The consequent hypoxia immediately affects the bodily structures, especially heart action, leading to bradycardia, slowing the pump action of the heart, compromising circulation, compounding the hypoxia.

Apnea is a manifestation of malfunction of the control centers in the brain that regulate respiration. It occurs spontaneously and automatically, and its occurrence cannot be controlled, nor can the attending hypoxia.

This infant weathered the apnea problem and did not die. Manifestly, though, he accrued cerebral damage, not enough to be lethal, but enough to produce cerebral damage causing lasting cerebral disability.

At 1 year the infant was functioning at a 7 month level; spastic quadriparetic cerebral palsy was diagnosed.

CT scan of the brain at 3 years showed dilated ventricles reflecting old deep periventricular damage, loss of tissue (Figure 465).

At 4 years the child had moderate mental retardation and a moderate degree of cerebral palsy.

Figure 465. CT scan of the head taken at 3 years shows moderate dilatation of the cerebral lateral ventricles, reflecting a loss of periventricular tissue.

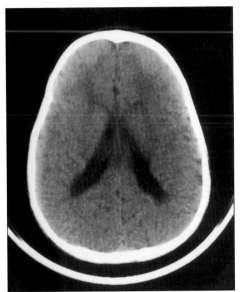

Fig. 465

A Case of   *Maternal chronic respiratory illness during pregnancy. Umbilical cord entanglement. Neonatal anemia; newborn with subacute cerebral damage. Infant developed cerebral palsy, seizure disorder, and microcephaly.*

The mother had chronic respiratory tract disease, ongoing problems of hay fever, asthma, URI. There were gastrointestinal problems with nausea and vomiting. Recurrent vaginal bleeding occurred. She became anemic.

Delivery occurred at 42 weeks of gestation.

At delivery, the umbilical cord was entangled around the foot of the fetus. With the occurrence of cord entanglement weeks or months before labor, the fetus may be subjected to hypoxia, with resulting total asphyxia and death of the fetus. Or, during the gestation, the fetus may be subjected to intermittent hypoxia, on and off, as the entanglement tightens and loosens. The fetus becomes weakened, registering loss of fetal activity, as occurred in the present case 7 weeks before delivery and again the day before delivery.

This infant at birth was enfeebled, severely anemic. Anemia causes hypoxia.

Although depressed at birth, the newborn infant soon improved — he had spontaneous respiration, was responsive, his vital function was stable. His improvement was interrupted by the early onset of seizures. The early onset of seizures in the newborn does not automatically make certain that the causal mechanism is related to perinatal processes. At times, neonatal seizures are due to cerebral damage incurred in early fetal life, present at birth.

In the months and years after birth the infant showed increasing evidence of severe diffuse cerebral damage and developed cerebral palsy, was severely mentally retarded, had a seizure disorder.

When was the cerebral damage incurred? During labor and delivery? Or at a time during intrauterine life, long before birth?

Clinical findings indicated that this newborn did not have fresh acute brain damage at birth. Acute cerebral damage, if present, would have caused cerebral swelling. Cerebral swelling would have caused bulging fontanelles — this was not present, the fontanelles remained soft and flat.

As noted, acute hypoxic damage causes cerebral edema, swelling; this edematous swelling is evident in the CT scans as decreased size of the ventricles. In the present case, the CT scans taken neonatally showed large ventricles. This scan shows evidence of far-advanced cerebral damage, of subacute nature, areas of decreased density, loss of substance in the white matter (Figure 466).

The subsequent CT scans (Figures 467, 468, 469) show progressive pathologic changes, progressive destruction of the cerebral structure, the transition of the neonatal cerebral damage to the chronic pattern of cerebral damage (page 189). This loss of cerebral structure was reflected clinically in the development of cerebral palsy, mental retardation, seizure disorder, and microcephaly.

Figure 466. CT scan of the brain at 9 days shows evidence of far-advanced cerebral damage, reflecting old, subacute hypoxic injury. The white matter shows confluent patches of decreased density, decreased substance; focal dense areas indicate localized old hemorrhagic damage. Ventricles are large, reflecting old periventricular loss of tissue.

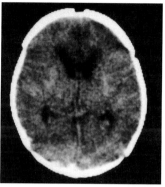

Fig. 466

Figure 467. CT scan of brain at 5 weeks. The cerebrum shows increased translucency of the white matter, loss of substance throughout the cerebrum.

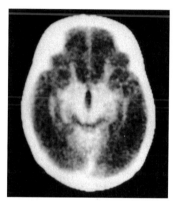

Fig. 467

Figure 468. CT scan of brain at 3 months; the cerebral white matter is of increased translucency, indicating progressive loss of substance. Ventricles are large. The cerebral walls appear composed of large cystic spaces separated by thin web-like septa.

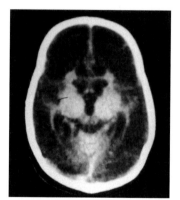

Fig. 468

Figure 469. CT scan of brain at 1 1/2 years. Almost total depletion of cerebral tissue. The preserved structure appears to be mainly the thalamus and adjoining tissue.

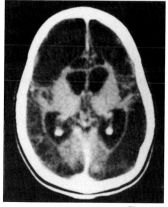

Fig. 469

A Case of   **Newborn with DIC (disseminated intravascular coagulopathy). Mother had acute infections, anemia. Infant developed spastic cerebral palsy, mental retardation, and seizure disorder. CT scan of brain showed ex vacuo hydrocephalus.**

The mother had obvious medical problems during this pregnancy. She had infections that required antibiotic treatment. She became anemic.

This newborn showed the effects of intrauterine compromise relevant to the mother's medical problems. Maternal illness exercises an adversive effect on the fetus; reflecting this, the fetus did not tolerate the ordinary stress of labor and showed some abnormalities in the monitor record. Likewise the enfeebled fetus, the newborn, was depressed at birth. However, he responded to resuscitation care and was soon improved. During the first day, with fair muscle tone, with adequate respiration, lung fields clear, the newborn was reported as resting quietly.

The infant in this case did not present the clinical picture of a newborn with acute diffuse hypoxic cerebral damage. Infants with acute hypoxic brain damage remain comatose for prolonged periods, with respiratory depression and congestive heart failure. This newborn was not like that; his clinical course was consistent with that of an enfeebled newborn who had incurred hypoxic cerebral damage during premature fetal life (related to maternal health factors) and was born with old, subacute damage in the deep structures of the cerebrum, affecting basal ganglia and resulting in the development of cerebral palsy.

Although improved, the enfeebled infant, soon after birth, developed anemia, hyperbilirubinemia (jaundice), platelet deficiency, and hemorrhages — blood oozing from skin punctures, and blood in the urine and trachea. These are characteristic manifestations of DIC, disseminated intravascular coagulopathy (page 114).

In DIC, platelets become clogged in blood vessels, become deficient. Platelet deficiency leads to hemorrhages. Red blood cells are broken down excessively; the hemoglobin in the red cells becomes converted to a yellow pigment, bilirubin, and, being in excess, jaundice results.

DIC occurs in adults as well as infants and commonly occurs in the enfeebled, after prolonged bodily stress and deprivation.

This infant had been born at 37 weeks of gestation by midforceps delivery.

There was some concern that the use of the forceps had caused trauma to the head, caused brain damage that resulted in cerebral palsy.

This is a belief that was widely held in times past. In recent times, research in the NIH Collaborative Perinatal Project (page 160) — by myself and others in pathology, and clinically by Niswander and by Nelson and Ellenberg (page 161) — has plainly disproved the idea that forceps delivery at term causes cerebral palsy. Cerebral palsy is due to hypoxic cerebral damage incurred by the premature immature brain.

The CT scan taken at 4 years in this case shows evidence of deep cerebral damage, affecting periventricular white matter and basal ganglia. There is asymmetrical enlargement of the lateral ventricles, greater on the left (Figure

470a). The frontal lobes show decreased density, indicating loss of tissue substance (Figure 470b).

The child at 5 1/2 years had spastic cerebral palsy, mild mental retardation, and a seizure disorder.

Figure 470(a). CT of the head taken at 4 years shows enlargement of the lateral ventricles, greater on the left, reflecting loss of substance in the periventricular strata, ex vacuo hydrocephalus. **(b).** The white matter of the frontal lobe (centrum semiovale) appears of low attenuation, suggesting loss of tissue substance, leukoencephalopathy.

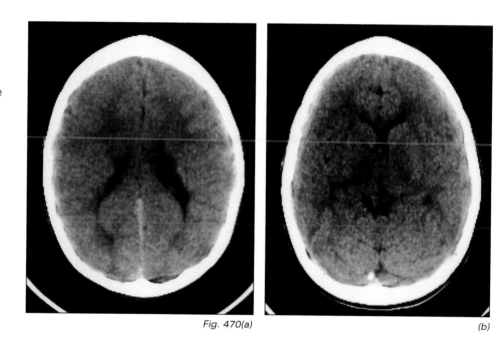

Fig. 470(a)   (b)

A Case of   *Maternal prediabetes, obesity, hypertension, vaginal bleeding. Newborn dysmaturity, anemia, cerebral infarction leading to porencephaly. Infant developed asymmetrical cerebral palsy, mental retardation, and a seizure disorder.*

This mother, with her morbid obesity, hypertension, and prediabetic condition, had a poor reproductive record; of three pregnancies, one (this case) was complicated by vaginal bleeding; a second pregnancy yielded a macrosomic baby (9 pounds 13 ounces); a third pregnancy, with vaginal bleeding, terminated in a miscarriage.

The mother gained 54 pounds during this pregnancy, weighing 251 pounds at term. Clinically, obesity during pregnancy is adversive to the mother and her fetus (page 47).

The mother had vaginal bleeding early on, over a period of 3 weeks. Bleeding during pregnancy is mainly due to pathologic processes affecting the placenta, processes potentially compromising the fetus, causing fetal hypoxia. The significance of the vaginal bleeding that occurred is reflected in the fact that, at a later pregnancy, vaginal bleeding leading to spontaneous abortion occurred.

The mother became anemic.

Together with her obesity, she became hypertensive and showed manifestations of prediabetes.

In the present case, the newborn infant showed the effects of adversive intrauterine processes. He was anemic and dysmature. Although depressed at delivery, he rapidly improved, and his Apgar score rose to 9 at five minutes. He was soon active, had good reflexes, and was admitted to the regular nursery. There was no bulging of the fontanelles. (Bulging indicates cerebral swelling, cerebral edema, acute brain damage. This was absent in this case.)

His progress was interrupted when, at 1 hour after birth, he had an episode of apnea and bradycardia, considered "seizure apnea." Soon after, frank seizures developed.

There is increasing clinical opinion that when seizures appear soon after birth in a previously active infant, the process is not attributable to acute asphyxial brain damage, but rather that the cause must be sought in other pathologic mechanisms (page 208).

CT studies of the brain on day 4 show evidence of focal hemorrhagic damage in the cerebrum (Figure 471). The cerebral ventricles were small, patent (Figure 472).

The question arose as to whether the hemorrhagic lesions were recent, fresh, or of a subacute nature incurred remotely, during fetal life.

In analyzing this question it is important to take into account both clinical and pathologic factors, the good clinical performance of the infant after delivery, the absence of bulging fontanelles, and the patent cerebral ventricles in the CT scan.

Infants born with massive *acute* cerebral damage are comatose at birth, and remain comatose for prolonged periods. This was not the pattern in the present case. This infant was active and alert soon after delivery. If there had been acute hypoxic cerebral damage, this pathologic cerebral process would have caused cerebral swelling; cerebral swelling would have caused bulging fontanelles and compression obliteration of the ventricles. This did not occur in this case. The fontanelles were soft and flat. The CT scan showed patent ventricles. Taking these factors into account, it was conclusive that the hemorrhagic lesions evident in the neonatal CT scans were not acute but were subacute pathologically, the residue of damage that originated early in fetal life.

This infant developed right-sided asymmetrical cerebral palsy (page 182). Relevant to this, the MRI taken at 6 years (Figure 473) shows a large porencephalic cyst in the left cerebrum that corresponds to the large infarctional lesion evident in neonatal CT scan (Figure 471) (page 28). The cerebral damage appearing on one side of the cerebrum accounts for the asymmetry of the neurologic disability.

This case demonstrates the transition of a localized cerebral infarct, present at birth, to a porencephalic cyst evident years later.

Figure 471. CT scan of brain taken at 4 days shows a large area of density in the left posterior region, consistent with hemorrhagic infarction. Smaller areas of density, areas of infarction, are present in the frontal area.

Figure 472. Mottled areas of density, hemorrhagic damage in the cerebrum. The lateral ventricles are patent and an open cavum septi pellucida is present, indicating an absence of cerebral edema. CT scan, as in Figure 471, at 4 days.

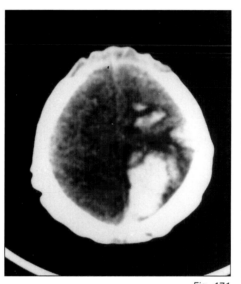

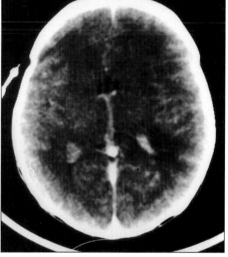

Fig. 471   *Fig. 472*

Figure 473. MRI of the brain at 6 years. The parieto-occipital region shows a sharply demarcated translucent cystic structure, a porencephalic cyst, that extends from the deep strata out to the surface of the cerebrum. The cystic defect corresponds to the area of hemorrhagic infarction evident in Figure 471. Clinically, the cystic lesion is associated with asymmetrical cerebral palsy and mental retardation and seizure disorder.

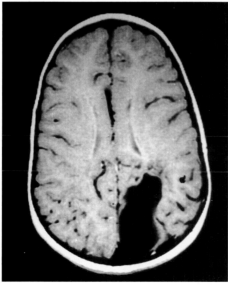

Fig. 473

A Case of   ***Maternal profound obesity, with hypertension and manifestations of prediabetes; acute respiratory viral infection. The postmature, dysmature, microcephalic newborn later developed cerebral palsy, epilepsy, and mental retardation.***

This mother had profound obesity; at a height of five feet, she weighed over 200 pounds during this pregnancy. Profound obesity is a hazard for both the mother and the fetus (page 47).

The mother was acutely ill during pregnancy, with sore throat, upper respiratory infection. Acute maternal illness has a compromising effect on the fetus (page 36).

This mother had manifestations of latent prediabetes — family history of diabetes (father), obesity, mild hypertension. Pathologically, the metabolic disturbances of prediabetics are adversive to a fetus.

The newborn infant was not only post-term, overdue, but was also *dysmature,* small for dates, evidencing intrauterine growth retardation.

In the present case it was thought by some that the cerebral damage in this child was incurred acutely during the intranatal period. This is inconsistent with the clinical course in this case. The clinical picture was not that of a newborn that had incurred fresh acute hypoxic cerebral damage in the intranatal period. Newborn infants with acute cerebral hypoxic damage present a characteristic clinical pattern, with persisting coma, cyanosis, respiratory depression, congestive heart failure. This pattern did not occur in the present case. The newborn infant responded to care given in the delivery room and was soon breathing spontaneously.

The postnatal pattern in the present case is characteristic of infants who have incurred brain damage early in fetal life and survive to term. These fetuses, harboring old, subacute cerebral damage, are enfeebled and do not tolerate the ordinary stress of labor, and are born depressed. In contrast to infants with *acute* cerebral damage, these infants with old cerebral damage usually respond to resuscitation in the delivery room, with spontaneous respirations, skin pink, and soon after, in the nursery, they are alert and active, as occurred in the present case (page 166).

The infant's improvement was compromised by the development of seizures at 10 hours on the first day.

CT scans of the head, taken on the second day of life, showed evidence of cerebral edema (cerebral swelling), with the ventricles consequently not being visualized (compressed) (Figure 474).

The CT scan was taken at a time when the infant was having seizures. The cerebral edema evident in the CT scans is attributable to the effects of the seizures.

Microcephaly was present at birth. This microcephaly is substantial evidence that the process of brain damage began long before birth: With brain damage occurring at an early time in fetal life, the brain fails to grow in size, the head growth is decreased because the brain, damaged, remains small (page 31).

The infant's microcephaly became more and more apparent in the following years. The infant developed cerebral palsy, reflecting early fetal damage to deep cerebral structures, to basal ganglia; seizure disorder and mental retardation were present, reflecting the extension of deep cerebral damage to the surface, to the cortex.

CT scan at 3 months showed the cerebral ventricles moderately dilated, reflecting loss of deep periventricular tissue (ex vacuo hydrocephalus) (Figure 475).

Deep cerebral damage that occurs during premature fetal life is due to gradual devitalization of the periventricular strata. The devitalized tissue may or may not be visualized by the CT scan at birth.

As the devitalized periventricular tissue is absorbed, the degree of ventricular enlargement progresses over a period of months—forming ex vacuo hydrocephalus.

Pathologically, this pattern of changes, a microcephalic cerebrum with enlarged hydrocephalic ventricles, is characteristic of cases of deep cerebral damage originating in early fetal life that leads to cerebral palsy.

Figure 474. CT scan of the brain taken on day 2 showing evidence of cerebral edema (cerebral swelling), with the ventricles consequently not visualized (compressed). Cerebral edema due to seizures.

Figure 475. CT scan of the brain at 3 months. Ventricles moderately dilated; deep periventricular cerebral tissue, previously devitalized, gradually absorbed, creating a moderate degree of ex vacuo hydrocephalus.

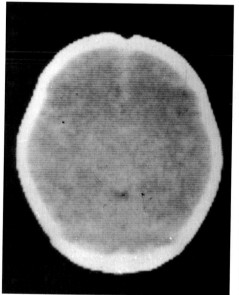

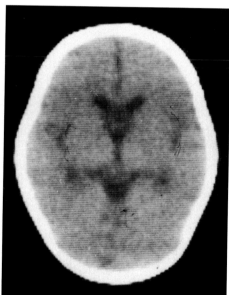

Fig. 474

Fig. 475

A Case of **A teenage pregnancy, maternal hypotension, anemia, and pretoxemia; decreased fetal activity. Depression of the newborn, early onset of seizures. Infant developed cerebral palsy, mental retardation, and seizure disorder.**

This 17-year-old single mother was anemic and hypotensive. Hypotension results in inadequate profusion of blood to the body organs, to the uterus, to the placenta. Decreased blood flow renders the fetus hypoxic. The mother became pretoxemic.

Decreased fetal activity occurred (page 169).

The infant, born at 42 weeks' gestation, appeared postmature. He was depressed at birth and was small for gestational age. He soon improved, with stable vital signs, good respiratory function; the infant was pink, crying, and responsive. However, within 5 hours seizures occurred requiring phenobarbital sedation.

Ultrasound of the brain on the first day demonstrated normal size of ventricles. This rules out the presence of *acute* cerebral damage; when acute fresh cerebral damage is present, the cerebrum becomes edematous, swollen, causing compression of the ventricles.

Pathologically, acute fresh brain damage, incurred during early fetal life, after a period of time "quiets down," with the cerebral edema receding and the ventricles returning to normal size. However, the damage to the cerebral tissue around the ventricles, irreversible, in time becomes of a subacute (old) form pathologically. In cases of subacute cerebral damage present at birth, tissue alterations in the cerebrum may be far advanced, but not visualized in the sonogram.

With the presence of acute brain damage at birth ruled out by the sonogram, and taking into consideration the adverse pregnancy factors in the case, the conclusion emerges that the cerebral damage, latent at birth, was incurred early in fetal life.

The CT scan taken at 6 years correlates with the clinical development of cerebral palsy and other cerebral disabilities in this child (Figure 476). The white matter is decreased, to a severe degree, diffusely through the cerebrum; a cystic cavity is present in the white matter of the left frontal lobe.

Figure 476. CT scan of the brain at 6 years. The cerebral white matter is much decreased, and in the left frontal lobe there is a large cavity. The loss of white matter around the ventricles results in ex vacuo hydrocephalus.

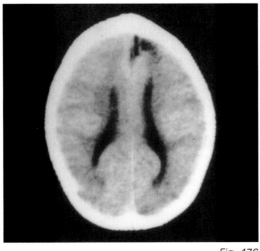

Fig. 476

A Case of   *Maternal acute influenzal infection with fever; nuchal cord. Newborn with intrauterine growth retardation; severe deep cerebral damage. Infant developed cerebral palsy, mental retardation, seizure disorder.*

This mother had an acute viral infection at 14 weeks of pregnancy, influenza with fever.

With acute infectious disease such as the flu, accompanied by clinical toxicity and fever, the basal metabolic processes of the mother, the oxygen requirements of the mother, are increased — leading to a relative decrease in oxygen available to the fetus, fetal hypoxia (page 42).

The mother had a period of disturbed bodily metabolism with rapid weight increase due to fluid retention, edema, a condition of mild toxemia.

Birth occurred at term.

In addition to the maternal factors, the fetus was exposed during intrauterine life to the hypoxia-producing complication of a tight nuchal cord.

That this fetus was affected by adversive processes during intrauterine life is indicated by the fact that the fetus, newborn, was underweight, indicating chronic intrauterine deprivation, intrauterine growth retardation.

The enfeebled fetus was unable to tolerate the ordinary stress of labor, had abnormal fetal monitor signs, and was born depressed.

The newborn infant soon improved, was breathing spontaneously. The infant was considered to be "doing well."

This is not the picture of a newborn with severe acute cerebral damage incurred during birth or in the delivery room. Infants with acute cerebral damage at birth have a specific clinical pattern: they are depressed at birth and stay that way for hours or days, comatose, with depressed vital function.

The newborn in this case was not that way. The pattern in the present case is reflective of an infant with chronic intrauterine nutritional deprivation, chronic hypoxia, bearing latent *subacute* cerebral damage (Figure 477) that became manifest in later infancy as cerebral palsy and severe mental retardation and seizure disorder.

The sequence of brain CT scans in this case shows an increasing loss of deep cerebral substance. The first CT scan, at 26 hours, shows extensive loss of deep cerebral substance, in the periventricular strata, damage of an advanced degree (Figure 477).

The follow-up CT scans taken at 9 days, at 6 weeks, at 7 months and at 4 years show the advancing pathologic changes, beginning with the early damage in Figure 477; as the devitalized white matter is gradually absorbed, the ventricles become gradually enlarged (Figures 478, 479, 480, 481).

Pertinently, in the early CT scans, with extensive deep cerebral damage evident, the surface layers of the cerebrum are present, not destroyed. This form of damage, wiping out the deep layers but not the surface layers, is characteristic of the pattern of hypoxic cerebral damage originating when the cerebrum is immature, premature.

The imaging studies present a demonstration of the transition from the subacute pattern of damage evident neonatally to the pattern of chronic damage present years later, associated clinically with cerebral palsy and other neurologic disabilities (page 189).

Figure 477. CT scan of the head taken on day 2. The white matter is decreased, indicating far advanced subacute damage.

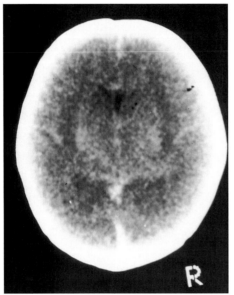

Fig. 477

Figure 478. CT scan of the head at 9 days. The cerebrum shows decreased white matter, destruction of white matter in the deep periventricular strata, most severe in the frontal area. The cortical and subcortical tissue is relatively preserved. The ventricles are moderately enlarged, the consequence of periventricular loss of tissue.

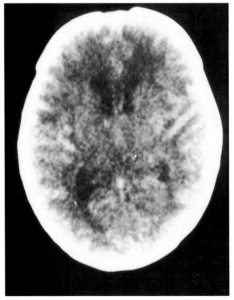

Fig. 478

Figure 479. CT scan at 6 weeks. Cerebrum shows loss of substance, most pronounced in the frontal lobes. Lateral ventricles much increased, more on the left than the right.

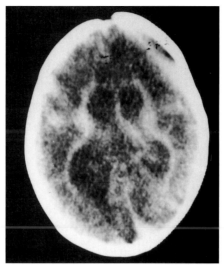

Fig. 479

Figure 480. CT scan of the head taken at 7 months evidencing far-advanced loss of white matter in the frontal region, with only a thin rim of cortical and subcortical tissue remaining. Posteriorly the disintegration of the white matter is pronounced but less severe than frontally. The ventricles are very large due to loss of cerebral substance with ex vacuo expansion of the ventricles resulting.

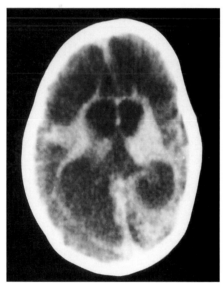

Fig. 480

Figure 481. CT scan of the head taken at 4 years shows decreased density through the white matter of the cerebrum leaving little difference in density between the white matter and the lateral ventricles. The lateral ventricles are enlarged.

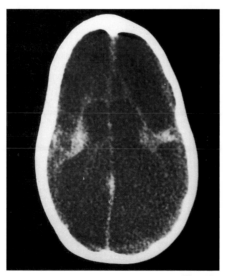

Fig. 481

A Case of ***IUD present during pregnancy; premature labor.
Postnatal hyaline membrane disease and apnea.
Infant later developed cerebral palsy.***

At 32 weeks of pregnancy, spontaneous rupture of membranes occurred; together with the leaking amniotic fluid, an IUD was expelled.

A month earlier, the mother had been treated for toxemia, with manifestations of sudden weight increase, edema, and rising blood pressure. During the 2 weeks prior to delivery the mother had "severe cramps."

The rupture of membranes and the extrusion of the IUD occurred 36 hours before delivery. Amniotic fluid remained clear. There was no evidence of intrauterine infection, no sepsis in the mother or in the newborn infant.

The newborn infant was somewhat depressed but soon improved, with an Apgar score of 4 and 7, a score considered good for a small premature infant. Weight was 1,500 grams, about average for 32 weeks' gestation.

The condition of the premature infant deteriorated postnatally, with the clinical course punctuated by hypoxia-producing complications of hyaline membrane disease and recurrent apnea; congestive heart failure developed; anemia was treated with transfusion.

The infant became obtunded, evidencing hypoxic cerebral damage.

The infant survived.

Subsequently, as a consequence of the postnatal hypoxic complications, the infant developed manifestations of cerebral palsy and was retarded mentally.

The question arises as to the relationship between the presence of the gestational IUD and the occurrence of premature labor. Experience demonstrates that in most pregnancies with an IUD present, the pregnancy goes to term without apparent effect on the fetus, on the newborn. However, the literature indicates that the presence of an IUD increases the risk of premature labor, at times of septic abortion. In the present case there was no sepsis. Whether the premature labor was due to the presence of the IUD, or due to other factors in the gestation, is open to question (page 88).

A Case of   *Maternal infection, chorioamnionitis. Newborn with intrauterine pneumonia, fetal-neonatal anemia. Infant later developed cerebral palsy, mental retardation, seizure disorder, and microcephaly.*

This pregnancy was complicated by maternal medical problems that affected the fetus, problems that began long before the delivery, that contributed to chronic intrauterine hypoxia, causing brain damage in the premature immature fetus.

The mother had a metabolic problem, gained excessive weight during the gestation. The weight gain was partly attributable, together with the onset of hypertension, to the development of toxemia manifestations during the last months of pregnancy. Toxemia is an hypoxia-producing pathologic process adversely affecting the fetus.

In midpregnancy this mother had a "cold," apparently a viral infection. The duration, the severity, of the infection was not indicated, but it was serious enough to have antibiotics prescribed. Viral infection during pregnancy is a hazard both to the mother and to the fetus. With acute illness, with fever, the metabolic oxygen requirements of the mother are sharply increased, leaving the fetus oxygen-deprived, hypoxic.

Sepsis was evident in the mother at the time of labor and delivery. On admission to the hospital, she had fever and leucocytosis. The amniotic fluid was foul smelling, infected. Subsequently, the pathology examination of the placenta revealed chorioamnionitis (Figure 482), indicating bacterial infection, inflammation, involving the inner lining of the amniotic sac, contaminating the amniotic fluid around the fetus (page 88).

Chorioamnionitis, with bacteria present in the amnionic membrane and in the amniotic fluid, exposes the fetus to intrauterine infection, sepsis. The inflamed amniotic surface sheds bacteria and pus cells into the amniotic fluid. Aspiration by the fetus of infected amniotic fluid leads to lung infection, to pneumonia in the fetus and newborn (page 112).

This newborn was anemic. One of the causes of newborn anemia is infection, sepsis (page 96). Such anemia develops gradually in utero, over a period of weeks.

At birth, the hematocrit was reported as 39.5 percent. Average for a newborn is 61 percent. The hematocrit measures the quantity of red cells in the blood. In the present case, correspondingly, the hemoglobin level was decreased, 12.1 grams (average for a newborn is 19 grams).

Clinically, even prior to the hematology studies, the newborn infant was repeatedly described as very "pale." Pale means anemia.

Chronic anemia, in the fetus as in the adult human, causes chronic hypoxia. The red cell is the oxygen-carrying vehicle in the blood. The decrease in hematocrit means this fetus existed with less than the average amount of oxygen supply, chronic severe fetal hypoxia (page 95).

Chronic intrauterine hypoxia leads to fetal hypoxic visceral damage; with intrauterine hypoxia, the fetus accrues subacute and acute cerebral damage.

Pathologically, *acute* brain damage, when present, causes the brain to become edematous, swollen. Such cerebral edema, when present in the newborn, causes bulging fontanelles and is evidenced in the ultrasound and CT scan by compression of the ventricles.

In the newborn in this case the ventricles were patent; the radiologist reported the ventricles as being of normal size. Clinically, the fontanelles were not bulging. It is implausible to have severe, acute, fresh brain damage present and have ultrasound and clinical evidence of no cerebral swelling, no edema.

The sequence of cerebral structural changes demonstrated in the ultrasound and CT scan studies in this case is characteristic of the syndromic occurrence of deep cerebral damage incurred in the immature premature fetal period, with the fetus surviving to term, born with old, subacute periventricular tissue damage, not yet apparent by ultrasound, but becoming demonstrable in CT scans weeks and months, later, with development of enlarged ventricles, ex vacuo hydrocephalus (Figure 483).

In newborn ultrasound and CT studies of the brain, cerebral damage that is acute or subacute, in many cases, is not immediately evident, or is equivocal early on (page 31). After a period of time, the damage becomes evident in the CT scans. Pathologically, the reason for this is that, in the course of time, as the periventricular damage becomes old, the devitalized tissue becomes softened and is gradually absorbed over a period of many days, weeks; only then does the damage become demonstrable, evident as enlarged cerebral ventricles.

This infant managed to survive the effects of the pulmonary complications, but was left with accumulated cerebral damage incurred during early fetal life, damage causing the clinical manifestations of cerebral palsy, mental retardation, seizure disorder, and microcephaly.

Figure 482. Chorioamnionitis in this case; microscopic section of amniotic membrane showing thick deposits of small dark-staining inflammatory cells, polymorphonuclear leukocytes, "pus cells," the pathologic pattern that characterizes chorioamnionitis.

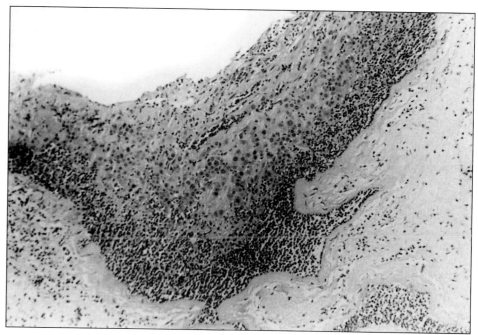

Fig. 482

Figure 483. CT scan taken at 5 months, showing ventricular enlargement reflecting loss of periventricular tissue; convolutional atrophy frontally and in the temporoparietal regions. These changes reflect cerebral atrophy, mainly affecting deep cerebral structures; clinically, infant with progressive microcephaly.

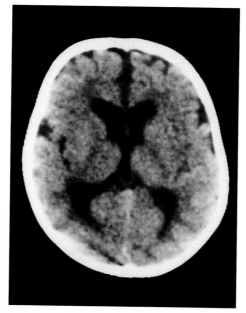

Fig. 483

A Case of **Spinal cord injury due to midforceps delivery with excessive traction. Infant tetraplegic at birth.**

In the present case, the resort to forceps delivery of the fetus, at a time when the fetal head was arrested at the +2, +3 station, was dictated by urgency, engendered by the monitor records of fetal bradycardia, fetal stress. The obstetrician opted to solve this problem by applying forceps rather than by performing a cesarean section (page 125).

The forceps extraction lasted a long time, with the forceps being applied over 15 minutes; fundal pressure was applied during the forceps extraction, and, admittedly, a lot of force was applied, pulling on the fetus' head (force quantitated at between "slight" and "foot-on-the-table pulling").

With reasonable medical probability there was a direct cause-and-effect relationship in this case between the delivery procedure and the presence at birth of manifest spinal cord injury.

Spinal injury during forceps delivery is due to excessive force of traction, rotation, flexion, or extension of the spinal structures. Excessive traction results in stretching and tearing of the spinal structures, with laceration of the meninges, nerve roots, and, in extreme cases, laceration of the spinal cord, partial or transectional tearing, as manifested in this case (page 134).

At birth, the infant was limp, without respiration. Eyes opened occasionally; there was no response to painful stimuli of the trunk or extremities; muscle tone was absent. Response to stimulation of cranial nerves was present; a good suck reflex and gag reflex were present. The infant grimaced; the extraocular muscles were normal. The neurologic exam concluded there was an upper cervical spinal cord injury. Postnatally, the infant was alert; there was no spontaneous movement of the extremities. He remained ventilator dependent, tetraplegic. At 1 year he appeared to have good cerebral function.

With spinal cord injury during delivery, location of the injury determines its effects. The location of the cord injury varies from case to case. In some cases, the damage is high, with stretching and tearing of the brain stem and upper cord; these lesions are lethal, lead to stillbirth. In other cases, the brain stem escapes damage, with the injury, as in this case, beginning in the upper cervical cord. If the damage at this level proves transectional, the infant has a chance to survive, but is rendered tetraplegic.

In the present case the MRI of the spine (Figure 484) at 2 months indicated absence of cord structure from the level of cervical 2 to 6. This accounts for the preservation of function of the brain stem and cranial nerves, but with the midcervical segmental loss of tissue, the infant remained tetraplegic.

Figure 484. MRI at 2 months; midsagittal section through the spinal canal demonstrating loss of cord structure from the level of cervical 2 to 6.

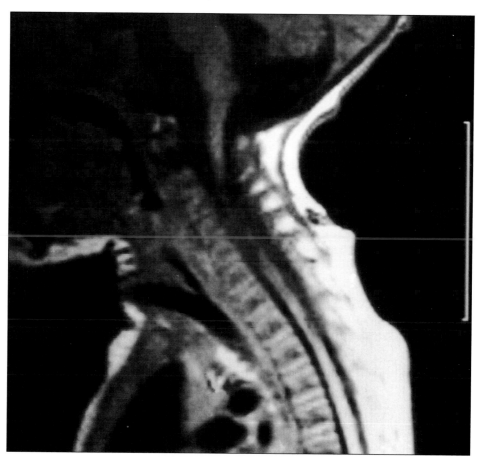

Fig. 484

A Case of ● *Maternal viral infections. Newborn with early onset seizures; xanthochromic spinal fluid. Infant developed cerebral palsy.*

This mother had a history of chronic recurrent upper respiratory disease. She was sick during this pregnancy, treated for acute tonsillitis at 4 weeks of gestation and treated for viral "flu syndrome" at 33 weeks.

Maternal illness causes fetal deprivation. The damaging effect on the fetus — the common denominator — is hypoxia. With acute febrile illness, the oxygen requirements of the mother are sharply increased, so that oxygenation of the fetus is depressed.

Labor developed at term. The fetus did not tolerate the stress of labor, with bradycardia appearing prior to delivery.

The infant was depressed at birth, was limp and cyanotic. He soon responded to resuscitation, with spontaneous respiration, crying, and improved muscle tone.

Seizure activity appeared at 4 hours of life. The early onset of seizures is consistent with the presence of old subacute cerebral damage, damage incurred during fetal life, damage attributable to adversive effects of the mother's illness during the pregnancy (page 207).

Spinal puncture done at 8 hours after birth yielded yellow, xanthochromic, fluid, further evidence that this newborn infant had old cerebral hemorrhagic damage (page 173).

The later development of cerebral palsy in this infant likewise indicates that the cerebral damage was incurred during early intrauterine life, when the fetus was immature. Cerebral palsy is the disease of prematurity, due to deep cerebral hypoxic damage, damage to periventricular tissue, to basal ganglia, incurred specifically in the premature fetus prior to 35 weeks' gestation, or in the premature newborn. It does not occur due to cerebral damage incurred at term. The presence of cerebral palsy is a time marker, indicating when the cerebral damage was incurred (page 190).

A Case of   *Premature twins. Twin A: placenta with infarcts; polycythemia; xanthochromic spinal fluid; microcephaly with subacute cerebral damage at birth. Infant developed severe cerebral palsy, mental retardation, and epilepsy. Twin B: no clinical problems reported.*

Delivery of twins (fraternal) occurred prematurely at 36 weeks.

This mother had had a "cold" at least once during this pregnancy. The mother had a period of excessive weight gain, up to 2 1/2 pounds per week for 2 months, excessive even for twin gestation, a weight gain reflective of an underlying metabolic disorder in the mother, a condition adversive to fetal well-being.

Birth was by vaginal delivery. Twin A was depressed and subsequently developed complications. Twin B, clinically, was in good condition at birth and without subsequent complications.

Examination of the placenta revealed two separate placental plates. Placenta A, from the affected newborn, revealed multifocal infarcts. This finding is of fundamental importance in interpreting the pathogenesis in this case. (The placenta of the other twin showed changes of minimal, equivocal nature.)

Placental infarction, as it occurred with twin A, means that portions of the placenta had been devitalized, creating placental insufficiency. This is a latent, silent pathologic process, causing chronic fetal deprivation, contributing to chronic intrauterine hypoxia (page 71).

This infant had polycythemia (*poly-*, many; *-cythemia*, blood cells) (page 104). The presence of polycythemia is measured by an increased level of hemoglobin (Hgb) and elevated hematocrit (Hct). This newborn, twin A, had Hgb of 21.8 grams (normal at 36 weeks is 15.5 grams). The Hct was 70.3 percent (normal at 36 weeks is 49 percent). Twin B had some elevation of the Hgb and Hct levels, but not to the severe degree that occurred in twin A.

Red cells are formed in the bone marrow. In polycythemia, as in the present case, excessive red cell formation is triggered by the presence of hypoxia. If the fetus is subjected to ongoing hypoxia, due to hypoxia-producing gestational factors, a degree of polycythemia may result. The red cells carry oxygen to the fetus; the increase in red cells in polycythemia is an effort to compensate, to increase oxygenation in the fetus.

The finding of xanthochromic (*xantho-*, yellow; *-chromia*, color) spinal fluid is of major importance in defining the time of incurrence of the cerebral damage. Xanthochromia of spinal fluid was found in the spinal fluid specimen at 14 hours after delivery (page 173). Xanthochromia, yellow coloration of the spinal fluid, is due to the presence of old hemorrhagic damage in the brain. With hemorrhage in the brain, with blood escaping into the ventricles, into the spinal fluid, red cells becomes lysed, broken down; the hemoglobin from the red cells first gives the spinal fluid a pink color. The hemoglobin gradually degenerates to a yellow pigment and gives the spinal fluid a yellow color —xanthochromia. (Just as a hemorrhagic black-and-blue bruise in the skin gradually becomes yellow-green after a time.)

This change in color takes many days, and continues to be present for weeks and months, when there is an old hemorrhagic lesion in the brain.

The finding of xanthochromic spinal fluid means there was present subacute damage, an old hemorrhagic lesion, in the brain. Subacute lesions tend to ooze blood into the cerebrospinal fluid for a long time. In such circumstances, as in this case, in addition to xanthochromia, the fluid contained some red blood cells.

The infant at birth was microcephalic, compared with the other twin.

The occurrence of neonatal microcephaly is rare. When it is present, it is hard evidence that the cerebrum was damaged long before birth, that the blighted brain then failed to grow normally during fetal life (page 31). This infant, microcephalic at birth, continued to be severely microcephalic.

CT scan taken on day 1 showed decreased density of the deep layers of cerebral white matter evidencing an advanced degree of damage, of subacute nature (Figure 485) (pages 24, 33).

CT scan of the brain taken at 5 days showed evidence of increased white matter loss, especially frontally (Figure 486). The lateral ventricles, viewed at other levels, were of normal size. CT scan taken at 1 month showed much enlarged lateral ventricles with extensive loss of white matter. The cerebrum was decreased, as if collapsing, leaving the subarachnoid space around the convolutions much increased (Figure 487).

It was thought by some that the brain damage was incurred during labor and delivery. However, the presence of microcephaly with advanced subacute cerebral damage at birth, with xanthochromic spinal fluid present, indicates that the brain damage present at birth was incurred a long time before birth.

Reflecting the severe cerebral damage evident in this microcephalic infant, the child at 5 years had severe spastic cerebral palsy, severe mental retardation, and a seizure disorder.

Figure 485. CT of the brain on day 1 shows deep strata of white matter of decreased density of a degree indicating old subacute damage; the cortical and subcortical layers appear relatively preserved. Lateral ventricles appear normal.

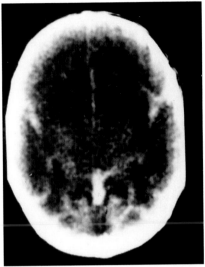

Fig. 485

Figure 486. CT scan of the brain at 5 days shows evidence of increased loss of white matter, most prominent frontally.

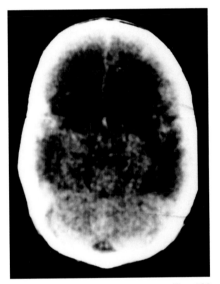

Fig. 486

Figure 487. CT scan of the brain at 1 month. The substance of the brain is much decreased, with far-advanced loss of cerebral white matter, leaving large lateral ventricles and increased subarachnoid space. A small density, apparently a calcified focus, is present in the subependymal tissue lateral to the left ventricle.

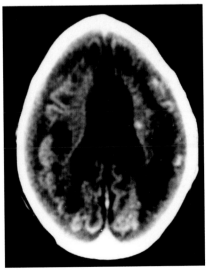

Fig. 487

A Case of **A very small premature; hyaline membrane disease. Surviving infant developed cerebral palsy and severe behavior disorder.**

This was a liveborn infant of 26 weeks' gestation. Spontaneous vaginal birth followed premature detachment of the placenta.

The infant was in good condition at birth, with an Apgar score of 5 and 7, considered very good for a small premature. Weight was 2 pounds 8 ounces (1,060 grams), somewhat above average for 26 weeks' gestation.

The infant suffered a succession of postnatal hypoxic complications — hyaline membrane disease, apnea, and congestive heart failure — but survived.

In the months following birth, increased muscle tone appeared in all extremities. At 14 months spastic cerebral palsy was diagnosed.

There were no seizures; the child was moderately retarded mentally.

A behavior disorder of increasing severity developed, with the child at 3 years described as having "a terrible temper." As with cerebral palsy and mental retardation, the behavior disorder, the psychopathy, was attributable to organic brain damage (page 212).

A Case of   *Maternal latent prediabetes. Macrosomic newborn; infant later developed cerebral palsy.*

This mother had many of the indicators of prediabetes (page 49). There was a family history of diabetes. As is common in diabetic conditions, the mother was obese, hypertensive, and had gained weight excessively (62 pounds) during the pregnancy. A glucose tolerance test yielded equivocal results.

Labor developed at 36 weeks of gestation. During delivery the fetus showed the effects of chronic intrauterine compromise, was unable to tolerate the stress of labor; fetal bradycardia developed.

The enfeebled infant was depressed at birth. However, he responded to attention given in the delivery room. His condition was noted to be "relatively OK" during the first 17 hours. He was active, had good respiration. Skin was pink. Neonatal reflexes were present.

The newborn infant weighed 8 pounds 3 ounces and, being of 36 weeks' gestation, was noted to be LGA (large for gestational age), macrosomic. An oversize baby, macrosomia, often is the first indication of the presence of maternal latent diabetes (page 48).

This newborn infant, although enfeebled, did not have clinical signs of acute cerebral damage. Infants with acute brain damage remain comatose, unresponsive, and limp for long periods. This newborn was not like that.

The clinical progress of this newborn was compromised by the early onset of seizures. Early onset of seizure activity, it is increasingly recognized clinically, does not occur in the presence of fresh acute (intranatal) cerebral damage, but is attributable to old subacute cerebral damage incurred during fetal life, long before birth (page 207).

This infant developed the dyskinesias of cerebral palsy, spastic quadriplegia. Cerebral palsy is known to be due to deep cerebral (basal ganglia) damage incurred at a time during the premature immature period of fetal life (page 178).

In retrospect, it is evident that metabolic dysfunction in this mother, pathologic processes of prediabetes, compromised the fetus, resulting in intrauterine accumulation of subacute cerebral damage, damage that postnatally caused the early onset of seizures and, in later infancy, resulted in cerebral palsy.

A Case of

Maternal chronic heart disease; low maternal weight gain. Newborn with neonatal microcephaly; IUGR. Infant later developed cerebral palsy, mental retardation, seizure disorder, microcephaly.

The mother in this case was sick; she had cardiac disease, chronic rheumatic valvular disease with a history of past hospitalizations and treatment with digitalis for congestive heart failure. Heart disorders lead to defective oxygenation of the mother and the fetus (page 51).

The mother's health was further undermined by a nutritional problem; she gained less than 1 pound per month during the last 5 months of the pregnancy.

Any prolonged chronic illness in the pregnant woman exercises its effects on the fetus, at times leading to intrauterine fetal deprivation, to IUGR.

IUGR was evident in the present case, with the term newborn infant weighing 4 pounds 13 ounces (2,183 grams), in the lower tenth percentile (page 94).

Intrauterine growth retardation is associated with deprivation of oxygenation as well as nutrition during fetal life, so that affected newborn have varying degrees of latent hypoxic cerebral damage at birth, damage that may remain silent postnatally and become manifest months after birth. Clinically, intrauterine growth retardation is associated with a subsequent high incidence of cerebral palsy, mental retardation, and other neurologic disabilities.

This term infant was microcephalic at birth, with head circumference of 30.5 centimeters (average at term, 33 to 34 centimeters). This attenuated head size reflects early fetal brain damage with failure of brain growth beginning weeks or months before delivery (page 31).

A Case of   *Maternal psychiatric disorder, narcotic addiction; vaginal bleeding; maternal anemia; abruptio placentae. Newborn with intrauterine growth retardation and microcephaly. Infant later developed cerebral palsy and mental retardation.*

This mother had health problems during pregnancy, problems known to have an adverse effect on the fetus (page 36). She had severe psychiatric stress during this pregnancy with a serious chronic narcotic addiction (page 53). There were recurrent episodes of vaginal bleeding, reflective of a pathologic placental defect that compromised the maternal-placental-fetal organization. With the bleeding, the mother became anemic, an hypoxia-producing factor for her and the fetus. The mother had chronic pelvic inflammatory disease, pathologically adversive to fetal genesis and development.

During pregnancy, illnesses in the mother, acute and chronic physical and emotional disorders, exercise an adversive effect on the fetus. The common denominator of these adversive processes is hypoxia — the fetus is subjected to varying degrees of oxygen deprivation that leads to an accruing of subacute cerebral damage in the fetuses that survive to term or near term. Newborn infants, so affected, are born harboring old, subacute cerebral damage.

At 37 1/2 weeks of the pregnancy, the mother was admitted to the hospital with heavy vaginal bleeding. An emergency cesarean section was done; a 90 percent abruption of the placenta was encountered (pages 66, 68).

The newborn infant showed the effects of intrauterine deprivation, IUGR, was small for dates, weighing 4 pounds 14 ounces (2,180 grams; average for 37 weeks' gestation, 2,800 grams).

This was an enfeebled sick fetus, unable to tolerate the stress of labor. The clinical course of this newborn is consistent with that of a chronically compromised fetus. Although he was depressed at birth, he soon improved, responded to care given, and is recorded to have been responsive, in good neurologic status, soon after birth. This newborn's performance was not that of an infant harboring acute stroke-like brain damage.

Neurologically, this child developed manifestations of global cerebral damage, disabilities reflecting damage to deep structures of the cerebrum (tissue of the periventricular white matter and basal ganglia) and damage to the cerebral surface (cortex). This pattern of fetal-neonatal damage, due to hypoxia-producing complications, does not occur in the term or near-mature fetus and newborn. It occurs specifically with hypoxia in the premature, immature fetus or newborn, prior to 35 weeks' gestation.

At the time of the hypoxic process in the premature brain, the cerebral damage may extend from the deep structures through the wall of the cerebrum, damaging the cortex, and later may cause (in addition to the cerebral palsy) mental deficiency and other developmental disabilities. This manifestly occurred in the present case.

Microcephaly was present in this newborn infant. The head circumference at birth was 12 1/2 inches or 31.25 centimeters. This is below the twenty-fifth percentile for gestational age of 37 weeks. The head size gradually showed decreased growth, and at 2 years 11 months measured 46.5 centimeters, below the second percentile. Microcephaly, common in cases of cerebral palsy, is the result of deep cerebral damage originating during premature immature fetal life, with consequent growth of the cerebrum compromised, reduced.

A Case of   *Vaginal bleeding; newborn sepsis, apnea. Infant later developed cerebral palsy, psychomotor retardation.*

The mother had vaginal bleeding during the first 3 months of this pregnancy. Recurrent bleeding during pregnancy is mainly due to pathologic processes affecting the placenta. Pathologic processes, such as partial detachment of the placenta, in their origin are often latent, subtle, so that the adversive effects on the fetus are far advanced by the time clinical symptoms of maternal bleeding occur. Throughout this silent latent period the fetus is being compromised, deprived, hypoxic (page 66).

Decreased fetal activity was noted by the mother (page 169). She reported that with her first pregnancy, "the baby (fetus) moved quite a lot but this baby (fetus) seemed to not move at all."

The mother was admitted at term for an elective repeat cesarean section.

The newborn infant was in good condition at birth, with an Apgar score of 7 and 8. However, within hours the infant became acutely ill, flaccid, unresponsive, with recurrent apnea, and was put on a ventilator. The infant became febrile with a temperature of 100.6 degrees. Sepsis was manifestly present in this newborn, complicating the first postnatal weeks, the source of the sepsis coming from the mother; the mother had fever, a spiking temperature postpartum, reflecting a latent infectious process in the mother.

The surviving infant at 7 months showed psychomotor retardation and was functioning at 2- to 4-month level. At 15 months, spastic cerebral palsy was diagnosed.

In summary, this fetus, newborn, was subjected to hypoxia-producing processes at two times, during fetal life and postnatally. First, during gestation, vaginal bleeding occurred, indicating a placental disorder. Pathologic processes affecting the placenta compromised oxygenation of the fetus, causing cerebral damage and, in this child, led to cerebral palsy.

Second, sepsis that developed postnatally, with apnea and fever, rendered the newborn infant hypoxic, contributing to cerebral cortical damage and, subsequently, to psychomotor retardation.

A Case of **Maternal cardiac disease; excessive pregnancy weight gain; placental infarction. Fetal-neonatal anemia. Infant developed cerebral palsy, mental retardation, seizure disorder, microcephaly.**

This mother had chronic hypoxia-producing health problems adversely affecting the fetus. She had a chronic cardiac disorder. She gained excessive weight.

The well-being of the fetus was also compromised by the presence of an (occult) latent placental infarct, revealed at delivery.

The cardiac problem in the mother, prolapse of the mitral valve, was clinically active, with arrhythmias and shortness of breath during the gestation. She was on antibiotics to prevent endocarditis. People with chronic valvular disease have varying degrees of cardiac insufficiency, chronic systemic hypoxia, affecting both the mother and the fetus.

Excessive weight gain, pregnancy obesity, developed in this mother, with a total weight gain of 65 pounds for this pregnancy.

Weight gain during pregnancy may in part be due to retention of fluid, with excessive swelling of the limbs. This was not a prominent factor in the present case.

Excessive maternal weight gain, of the degree in the present case, is usually of metabolic origin, due to endocrine dysfunctions such as in diabetic conditions (page 47).

Labor developed at 39 weeks of the pregnancy. This was a vaginal delivery. Bradycardia, indicating fetal distress, occurred during the last 20 minutes of the delivery,

The newborn infant was depressed at birth.

He was pale, anemic.

One of the important elements in defining the causal mechanism in this case is the fact that this fetus had been subjected to chronic anemia, with associated chronic hypoxia. At birth, the hematocrit was reported as 43.5 percent. Normal for newborn is 61 +/- 7.4 percent. The hematocrit measures the quantity of red cells in the blood. In the present case the quantity, the bulk mass, of red cells, was reduced by one-third.

Chronic anemia, in the fetus as in the adult human, causes chronic hypoxia. The red cell is the oxygen-carrying vehicle in the blood. The decrease in hematocrit by a third means this fetus existed with less than the average amount of oxygen.

The cause of the fetal-neonatal anemia is open to question. It was thought that with the placental infarction present in this case, a transplacental fetal-maternal transfusion may have occurred (page 97).

The question arose as to whether the fetus had incurred *acute* hypoxic brain damage during birth.

Although the infant was depressed at birth, he responded to resuscitation, had an Apgar score of 7 at five minutes, and was placed in the regular nursery. He was stable; his lung fields were clear; he had a good cry, good muscle tone. He was active, alert, soon held by the father. He was bathed and fed during the first morning. This is not the picture of a newborn with acute brain damage. Newborn infants with acute brain damage are comatose, limp, for prolonged periods, with ongoing depression of vital function. This newborn was not like that. The initial depression of the infant at delivery is attributable to the effects of chronic intrauterine compromise.

During pregnancy, medical problems in the mother, acute and chronic disorders, exercise an adverse effect on the fetus. The common denominator of these adversive processes is hypoxia—the fetus is subjected to varying degrees of oxygen deprivation, which leads to an accruing of subacute cerebral damage in the fetuses that survive to term or near term. Newborn infants, so affected, are born harboring old, subacute cerebral damage (page 24).

Subacute cerebral lesions, areas of devitalized tissue present at birth, often are not visible by ultrasound or CT scan at birth, becoming evident months later, together with the development of cerebral palsy and other cerebral disabilities.

Microcephaly with cerebral palsy, as in the present case, is due to failure of the cerebrum to grow consequent to the damage to the deep strata incurred during premature fetal life.

A Case of   *Nuchal cord, IUGR, neonatal anemia. Infant developed cerebral palsy, epilepsy, and mental retardation.*

Birth occurred at 41 1/2 weeks of gestation. A cesarean section was done due to the presence of a large uterine fibroid that inhibited vaginal delivery.

The newborn infant was pale and severely depressed, with an Apgar score of 1 and 3.

A nuchal cord, evident at delivery, manifestly had contributed to the newborn infant's initial depression (page 83).

The infant, weighing 6 pounds (2,722 grams) at 41 1/2 weeks of gestation, was noted to be SGA (small for gestational age), reflecting intrauterine growth retardation, IUGR (page 94).

Anemia, indicated by the pale appearance of the newborn, was confirmed in the laboratory; the hematocrit level was 48.9 percent (average for a newborn, 61 percent). The presence of anemia during fetal life, evident at birth, is reflective of adversive gestational conditions causing fetal-neonatal hypoxia.

Although depressed at birth, the infant soon became stable, with improved muscle tone, activity, and voluntary breathing, and at 15 hours was described as "alert and looking around." Fontanelles were soft, indicating absence of cerebral swelling. These clinical observations indicated an absence of acute stroke-like cerebral damage in the infant. Infants with acute cerebral damage remain depressed, unstable, comatose, for prolonged periods. This infant was not like that.

In summary, this enfeebled fetus, newborn, was affected by multiple adversive gestational factors — a nuchal cord, IUGR, anemia — factors responsible for the newborn infant's initial depression. The fact that the infant soon improved, became alert, ruled out the presence of acute cerebral damage.

The later development of cerebral palsy and other cerebral disabilities is attributable to the presence of old subacute cerebral damage, accumulated during intrauterine life.

A Case of   *Maternal excessive pregnancy weight gain, recurrent viral infection, vaginal bleeding. Newborn depressed; xanthochromic spinal fluid; early postnatal seizures. Infant developed cerebral palsy, mental retardation, seizure disorder, microcephaly.*

The mother had health problems during this pregnancy, problems known to have an adverse effect on the fetus: she gained excessive weight; she had viral-type "colds" with fever; she had vaginal bleeding.

Excessive weight gain occurred in this pregnancy. This mother was short, 5 feet 5 inches in height; her weight went up to 191 pounds at term. Excessive pregnancy weight gain is usually of metabolic origin, due to endocrine dysfunction, such as in latent diabetic conditions.

Viral-type respiratory infections with fever, as occurred repeatedly during this pregnancy, are a hazard to the mother and the fetus. With acute illness, with fever, the metabolic oxygen requirements of the mother are sharply increased, leaving the fetus oxygen-deprived.

Vaginal bleeding occurred, continuing for 5 days, bright red at times. Bleeding during pregnancy is mainly due to pathologic processes affecting the placenta, processes that potentially compromise the fetus, causing fetal hypoxia (page 44).

Spontaneous labor occurred at 38 weeks of the pregnancy. Delivery was vaginal, with low forceps.

The newborn showed the effects of chronic intrauterine compromise. The enfeebled sick fetus was depressed at birth. He responded to resuscitation, had an Apgar score of 7 at five minutes, and was placed in the regular nursery. During the first hour he was stable; lung fields were clear; he was recorded to have had a strong cry, good color, good muscle tone. He was considered "in fairly good condition" during the first postnatal hours. This is not the picture of a newborn with acute brain damage. Newborn infants with acute brain damage are comatose, limp, for prolonged periods, with ongoing depression of vital function. This newborn was not like that.

The clinical course of this newborn was compromised by the early onset of seizure manifestations during the first day, a complication requiring heavy sedation with phenobarbital, rendering the infant neurologically depressed for days. Clinically, early onset of seizures in the newborn is increasingly recognized to be due to causes other than acute brain damage.

Health problems in the mother, acute and chronic disorders, exercise an adverse effect on the fetus. The common denominator of these adverse processes is hypoxia — the fetus is subjected to varying degrees of oxygen deprivation, which leads to an accruing of subacute cerebral damage in the fetuses that survive to term or near term. Newborn infants, so affected, are born harboring old, subacute cerebral damage.

The infant in this case presented substantial evidence of harboring old, subacute hemorrhagic cerebral damage at birth. Xanthochromic, yellow, spinal fluid was revealed by spinal puncture soon after delivery; yellow discoloration of spinal fluid occurs in the presence of old hemorrhagic subacute cerebral lesions; the red hemoglobin in the blood decomposes, forming a yellow pigment (page 173).

This infant developed the dyskinesia of cerebral palsy. Cerebral palsy is known to be due to deep cerebral damage (basal ganglia) incurred at a time during premature immature fetal life prior to 34 or 35 weeks of gestation. It does not occur related to events of labor and delivery in mature birth (Chapter 3).

Deep damage incurred in the premature brain, causing cerebral palsy, at times extends to the cerebral surface, to the cortex, resulting in cortical manifestations of mental retardation and epilepsy.

Microcephaly was evident in early infancy. With deep brain damage occurring during fetal life, with destruction of periventricular tissue, the brain is decreased in size, fails to grow normally, leading to microcephaly.

A Case of   *A mother with poor reproductive history; vaginal bleeding; maternal anemia. Premature birth; newborn with IUGR, apnea, hyperbilirubinemia. Infant later developed cerebral palsy, seizure disorder, mental retardation, microcephaly.*

A poor reproductive history is a significant factor in a pregnancy, ominous for the well-being of the fetus. This mother did not have a healthy reproductive capability. Prior to the pregnancy in the present case, she had had three abortions; there was one neonatal death. Subsequent to the present case, she had two more premature deliveries, one at 34 weeks' gestation (newborn death) and another birth at 32 weeks of gestation. The literature indicates that with a clinical history of poor reproductive performance of the mother in past pregnancies, as in the present case, there is an increased incidence of cerebral palsy (page 41).

Vaginal bleeding developed at 22 weeks of this pregnancy, requiring hospitalization. Bleeding during pregnancy is mainly due to pathologic processes affecting the placenta, processes that potentially compromise the fetus, causing fetal hypoxia. Parenthetically, in infants surviving, in cases with a history of maternal bleeding during pregnancy, there is a high incidence of cerebral palsy and related cerebral difficulties (page 69).

Anemia developed in the mother subsequent to the vaginal bleeding. Anemia, as in this case, compromises oxygenation of the mother, with a resulting decreased oxygen supply to the placenta and to the fetus.

Premature labor (consistent with the mother's poor reproductive pattern) developed at 33 weeks of gestation, followed by spontaneous vaginal birth.

The newborn infant was in good condition at birth, with an Apgar score of 8 and 8.

IUGR, intrauterine growth retardation, was evident, reflecting the effects of adverse gestational processes. With a birth weight of 1,559 grams (3 1/2 pounds) the infant was below the twentieth percentile for 33 weeks' gestation.

Apnea with bradycardia, an hypoxia-producing postnatal complication common in prematures, developed in recurring episodes on day 2. In the premature infant, apnea (hypoxia) causes deep cerebral damage, damage to periventricular structures, basal ganglia.

Hyperbilirubinemia, an increase in bilirubin in the blood, common in prematures, developed in this case. Hyperbilirubinemia, resulting from excessive breakdown of red cells, causes jaundice, yellow staining of the skin and other bodily tissues.

Anemia developed consequent to the excessive breakdown of red cells. Anemia contributed to postnatal hypoxia in this infant.

Cerebral palsy developed later in infancy, the consequence of hypoxic processes during intrauterine life and postnatally during the period of prematurity.

Cerebral palsy is caused by damage to the basal ganglia, located deep in the brain, incurred in the immature premature brain. The deep damage incurred in the premature brain at times extends to the cerebral surface, to the cortex, resulting in cortical manifestations of mental retardation and epilepsy. Microcephaly developed in this child as a consequence of failure of the (damaged) brain to grow.

A Case of *Maternal diabetes; poor reproductive history; macrosomic newborn. Infant developed cerebral palsy, seizure disorder, and mental retardation.*

This mother had an oncoming diabetic condition during this pregnancy, with metabolic processes that adversely affected the fetus, indicated in the delivery of an oversized (macrosomic) newborn — a pattern characteristic of diabetic gestational conditions. The mother had a family history of diabetes.

She had no outward manifestations of diabetes during this pregnancy; her urinalyses were negative for glucose, the incipient diabetes being clinically occult.

This term newborn infant weighed 9 pounds 1 ounce. The large size of this newborn triggered suspicion of latent diabetes in this mother; an abnormal glucose tolerance test the day of delivery likewise was indicative of latent diabetes.

Macrosomia, an oversized neonate, often is the first sign of latent diabetes in a mother (page 48). This mother manifestly had a smoldering diabetic condition that could not be confirmed during this pregnancy. (However, the mother, 2 years later, was found to have overt, advanced diabetes following a succession of two oversized babies.)

As in this case, in people who become diabetic, the bodily metabolic dysfunctions have origin many years before the diabetes becomes clinical. In mothers, large babies are the hallmark of latent diabetes.

Maternal prediabetes (or diabetes) effects an unfavorable uterine environment, exercises a damaging effect on the fetus, extending over the entire length of the gestational period. In these circumstances there is a high incidence of malformations and stillbirth.

Relevantly, this mother had a poor reproductive history; she had had two previous stillbirths and an infant born with a malformation of the abdominal wall. Spontaneous abortion is common in diabetic conditions.

In mothers with diabetic conditions, the pathologic mechanism causing stillbirths and malformations, the mechanism causing the injurious effects on the fetus, is not known. Often the newborn infant, born alive, oversized, "just doesn't do well."

This was the circumstance in the present case. This sick fetus, enfeebled, compromised, by adversive conditions during fetal life due to maternal problems, did not tolerate the stress of labor and was depressed at birth, with a low Apgar score. After resuscitation care, he improved, with spontaneous respiration and good color. The progress was interrupted by the development of seizures.

The fact that seizures occur soon after birth does not mean that the causal mechanism is related to perinatal processes. With cortical damage incurred due to hypoxia during the premature period of fetal life, with damage originating deep in the cerebrum and extending to the cortical surface, with the fetus surviving to term, the lesions in the cortex become subacute, capable of causing seizure activity soon after birth (page 17).

This infant developed cerebral palsy. Cerebral palsy is due to damage in the basal ganglia, located in the deep portion of the cerebrum (page 178). Damage to the deep structures to the basal ganglia, often occurs during intrauterine life, to the premature immature fetus, due to hypoxia-producing complications during pregnancy. At the time of the hypoxic process in the premature fetus, the cerebral damage may extend from the deep structures through the wall of the cerebrum, damaging the cortex, and later may cause (in addition to cerebral palsy) seizures and mental deficiency, as in the present case.

Clinical studies have shown that in offspring of mothers with diabetic conditions, the incidence of cerebral palsy and epilepsy is three to five times higher than in the general population.

A Case of   *Maternal recurrent viral infections, obesity, toxemia. Neonatal seizures; spinal fluid xanthochromic. Infant later developed cerebral palsy, seizure disorder, mental retardation, microcephaly.*

This mother was sick during pregnancy with viral-type infections, with flu at 8 weeks and sore throat at 24 weeks.

Maternal illness causes fetal deprivation. The damaging effect on the fetus, the common denominator, is hypoxia. With acute febrile illness, the oxygen requirements of the mother are sharply increased, so that oxygenation of the fetus is depressed. Likewise with other maternal illnesses.

Maternal obesity was a factor in this case. This five-foot-tall mother weighed 180 pounds at term. She developed signs of toxemia, with hypertension prior to labor.

Obesity developing during pregnancy is a reflection of disturbed bodily metabolism and predisposes to the development of hypertension and toxemia, as occurred in this case.

Labor developed at term. After prolonged labor, with failure of the fetus to descend, a cesarean section was done.

The infant was depressed at birth but gradually improved. At 4 hours, vital signs were stable, respirations were good, skin was pink; there was a good cry; tone and activity improved. Fontanelles remained flat.

The infant's condition was compromised by the sudden unexpected onset of seizures at 15 hours.

Spinal fluid, examined at 17 hours, was xanthochromic, indicating the presence of old, subacute, hemorrhagic damage in the brain (page 173).

In retrospect, in correlating clinical factors with underlying pathologic processes, the conclusion emerges that this fetus accumulated hypoxic cerebral damage during intrauterine life due to adverse maternal gestational factors, with the newborn infant harboring latent subacute cerebral damage. This was confirmed by the finding of xanthochromic spinal fluid.

The fact that the baby improved after delivery, was active and stable, is evidence that there was no acute cerebral damage. Infants with acute cerebral damage remain limp, comatose, and unstable for prolonged periods. This infant was not like that.

The clinical pattern is consistent with the presence of latent subacute cerebral damage, present at birth, accounting for the early onset of seizures and the development later of cerebral palsy with microcephaly and mental retardation.

A Case of **Twin pregnancy; second twin with long umbilical cord; apparent entanglement of the cord. Infant later developed cerebral palsy, seizure disorder, mental retardation, and microcephaly.**

In the present case, in which male dizygotic twins were delivered at 43 weeks' gestation (delivered by cesarean section because of failure of labor to progress after 11 hours), the first twin at birth was in good condition and no manifest abnormal neurologic disability developed. The second twin was asphyxial at birth, with a low Apgar score; later he developed cerebral palsy and other cerebral disabilities. There was no substantial difference in size; the first weighed 8 pounds 4 ounces, the second, a pound less. There were no signs of twin transfusion syndrome.

The one outstanding difference between the twins was the presence in the second twin of a long cord, of more than 90 centimeters (average cord length is 50 to 60 centimeters).

The umbilical cord in this case was not only long, but it also showed local pathologic changes. The operating room nurse noticed that the cord near the fetus looked "mushy," and the neonatologist noted that the cord at the umbilicus was bruised and hemorrhagic.

A long cord predisposes to entanglements, with the cord becoming wrapped around a limb or the neck (page 80).

It is apparent that the damaged, "mushy," hemorrhagic segment of the umbilical cord was the result of an entanglement present during intrauterine life. Entanglement leads to injury of the cord and cord compression; the resulting interference with cord circulation leads to fetal hypoxia. The entanglement may occur early in fetal life, tightening and loosening, with the effects being intermittent, with the fetus subjected to varying severity of nutritional and oxygen deprivation, accruing acute and subacute hypoxic cerebral damage, with surviving infants, as a consequence, later developing cerebral palsy and other cerebral disabilities.

A Case of   *Maternal recurrent viral infections; excessive weight gain. Neonatal anemia; xanthochromic spinal fluid. Infant developed cerebral palsy and mental retardation.*

The mother was sick during this pregnancy, with at least two episodes of viral-type upper respiratory infection. Viral infection during pregnancy is a hazard both to the mother and to the fetus. With acute illness, with fever, the metabolic oxygen requirements of the mother are sharply increased, leaving the fetus oxygen deprived, hypoxic (page 42).

Excessive weight gain occurred. This mother went from a pregravid weight of 165 pounds to 218 pounds at term, a gain of 53 pounds. Excessive maternal weight gain, of the degree in the present case, is usually of metabolic origin, due to endocrine dysfunctions such as in diabetic conditions.

Labor developed at 41 weeks of gestation. Delivery was vaginal, with low forceps.

The newborn infant had a good Apgar score. She did well initially, was described as having a strong cry; color was pink, she was moving all extremities. Fontanelles were flat. Lung fields were clear. Plainly, this was not the clinical picture of a newborn infant with fresh acute brain damage.

The mother developed signs of postpartum sepsis, with fever, at 3 hours after delivery. Soon after, it was noted that the newborn infant had become less active and was pale; it was thought that the infant had become septic.

It was apparent that the pale infant was anemic. Her hematocrit was 42.3 percent (normal at term, 61 percent). It was evident that the anemia present in this newborn had its origin during fetal life. Prolonged anemia, in the fetus as in the adult human, causes chronic hypoxia. The red cell is the oxygen-carrying vehicle of the blood. The decrease in hematocrit means that this fetus existed with less than the needed oxygen going to the brain.

Postnatally, on the afternoon of the first day, with the decline in the infant's condition, with sepsis suspected, a spinal puncture was done. The spinal fluid was xanthochromic, yellow. The presence of xanthochromic spinal fluid indicated that cerebral hemorrhagic damage was present and that the damage was old, pathologically subacute (page 173).

In summary, the fetus in this case, compromised by adverse hypoxia-producing maternal factors, and by intrauterine anemia, was born enfeebled, with latent subacute hypoxic cerebral damage. That the damage was subacute was confirmed by the finding of xanthochromic spinal fluid. The latent subacute cerebral damage, present at birth, later led to cerebral palsy and mental retardation.

A Case of   **Neonatal spasticity, with contractures. Teenage pregnancy, maternal emotional stress, pelvic inflammatory disease, chlamydia infection. Nuchal cord; neonatal early onset of seizures. Infant developed severe cerebral palsy, mental retardation, and microcephaly.**

The present case is singular in that this newborn infant was hypertonic, spastic, at birth and showed frank contractures of the limbs directly after birth. These disabilities reflect damage to deep cerebral structures, to basal ganglia, incurred in early fetal life due to pathologic hypoxia-producing gestational processes (page 184).

This gestation was complicated by maternal and fetal conditions that compromised the well-being of the fetus, the newborn.

Emotional stress, maternal instability, was manifest in this pregnancy. This was a teenage girl, finding herself pregnant, unmarried. There is substantial evidence, clinical and experimental, that maternal anxiety affects the fetus (page 53).

The prenatal information in this case was sparse. The mother came in for the initial prenatal examination at 13 weeks of pregnancy because she had abdominal pain, due to pelvic inflammatory disease; culture for gonorrhea was positive; culture for chlamydia was also positive. Chlamydia infection during pregnancy is known to be adversive to the fetus.

Nuchal cord was present at delivery, another potentially adversive condition for the fetus. A nuchal cord may be present for months, with origin early in fetal life. The hypoxia-producing effects of a nuchal cord during intrauterine life may be intermittent, occurring early in gestation, with the cord becoming tightened and loosened from time to time. The effects, accordingly, may be sublethal, with hypoxic visceral damage being accrued.

Gestation in this case was 41 weeks. Delivery was spontaneous, vaginal.

The newborn infant was in stable condition soon after delivery, with an Apgar score of 7 at five minutes. At 1 hour, he was pink, active; lungs were clear. At 3 hours, he was bathed. In the following hours, he was active, had a good suck reflex, and was in the room with his mother. This is not the clinical picture of a newborn infant harboring fresh acute cerebral damage. Infants born with acute hypoxic cerebral damage remain limp, not moving, are comatose, with unstable vital function, and they stay that way for prolonged periods. The newborn in this case was not like that after delivery.

The clinical pattern in this case is consistent with the syndromic pattern of latent subacute cerebral damage present at birth, damage incurred a period of time prior to birth, damage related to adversive pathologic processes during gestation.

Seizure activity developed unexpectedly at 22 hours after birth, interrupting the infant's stable condition. With cerebral damage incurred during the premature period, with the damage originating deep in the cerebrum and extending to the cortical surface, with the fetus surviving to term, the lesions in the cortex become subacute, and are capable of causing seizure activity soon after birth.

Deep damage incurred in the premature brain extending to the cerebral surface, to the cortex, results in cortical manifestations of mental retardation and other disabilities, as occurred in the present case.

Cerebral palsy is due to hypoxic damage to the deep cerebral structure, to basal ganglia, incurred at a time when the fetal brain is premature, immature. This deep damage, in most cases, remains latent, not evident at birth. In most cases it takes a period of time, months, until motor disabilities, spasticity, caused by the deep cerebral damage become manifest as cerebral palsy. It is conclusive that in this infant, already spastic at birth, the underlying cerebral damage was incurred months before birth.

A Case of **_Maternal chronic cardiac disease; placental insufficiency; toxemia. Infant developed cerebral palsy, mental retardation, seizure disorder._**

This mother had had acute rheumatic heart disease early in life. Rheumatic fever damages the valves of the heart and the muscle, the myocardium. Scarring of the valves, particularly the mitral valve, causes heart murmur, "leakage" of the valve, chronically compromising the pump function of the heart. Valve replacement in this woman improved her cardiac function. The total effect of the old rheumatic heart disease, of the degree manifested in this woman, is a chronic marginal cardiac performance. This, plus the hypertension that developed, no doubt further compromised the oxygenation machinery of the mother, and oxygenation of the fetus (page 51).

This infant was small and initially was thought to be immature. However, there was substantial evidence that the infant was indeed of at least 37 weeks' gestation, established by the facts that (1) the testes were descended, and (2) the footprint pattern of the newborn infant was consistent with that of a near-mature newborn.

In the male newborn, a most reliable determinant of gestational age is the location of the testes: The testes are formed in the abdomen and gradually descend into the scrotal sac near term. Presence of the testes in the scrotum was evidence of maturity.

The footprint of a fetus becomes increasingly complex as the fetus matures. In the present case, the pattern of the footprint, with creases in the sole extending to the heel, was consistent with a near-mature infant.

Intrauterine growth retardation was evident in this newborn infant. The baby weighed 3 pounds 3 ounces (1,434 grams) at birth, far below the tenth percentile. The average weight at 37 weeks is 2,800 grams (page 94).

Placental insufficiency was evident. The placenta was (1) of abnormal form, bipartite, and (2) small; the placenta, at or near term, averages 450 to 500 grams; the placenta in this case weighed 280 grams.

What is the relationship between the small placenta and the small size of the fetus, the newborn?

The abnormal form of the placenta in this case, with two portions of the placental plate separated by a thin membranous part, may be a formative abnormality. At times, however, the thin part of the placenta is the result of an old infarction; with placental infarction early in gestation, the size, the weight of the placenta, is decreased. An inordinately small placenta, due to infarction or other pathologic process, leads to fetal deprivation of nutrition and oxygenation.

It should be recognized, however, that the placenta is a fetal structure, part of the fetus. During gestation, when there are adversive conditions affecting the gestation (maternal factors, as in this case), both the fetus and the placenta are affected. Adversive processes that lead to retardation of fetal growth at the same time may lead to retardation of placental growth, placental insufficiency (page 76).

Toxemia developed at 34 weeks of pregnancy, and the mother was admitted to the hospital. She complained of headache and dizziness, and she developed hypertension of 150/90, albuminuria 3+, peripheral edema, elevation of hepatic enzymes — characteristic manifestations of toxemia of pregnancy. Toxemia of pregnancy broadly affects the maternal-placental-fetal complex. The visceral changes in this disease compromise maternal kidney, liver, cardiovascular, and other visceral functions, beginning in a prelusive period, at a time before signs and symptoms appear in the mother. The adversive effects on the mother and fetus begin before albuminuria and hypertension appear. Maternal renal, hepatic, and other metabolic disturbances that occur with toxemia affect not only the mother but also the well-being of the fetus. The compromise of the uteroplacental circulation that occurs contributes to the occurrence of intrauterine hypoxia.

Delivery was spontaneous, vaginal, with low forceps. The fetus in this case, chronically compromised by adversive gestational factors, was enfeebled and did not tolerate the stress of labor. The newborn infant was severely depressed. However, he soon improved. At a half hour, he was alert, with good color and good cry. Lungs were clear. This is plainly not the picture of a newborn with a head full of acute cerebral damage. Infants who are born with acute cerebral damage are comatose at birth, and remain comatose, with reduced vital function, for prolonged periods. This was not the pattern in the present case.

The clinical pattern in this case is compatible with latent subacute cerebral damage present at birth, damage accrued during early intrauterine life, damage later manifested as cerebral palsy, mental retardation, and seizure disorder, as occurred in the present case.

A Case of **_Cytomegalic viral disease; nuchal cord. Infant later developed cerebral palsy and other cerebral disabilities._**

The circumstances of this pregnancy were not optimal. The mother was a teenage primipara with no prenatal care during the first 22 weeks of pregnancy. The mother had health problems, with periods of weight loss and with low weight gain, 15 pounds, during the pregnancy.

This was a term gestation; vaginal delivery after prolonged labor.

Nuchal cord was present at delivery, with three loops of cord around the neck.

The newborn infant was depressed at birth but soon improved. At 3 hours the infant was active, with good color; fontanelles were soft. During the first evening the baby was "doing well" and was out to the mother.

This is not the clinical picture of a newborn with acute brain damage. Newborn infants who have acute brain damage show it. They do not soon improve; they stay comatose, depressed, flaccid, with bulging tense fontanelles, with unstable vital signs, for prolonged periods. The infant in the present case was not like that.

The effects of the nuchal cord present at birth are open to question. The postdelivery depression of the infant may have been due to the nuchal cord. If present for a prolonged time during intrauterine life, the nuchal cord may have contributed to the accumulation of fetal hypoxic cerebral damage.

Jaundice, hyperbilirubinemia, was noted soon after birth; bilirubin rose to 17 on day 4. The infant's condition deteriorated, and by day 4 he had become lethargic and floppy. Physical examination revealed hepatosplenomegaly, with the liver enlarged to 7 centimeters below the right costal margin.

Pathologically there are four common causes of hepatosplenomegaly with jaundice in the newborn: (1) congestive heart failure; (2) isoimmune reaction due to Rh incompatibility (erythroblastosis); (3) systemic sepsis associated with acute processes such as pneumonia, urinary tract infection; (4) specific acute neonatal infection, commonly cytomegalovirus disease.

In this case there was no clinical evidence of congestive heart failure or erythroblastosis; there was no septic process diagnosed, such as pneumonia. There _were_ in this case elements consistent with cytomegalovirus disease. Cytomegalic viral infection is characterized by enlargement of the liver and spleen, hyperbilirubinemia, and neurologically by lethargy and weakness (page 118).

The infant improved during the second week and was discharged on day 10.

During the first 3 months developmental delays became evident. Spastic cerebral palsy with athetosis was diagnosed. In early childhood, microcephaly was evident; seizure disorder and mental retardation were present.

In summary, considered retrospectively, this was a sick fetus, compromised by adverse maternal factors, by the presence of a nuchal cord, and by postnatal signs of cytomegalic viral disease. The fact that the newborn infant improved after delivery, was doing well during the first day, is evidence that acute cerebral damage was not present neonatally. The clinical course in the present case is compatible with the presence of latent subacute cerebral damage, present at birth, due to adverse processes during intrauterine life.

A Case of   *Teenage mother with pregnancy low weight gain; maternal anemia. Neonatal depression; early onset seizures; IUGR. Infant developed cerebral palsy, mental retardation, and seizure disorder.*

The mother was 17 years old, a primipara, an unmarried school girl—a clinical pattern conducive to emotional stress. These maternal factors are adversive to the well-being of the fetus. Malnutrition was recorded; the mother was on a one-meal-a-day routine. She lost weight during this pregnancy (page 46). She became anemic.

Duration of gestation was uncertain. Presentation was cephalic; delivery was spontaneous, vaginal.

The newborn infant was depressed, with an Apgar score of 2 and 5. The infant responded to resuscitation; he was intubated, bagged, and an umbilical catheter was placed.

Weight at birth was 3,100 grams (6 pounds 14 ounces).

Postmaturity was evident on physical examination; the skin was dry and peeling. Skin was wrinkled; there was little subcutaneous adipose tissue.

The birth weight of 3,100 grams is marginal for a postmature newborn, and taken together with the postmature physical features of the infant, this reflects a measure of intrauterine deprivation, IUGR.

Seizure activity with episodes of apnea began at 3 hours of life. Seizures were controlled with medication. The infant gradually improved and was discharged at 3 weeks.

The infant failed to thrive. At 3 months, spastic cerebral palsy was diagnosed. Seizure disorder continued. Mental retardation was evident in infancy; at age 5 years the child was functioning at a 2-year-old's developmental level.

In summary, adversive maternal gestational physical and emotional factors in this case — a teenage, malnourished, anemic mother — impacted on the fetus, resulting in a feeble depressed newborn.

During pregnancy, health problems in the mother, acute and chronic physical and emotional factors, exercise an adversive effect on the fetus. The common denominator of these adversive processes is hypoxia — the fetus is subjected to varying degrees of oxygen deprivation, which leads to an accruing of subacute cerebral damage in fetuses who survive to term or near term. Thus, infants so affected are born harboring old, subacute cerebral damage. The presence of subacute cerebral damage may remain latent in early infancy, ultimately becoming manifest as cerebral palsy and other cerebral disabilities.

The development of cerebral palsy, as in this case, reflects hypoxic cerebral damage incurred during early fetal life, affecting deep structures of the cerebrum. Extension of the deep cerebral damage outward to the cortex results in cortical disabilities of mental retardation and seizure disorder, as occurred in this infant.

A Case of   *Maternal latent diabetes, obesity, viral infection. Macrosomic newborn; neonatal depression; apnea; xanthochromic spinal fluid. Infant developed cerebral palsy, seizure disorder, and mental retardation.*

Maternal health problems were evident in this case, problems adversive to fetal well-being. This mother had an ongoing metabolic disorder, with obesity and excessive pregnancy weight gain. The newborn was macrosomic, excessively large—characteristic of offspring of mothers with diabetic conditions. In addition to macrosomia, the factors of maternal obesity and excessive pregnancy weight gain indicated prediabetes. The underlying diabetic metabolic disorder was confirmed 3 years later in a second pregnancy, when the mother spilled sugar in the urine and had a positive glucose tolerance test, manifestations of overt diabetes. This second baby also was macrosomic (page 48).

Regarding the mother's obesity, this mother was morbidly obese, with weight up to 279 pounds. Marked obesity is a hazard to the pregnant mother and her fetus. Morbid obesity is reflective of a disturbed metabolism. Obesity predisposes to diabetes; this proved to be the case with this mother, with the development of frank diabetes in her second pregnancy.

The mother had excessive weight gain during this pregnancy. Her weight increased from 236 pounds, prepregnancy, to 279 pounds at delivery, a gain of 43 pounds, about 15 pounds above optimal pregnancy weight gain.

In people who become diabetic, as in this mother, the bodily dysfunctions have origin many years before the diabetes becomes overt. Maternal prediabetes (or diabetes) effects an unfavorable uterine environment and exercises a damaging effect on the fetus, extending over the entire length of the gestational period (page 49).

A viral-type upper respiratory infection with cough and sore throat occurred at 16 weeks of this pregnancy. Viral infection during pregnancy is a hazard both to the mother and to the fetus. Pregnant women clinically have increased susceptibility to viral infections, to influenza, upper respiratory infections, viral sore throat. With acute illness, with fever, the metabolic oxygen requirements of the mother are sharply increased, leaving the fetus oxygen-deprived, hypoxic. In my own pathology experience, in cases of maternal flu with miscarriage, autopsy examination has revealed hypoxic cerebral damage in the aborted fetuses.

This pregnancy was thought to be at term or slightly post-term, at 43 weeks by dates. Labor was desultory, and because of failure to progress after 10 hours of labor, a cesarean section was done.

The infant was severely depressed at birth; she failed to respond to treatment. Neurologically it was apparent that intracerebral damage was present.

Xanthochromic spinal fluid was revealed by spinal tap at 2 hours after delivery. The finding of xanthochromic (*xantho-,* yellow; *-chromia,* color) spinal fluid in this case is of major importance in defining the time of incurrence of the cerebral damage. Xanthochromia, yellow coloration of the spinal fluid, is due to the presence of *old* hemorrhagic damage in the brain (page 173).

With hemorrhage in the brain, with blood escaping into the ventricles, into the spinal fluid, red cells become lysed, broken down; the hemoglobin from the red cells first gives the spinal fluid a pink color. The hemoglobin gradually degenerates to a yellow pigment and gives the spinal fluid a yellow color — xanthochromia. This change in color takes many days, and continues to be present for weeks and months, when there is an old hemorrhagic lesion in the brain. The finding of xanthochromic spinal fluid indicates the presence of subacute damage, an old hemorrhagic lesion, in the brain.

Ultrasound studies on day 3 confirmed the presence of intracerebral damage and revealed evidence of deep cerebral hemorrhage.

Anemia of a severe degree was evident in the newborn, confirmed in hematology tests done after delivery. The hemoglobin level was 12.2 grams (normal is 19 grams). The hematocrit was 37.1 percent (normal, 61 percent). The infant was transfused soon after birth (page 95).

The anemia in this newborn infant had its origin during fetal life. The presence of fetal-neonatal anemia is one of the main elements in defining the causal mechanism of the brain damage in this case. Anemia, in the fetus as in the adult human, causes chronic hypoxia. Intrauterine hypoxia leads to hypoxic visceral damage in the fetus. The brain is the most sensitive target tissue in the body; with chronic intrauterine hypoxia, the fetus accrues acute and subacute cerebral damage.

The cause of the fetal-neonatal anemia is open to question. Most likely this was a case of fetal-maternal transfusion syndrome (page 97).

Macrosomia, LGA, large-for-gestational-age, was diagnosed, with the newborn infant weighing 8 pounds 8 3/4 ounces (3,800 grams). The macrosomia of this newborn is attributable to the mother's disordered metabolism, to latent prediabetes.

Macrosomic infants are feeble, do not do well. Big does not mean strong, robust. Some are stillborn or die soon after birth. The pathologic mechanism causing the injurious effects in the fetus is not known. In surviving infants there is a high incidence of epilepsy and cerebral palsy.

In summary, cerebral damage was accumulated during intrauterine life, due to adverse effects of maternal prediabetes and other maternal factors and complicated by fetal-neonatal anemia. The cerebral damage, subacute at birth, later resulted in cerebral palsy and other cerebral disabilities.

A Case of   *Maternal illness, with anemia, chronic hypotension, viral infection, emotional stress. Neonatal depression, anemia. Infant developed cerebral palsy and mental retardation.*

The prenatal record of this mother indicated that this was less than a robust pregnancy. The mother was sick during this pregnancy; she was treated for emotional distress; she was hypotensive, had a febrile flu episode, and became anemic.

With gestational problems present during fetal life, the common denominator of these adverse processes is *hypoxia* — the fetus is subjected to varying degrees of oxygen deprivation which leads to an accruing of subacute cerebral damage in the fetuses that survive to term.

Emotional stress was a prominent factor during this pregnancy. The mother complained of various gastrointestinal symptoms, diagnosed as irritable bowel syndrome, thought to be due to stress. She stated she "fights with her husband all the time" because she did not feel well. She was treated with antidepressant medication. There is increasing evidence clinically and experimentally that maternal emotional stress, in the same way as physical illness, has adverse effects on the fetus (page 53).

Hypotension was present in the mother during this pregnancy, with blood pressure levels ranging 20 to 50 millimeters below average. With regard to the effect of hypotension on the uterus during pregnancy, just as there was inadequate blood going to the brain, there would correspondingly be inadequate arterial perfusion to the uterus, to the placenta. This hypotensive lack of perfusion is increased when the mother is lying down, during the hours of sleep; the condition is well known obstetrically. Hypotension clinically is associated with symptoms of fatigue, fainting. Hypotension may apparently be tolerated during pregnancy; however, combined with periods of stress, infection, and other complications of pregnancy, hypotension becomes a hazard to both mother and fetus.

A viral-type upper respiratory infection affected the mother over a protracted period during the first trimester. She had fever, and she reported she had been "very tired" and had lost weight. With viral infection, with fever, the mother's metabolism is elevated, the oxygen requirements of the mother are sharply increased, so that oxygenation of the fetus is depressed. Viral infection during pregnancy is a hazard both to the mother and to the fetus.

Anemia developed in this mother following her illness. Anemia involves a decrease in the hemoglobin in the blood. Hemoglobin is the oxygen-carrying vehicle in the blood. Anemia compromises oxygenation of the mother, with resulting decreased oxygen supply to the placenta and to the fetus.

Fetal movements were decreased during the last 2 weeks, according to the mother. Decreased fetal activity reflects fetal compromise, fetal enfeeblement, the result of adverse gestational processes impacting on the fetus.

Labor ensued at 41 weeks of gestation. This was a breech delivery; entrapment of the aftercoming head developed, with some delay in delivering the head.

The newborn, although severely depressed at birth, responded to resuscitation and soon improved. During the first afternoon lungs were clear. Muscle tone improved. Pupils reacted to light. Fontanelles were soft and flat. Blood pressure and pulse were stable.

Anemia was evident at birth; the newborn infant was pale. Anemia was confirmed in the newborn hematology reports, with the hemoglobin level at 14 grams (normal, 19 grams) and the hematocrit level at 44.3 percent (normal, 61 percent).

Chronic anemia, in the fetus as in the adult human, causes chronic hypoxia. The decrease in hematocrit means this fetus existed with less than the average amount of oxygen supply, chronic fetal hypoxia. Intrauterine hypoxia leads to fetal hypoxic visceral damage; with intrauterine hypoxia, the fetus accrues subacute cerebral damage.

The infant was transfused and improved.

Regarding the cause of the anemia, it was thought that, with other causes excluded clinically, this was an example of the fetal-maternal transfusion syndrome (page 97).

Seizure activity developed soon after birth.

The question arises as to whether such seizure activity reflected the presence of acute cerebral damage, or whether the seizure activity was due to cerebral damage incurred before birth, due to hypoxic cerebral damage during fetal life prior to term.

With cerebral damage incurred during the early premature period, with the damage originating deep in the cerebrum and extending to the cortical surface, with the fetus surviving to term, the lesions in the cortex become subacute and are capable of causing seizure activity soon after birth (Chapter 5).

Regarding the origin of the cerebral damage in this case, it is apparent that the damage was due to adversive intrauterine factors ongoing during the gestation, related to the mother's clinical problems — that the newborn infant had latent subacute cerebral damage present at birth, damage that later was manifested as cerebral palsy and mental retardation (Chapter 3).

A Case of **_Maternal prediabetes. Newborn infant with cardiac hypertrophy; neonatal death._**

This case demonstrates a rare but specific fetal cardiac abnormality, cardiac hypertrophy, linked to a maternal diabetic condition.

The mother presented cardinal signs of latent prediabetes: a family history of diabetes, obesity, elevated blood sugar, and macrosomic babies.

In mothers who become diabetic, the bodily dysfunctions originate many years before the diabetes. Maternal prediabetes (or diabetes) effects an unfavorable uterine environment, exercises a damaging effect on the fetus, extending over the entire length of the gestational period. In these circumstances there is a high incidence of malformations and stillbirths. In mothers with a diabetic process, the pathologic mechanism causing injurious effects on the fetus is not known.

Obesity is a common factor associated with maternal diabetic conditions. This mother was morbidly obese; with a height of 5 feet 1 inch, she went from a pregravid weight of 185 pounds to 215 pounds at delivery.

Obesity is a hazard to the pregnant mother and her fetus. Morbid obesity is reflective of a disturbed metabolism. Metabolic disorders in the mother exercise an adverse effect in the fetus. Obesity predisposes to diabetes, which may be unveiled during pregnancy, as occurred in this case.

Macrosomic babies, weighing near 9 pounds, had previously been born to this mother in two previous pregnancies. The infant in the present case weighed 9 pounds 14 1/2 ounces (4,300 grams), obviously macrosomic. Macrosomia in offspring is commonly the first sign of latent prediabetes in the mother (page 48).

The present case was a term birth: cephalic presentation and vaginal delivery.

The newborn infant, although macrosomic, was in fair condition, with an Apgar score of 5 and 7. At 20 minutes he was alert and active. However, gradual physical deterioration occurred, with increasing cardiac manifestations, with bradycardia, and with inexorable cardiac failure. Death occurred on day 14.

Autopsy revealed findings of congestive heart failure with hydrothorax and visceral congestion.

Cardiac hypertrophy, a heart malformation, was the most important finding at autopsy. This malformation of the heart is a well-recognized clinical and pathologic entity. This cardiac abnormality is commonly linked to the presence of a diabetic condition in the mother.

The heart was large, weighing 42 grams; the average weight of the heart in an infant of 4,300 grams (as in this case) is 28 grams; this heart was 50 percent heavier than normal. The ventricle walls were 5 to 10 millimeters in thickness, two to three times the usual thickness.

In such cases, although the heart muscle is overgrown, paradoxically the muscle performs inefficiently, and this leads to cardiac failure.

In adults there is a form of cardiac abnormality like that in the present case, termed "idiopathic hypertrophic myocardiopathy." In some of these cases, death occurs unexpectedly, suddenly; in others, the terminal period may be prolonged, with congestive heart failure developing toward the end.

A Case of **Microcephaly in a newborn; IUGR; xanthochromic spinal fluid. Infant developed cerebral palsy, mental retardation, and seizure disorder.**

Of primary interest in this case was the fact that this infant was microcephalic at birth. The baby's small head was noted at delivery by the obstetrician. The circumference of the head was 31.75 centimeters, between the fifth and tenth percentiles for a term newborn.

Microcephaly present at birth is substantial evidence that the process of brain damage began long before birth: With brain damage occurring at an early time in fetal life, the brain fails to grow in size, encephaloclastic microcephaly (page 31). The head growth in turn is retarded because the damaged fetal brain remains small. Microcephaly continued to be present in infancy, the head size at 2 years, at 38.9 centimetrers, remaining below the fifth percentile.

This baby, born at term, weighing 2,270 grams (5 pounds 7 ounces), was small for gestational age (IUGR), below the tenth percentile for weight. IUGR reflects intrauterine malnutrition and hypoxia, the result of adversive gestational processes. In the present case, the cause of the intrauterine deprivation was not clear. There was a paucity of prenatal information. It was evident, however, that this had not been a robust pregnancy, with the mother becoming anemic and failing to gain weight appropriately in the third trimester.

Labor occurred at 39 weeks of the pregnancy. Fetal distress was evident clinically. Cesarean section was done.

The newborn infant was depressed at birth and remained with little improvement in the early postnatal hours.

CT scans done early on day 1 revealed evidence of periventricular infarctional damage.

Spinal fluid examination on day 1 revealed xanthochromic spinal fluid, indicating that the deep periventricular cerebral damage was old, subacute pathologically, not recent, damage incurred during early intrauterine life (page 173).

Early postnatal onset of seizures occurred. There is increasing clinical and pathologic evidence that early seizure onset is due to brain damage incurred a long time prior to labor (page 208).

This infant later developed the dyskinesias of cerebral palsy. Cerebral palsy is known to be due to deep (basal ganglia) cerebral damage incurred at a time during premature, immature, fetal life. At times the deep cerebral damage extends outward to the cerebral cortex, resulting in mental retardation and seizure disorder, as occurred in this case.

A Case of   *Twin transfusion syndrome with death of one twin. The surviving twin developed cerebral palsy, mental retardation, seizure disorder, and microcephaly.*

This case is concerned with the second of twins born at 36 to 37 weeks' gestation. The first twin was stillborn. The surviving child developed spastic athetoid cerebral palsy, mental retardation, and epilepsy.

Cases of twin gestation with one infant stillborn and one surviving, in most instances, have to do with the fetus-to-fetus placental transfusion syndrome (page 97).

In the fetus-to-fetus transfusion syndrome, one fetus is the donor, the other, the recipient.

The donor tends to be smaller; blood loss to the other fetus may cause fetal anemia in the donor; if the process is long, protracted, the donor tends to compensate for the loss of blood. In the present case the surviving small fetus (5 pounds 8 ounces) was the donor fetus.

The other fetus, stillborn, was the recipient. The hazard to this fetus is the danger that the abnormal inflow of blood coming from the donor may overload the circulatory system of the recipient fetus and cause congestive heart failure, so that this newborn is bloated, plethoric. The stillborn infant in the present case, the larger one (6 pounds 11 ounces), at autopsy showed this — the presence of excessive fluid in the body cavities (ascites and hydrothorax) and visceral congestion, findings characteristic of congestive heart failure.

Paradoxically, the death of the larger fetus ended the process of fetal transfusion, ended the drain of blood from the smaller fetus — and saved its life. In this sequence, the fetal life of the surviving infant was divided into three periods: the first part, with normal development; the middle part, during which the placental transfusion syndrome was ongoing, in which the fetus was compromised, hypoxic; and the last period — after the death of the other twin and the cessation of the transfusion process — more or less a time of recovery for the smaller fetus.

The second twin was delivered by cesarean section, made necessary by the fact that the fetus presented as a footling breech, a condition likely to lead to more serious complications.

The surviving smaller fetus, debilitated by the placental transfusion process, rendered anemic, hypoxic, was subjected to cerebral hypoxic damage during intrauterine life. In such circumstances, if the fetus survives, the cerebral lesions, at first acute, later become subacute, undergoing "healing" with scarring. The presence of such latent subacute lesions, not manifest at birth, accounts for many cases of cerebral palsy that develop in cases of term or of near-term delivery.

The compromised fetus, newborn, in this case was depressed at birth. However, as is characteristic in such circumstances, in such infants, debilitated and harboring subacute brain damage — they respond well to postdelivery care and, as in the present case, are active, alert, breast-feeding during the first days after delivery.

If this infant had incurred fresh, acute brain damage in the prenatal period and during labor, she would not have responded and been active, alert, nursing on the first day.

Microcephaly was present at birth (head circumference was 30.25 centimeters. at birth; this is in the tenth percentile). This is substantial evidence that the process of brain damage began long before birth; with brain damage occurring at an early time in fetal life, the brain fails to grow. The head growth is retarded because the brain, damaged, remains small.

The occurrence of cerebral palsy in this case is firm evidence that the cerebral damage had its origin a long time before delivery. Cerebral palsy is a time marker with regard to the time of incurrence of the brain damage. Cerebral palsy is due to deep cerebral (basal ganglia) damage incurred consistently in the fetus (or newborn) prior to 35 weeks of gestation. Deep cerebral damage does not occur in the mature or near-mature fetus. Deep cerebral damage incurred in the premature period may extend globally, diffusely, through the cerebral hemisphere to the surface, to the cortex, causing mental retardation and epilepsy.

A Case of **Hyperemesis gravidarum; maternal excessive pregnancy weight gain; anemia; prediabetes. Newborn macrosomia; anemia. Infant developed cerebral palsy and mental retardation.**

Although the record stated that this was an "uncomplicated" gestation, the fact is, this mother was sick in this pregnancy with unremitting vomiting (hyperemesis gravidarum). There was evidence of a latent diabetic condition. The mother gained excessive weight. The mother was anemic. All these health problems are known to be hostile to the well-being of the fetus.

Persistent vomiting (hyperemesis gravidarum) occurred in this pregnancy (page 45). The mother reported that she had nausea and vomiting all through this pregnancy, vomiting "three, four times a day." Vomiting leads to dehydration, electrolyte imbalance, and acid-base disturbances. Persistent vomiting is an exhausting, stressful pregnancy complication. This, like any kind of maternal stress during pregnancy, physical or emotional, directly affects the maternal-fetal complex, compromising the fetus. Women who are affected by persistent vomiting during pregnancy commonly have well-defined psychopathology of emotion.

Anemia became apparent in the mother. Hematology studies indicated that the mother had hypochromic anemia, with a hematocrit of 31 percent (normal, 42 percent). Although the red cells were only mildly reduced in number, the individual red cells lacked hemoglobin (hypochromia). It was evident that the anemia in this mother was a chronic condition; hematology studies indicated qualitative findings of microcytosis (red cells smaller than normal), poikilocytosis (cells of varied size and shape), and hypochromia; these are red-cell alterations that do not develop acutely, but take a long time to develop.

Excessive pregnancy weight gain occurred in this mother, paradoxically, despite the vomiting. She gained 61 pounds. (The average optimal weight gain during pregnancy is 20 to 25 pounds.) Pregnancy obesity is a hazard to both mother and fetus; it is reflective of a disturbed metabolism and predisposes to diabetes.

Latent diabetes was suspected in this case. The mother was found to have glycosuria at least four times during the prenatal period. This, together with the factor of excessive weight gain and the fact that she ultimately gave birth to a macrosomic baby, all pointed to prediabetes. There is a tendency to arbitrarily minimize the significance of this diabetic condition during pregnancy. The fact is, however, that in women with pregnancy diabetic signs, over 50 percent develop overt diabetes later in life.

In people who develop diabetes, the bodily metabolic dysfunctions have origin many years before the diabetes becomes clinically overt. The pathologic bodily processes of maternal diabetic conditions create an unfavorable intrauterine environment, exercising damaging effects on the fetus, extending over the length of the gestation, from embryonic life to term.

Labor onset occurred at 38 weeks of gestation. Presentation was cephalic. Delivery was vaginal.

Newborn depression of moderate degree was evident, with an Apgar score of 6 and 5. The enfeebled newborn improved slowly.

Macrosomia was apparent in the baby at birth. This infant was large, heavy and long. The baby weighed 3,770 grams (8 pounds 5 ounces), over the ninetieth percentile by weight for an infant of 38 weeks' gestation

The macrosomia of this baby is related to the mother's disordered metabolism, her pregnancy excessive weight gain. The latter, together with the macrosomic offspring, are indicative, characteristic, of the disordered metabolism of latent prediabetes.

Macrosomic babies, as in this case, are feeble, do not do well. Big does not mean strong, robust. Some are stillborn or die soon after birth. Macrosomic babies who survive have an increased incidence of cerebral palsy.

This newborn infant was anemic at birth. The anemia was evident clinically, outwardly, with the newborn infant described as "pale pink." This clinical observation of anemia was confirmed in the laboratory hematology tests: red cell count was 4.06 million (normal, 5.14 million); hemoglobin was 14.0 grams (normal, 19 grams); hematocrit was 42.5 percent (normal, 61 percent). The hematocrit measures the bulk quantity of red cells in the blood.

Regarding the cause of the fetal-neonatal anemia, it is likely that this case was an example of fetal-maternal transfusion. The transfer of blood from fetal to maternal circulation occurs regularly, to some degree, in all gestations. The degree, the amount of transfusion, varies but is severe in some instances (page 97).

Anemia, in the fetus as in the adult human, causes chronic hypoxia. The red cell is the oxygen-carrying vehicle of the blood. The decrease in hematocrit means that this fetus existed with less than the needed oxygen going to the brain. Intrauterine hypoxia leads to fetal hypoxic visceral damage. The brain is the most sensitive target tissue in the body; with chronic intrauterine hypoxia, the fetus accrues subacute and acute cerebral damage. The initial examination of the newborn in this case revealed a neurologically responsive infant with Moro, suck, and grasp reflexes present. This is not the clinical picture of a newborn infant harboring acute diffuse cerebral damage. Infants with acute brain damage remain comatose, unresponsive, and limp for long periods. This newborn was not like that.

This infant developed cerebral palsy, a defect in motor function caused by damage to the basal ganglia, located deep in the brain. This deep damage occurs consistently, specifically, only in the immature premature brain, during early fetal life. The cerebral damage is commonly due to hypoxia-producing maternal and fetal pathologic processes during gestation. The cerebral damage, at first acute, gradually becomes old, subacute. If the fetus survives to term, the infant is born with old, latent, subacute brain damage.

Deep damage incurred in the premature brain (causing cerebral palsy) at times extends to the cerebral surface, to the cortex, resulting in cortical manifestations of mental retardation and seizure disorder.

Clinically and pathologically, this is the pattern that evolved in the present case.

A Case of   *Maternal psychiatric stress, viral infection, anemia, hypotension, excessive weight gain. Neonatal depression, neonatal seizures. Infant later developed cerebral palsy and mental retardation.*

The mother had emotional stress and physical health problems during this pregnancy that created an adverse environment for the fetus.

Psychiatric stress was ongoing during this pregnancy for this unmarried college student.

There is increasing evidence clinically and experimentally that maternal emotional stress, in the same way as physical illness, has adverse effects on the fetus (page 53).

Hypotension, low blood pressure, was recorded for this mother through the prenatal period. This mother had diastolic blood pressure ranging around 40 to 60 (normal is 80). Systolic pressure ranged around 90 (normal is 120). Translating this to the effect on the uterus, just as there was inadequate blood going to the brain, there would correspondingly be inadequate arterial perfusion to the uterus, to the placenta — fetal hypoxia. The hypotensive lack of perfusion is increased in the mother during the hours of sleep; the condition is well known obstetrically. Hypotension clinically is associated with symptoms of fatigue, fainting. Hypotension may apparently be tolerated during pregnancy; however, combined with periods of stress, infection, and other complications of pregnancy, hypotension becomes a hazard to both mother and fetus (page 53).

Excessive weight gain occurred during periods of this pregnancy despite, or because of, the mother's emotional problems. In the last trimester, in a period of 11 1/2 weeks, this mother gained 22 pounds, an average of almost 2 pounds per week. The appropriate weight gain during the last trimester is about 3/4 pound per week.

Excessive maternal weight gain, of the degree in the present case, at times is of metabolic origin, due to endocrine dysfunctions. Pregnancy obesity exercises an adverse effect on the fetus (page 47).

A viral infection occurred during midpregnancy; this mother indicated she was "tired a lot" and subsequently came down with a cold, the flu, that lasted for weeks. Pregnant women clinically have increased susceptibility to viral infections, to influenza, upper respiratory infections, viral sore throat. With acute illness, with fever, the metabolic oxygen requirements of the mother are sharply increased, leaving the fetus oxygen deprived, hypoxic. In cases of maternal flu with miscarriage, autopsy studies have revealed hypoxic cerebral damage in the aborted fetus.

Anemia developed during the period of the mother's viral infection. Anemia, as in this case, compromises oxygenation of the mother, with resulting decreased oxygen supply to the placenta and to the fetus. Such oxygen deprivation may lead to intrauterine fetal death or may be sublethal and cause fetal deprivation with lasting cerebral damage.

Labor occurred at term. Presentation was cephalic. Delivery was spontaneous, vaginal.

Depression of this infant at delivery was of severe degree. The newborn infant was limp, with an Apgar score of 2 and 2. She soon improved, breathing spontaneously. At 25 minutes, eyes were open, color was pink, muscle tone had improved. Fontanelles were soft, indicating there was no cerebral edema. During the first afternoon she took an oral feeding of glucose. Later, the first evening, she was bathed and transferred to the regular nursery.

This is not the clinical picture of a newborn infant harboring fresh acute cerebral damage incurred intranatally, as thought initially. Infants born with acute hypoxic cerebral damage remain limp, not moving, are comatose, with unstable vital function, and stay that way for prolonged periods. The newborn in this case was not like that after delivery.

The clinical pattern in this case is consistent with the syndromic pattern of latent subacute cerebral damage present at birth, damage incurred a period of time prior to birth, damage related to adversive pathologic processes during gestation.

This newborn infant's improvement was interrupted by the early onset of seizure activity a short time after birth. The seizure activity is attributable to brain damage incurred in the fetal brain antenatally, weeks or months before birth. In the premature immature fetus, brain damage beginning deep in the cerebrum (causing cerebral palsy) may extend to the cortex, causing seizure disorder and mental retardation, as in the present case.

With cerebral damage incurred during the early premature period, with the damage originating deep in the cerebrum and extending to the cortical surface, with the fetus surviving to term, the lesions in the cortex become subacute, and are capable of causing seizure activity soon after birth.

In summary, it was evident that the initial postdelivery depression of the infant, and the early onset of seizure activity, and the later development of cerebral palsy and mental retardation are attributable to cerebral subacute hypoxic damage accrued during early fetal life, damage due to hypoxia-producing gestational processes.

A Case of   *Maternal obesity, vaginal bleeding, viral infection;*
               nuchal cord. Newborn with polycythemia. Infant
               developed cerebral palsy and mental retardation.

Obesity is a hazard to the pregnant mother and her fetus. The mother in the present case was morbidly obese, 298 pounds at delivery. Morbid obesity (over 280 pounds) is reflective of a disturbed metabolism. In the present case, the mother's weight was unstable, with rapid gains and losses (page 47).

Vaginal bleeding occurred during the fifth month of pregnancy. Bleeding during pregnancy is mainly due to pathologic processes affecting the placenta; the most common cause is premature detachment of the placenta. The amount of vaginal bleeding is not necessarily proportional to the degree of placental disease or to the severity of fetal damage. There is a known high incidence of stillbirth associated with maternal bleeding, with the fetus at autopsy showing hypoxic cerebral damage.

Parenthetically, in infants surviving — in cases with history of maternal bleeding during pregnancy — there is a high incidence of cerebral palsy and related cerebral disabilities.

A viral-type upper respiratory infection occurred at 35 weeks of the gestation. The mother had a fever of 102 degrees. With acute febrile illness, the oxygen requirements of the mother are sharply increased, so that oxygenation of the fetus is depressed; likewise with other maternal febrile illnesses.

Labor occurred at term. Presentation was vertex; delivery was vaginal, augmented with Pitocin.

A nuchal cord wrapped two times tight around the neck, was present at delivery. Whether or not this caused intranatal hypoxia was open to question; an hypoxia-producing effect during fetal life could not be ruled out (page 83).

The infant was in good condition at birth, with an Apgar score of 7 and 10. However, the neurologic condition of the infant began to deteriorate during the first day, with increasing lethargy. Periods of cyanosis appeared, requiring oxygen ventilation.

Polycythemia was evident, based on hematologic studies on day 1 (page 104). Polycythemia is the condition in which the red cells in the blood are present in excessive concentration; with this red cell increase, there is elevation of the hemoglobin and hematocrit levels in the blood.

The newborn infant in this case had a red cell count (RBC) of 6 million (average at term is 5.2 million); the hemoglobin was 22.6 grams (average at term is 19.0 grams); the hematocrit was 65.7 percent (average at term is 61 percent).

In the type of polycythemia in the present case, excessive red cell formation is triggered by the presence of intrauterine hypoxia. During gestation, if the fetus is subjected to ongoing hypoxia, due to adversive hypoxia-producing maternal factors, a degree of polycythemia may result. The red cells carry oxygen to the fetus; the increase in red cells in polycythemia is an effort to increase oxygenation to the fetus. With polycythemia, the increased concentration of red cells in the blood causes increased blood viscosity. The sludging, thickening, of the blood in small blood vessels compromises visceral function, especially the nervous system. Pulmonary compromise leads to cyanosis and dyspnea.

Polycythemia does not come on suddenly. Plainly, the presence of polycythemia in this infant at birth indicated that polycythemia was present during intrauterine life and that the fetus was subjected to ongoing chronic hypoxia in the weeks, months, prior to birth.

Postnatally, the infant soon improved despite the adversive gestational factors. On day 3 the infant was stable, breast-feeding, and on day 5 he was discharged.

During early infancy, motor defects of hypotonic cerebral palsy and severe mental retardation were evident.

The development of these cerebral disabilities is attributable to hypoxic cerebral damage incurred during fetal life, due to adversive maternal pregnancy factors, to the presence of a nuchal cord, and to the polycythemic condition.

A Case of   *Maternal hypertension, toxemia; nuchal cord. Infant developed cerebral palsy, mental retardation, and epilepsy.*

This was a complicated pregnancy. The mother, early on cautioned about inappropriate weight gain, went on to develop hypertension of early toxemia.

Additionally, the gestation was complicated by the presence of a nuchal cord.

Regarding the mother's hypertension and toxemia, her blood pressure in the first trimester was 120/72. She gained weight inappropriately, putting on some 40 pounds by 36 weeks of pregnancy, and coincidentally had a gradual rise in blood pressure. She developed albuminuria and peripheral edema, with blood pressure rising to 150/100. With these signs of toxemia, she was hospitalized (page 51). That the hypertension in this mother was a substantial complication is evidenced by the fact that her blood pressure remained elevated during the postpartum period, ranging up to 102 diastolic on the sixth day after delivery.

The mother was admitted at term in active labor. Presentation was vertex. Delivery was vaginal, after prolonged labor, with Pitocin augmentation.

The fetus, the newborn, showed the effects of the chronic adverse gestational processes. The enfeebled fetus was unable to tolerate the stress of labor; the newborn infant was depressed at birth. However, soon after delivery, the infant began to improve. During the first day lung fields were clear; pulse, blood pressure, and respiration were soon stable. Tone improved. Reflexes improved. The newborn infant was crying, sucking on a pacifier, and was visited and held by the mother early on the first day.

Clinically and pathologically, this is not the picture of a newborn with acute cerebral damage. Infants with acute fresh cerebral damage at birth *show it;* these infants remain comatose, limp, unstable, on ventilator care, for hours and days after birth. The infant in this case was not like that.

The early course of this newborn was compromised by the early onset of seizure activity. It is increasingly realized clinically that early onset of seizures in the newborn is not due to acute brain damage, that such seizures are attributable to antecedent early fetal cerebral damage.

With gestational problems present during fetal life — with maternal illness, with nuchal cord present — the common denominator of these adverse processes is *hypoxia.* Fetuses are subjected to varying degrees of oxygen deprivation leading to an accruing of subacute cerebral damage in the fetuses that survive to term. Newborn infants so affected, underweight, enfeebled, are born harboring old, subacute cerebral damage. The subacute damage present at birth, latent, silent, later becomes manifest as cerebral palsy and other cerebral disabilities (Chapter 3).

A Case of   *Maternal chronic respiratory disorder, acute viral infection, excessive pregnancy weight gain. IUGR; infant developed cerebral palsy and mental retardation.*

This mother had a long history of chronic pulmonary allergy disease of the nature of asthma. During this pregnancy she received ongoing treatment for this respiratory disorder. The illness was punctuated by episodes of viral-type upper respiratory infection, "colds."

Pulmonary disorders cause respiratory insufficiency, hypoxia, especially when complicated by acute respiratory infection. During pregnancy, body metabolism, the oxygen requirements of the body, is increased up to 25 percent. Further, with acute viral illness, with fever, the metabolic oxygen requirements of the mother are sharply increased, leaving the fetus oxygen deprived, hypoxic.

Excessive maternal weight gain occurred during this pregnancy. During the last 22 weeks the mother gained an average of 1 1/2 pounds per week (optimal weight gain, 3/4 pound per week).

Excessive maternal weight gain, of the degree in the present case, is usually of metabolic origin, due to endocrine dysfunctions; metabolic disorders such as diabetes exercise an adversive effect on the fetus. It is relevant to note that this mother in her subsequent pregnancy 5 years later, developed gestational diabetes.

Birth occurred at term.

Dysmaturity, intrauterine growth retardation (IUGR), was evident at birth, indicating fetal nutritional deprivation. The baby was long and thin. Weight was 2,725 grams (6 pounds), in the fifteenth percentile for term. The Ponderal index, the weight-length ratio, a measure of fetal nutrition, was 2.5, in the tenth percentile (page 94).

Depression of severe degree was present in this infant at delivery. Although cyanotic and limp, she quickly improved, and was active and crying at 5 minutes, with an Apgar of 9. The initial depression of this newborn is attributable to intrauterine deprivation, enfeeblement. This was a chronically weakened fetus, newborn. At 1 hour after delivery, the skin was pink, lungs were clear, fontanelles were soft and the infant was bathed and put to breast-feeding the first morning. The finding of soft fontanelles means there was no bulging, swelling, of the brain, no cerebral edema, no acute cerebral damage. Newborn infants who have acute brain damage are depressed at delivery and do not soon improve; they stay depressed, comatose, flaccid, with respiratory failure, congestive heart failure, bulging fontanelles. This newborn infant was not like that.

The clinical pattern in the present case is compatible with the presence of latent subacute cerebral damage at birth, damage due to adversive processes during gestation, damage that later brought about the development of cerebral palsy and mental retardation.

A Case of   *Maternal low weight gain, viral infection; nuchal cord. IUGR; infant later developed cerebral palsy, mental retardation, and seizure disorder.*

This was a complicated pregnancy. This mother was sick and had a nutrition problem.

Maternal low weight gain occurred. Ordinarily, weight gain in pregnancy is 25 to 30 pounds. This mother gained 16 pounds. Low weight gain indicates disordered maternal nutrition and metabolism. Low maternal weight gain compromises fetal well-being, compromises fetal nutrition. It is associated with impaired neonatal outcome. The present case is an example of this (page 46).

A viral infection, the flu, occurred during the midtrimester. Viral infection during pregnancy is a hazard both to the mother and to the fetus. Pregnant women clinically have increased susceptibility to viral infections, to influenza, upper respiratory infections, viral sore throat. Flu epidemics in times past resulted in a maternal mortality of up to 50 percent in pregnant women. With acute illness, the metabolic oxygen requirements of the mother are sharply increased, leaving the fetus oxygen deprived, hypoxic. In cases of maternal flu with miscarriage, often hypoxic cerebral damage in the aborted fetus is evident at autopsy.

Birth occurred at 42 weeks of pregnancy, a spontaneous vaginal delivery.

Nuchal cord, the umbilical cord wrapped tightly around the neck of the fetus, was present at delivery.

In many cases, the umbilical cord becomes wound around the neck early on, months before term. At times, intrauterine death of the small fetuses occurs, with the umbilical cord tight around the neck. In other cases, the hypoxia-producing effects of the entanglement during intrauterine life may be intermittent, occurring early in gestation, with the cord becoming tightened and loosened from time to time. The effects, accordingly, may be sublethal, with hypoxic acute and subacute cerebral damage being accrued.

Depression of the infant was of a pronounced degree at birth.

Intrauterine growth retardation (IUGR), dysmaturity, was evident. This newborn infant, at 42 weeks of gestation, weighing 6 pounds 1 ounce (2,740 grams), was more than 1 pound underweight, was in the fifteenth percentile for weight. The length of the infant was 51 centimeters; the factor of length is important, in that 51 centimeters puts this infant in the seventy-fifth percentile for length. With the weight of the infant at the fifteenth percentile and the length at the seventy-fifth percentile — this was a long thin baby, reflecting intrauterine deprivation, dysmaturity.

The Ponderal Index, the weight-length ratio, is a measure of fetal nutrition. It is calculated as the weight in grams times 100, divided by the length in centimeters cubed (multiplied to the third power). In the present case the PI was 2.07, far below the tenth percentile. The low Ponderal Index indicates this fetus was chronically deprived, malnourished, dysmature.

Dysmature babies do not tolerate labor and delivery well and, as in this case, are born depressed. Although depressed at birth, this infant gradually responded to treatment. At 2 hours he appeared stable. At 5 hours he was in no respiratory distress, lung fields were clear; color became pink, tone increased; he was moving all extremities, had good suck reflex. At 18 hours the infant was alert and active. Fontanelles were flat. Pathologically, the presence of soft flat fontanelles rules out the presence of acute brain damage in this newborn infant (page 167).

The performance of this infant in the hours after birth, gradually improving, is not the pattern of an infant with acute stroke-like brain damage. Newborn infants who have *acute* diffuse brain damage are depressed at delivery and do not soon improve; they stay depressed for a long time, comatose, flaccid, with unstable vital signs, with bulging fontanelles. This newborn was not like that. The clinical pattern in the present case, with the infant beginning to improve after delivery, is compatible with the presence of latent *subacute* cerebral damage at birth. Infants who are born harboring subacute cerebral damage, characteristically depressed at birth, respond to attention given with improvement in vital function.

Seizure activity that began soon after delivery interrupted the infant's improvement. Regarding the pathogenesis of the seizures, with cerebral damage incurred during the early premature period, with the damage originating deep in the cerebrum and extending to the cortical surface, with the fetus surviving to term, the lesions in the cortex become subacute, and are capable of causing seizure activity soon after birth. There is increasing clinical opinion that when seizures appear soon after birth, the process is not attributable to acute intranatal asphyxial brain damage, but rather, the cause must be sought in pathologic processes, brain damage, prior to birth.

Fetal dysmaturity is associated with inadequate fetal nutrition and inadequate oxygenation. Chronic intrauterine hypoxia leads to the accruing of fetal brain damage, silent at birth—old subacute cerebral damage demonstrated pathologically at autopsy in cases of stillborn dysmature infants. In infants surviving, the latent cerebral damage ultimately is manifested as cerebral palsy, mental retardation, and seizure disorder.

A Case of   *Anemia in the newborn; IUGR. Maternal low pregnancy weight gain. Infant with cerebral damage present at birth; later developed cerebral palsy, mental retardation, seizure disorder.*

Anemia of severe degree was evident in this infant at birth (page 95). The newborn infant was described as "very pale." Presence of severe anemia was confirmed in the hematology studies done immediately after delivery. The red cell count (RBC) was 1.67 million (normal, 5.1); hemoglobin was 6.8 grams (normal, 19 grams); hematocrit was 20.3 percent (normal, 61 percent).

Transfusion of packed red blood cells was given to the infant at 3 hours after birth and repeated during the first day.

The anemia pathologically proved to be of a chronic nature in the fetus.

Chronic anemia, in the fetus as in the adult human, causes chronic hypoxia. The red cell is the oxygen carrying vehicle in the blood. The decrease in hematocrit to one-third means this fetus existed with much less than the average amount of oxygen supply, chronic severe fetal hypoxia.

The fact that this was a chronic anemia is indicated by the hematology report of greatly increased numbers of nucleated red cells (NRC) present in the newborn blood count (page 96). At birth the nucleated red cell count was 100 (normal for a newborn is 0 to 24).

The cause of the anemia, clinically unclear, may have been due to fetal-maternal transfusion.

This case, in addition to the hypoxia-producing fetal-neonatal anemia, presented maternal factors known to be adversive to the well-being of the fetus.

A poor reproductive record was evidenced in the mother's previous pregnancies. This mother produced babies that were small, infants that were weak, enfeebled. Her first pregnancy was complicated by vaginal bleeding, requiring a cesarean section. The second baby was small, 2,420 grams. With the third baby, this case, the mother had low weight gain during pregnancy.

Plainly, this mother exhibited ineffective biologic processes for producing healthy infants. With a clinical history of poor reproductive performance of the mother in past pregnancies, as in the present case, there is an increased incidence of cerebral palsy in the offspring.

Low pregnancy weight gain, inappropriate weight gain, was evident in the mother's prenatal record. During the last 6 months of pregnancy, the last two trimesters, she gained 10 1/2 pounds. The usual weight gain during the last two trimesters is about 20 pounds. This mother not only had a low pregnancy weight gain but also showed periods of stasis and loss of weight during this pregnancy.

Low weight gain indicates a disordered maternal metabolism with consequent poor fetal nutrition, poor fetal oxygenation. Low maternal weight gain is an ominous sign. Low maternal weight gain compromises fetal well being and is associated with impaired neonatal outcome (page 46).

Dysmaturity, low birth weight, was evident in this anemic, feeble newborn. This was a long thin baby, typical of dysmaturity, intrauterine deprivation (IUGR).

The weight of this newborn infant, at 2,720 grams (6 pounds), was in the tenth percentile, about a pound underweight for a term newborn.

The Ponderal Index, the weight-length ratio, is a measure of fetal nutrition (page 94). In the present case the Ponderal Index was 2.3, in the fifteenth percentile. The low PI reflects chronic intrauterine malnutrition, dysmaturity.

Depression of the infant, of severe degree, was present at birth. However, after being transfused the infant improved. Vital function was stable. Fontanelles were flat.

Seizure activity began late on the first day, associated with depression of the infant's neurologic function.

CT and ultrasound studies of the brain at this time showed far-advanced cerebral damage. The CT scan at 17 hours showed decreased density of the cerebral white matter, especially in the frontal regions (Figure 488). Significantly, however, the lateral ventricles were patent. The patent ventricles, together with the clinical observation of flat fontanelles, are evidence that cerebral edema was not present and that the damage in the cerebrum was not of an acute nature, but was old, subacute pathologically.

Figure 489, the CT scan of the brain at 14 days, shows evidence of far-advanced, severe frontal cerebral damage, damage that corresponds to that seen on day 1.

The cerebral damage present at birth, damage of old subacute nature, is attributable to adverse gestational processes that impacted on this fetus, on the fetal cerebrum.

This child developed the dyskinesias of cerebral palsy together with seizure disorder and mental retardation. Cerebral palsy is known to be due to deep cerebral damage (basal ganglia) incurred at a time during premature immature fetal life prior to 34 or 35 weeks (Chapter 3).

Figure 488. CT scan of the brain on day 1. Decreased density in the cerebrum, most pronounced in the frontal regions, evidencing far-advanced old subacute hypoxic damage. Lateral ventricles patent, indicating absence of cerebral edema, absence of acute cerebral damage.

Figure 489. CT scan of brain at 14 days. Pronounced decreased density in the frontal areas, indicating severe loss of cerebral substance; pattern of damage corresponds to that evident at birth (Figure 488).

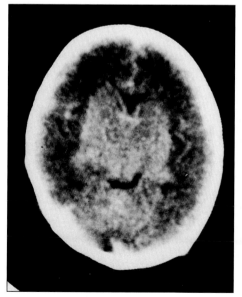

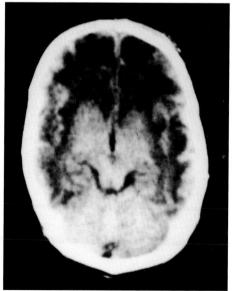

Fig. 488

Fig. 489

A Case of **Macrosomia and anemia in a newborn. Maternal obesity, hypothyroidism, prediabetes. Infant developed cerebral palsy, mental retardation, and seizure disorder.**

Macrosomia of severe degree was present; the newborn infant weighed 5,320 grams (11 pounds 12 ounces). The baby was large, heavy, and long. As to the cause of this baby's macrosomia, often the delivery of an oversize baby is the first sign of latent diabetes in the mother.

Macrosomic babies, as in this case, are feeble, do not do well. Big does not mean strong, robust. Some are stillborn or die soon after birth. Macrosomic babies are commonly the offspring of mothers with diabetic conditions, and related to this, there is an increased incidence of cerebral palsy in these infants.

The mother in this case presented significant medical problems adverse to the well-being of the fetus.

Obesity, excessive pregnancy weight gain, developed; this mother, 5 feet 5 inches tall, weighed 196 pounds at delivery.

Pathologically there are two endocrine disorders, metabolic dysfunctions, associated with maternal excessive weight gain: diabetic conditions and thyroid disease. Both of these conditions were evidenced in this case.

Diabetes was not overt in this mother; however, she presented three key premonitory signs of latent diabetes: a family history of diabetes, obesity, and a macrosomic baby (page 49).

Thyroid disease of long standing was present in this mother. She was being treated for nodular goiter. Goiter of this type usually results in decreased formation of thyroxin by the thyroid, bodily hypothyroidism. This was not an incidental matter, but was a substantial problem in this case, evidenced by the fact that not only the mother, but also her mother and grandmother had this thyroid disease.

Thyroid disease, hypothyroidism, at times compromises gestation. The thyroid regulates metabolism. With hypothyroidism present, the metabolic demand of the mother, the oxygen requirement of the mother, is not maintained, and the mother and the fetus are rendered hypoxic.

Labor developed spontaneously at 39 weeks. This was a difficult midforceps delivery of a very large baby.

The infant at delivery was depressed, limp, pale, almost lifeless. The infant was maintained on a ventilator. The infant remained in poor condition; congestive heart failure developed.

Anemia, evident clinically at delivery, was confirmed in the hematology studies soon after birth. The hematocrit at 2 hours was 44 percent (normal, 61 percent). Hemoglobin level was 13 grams (normal, 19 grams). The anemia required multiple transfusions.

The anemia, pathologically, was of chronic form. Chronic anemia, in the fetus as in the adult human, causes chronic hypoxia. The red cell is the oxygen-carrying vehicle in the blood. The decrease in hematocrit means this fetus existed with less than the average amount of oxygen supply, chronic fetal hypoxia.

The fact that this was a chronic anemia is indicated by the hematology report of 381 nucleated red cells, meaning 381 nucleated red cells per 100 white blood cells. Normally, term newborn infants have an average of 8 to 20 nucleated red blood cells per 100 white blood cells. The presence of excessive nucleated red cells in the blood means the anemia was of long standing during fetal life (page 96).

The cause of the anemia remained undetermined, with fetal-maternal transfusion a possibility (page 97).

In conclusion, it is evident that adversive gestational processes, the intrauterine hypoxia-producing anemia and the maternal metabolic disorders, resulted in an enfeebled macrosomic newborn with latent accrued subacute hypoxic cerebral damage present at birth, damage that later led to cerebral palsy, mental retardation, and seizure disorder.

A Case of   *Spinal cord injury; face presentation; tetraplegia at birth.*

Malposition of the fetus, face presentation, was apparent prenatally, with subsequent loss of fetal activity.

Face presentation causes the spinal column to be bent backwards excessively, in extreme hyperextension.

Face presentation occurs in .2 to .4 percent of deliveries.

Spinal cord injury occurs with face presentation due to the hyperextension of the spine. Hyperextension causes stretching of the cord and narrowing of the spinal canal, with compression of the cord. With hyperextension of the spine, the upper cervical and midcervical portions of the cord are damaged by the stretching of the cord and by the narrowing of the spinal canal due to the distortion of the spinal axis. The cord becomes mangled, transected.

Loss of fetal activity occurred prenatally. The mother reported that the fetus was "hyperactive" 4 days before delivery and this was followed by decreased fetal activity for 2 or 3 days. This hyperactivity may have signaled fetal distress at the onset of the spinal distortion, the spinal cord damage. By the time that fetal activity was lost, 2 or 3 days before delivery, the spinal cord had probably become irreversibly damaged, rendering the fetus paralyzed.

As with other latent, silent, life-threatening intrauterine complications, such as formation of a tight umbilical cord knot, the damage to the fetus is far advanced before the intrauterine pathologic process shows any manifestation — loss of fetal activity.

Labor developed spontaneously at term, and the mother delivered vaginally after some difficulty in extracting the baby.

Tetraplegia was evident at delivery.

The infant was resuscitated with positive pressure oxygen. The Apgar score was 3 at five minutes (1 for heart action, 2 for color). The infant cried at two minutes. Neurologic examination indicated the cranial nerves were intact; there were vigorous facial movements.

Tracheostomy was done; the infant was maintained on the ventilator. Following pneumonia, death occurred at 6 months.

At autopsy, the spinal cord showed a segment of the midcervical cord obliterated, replaced by scar tissue. Pathologic examination of the damaged segment showed complete loss of cord structure with replacement by granulation tissue. The upper cervical spinal cord and the brain stem were intact.

In cases of face presentation, with hyperextension, with spinal cord injury, survival is possible if the segment of the cervical damage is relatively low, so that the vital (regulatory) centers in the uppermost part of the cord and medulla escape damage.

Spinal injury at times is due to forceful extraction and torsion of the head during delivery, as occurred in the past when high and middle forceps delivery was done. Most of the cord damage in such circumstances was located in the upper cervical segment and at times involved the adjoining brain stem. With laceration of cord and brain stem, the process is immediately lethal.

The pattern of spinal cord damage, with the upper cervical cord and brain stem intact and middle cervical cord destroyed, usually results from endogenous processes, as with hyperextension in face presentation. This is what happened in the present case (page 134).

A Case of   *Uncontrolled maternal diabetes. Macrosomic newborn. Infant later developed cerebral palsy, mental retardation, and seizure disorder.*

Diabetes mellitus in this mother was of long standing. Diabetes was diagnosed at her first pregnancy; she was then 17 years old, hypertensive, and obese, weighing 215 pounds at delivery. She produced a macrosomic 11 pound 7 ounce stillborn infant, delivered by cesarean section because of the large size of the fetus.

At age 18, 3 months after her first delivery, she became pregnant again (the pregnancy in the present case).

Teenage pregnancy and a short interval between pregnancies, as in this case, are factors adverse to the outcome of the gestation.

Diabetes, as in the first pregnancy, was a major problem in this second pregnancy. Control of the diabetes during this pregnancy was difficult; the mother often was out of diabetic control, especially during the stress of illness. The mother was sick, anemic, hospitalized twice during this pregnancy, with the diabetes out of control. This obese mother was manifestly not healthy during the last half of pregnancy; she failed to gain weight appropriately in this period.

Maternal illness exercises an adverse effect on the fetus, causing fetal hypoxia, at times leading to miscarriage—or the fetus is blighted, born with old, subacute brain damage.

Maternal disorders cause fetal deprivation. The damaging effect on the fetus—the common denominator—is hypoxia. With acute and chronic maternal disorders, the oxygen requirements of the mother are increased, so that oxygenation of the fetus is depressed. With intrauterine hypoxia, the fetus accumulates hypoxic cerebral damage. The surviving fetus is born with latent subacute cerebral damage.

Obesity, as in the present case, is a regular concomitant factor in the development of diabetes. This mother's diabetes was compounded metabolically by her weight problem. She was on a 1,000 to 1,200 calorie diet but failed to stay on the diet. She was hospitalized because of increasing excessive weight gain. Weight loss occurred during the week of hospitalization; after discharge from the hospital she gained 9 1/2 pounds in 1 week. Obesity is a hazard to both mother and fetus.

Delivery by repeat caesarean section was done at 36 weeks of pregnancy because of the large size of the fetus evident clinically.

Macrosomia—with the baby weighing 8 pounds 4 ounces (3,712 grams) at 36 weeks of gestation—was evident at birth. The average birth weight at this gestational age is 2,600 grams (5 pounds 12 ounces). This macrosomic newborn was above the ninetieth percentile for weight.

Macrosomic babies are feeble. Big does not mean strong, robust. Some are stillborn or die soon after birth. Macrosomic babies are commonly the offspring of mothers with diabetic conditions, and related to this, there is an increased incidence of cerebral palsy in these infants. This clinical pattern evolved in the present case (page 48).

Depression of moderate degree was evident in this macrosomic newborn infant, but she responded quickly. She had a spontaneous cry at birth. Spontaneous respiration was present at 1 minute. At 16 minutes she was admitted to the nursery "in fairly good condition." At 2 hours the infant was fed, and took the feeding well. The next day, at 18 1/2 hours of age, the infant was bathed.

In the light of the clinical pattern of this newborn, the conclusion emerges that this newborn infant did not have acute hypoxic cerebral damage. Infants who are born with acute cerebral damage are comatose at birth, and remain comatose for prolonged periods. This was not the pattern in the present case.

The clinical course in this case is consistent with the syndrome of subacute cerebral damage present at birth, with old, subacute, cerebral hypoxic damage, damage incurred a long time before birth, not evident at birth but becoming manifest as cerebral palsy and mental retardation months, years, later.

A Case of **Maternal diabetes; viral infection during pregnancy. Newborn with anemia. Infant developed cerebral palsy, seizure disorder, mental retardation.**

Diabetes mellitus, in addition to the advanced age of the mother and multiparity, were regarded as risk factors in this case. The mother was 37 years old at this pregnancy. She had had three previous pregnancies during which diabetes was diagnosed.

Maternal diabetes effects an unfavorable uterine environment, exercises a damaging effect on the fetus, extending over the entire length of the gestational period. In these circumstances there is a high incidence of stillbirths.

In mothers with diabetes, the pathologic mechanism causing the injurious effects on the fetus is not well understood. Often infants of mothers with a diabetic condition, even with optimal diabetic control, "just don't do well." In surviving infants there is a high incidence of epilepsy and cerebral palsy.

A viral-type upper respiratory infection (URI) occurred at 30 weeks of pregnancy in this case. The mother was sick with this cold, with sore throat, chest pain, for 2 weeks. In the following 2 weeks she failed to gain weight appropriately.

Viral infection during pregnancy is a hazard both to the mother and to the fetus. Pregnant women clinically have increased susceptibility to viral infections. With acute illness, with fever, the metabolic oxygen requirements of the mother are sharply increased, leaving the fetus oxygen-deprived, hypoxic.

Labor occurred spontaneously at 39 weeks of pregnancy. Presentation was vertex. After 5 hours of labor, Pitocin augmentation was started. Late deceleration developed. With a diagnosis of fetal distress, a cesarean section was done.

The newborn infant was limp and apneic. He improved slowly.

Anemia was present at birth. This newborn infant was noted to be pale. Pale means anemia. Anemia was confirmed in the newborn hematology reports. At birth the red blood cell count (RBC) was 4.28 million (normal, 5.14 million). The hemoglobin level was 15.5 grams (normal, 19 grams). The hematocrit level was 47.2 percent (normal, 61 percent).

Chronic anemia, in the fetus as in the adult human, causes chronic hypoxia. The red cell is the oxygen-carrying vehicle in the blood. The decrease in hematocrit means this fetus existed with less than the average amount of oxygen supply, chronic fetal hypoxia.

The fact that this was a chronic anemia is indicated by the hematology report of "44 NRC per 100 cells," meaning 44 nucleated red cells per 100 white blood cells. Normally, term newborn infants have an average of 8 nucleated red blood cells per 100 white blood cells. In the present case there were more than five times the average number of nucleated red blood cells in the blood of this newborn. Nucleated red cells in excessive number in the fetal blood means there has been chronic fetal anemia (page 96).

The anemia that developed in this fetus is attributable to the mother's diabetes and to other adverse gestational factors.

What was the cause of the depression in this newborn infant? Was the neurologic depression due to fresh, acute brain damage incurred during birth? A newborn infant who has fresh cerebral damage has specific physical evidence of the brain damage: The hypoxic, damaged cerebrum becomes edematous, swollen. Fontanelles become bulging, turgid, and stay that way for many days. This baby did not have bulging fontanelles.

CT scans in cases with acute brain damage show evidence of cerebral swelling — persisting compression, obliteration, of the cerebral ventricles. The CT scan taken neonatally in this case showed normal patent ventricles, no evidence of cerebral damage, no edema.

This newborn infant's clinical course was compromised — not by acute brain damage — but by ongoing debilitation caused by adversive maternal gestational factors and by (fetal) neonatal anemia.

The baby's improvement was impeded by the early onset of seizures. The occurrence of seizures in the newborn period does not mean that the underlying cerebral damage was incurred during labor and delivery. There is increasing clinical opinion that when seizures appear soon after birth, the process is not attributable to acute intranatal asphyxial brain damage, but rather, the cause must be sought in pathologic processes, brain damage, prior to birth. With cerebral damage incurred during the early premature period, with the damage originating deep in the cerebrum and extending to the cortical surface, with the fetus surviving to term, the lesions in the cortex become subacute, and are capable of causing seizure activity soon after birth.

The clinical pattern in the present case, with the infant beginning to improve after delivery, with the occurrence of early onset of seizures, with the later development of cerebral palsy and mental retardation, is compatible with the presence of latent *subacute* cerebral damage at birth, damage incurred during early fetal life.

A Case of   *Maternal illness during pregnancy, acute appendicitis with surgery; severe viral infection. Infant developed cerebral palsy, mental retardation, and seizure disorder.*

The mother had serious medical problems during this pregnancy, problems adversive to the well-being of the fetus.

Appendicitis developed in this mother at midpregnancy. Acute inflammatory disease, such as acute appendicitis, during pregnancy is a hazard to both the mother and the fetus. Clinically, pathologically, this is a process of stress, the stress of the infectious disease and the stress of a surgical operation requiring anesthesia and sedation.

The physical bodily effects of the attack of appendicitis, the stress factor in this case, is evidenced by the fact that the mother, at midpregnancy at this time, became anemic and failed to gain weight appropriately in this period.

In pregnancy complicated by acute appendicitis, while the prognosis in such cases, in the present day, is generally good, the fetal loss rate in most series is reported to be about 15 percent. Clinical studies have shown that appendicitis increases the fetal death rate.

With gestational problems present during fetal life, the common denominator of these adversive processes is hypoxia—the fetus is subjected to varying degrees of oxygen deprivation, which leads to an accruing of subacute cerebral damage in the fetuses surviving to term.

A viral infection occurred following the appendicitis, "a very bad cold." With viral infections, with fever, the mother's metabolism is elevated and the oxygen requirements of the mother are sharply increased, so that oxygenation of the fetus is depressed.

Labor developed at 42 weeks of the pregnancy. Presentation was cephalic. Spontaneous vaginal delivery occurred after 4 hours of labor.

The newborn infant was in good condition at birth, with an Apgar score of 6 and 7. The infant had physical features of postmaturity, with peeling skin.

The adversive conditions of the gestation manifestly affected the newborn infant. The baby was somewhat anemic, enfeebled.

During the first several hours this infant was considered to be in fair clinical condition; she was active, had a strong cry and good heart tones; lungs were normal. This is not the clinical pattern of a newborn with acute diffuse cerebral damage. Newborn infants who have acute diffuse brain damage are depressed at delivery and do not soon improve; they stay depressed, comatose, flaccid, with unstable vital signs.

Regarding the initial postdelivery depression in this case, considered retrospectively this was a chronically deprived, anemic, enfeebled fetus, unable to tolerate the stress of birth; however, the newborn responded to care and was soon improved. The clinical pattern in the present case, with the infant beginning to improve after delivery, is compatible with the presence of latent subacute cerebral damage at birth (page 166).

Seizure activity that began soon after delivery interrupted the infant's improvement. There is increasing clinical opinion that when seizures appear soon after birth, the process is not attributable to acute intranatal asphyxial brain damage, but rather, the cause must be sought in pathologic processes, brain damage, prior to birth (page 207).

This child developed cerebral palsy. Cerebral palsy is a "dyskinesia," a defect in motor function caused by damage to a certain part of the brain, the basal ganglia, located deep in the brain. This deep damage occurs consistently, specifically, only in the immature premature brain, during early fetal life. When the fetus is damaged during early fetal life, if the fetus survives to term, the infant is born with old subacute brain damage. Deep damage incurred in the premature brain (causing cerebral palsy) at times extends to the cerebral surface, to the cortex, resulting in cortical manifestations of mental retardation and seizure disorder.

A Case of **Newborn with IUGR; neonatal microcephaly; spinal fluid xanthochromia. Infant developed cerebral palsy, seizure disorder, mental retardation.**

This newborn infant presented physical signs of severe deprivation during intrauterine life, dysmaturity (IUGR) and microcephaly at birth. The cause of the fetal intrauterine deprivation was not revealed in the mother's medical records. There was little information about the mother's health during the first trimester of this pregnancy. According to the records, the mother did not indicate any acute illnesses, colds, flu, that may have occurred during the 39 weeks of this pregnancy. Often mothers hesitate to report periods of bleeding, viral infections, or they forget. Were there episodes of maternal illness that went unreported? The severity of the maternal illness does not necessarily correspond to the degree of fetal damage. Even a mild illness may prove disastrous for the fetus.

Although the prenatal maternal record in this case provided no relevant clue to adverse processes causing fetal compromise—the effects were plainly evident in the enfeebled, malnourished fetus, unable to tolerate labor, with the newborn in the delivery room depressed, with a low Apgar score.

Dysmaturity, a classic example of intrauterine growth retardation, was present in this case. This newborn infant, while presenting conclusive physical evidence of maturity, weighed 2,620 grams, was underweight, reflecting chronic intrauterine nutritional deprivation (IUGR).

The length of this newborn was 20.5 inches (51 centimeters), placing him in the upper ninetieth percentile for body length for 39 weeks. In contrast, the body weight, at 2,620 grams, put him in the lower fifthteenth percentile for weight. The present case is an example of "disproportionate intrauterine growth retardation," a form of dysmaturity in which the newborn is long and thin.

Thymic atrophy was revealed in the x-ray of the chest in this newborn. The thymus is a thick spongy structure that lies in the upper part of the thorax, beneath the sternum. It is normally relatively large in the healthy fetus and newborn. In the present case, the small size of the thymus attracted the attention of the radiologist, who stated, "The thymus appears small," in reviewing the x-ray. The thymus in the fetus becomes small, atrophied, "thymic involution," after exposure to prolonged adverse conditions during intrauterine life. The finding of thymic atrophy in the present case is another piece of evidence indicating that the fetus was subjected to adverse conditions during premature life.

Microcephaly was evident in the newborn. The head circumference was 31 centimeters (normal for 39 weeks gestation is 33.5 centimeters), in the tenth percentile. Microcephaly present at birth (in cases that later develop cerebral palsy) is the result of deep cerebral damage originating during premature immature fetal life, with consequent growth of the cerebrum compromised, reduced.

Depression of severe degree was present in this newborn, with an Apgar score of 1 and 1. However, the infant soon improved, soon had spontaneous respiration with good air exchange. At 15 minutes, muscle tone was improved. At 50 minutes, the skin was pink. The infant steadily improved, showing good reflexes and moving his extremities. Fontanelles remained soft.

In light of this clinical pattern, it was conclusive that this newborn infant did not have acute hypoxic cerebral damage. Infants who are born with massive acute cerebral damage are comatose at birth, and remain comatose for prolonged periods, days, with respiratory depression and congestive heart failure. This was not the pattern in the present case.

Seizure activity in the first day interrupted the improvement of this newborn. He deteriorated neurologically.

Xanthochromic spinal fluid was found on spinal puncture subsequently on the first day. The finding of xanthochromic (*xantho-*, yellow; *-chromia*, color) spinal fluid is of major importance in defining the time of incurrence of the cerebral damage. Xanthochromia of the spinal fluid is due to the presence of old hemorrhagic damage in the brain (page 173).

With hemorrhage in the brain, with blood escaping into the ventricles, into the spinal fluid, red cells become lysed, broken down; the hemoglobin from the red cells first gives spinal fluid a pink color. The hemoglobin gradually degenerates to a yellow pigment and gives the spinal fluid a yellow color — xanthochromia. This change in color takes many days. The finding of xanthochromia is firm evidence that the brain damage in this fetus, this infant, occurred a long time before labor and delivery.

This child developed cerebral palsy. Pathologically, brain damage that leads to manifestations of cerebral palsy is due to hypoxic damage of deep cerebral structures, damage that takes place specifically in the premature period of fetal life, months before term (Chapter 3).

Deep cerebral damage that occurs during the premature immature period of fetal life at times extends outward to the surface, to the cortex, so that in such cases cortical manifestations of mental retardation and epilepsy are superimposed on the cerebral palsy.

The present case is consistent with the syndrome of subacute cerebral damage present at birth, damage incurred a long time before birth, damage capable of triggering early neonatal onset of seizures, damage responsible for microcephaly at birth, damage manifest months, years, later as cerebral palsy, mental retardation, and other cerebral disability.

A Case of   ***Maternal prediabetes, obesity; teenage pregnancy. Macrosomic newborn. Infant later developed cerebral palsy, mental retardation, seizure disorder.***

Prediabetes, latent diabetes, was evidenced in this mother. Familial diabetes, involving many of her relatives, was noted. Characteristic of prediabetic mothers, she developed pregnancy obesity and she delivered an oversize macrosomic baby.

In people who become diabetic the bodily metabolic dysfunctions have their origin many years before the diabetes becomes clinical. Large babies are the hallmark of latent diabetes, often the first sign of an underlying diabetic condition.

Maternal prediabetes (or diabetes) effects unfavorable intrauterine conditions, exercises a damaging effect on the fetus, extending over the entire length of the gestational period. In these circumstances there is a high incidence of stillbirths. The precise mechanism causing this injurious effect on the fetus is not known. In surviving infants there is a high incidence of cerebral palsy.

Obesity, increasing during the pregnancy, was an explicit metabolic abnormality in the mother. This mother, 5 feet 2 inches tall, went from a pregravid weight of 135 pounds to a weight of 170 pounds at term. Normally weight gain during pregnancy is 20 to 25 pounds. Excessive weight gain during pregnancy is common in diabetic conditions.

Teenage pregnancy was a factor in this case. The mother was young, 15 years old, at the beginning of this pregnancy, a factor in itself unfavorable to the mother and the fetus. There is an increased incidence of fetal and neonatal morbidity and mortality with young teenage mothers.

Emotional stress manifestly was an adversive influence. This mother, finding herself pregnant—a teenage girl, unmarried—confronted substantial emotional stress in the circumstance of this pregnancy. Maternal stress can and does affect the condition of the fetus (page 53).

Delivery occurred at term, after prolonged labor, with oxytocin augmentation, a vaginal delivery with vacuum extraction of a large baby.

Macrosomia, excessive size of the infant, was obvious at delivery. This baby was large, heavy and long. The baby weighed 9 1/2 pounds (4,259 grams), over the ninetieth percentile for weight (average newborn term weight, 3,200 grams, or 7 to 7 1/2 pounds). The baby was long, 61 centimeters (23 inches) over the ninetieth percentile.

The macrosomia of this baby is attributable to this mother's disordered metabolism, her latent prediabetes.

Macrosomic babies, as in this case, are feeble, do not do well. Big does not mean strong, robust. Some are stillborn or die soon after birth. Macrosomic babies, commonly the offspring of mothers with diabetic conditions, have an increased incidence of cerebral palsy in later infancy.

Depression of vital function was present at birth, with an Apgar score of 2 and 3. Depression in the newborn has two different causal mechanisms, two patterns. At times the underlying pathogenesis is related to hypoxic acute cerebral damage incurred during labor and delivery. In other instances the newborn depression is primarily due to the presence of old, subacute cerebral damage incurred weeks or months prior to labor, with the previously compromised fetus unable to tolerate the ordinary stress of labor.

The postnatal course of infants born with hypoxic brain damage is of two types, depending on whether the cerebral damage is acute or subacute. Infants who are born with massive *acute* cerebral damage are comatose at birth, and remain comatose for prolonged periods, days, with respiratory depression and congestive heart failure. This was not the pattern in the present case. Infants born harboring *subacute* cerebral damage, depressed at delivery, soon respond and are improved in the hours after birth. This was the pattern in the present case. This newborn infant responded to care in the delivery room and after 3 hours he was described as active and kicking.

This infant later developed cerebral palsy, mental retardation, and seizure disorder. Cerebral palsy is due to damage to deep cerebral structures, damage to basal ganglia, incurred specifically in the premature immature fetal brain. Cerebral damage in the premature fetus at times extends from the deep cerebral structures through the cerebrum to the surface (cortex). Infants surviving are subject to the development of cerebral palsy, due to deep cerebral damage, plus superimposed cortical manifestations, seizure disorder and mental retardation.

A Case of   *Prediabetic obese mother; twin pregnancy; premature delivery at 35 weeks. One twin with massive intraventricular hemorrhage. This infant later developed cerebral palsy, mental retardation, and seizure disorder.*

This was not an optimal pregnancy circumstance: a twin pregnancy, the mother with a diabetic condition, morbidly obese, gaining weight excessively, and with a period of viral infection, a "cold," during midpregnancy.

Prediabetes manifestations were evidenced in this mother. Familial diabetes was reported in the mother's history, with several relatives known to be diabetic. Her husband (the father of the infant in this case) was diabetic. During this pregnancy the mother continued to have an elevated blood glucose level and had a positive glucose tolerance test.

In people who become diabetic, the bodily dysfunctions have origin many years before the diabetes becomes manifest. Maternal prediabetes (or diabetes) effects an unfavorable uterine environment, exercises a damaging effect on the fetus, extending over the entire length of the gestational period. In these circumstances there is a high incidence of stillbirth. In mothers with a diabetic process, the pathologic mechanism causing the injurious effects on the fetus is not known. Often the newborn infant "just doesn't do well." In surviving infants there is a high incidence of cerebral palsy.

Obesity, common in mothers with diabetic conditions, was present in this mother. This 5 foot 2 1/2 inch mother, prior to this pregnancy, weighed 200 pounds. Excessive weight gain occurred, with the mother at 35 weeks of pregnancy weighing 232 pounds (usual weight gain at 35 weeks is about 17 pounds). Pregnancy obesity is reflective of defective maternal metabolic function, adversive to the well-being of the fetus.

A viral-type upper respiratory infection occurred, lasting for a period of a week in midpregnancy.

Any kind of maternal illness during pregnancy, physical or emotional illness, directly affects the maternal-placental-fetal complex, compromising the fetus. Pathologically, the causal process exercises its effects through the common denominator of intrauterine hypoxia. The severity of the maternal illness does not necessarily correspond to the degree of fetal damage. A mild maternal illness may prove disastrous for the fetus.

Labor developed after spontaneous rupture of membranes, at 35 weeks of gestation.

The first twin (this case), with a cephalic presentation, was delivered vaginally. This twin, a male, was in poor condition at birth, with an Apgar score of 3 and 7. Weight was 2,174 grams (4 pounds 13 ounces).

The second twin, with a footling presentation, was delivered by cesarean section. This infant, a female in good condition at birth, weighing 2,180 grams (4 pounds 13 ounces), was discharged on day 6.

The placenta examination indicated a diamniotic, dichorionic placenta.

With regard to twin gestation as a factor in this case, it is a common observation that with twinning, the two infants come out and develop differently, physically and mentally. During intrauterine life, adversive gestational factors at times affect one fetus more than the other. As with adults during a flu epidemic, one member of the family is affected, another member not affected. In this direction, in the present case, one twin, the infant in this case, was enfeebled and proved more vulnerable to pathologic processes than the other.

The depression in the first twin, the infant in this case, persisted, with the infant responding poorly after birth. At 3 hours after birth his condition deteriorated; he became pale and hypotensive, in severe shock. The hematocrit, previously 60, dropped to 46.3, a precipitous development of anemia.

The rapid development of anemia and hypotension, shock, in the newborn signals the occurrence of internal hemorrhage. In premature newborn infants, commonly the internal hemorrhage is intracerebral.

This occurred in the present case. The CT scan of the brain showed large bilateral intraventricular hemorrhage (Figure 490).

Intraventricular hemorrhage is a pathologic process that occurs predominantly in the premature fetus and newborn infant. Pathologically, the intraventricular hemorrhage is due to hemorrhagic infarction of periventricular tissue (page 13).

At times, hemorrhagic infarction in the periventricular tissue breaks through into the lateral ventricles causing intraventricular hemorrhage. Clot formation in the intraventricular drainage system may lead to obstruction of cerebrospinal fluid outflow, with consequent development of obstructive hydrocephalus, as occurred in the present case (Figure 491).

The cerebral palsy that developed in this infant is attributable to the periventricular cerebral damage, damage to basal ganglia. Extension of the damage to the cerebral surface resulted in cortical manifestations of mental retardation and seizure disorders.

Figure 490. Intraventricular hemorrhage (CT scan of brain at 25 hours). In the upper portion of the scan, on each side near the midline, there are large opaque areas, intraventricular hemorrhages in the lateral ventricles. Below, in the posterior and inferior horns of the lateral ventricles, are similar opaque deposits of intraventricular hemorrhage.

Figure 491. Obstructive hydrocephalus following intraventricular hemorrhage. Sonogram at 20 days. Dilated lateral ventricles appear as large translucent chambers. In the adjoining periventricular tissue there are irregular translucent cystic defects, indicating areas of damaged, destroyed tissue.

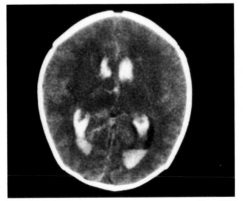

Fig. 490

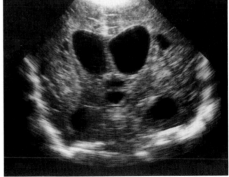

Fig. 491

A Case of   *Maternal hyperemesis gravidarum, vaginal bleeding, recurrent upper respiratory infections. Newborn with multiple malformations. Infant developed cerebral palsy, mental retardation, seizure disorder.*

The mother in this case was chronically sick, with nausea and vomiting serious enough to require hospitalization. At this same time she had vaginal bleeding. Later she was found to be anemic. She had upper respiratory infections — sore throat, flu — lasting for weeks and requiring treatment. The ongoing poor health of the mother during this pregnancy was indicated in the record, that noted "bed rest during the first 4–5 months" of the pregnancy.

The maternal-fetal organic relationship is delicately balanced. Essentially, whatever happens to the mother affects the fetus. Maternal pathologic processes exercise an adverse effect on the fetus, causing fetal hypoxia, at times leading to miscarriage — or, if the fetus is blighted, the infant is born with old, subacute cerebral damage.

Hyperemesis gravidarum, "malignant vomiting of pregnancy," was a major problem for this mother. Nausea and vomiting persisted through the pregnancy, with the mother stating she had "morning sickness — 24 hours a day, all 9 months."

Persistent vomiting, with loss of gastric secretions, loss of gastric acid, leads to electrolyte imbalance, to acute ketosis, dehydration. The mother became weakened, unable to retain food or fluids. She was hospitalized for 2 months in the first trimester.

At this time vaginal bleeding with abdominal cramps occurred, with signs of a threatened miscarriage. The mother became anemic.

Ultrasound of the uterus demonstrated loss of fetal movement. The absence of fetal movement is interpreted as a sign of fetal debility.

Recurrent respiratory infections, viral-type infections, occurred during this pregnancy. At 3 months of pregnancy she had the "flu" that lasted for weeks; she lost weight at this time. Sore throat and flu symptoms occurred again at 6 months of pregnancy.

Viral infection during pregnancy is a hazard both to the mother and to the fetus. Pregnant women clinically have increased susceptibility to viral infections. With acute illness, with fever, the metabolic oxygen requirements of the mother are sharply increased, leaving the fetus oxygen deprived, hypoxic.

Labor developed at 41 weeks of gestation. After prolonged labor, with lack of progress, cesarean section was performed.

Depression of the infant was present at birth. Although depressed, with a one-minute Apgar score of 2, she quickly responded, had an Apgar score of 8 at five minutes. The initial depression was attributable to the enfeebled condition of the fetus, subjected to adverse conditions during fetal life. After resuscitation, she improved. She was recorded as being "fairly well" on day 1, nursing well, and "alert and active" on day 2. On day 4 she was noted to be "neurologically normal."

Seizure activity appeared during the second week. There is substantial basis for concluding that the seizures were not due to acute cerebral damage, but were due to cerebral lesions incurred long before birth, incurred during early fetal life (Chapter 5).

This infant developed cerebral palsy. Cerebral palsy is known to be due to deep cerebral (basal ganglia) damage incurred at a time during premature immature fetal life prior to 34 or 35 weeks (Chapter 3).

At the time of the hypoxic process in the premature, the cerebral damage may extend from the deep structures through the wall of the cerebrum, damaging the cortex, and later cause mental deficiency and seizure disorder, as in the present case.

Multiple malformations, a constellation of bodily abnormalities, were present in this infant: abnormal facial structures, with hypertelorism (widely spaced eyes), hypoplastic jaw, big tongue, flat nasal bridge, trigger fingers, chest deformity, deformity of the bones of the left arm, possible cardiac defect (pulmonic stenosis), microcephaly.

Malformations are of two main types: genetic and induced. Genetic causes refer to inherent defects, transmitted through abnormal genes. Genetic studies done in this case essentially ruled out a genetic cause.

Induced malformations are due to exposure of the mother during early pregnancy to external factors — such as chemicals, maternal illness, irradiation — that affect the development of the embryo. When the embryo or early fetus is exposed to a noxious process, those bodily structures that are actively undergoing formation at that point in time are specifically highly susceptible to injury, with the consequence that if the organism survives, it will have defects in the structures previously insulted (page 141).

The period of 6 to 8 weeks of gestation is precisely the time at which formation occurs of the skeletal structures, the bones of the face and limbs; simultaneously, at this time, the heart and the brain are being formed. Accordingly, an adversive condition, an insult to the organism at this time, predisposes these structures to defective formation, creating a constellation of malformations in the fetus.

This mother was acutely sick during the second month. The clinical assessment in this case indicated that the malformations in this child "seem to be due to an embryopathy."

Microcephaly developed in this infant. Although the size of the head was normal at birth, the head failed to increase in size with age, and later by the eleventh month, with the head circumference of 42 centimeters (below the fifth percentile), the infant was plainly microcephalic.

Microcephaly, common in cases of cerebral palsy, is the result of deep cerebral damage originating during premature immature life, with consequent growth of the cerebrum reduced.

A Case of **_Maternal morbid obesity, gestational diabetes; nuchal cord. Infant developed cerebral palsy, mental retardation, and seizure disorder._**

Obesity was a problem in this pregnancy. This mother, at 5 feet 3 inches tall, weighed 268 pounds at term, morbidly obese. Obesity, a hazard to the pregnant mother and her fetus, is reflective of a disturbed bodily metabolism. Obesity predisposes to diabetes, common in people who develop diabetes.

Gestational diabetes was diagnosed in this mother. In people who become diabetic, the related bodily metabolic dysfunctions have origin many years before the diabetes becomes manifested. Metabolic disorders, diabetic processes, effect an unfavorable uterine environment, exercise a damaging effect on the fetus, extending over the entire length of the gestational period. The mechanism causing the injurious effects on the fetus is not known. In surviving infants there is a high incidence of cerebral palsy.

Labor developed at term; presentation was cephalic. Labor was desultory. After 19 hours, with failure to progress and with signs of fetal distress appearing, cesarean section was done.

Nuchal cord, the umbilical cord wrapped four times around the neck of the fetus, was present at delivery.

In many cases, the umbilical cord becomes wound around the neck early on, months before term. I have autopsied many cases of intrauterine death, small fetuses, with tight nuchal cord. The hypoxia that occurs with nuchal cord is not due to "choking," not due to pressure on the neck; rather, the fetal hypoxia is due to the compression of the cord — compression of the blood vessels in the cord obstructs the flow of blood to the fetus.

Depression of the infant was present at delivery. That the adversive maternal and fetal gestational problems impacted unfavorably on the fetus was evidenced by the fact that the fetus, the newborn, showed the effects of chronic compromise, was enfeebled. This fetus was unable to tolerate the stress of parturition but, although depressed at birth, the newborn responded to treatment, with an Apgar score of 6 at five minutes. She slowly improved, soon had good heart action, was pink, and within hours vital function and muscle tone improved, with the baby moving all extremities, responding to stimuli.

There was no substantial evidence of cerebral edema, no cerebral swelling, no bulging fontanelles in this newborn; the ultrasound studies on day 1 showed cerebral ventricles patent, ruling out edema, cerebral swelling.

Pathologically, this was not the picture of a newborn with acute cerebral damage. Infants with acute fresh cerebral damage at birth show it. These infants have cerebral edema, bulging fontanelles, and abnormal scans. They remain depressed for prolonged periods. The infant in this case was not like that.

Seizure activity appeared, however, at 4 hours after birth. The improved clinical course of the newborn was compromised by the onset of seizures. It is increasingly realized clinically that the early onset of seizures in the newborn is not due to acute brain damage, that such seizures are attributable to antecedent early fetal cerebral damage.

Cerebral palsy developed in this infant. Cerebral palsy is known to be due to deep cerebral (basal ganglia) damage incurred at a time during premature immature fetal life (Chapter 3).

At times the deep cerebral damage in the premature fetus extends outward to the cerebral cortex causing mental retardation and seizure disorder.

The conclusion emerges that the cerebral damage, responsible for the infant's disabilities, was due not to acute cerebral damage at birth but to subacute damage originating during premature immature fetal life, the consequence of adversive maternal and fetal (nuchal cord) hypoxia-producing processes during early intrauterine life.

A Case of **Vaginal bleeding, maternal low weight gain. Nuchal cord; IUGR. Infant developed cerebral palsy, mental retardation, and seizure disorder.**

This was a complicated pregnancy, with a mother having vaginal bleeding of serious degree, with a mother who failed to gain weight appropriately and, superimposed on this, at delivery, the fetus with a tight nuchal cord. These are hypoxia-producing factors adverse to the well-being of the fetus.

Vaginal bleeding that occurred in this case was of considerable amount, described as menstrual-like. This was not of the nature of "spotting" that sometimes occurs early in pregnancy. Rather, this vaginal bleeding occurred well along in the gestation, at 8 weeks, and was of the character of a threatened spontaneous abortion. The obstetrician warned the mother that he regarded the condition serious, a threatened miscarriage.

Bleeding during pregnancy is mainly due to pathologic processes affecting the placenta, processes that potentially compromise the fetus, causing fetal hypoxia. The most common cause is partial detachment of the placenta from the uterine wall. Partial detachment of the placenta, in its origin, is often latent, subtle, so that the adverse effects on the fetus are far advanced by the time clinical symptoms of maternal bleeding occur. Throughout this silent latent period the fetus is being compromised, deprived, hypoxic. There is a known high incidence of stillbirth associated with maternal bleeding, with the fetuses at autopsy showing hypoxic cerebral damage.

Parenthetically, in infants surviving, in cases with history of maternal bleeding during pregnancy, there is a high incidence of cerebral palsy and related cerebral disabilities.

Low maternal weight gain that occurred in this case is an indication of a significant gestational metabolic problem. This mother gained 7 pounds during the last two trimesters. During the last two-thirds of pregnancy, the average weight gain is 20 pounds.

Low maternal weight gain compromises fetal well-being and is associated with impaired neonatal outcome. The present case is an example of this (page 46).

Labor occurred spontaneously at a time past term, at 42 to 44 weeks of pregnancy. After prolonged labor, with failure of the parturition to progress and with signs of fetal distress developing, a cesarean section was done.

Postmaturity was a factor in this case. According to information from the mother, by dates, this pregnancy was 42 to 44 weeks. Supporting this interpretation was the clinical assessment of the newborn infant, that "the baby appeared postmature." The clinical appraisal of postmaturity was based on the overall appearance, peeling skin, hair growth, foot creases, nail growth—criteria that are substantially reliable.

The factor of postmaturity was of significance with reference to the relatively low birth weight of the infant.

Low birth weight (intrauterine growth retardation, dysmaturity) was evident in this infant. This infant, of 42 to 44 weeks of gestation, weighing 6 pounds 15 ounces (3,144 grams), was in the lower tenth percentile for birth weight.

Low birth weight, as in the present case, often occurs in association with low maternal weight gain during pregnancy. Intrauterine growth retardation is associated with deprivation of nutrition and oxygenation during fetal life, so that affected newborns have varying degrees of latent hypoxic cerebral damage at birth. Clinically, intrauterine growth retardation is associated with a high incidence of cerebral palsy and other neurological disabilities.

Dysmature newborns are weaklings constitutionally and do not tolerate well the ordinary stress of labor, so they tend to be depressed at birth. IUGR infants usually have a low Apgar score.

Nuchal cord was present at delivery, with the umbilical cord described as being wound three times "snug" around the neck.

The hypoxia-producing effects of nuchal entanglement during intrauterine life may be intermittent, beginning early in gestation, with the cord becoming tightened and loosened from time to time. The effects, accordingly, may be sublethal, with hypoxic cerebral damage of subacute nature being accrued. In other cases, the effects are lethal, leading to fetal death. At autopsy, the brain specimens in these cases show varying severity of hypoxic cerebral damage.

In cases of tight nuchal cord, if the fetus survives, the newborn infant is usually depressed.

Depression of vital function was severe in this infant at delivery, with an Apgar score of 2 and 4. The infant was resuscitated with oxygen and positive pressure ventilation.

Respiratory distress developed. Pneumothorax was found, and this was evacuated, with improvement of respiration.

Neurologically the infant gradually improved. At 5 hours vital signs were stable; good reflexes were elicited; eyes were open, looking about; there were spontaneous movements of the extremities. Fontanelles were soft.

Clinically, in this case, the question arises as to the cause of the postdelivery neurological depression of the newborn.

Depression of the newborn at delivery at times is related to acute cerebral damage incurred during labor and delivery. In other instances, the newborn depression is primarily due to the presence of old, subacute cerebral damage incurred weeks or months prior to labor, with the previously compromised fetus unable to tolerate the ordinary stress of labor.

Infants born with massive fresh, acute hypoxic cerebral damage have a consistent clinical pattern: They remain limp and comatose for prolonged periods. The infant in the present case did not have this pattern. She responded well to the attention given in the delivery room and improved neurologically.

The clinical pattern in this case reflects the pattern of a chronically debilitated weakling fetus and newborn with accrued old brain damage. In the present case, factors adverse to the well-being of this fetus are evident, extending through intrauterine life, including maternal vaginal bleeding early in pregnancy, low birth weight, and particularly the presence of nuchal cord. These are hypoxia-producing complications that lead to cerebral damage in the fetus. Fetuses that have incurred chronic injury during early fetal life, surviving marginally, react poorly to the stress of labor; the newborn infants are depressed at delivery, but characteristically they soon recover from the stress of labor, become responsive and improve neurologically. This was the clinical pattern in the present case. The conclusion emerges that the fetal distress and the postdelivery depression in this newborn were due to debility and to subacute cerebral damage accumulated during early fetal life.

Cerebral palsy and other cerebral disabilities developed in this infant. Cerebral palsy is due to damage to the basal ganglia located in the deep portion of the cerebrum, damage that occurs consistently in the premature (immature) fetus following gestational hypoxia-producing complications. The cerebral damage in the deep cerebral tissues consists of hemorrhagic infarction. Fetuses that survive to term are born harboring old, subacute lesions in the deep periventricular structures and later develop cerebral palsy. At the time of the hypoxic process in the premature period, the cerebral damage may extend from the deep structures through the wall of the cerebrum, damaging the cortex, and later may cause (in addition to the cerebral palsy) mental deficiency, epilepsy, and other developmental disabilities, as occurred in this case.

A Case of   *Pre-eclampsia; maternal low weight gain.*
Dysmature newborn. Infant later developed
cerebral palsy, mental retardation, and seizure disorder.

The mother was manifestly sick during the last months of this pregnancy: Preeclamptic toxemia with hypertension up to 164/110 occurred, requiring hospitalization (page 51).

Eclampsia affects all the organs of the body, especially the kidneys, liver, brain, and circulatory system. The placenta is damaged; vascular changes occur, compromising circulation, affecting oxygenation and nutrition of the fetus.

Low inappropriate weight gain occurred. Maternal weight gain during the last months of pregnancy should average 3/4 pound per week. In the present case, during the last months of pregnancy, during a period of 11 weeks, the mother gained a total of 1 1/2 pounds. Low maternal weight gain compromises fetal well-being and is associated with impaired neonatal outcome. The present case is an example of this (page 46).

Labor was induced. Pregnancy was at 42 weeks of gestation. Delivery was vaginal assisted with low forceps.

The infant at delivery was in good condition, with an Apgar score of 8 at five minutes. No resuscitation was necessary.

Dysmaturity was recognized clinically at birth by the overall abnormal appearance of the newborn, a long thin infant, and particularly by a noticeable lack of subcutaneous tissue. Dysmaturity is usually associated with some degree of low birth weight. This factor was evident in the present case. The infant weighed 7 1/2 pounds, somewhat less than expected for an infant of 42 weeks' gestation. The length of the baby was noticeably excessive, 53.3 centimeters (21 inches), in the ninetieth percentile.

Dysmaturity (IUGR) commonly occurs in association with low maternal weight gain during pregnancy, associated with deprivation of nutrition and oxygen during fetal life.

Dysmaturity is associated with a high incidence of cerebral damage, subacute damage accrued over a period of weeks, months, during fetal life, damage that leads to cerebral palsy, mental retardation, and epilepsy. This occurred in the present case. Cerebral palsy is due to deep damage, damage to cerebral basal ganglia. Extension of the deep damage to the cerebral surface, to the cortex, leads additionally to mental retardation and seizure disorder.

A Case of   *Twin transfusion syndrome. Poor reproductive record of mother. Premature delivery, stillbirth of one twin; surviving newborn with anemia, apnea. Infant later developed cerebral palsy, mental retardation, and a seizure disorder.*

This twin pregnancy was complicated by adversive maternal, fetal, and neonatal factors.

Poor reproductive function of the mother was recorded in this mother's background. Of the four pregnancies prior to the present case, two ended in spontaneous abortion in the first trimester. In the other two pregnancies the babies were small, manifesting intrauterine growth retardation.

This kind of reproductive record is ominous for the well-being of the fetus. With a clinical history of poor reproductive performance of the mother, as in the present case, there is an increase in incidence of cerebral palsy in the offspring.

Advanced age of the mother, 36 years old at this pregnancy, was another factor adversive to the gestation.

Fetal activity decreased during the 2 days prior to labor, indicating the presence of intrauterine processes adversive to the fetus (page 169).

Labor onset occurred at 31 1/2 weeks of gestation. After ultrasound examination revealed one fetus with loss of cardiac action, cesarean section was performed.

The first infant delivered was stillborn; weight 3 pounds 6 ounces. No autopsy was done.

The second twin was liveborn (the infant in this case).

The newborn twin had an Apgar score of 2 and 4. Weight was 4 pounds 5 ounces.

Anemia was evident at delivery. The infant was described as being "very pale." The hemoglobin level (blood taken in the delivery room) was 6.2 grams (normal for newborn at 32 weeks' gestation is 15 grams).

Anemia, in the fetus as in the adult human, causes hypoxia. The red cell is the oxygen-carrying vehicle of the blood. The decrease in hemoglobin to less than 50 percent of normal means that this fetus existed with less than half the average amount of oxygen supply.

The anemia in this twin is attributable to a placental transfusion process. In the fetus-to-fetus twin transfusion syndrome, one twin is the donor and becomes bled out, anemic. The recipient twin becomes polycythemic, with an excessive amount of red cells. Usually the donor fetus is smaller than the recipient twin; however, this difference in size varies. In the present case, the fetuses remained about the same size.

Respiratory distress syndrome (hyaline membrane disease) developed in this infant. Newborn infants of this degree of prematurity almost all, if not all, develop hyaline membrane disease. Hyaline membrane disease compromises the function of the lung in a manner similar to pneumonia, with the alveoli (air sacs) becoming filled with pathologic material, hindering the transfer of oxygen into the blood, rendering the infant hypoxic (page 106).

Apnea, recurrent episodes of arrested breathing, developed. The apnea problem could not be controlled and resulted in rapid deterioration on the ninth day. The problem of apnea is innate to the premature—the cause of this complication and effective treatment remain unsolved (page 105).

This infant survived and later developed cerebral palsy, mental retardation, and seizure disorder.

Cerebral palsy is due to damage to the basal ganglia located in the deep portion of the cerebrum. Damage to the deep structures, to the basal ganglia, often occurs in the premature fetal brain and premature newborn brain subjected to hypoxia-producing complications. At the time of the hypoxic process in the premature, the cerebral damage may extend from the deep structures through the wall of the cerebrum, damaging the cortex, and later may cause (in addition to the cerebral palsy) mental deficiency, epilepsy, and other developmental disabilities (Chapter 3).

Cerebral palsy is of increased incidence in cases of twin gestation. Twin births often occur prior to 35 weeks, often complicated by hypoxia-producing processes that lead to deep cerebral damage and consequent cerebral palsy. The occurrence of this kind of case—a twin gestation with one twin succumbing and at autopsy showing hypoxic cerebral damage and the surviving twin later developing cerebral palsy—has been observed by me and by other pathologists.

In summary, the cause of this infant's brain damage, which resulted in cerebral palsy and other cerebral disabilities, can be linked to hypoxia-producing, brain-damaging fetal-neonatal anemia, and to the postnatal apnea and respiratory distress syndrome.

A Case of   *Maternal diabetes, viral infection, low weight gain. Newborn with pneumothorax. Infant later developed cerebral palsy and mild mental retardation.*

Diabetes was diagnosed in this mother at age 19, 7 years before this pregnancy; this was class B diabetes, maintained on insulin medication.

Diabetes in the mother exercises diffuse adversive effects on the fetus. Newborn infants often are defective in structure and function. Control of diabetes during pregnancy often is difficult, and mothers often are out of diabetic control, especially during the stress of maternal illness. This mother was sick, hospitalized, with an upper respiratory infection at 7 1/2 months, with the diabetes out of control. This mother was manifestly not healthy during the last half of the pregnancy and failed to gain weight appropriately in this period.

With maternal diabetes, even with optimal diabetic control, at times the newborn infant simply does not do well, does not thrive. The underlying cause of the failure to thrive is not well understood. There is an increased incidence of miscarriage and neonatal death associated with maternal diabetes.

Poor reproductive function, recorded in this mother's background, is characteristic of mothers with diabetes. This mother was gravida 5, para 1. In prior years she had had 3 spontaneous abortions.

This kind of reproductive record is ominous for the well-being of the fetus. With a clinical history of poor reproductive performance of the mother, as in the present case, there is an increase in incidence of cerebral palsy in the offspring.

One previous pregnancy had yielded a macrosomic baby weighing 8 pounds 6 ounces. Macrosomic babies occur in about one-third of pregnancies of diabetic mothers.

Viral upper respiratory infection occurred. Pregnant women are particularly susceptible to viral infection. The effect on the fetus of such viral infection (URI, upper respiratory infection) varies, at times causing brain damage (by hypoxia), at times leading to fetal deaths. Acute maternal illness is associated with an increased maternal oxygen requirement and correspondingly renders the fetus hypoxic. As previously noted, this mother had a severe upper respiratory infection at 7 1/2 months of pregnancy, an illness that started with a "cold" and went on to bronchitis.

Seven and one-half months is a most critical time for the fetus in the development of the cerebrum. At this time in fetal life hypoxia-producing complications result in deep cerebral damage.

Decreased fetal activity was noted by the mother. The fetus during the mother's acute illness showed decreased activity and reactivity, indicating that the fetus was affected. There is substantial clinical and pathologic evidence that with maternal hypoxia-producing complications the asphyxiated fetus may gradually become comatose, paralyzed, manifested as a loss of fetal activity and reactivity.

Low maternal weight gain occurred in this pregnancy. In the last half of the pregnancy the mother gained 3 pounds. This record of low weight gain reflects poor maternal health during the last part of the pregnancy. Poor weight gain during pregnancy has been correlated with impaired neonatal outcome.

Delivery was by elective repeat cesarean section at 38 weeks of gestation. In the previous pregnancy, with the macrosomic baby, a primary cesarean section had been done.

The newborn infant was in good condition at delivery, with an Apgar score of 7 and 8, with spontaneous respiration.

The infant's condition gradually deteriorated, with grunting respiration and decreased muscle tone. On day 2 pneumothorax was diagnosed (page 111). A chest tube was inserted and the pneumothorax was reduced. The infant improved, became alert and active in the following days.

Cerebral palsy was diagnosed during the first year. Cerebral palsy is due to damage to the basal ganglia located in the deep part of the cerebrum. Damage to the deep structures, to the basal ganglia, occurs consistently in the premature (immature) fetus following gestational hypoxia-producing complications, such as occurred in the present case. The cerebral damage in the deep cerebral tissues consists of hemorrhagic infarction. If the fetus survives, the lesions, at first acute, undergo "healing" with scarring, become subacute. Fetuses that survive to term are born harboring old, subacute lesions in the deep periventricular structures; later, in infancy, cerebral palsy develops. At the time of the hypoxic process in the premature period, the cerebral damage may extend from the deep structures through the wall of the cerebrum, damaging the cortex, and later may cause (in addition to the cerebral palsy) mental deficiency, as occurred in the present case (Chapter 3).

A Case of **Maternal diabetes, low weight gain. Macrosomic newborn with cardiac hypertrophy. Infant later developed cerebral palsy, mental retardation, behavior disorder, and seizure disorder.**

This mother had serious pregnancy problems, pathologic processes that contributed to cerebral damage during early fetal life. The mother had diabetes uncontrolled during this pregnancy. She had a period of low weight gain during midpregnancy and became anemic. The adversive effects on the fetus caused by the mother's gestational problems were clinically evident in the newborn, with the presence of macrosomia and cardiomegaly.

Diabetes was a major hazard in this pregnancy. This was an insulin dependent diabetic mother with the diabetic condition often out of control during this pregnancy, and with diet not well maintained.

Diabetes exercises diffuse adversive effects on the fetus. Newborn infants often are defective in structure and function. Control of diabetes during pregnancy often is difficult, and mothers often are out of diabetic control. This mother was hospitalized at midpregnancy with the diabetes out of control. Periods of uncontrolled diabetes, with episodes of ketoacidosis, as occurred in this case, are known to exercise harmful effects on the fetus. Experimental studies have shown that ketoacidosis results in fetal hypoxia.

With maternal diabetes, even with optimal diabetic control, the newborn infant often does not do well, does not thrive. The underlying cause of the failure to thrive is not well understood. There is an increased incidence of fetal and neonatal death associated with maternal diabetes.

The incidence of cerebral palsy is noted to be three to five times greater in offspring of diabetic mothers than in nondiabetic mothers.

Low weight gain occurred during this pregnancy. In a period of 3 months, at midpregnancy, this mother's weight went from 141 to 143 1/2 pounds, a gain of 2 1/2 pounds. The average weight gain in midpregnancy optimally is 3/4 pound per week. Accordingly, in the 3-month period noted, the mother should have gained about 9 pounds, compared to the 2 1/2 pounds she gained.

This period of low weight gain was plainly a reflection of an unhealthy pregnancy course. This was a period of poor diabetic control for the mother, a recurrent problem that included an admission to the hospital when she became unresponsive, out of diabetic control.

Low weight gain, reflective of a disordered maternal metabolism, is an ominous sign, associated with impaired neonatal outcome.

Delivery, by repeat cesarean section, was done at 36 1/2 weeks of gestation. Ultrasound prior to delivery had revealed a macrosomic fetus. Fetal activity decreased late in gestation.

Macrosomia was evident in the delivery room. The infant was obviously oversized, with a weight of 8 pounds 3 ounces (3,714 grams), in the ninetieth percentile for 36 weeks' gestation.

Macrosomia in this infant was due to the maternal diabetes. Macrosomic babies, the hallmark of maternal diabetes, as in this case, are feeble. Big does not mean strong, robust. Some are stillborn or die soon after birth.

Depression of severe degree was present in this feeble macrosomic infant, with an Apgar score of 2 and 2. Muscle tone was poor; respirations were grunting.

Cardiac hypertrophy was diagnosed clinically. The initial chest x-ray had shown an enlarged heart. An echocardiogram indicated the enlarged heart was due, *not* to cardiac dilatation, but was due to myocardial hypertrophy, to overgrowth of the muscle of the heart.

This kind of heart abnormality occurs commonly in newborn infants of diabetic mothers. It is estimated that 30 percent of newborns of diabetic mothers have cardiomegaly. The cardiac enlargement in infants of diabetic mothers is analogous to "idiopathic hypertrophic cardiomyopathy" that develops in older children and adults. Although the heart muscle is overgrown, paradoxically the muscle performs inefficiently, often leading to congestive heart failure.

This infant, depressed at birth, responded to treatment and improved. She became pink and had fair muscle tone. Respirations improved, and at 2 hours, she had good tone, gag, cry, grasp, and Moro reflexes. Respirations were easy and quiet. The next morning, at 14 hours, she was on room air.

Postnatally the fontanelles remained soft and flat, no cerebral edema, evidence that there was no acute brain damage (page 167).

Newborn infants who have acute diffuse brain damage are depressed at delivery and do not soon improve; they stay depressed, comatose, flaccid, with respiratory failure, congestive heart failure, bulging fontanelles.

The infant in the present case was not like that.

The clinical pattern in this newborn infant is consistent with the syndrome of subacute cerebral damage incurred during early fetal life, hypoxic cerebral damage, the consequence of maternal diabetes out of control, and other adverse gestational factors affecting this fetus. Newborn infants with subacute cerebral damage are usually depressed at birth but improve and soon become stable and active, as in this case. Subacute cerebral damage, present at birth, is not manifest until later in infancy.

This infant developed cerebral palsy and other cerebral disabilities. Cerebral palsy is due to deep cerebral damage (basal ganglia) incurred at a time during premature immature fetal life prior to 34 or 35 weeks. It does not occur related to events of labor and delivery in mature birth.

Deep damage incurred in the premature brain causing cerebral palsy at times extends to the cerebral surface, to the cortex, resulting in cortical manifestations of mental retardation and epilepsy.

A Case of **Maternal obesity; low pregnancy weight gain. Nuchal cord at delivery; IUGR; newborn anemia; xanthochromic spinal fluid. Infant developed cerebral palsy, mental retardation, and other cerebral disabilities.**

This mother had health problems during pregnancy, all known to have an adversive effect on the fetus. The gestation was also threatened by the presence of a tight nuchal cord, revealed at delivery. The fetus showed the effect of chronic intrauterine compromise, was underweight, an enfeebled sick fetus, unable to tolerate the ordinary stress of labor; the infant was depressed at birth. Of importance pathologically was the finding of xanthochromic spinal fluid in this newborn infant.

Obesity, maternal morbid obesity, was a significant factor in this case. The mother weighed 224 pounds prior to delivery. Obesity is a hazard to the pregnant mother and her fetus, reflective of a disturbed metabolism. Metabolic disorders in the mother exercise an adversive effect on the fetus.

Obesity predisposes to hypertension. This mother developed frank hypertension. The systemic effects of hypertension have an adversive effect on both the mother and the fetus, and often hypertension is the prodromal sign of toxemia.

Low pregnancy weight gain occurred. The record indicated that the mother gained 10 pounds during this pregnancy. In the last 14 weeks of this pregnancy, weight gain was 1 pound. Maternal weight gain during the last months of pregnancy should average 1/2 to 3/4 pounds per week. In comparison, in her three previous pregnancies, the mother gained weight in a normal range.

The low weight gain in this last pregnancy indicated a disordered maternal metabolism with consequent poor fetal nutrition, a case of IUGR. This kind of fetal deprivation is well described in the literature. Obese gravida who gain less that 12 pounds during gestation have a high incidence of IUGR infants.

The mother was a multipara with three term liveborn infants. Delivery in the present case occurred at 42 weeks of gestation; this was a spontaneous vaginal birth.

Nuchal cord was present at birth, wound tightly around the neck. This was described by the obstetrician as a "strong nuchal cord."

In some cases, the umbilical cord becomes wound around the neck early on, months before term. I have autopsied many cases of intrauterine death, small fetuses, with tight nuchal cord.

The hypoxia that occurs with nuchal cord is not due to "choking," not due to pressure on the neck; rather, the fetal hypoxia is due to compression of the cord causing obstruction of blood flow to the fetus (page 83).

Depression of a severe degree was present at birth, with the infant limp and unresponsive. Physical features of postmaturity were present. The infant slowly began to improve. Fontanelles remained soft.

Intrauterine growth retardation of the infant was evident clinically. This newborn infant, weighing 6 pounds 7 ounces (2,900 grams), was underweight, in the fifteenth percentile for 42 weeks' gestation. This mother's previous pregnancies had yielded newborn infants who ranged up to 8 pounds 6 ounces.

Big mothers, like the mother in this case, regularly produce big babies. The fact that this infant was small means there was something wrong going on, adversive intrauterine conditions, leading to chronic fetal deprivation.

IUGR newborns are constitutionally weaklings and do not tolerate well the ordinary stress of labor, so that they tend to be depressed at birth, but respond, as did the infant in this case.

Anemia was present in this newborn. The hematocrit was 47.3 percent; normal is 61 percent at term. The hematocrit measures the bulk quantity of red cells in the blood.

Anemia, in the fetus as in the adult human, causes chronic hypoxia. The red cell is the oxygen-carrying vehicle of the blood. The decrease in hematocrit means that this fetus existed with less than the needed oxygen going to the brain.

Intrauterine hypoxia leads to fetal hypoxic damage. The brain is the most sensitive target tissue in the body; with chronic intrauterine hypoxia, the fetus accrues subacute and acute cerebral damage.

The cause of the anemia was not clear. Fetal malnutrition, fetal debility, as occurred in the present case, is a plausible contributory cause.

Clinical improvement in the newborn infant was compromised by the early onset of seizures at 4 hours after birth.

Early onset of seizure activity, it is increasingly recognized clinically, is attributable to old subacute cerebral damage, incurred during fetal life, before birth (Chapter 5).

Evidence of old hemorrhagic brain damage was indicated in the results of spinal fluid examination.

Xanthochromic spinal fluid was found in the spinal tap done at 5 hours. Xanthochromia, yellow discoloration of the spinal fluid, is due to the presence of old hemorrhagic damage in the brain. With hemorrhage in the brain, with blood escaping into the ventricles, into the spinal fluid, red cells become lysed, broken down; the hemoglobin from the red cells first gives the spinal fluid a pink color. Over a period of days, the pink hemoglobin gradually degenerates to a yellow pigment and gives the spinal fluid a yellow color — xanthochromia. The finding of xanthochromia is firm evidence that brain damage in this fetus, this infant, occurred a long time before labor and delivery (page 173).

This infant developed cerebral palsy, mental retardation, seizure disorder, blindness, and microcephaly.

Cerebral palsy is due to damage in the basal ganglia, located in the deep portion of the cerebrum. Damage to the deep structures, to the basal ganglia, occurs in premature newborn infants due to hypoxia-producing complications prenatally. At the time of the hypoxic process in the premature, the cerebral damage may extend from the deep structures, through the wall of the cerebrum, damaging the cortex, and later may cause (in addition to cerebral palsy) mental deficiency and other developmental deficiencies, mental retardation, blindness, and seizure disorder.

Microcephaly of severe degree developed in this infant. Microcephaly, common in cases of cerebral palsy, is the result of deep cerebral damage originating during premature immature fetal life, with consequent growth of the cerebrum compromised, attenuated.

A Case of   **Basal ganglia calcification in the newborn; later development of ex vacuo hydrocephalus; cerebral palsy. Maternal heroin addiction, psychiatric stress, gestational diabetes.**

Calcification of the basal ganglia was evident in this infant in CT scans of the brain at 21 days after birth. Spasticity of the extremities was evident in the neonatal neurologic examination.

In the background of the case there were significant maternal pregnancy problems, problems of drug addiction, alcoholism, gestational diabetes, and emotional stress, processes that exercised their damaging effects on the fetus.

Heroin addiction in this mother began 2 years prior to this pregnancy. Whether or not heroin, morphine substances, directly damage the fetal brain is open to question. However, in mothers who are heroin addicts, commonly there are concomitant medical, nutritional, and emotional problems adversive to the well-being of the fetus.

Alcoholism additionally complicated this pregnancy, contributed to the enfeeblement of this newborn (page 57).

Gestational diabetes was diagnosed in this mother. There was a family history of diabetes. Maternal diabetic conditions have a compromising effect on the fetus, the newborn.

Psychiatric stress was manifestly present in this pregnancy. This mother was single, an addict, with a history of multiple abortions. Early in this pregnancy she was treated with "mild tranquilizers." There is increasing evidence clinically and experimentally, that maternal emotional stress, in the same way as physical illness, has adverse effects on the fetus.

Labor developed at term. The fetal monitor record indicated fetal distress. A cesarean section was done.

Depression of the newborn was severe. This was an enfeebled sick newborn, reflecting the impact of maternal gestational factors. The Apgar score was 1 and 4. The infant remained unstable, maintained on ventilator support for a long period. The neurologic status of the infant was poor, with decreased responsiveness, with decreased root and suck reflexes. During the first week it was noted that there was increased muscle tone, hypertonia, in the extremities. Hypertonia, as in this case, reflects damage to the basal ganglia of the cerebrum.

Deep cerebral damage, basal ganglia damage, leading to spasticity, to cerebral palsy, is due to hypoxia-producing maternal and other adversive gestational processes affecting the immature fetus.

When deep cerebral hypoxic damage occurs, the necrotic tissue, after a period of months, after scar tissue has formed, may become impregnated with calcium. As occurred in the present case, the infant is born with deep cerebral (basal ganglia) calcification (Figure 492).

In the present case, postnatally the infant failed to thrive. He became increasingly hypertonic, with the diagnosis of spastic cerebral palsy made at 10 months.

Follow-up CT studies of the brain showed increasing enlargement of the cerebral lateral ventricles due to loss of periventricular white matter.

The infant gradually deteriorated and died at 11 months.

The brain at autopsy presented the effects of far-advanced chronic hypoxic cerebral damage, with the cerebral walls thinned, with the ventricles enlarged: ex vacuo hydrocephalus (Figure 493) (page 29).

Figure 492. Calcification of basal ganglia. Densities in the periventricular cerebral tissue bordering the lateral ventricles, in the region of the basal ganglia (dentate nuclei). Lateral ventricles enlarged. CT scan of brain 20 days after birth. Spasticity of extremities present neonatally.

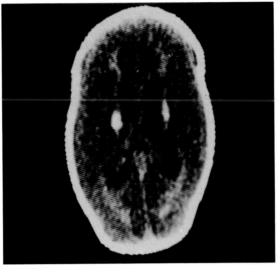

Fig. 492

Figure 493. Ex vacuo hydrocephalus of the cerebrum. Enlargement of ventricles due to loss of periventricular tissue. Hemispheric walls irregularly thinned; spongy cystic tissue in parts of remaining cerebral walls. Infant with cerebral palsy; death at 11 months. Frontal section of brain; autopsy specimen.

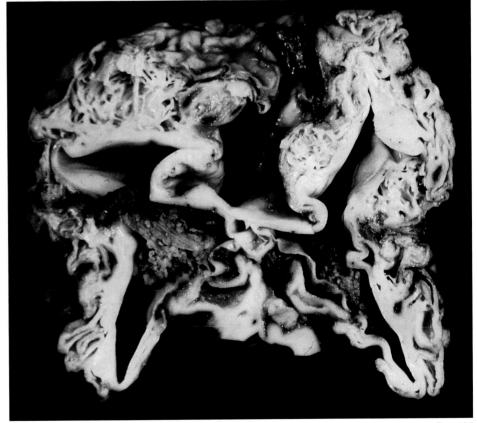

Fig. 493

A Case of **Maternal thyroid disorder; maternal excessive pregnancy weight gain. Infant developed cerebral palsy, mental retardation, seizure disorder.**

Excessive weight gain in this pregnancy reflected a major problem with bodily metabolism. This mother had a pregnancy weight gain of 50 pounds.

Excessive weight gain is associated with endocrine disorders, with diabetic conditions, pituitary disorder, and in this case is attributable to the mother's thyroid problem.

The optimal weight gain is about 20 pounds during pregnancy. When maternal weight gain is greater than 32 pounds, prenatal mortality increases.

Thyroid disease, carcinoma of the thyroid, was diagnosed two years previously in this mother, and a thyroidectomy was done. She subsequently was maintained on supplemental thyroid medication.

The thyroid exercises a major role in maintaining a normal gestation. The hazards to the fetus of maternal hypothyroidism or hyperthyroidism are well known. Although the mother appeared to be in thyroid balance, on thyroid medication, at the onset of pregnancy, the dilemma was, whether she needed more thyroid medication, which would risk creating hyperthyroidism, or whether she could be left alone regarding the thyroid dosage. As the gestation progressed, she showed no specific manifestations of hypothyroidism. Her blood pressure and other vital signs recorded during pregnancy were normal (blood pressure and heart rate are usually affected with thyroid imbalance).

However, one factor that stood out was the development of excessive weight gain, pregnancy obesity. Obesity is one of the primary signs of hypothyroidism. In the present case this condition proved a hazard, damaging to the fetus.

Maternal disorders cause fetal deprivation. The damaging effect on the fetus, the common denominator, is hypoxia. With acute and chronic maternal disorders, the oxygen requirements of the mother are increased, so that oxygenation of the fetus is depressed.

Labor developed at 42 weeks of the pregnancy. During descent of the fetus prolapse of the cord occurred. The infant was delivered by cesarean section.

Depression of the infant was present at delivery, but she responded to resuscitative care. The Apgar score, initially 4, rose to 8 at five minutes, with good respiratory effort and good muscle tone. At 4 hours, her cry was recorded as normal. At 9 hours after birth, responses were normal and at 17 hours she was "active and crying." Fontanelles were soft, indicating there was no brain swelling.

Her postnatal progress was interrupted by the onset of seizure activity during the afternoon of the first day.

Taking into consideration the good clinical course during the early postnatal period, it was conclusive that this newborn infant did not have acute hypoxic cerebral damage at the time of the onset of seizure activity. She could, however, with this clinical picture, have residues of old, subacute cerebral damage, damage incurred a long time before birth due to adversive gestational processes, damage not evident at birth, triggering the early onset of seizures, and becoming manifest as cerebral palsy, mental retardation, and seizure disorder months, years, later.

A Case of   *Pregnancy low weight gain; placental abruption.*
Newborn anemia. Infant developed cerebral
palsy, mental retardation, seizure disorder,
and microcephaly.

Two major problems that occurred during this pregnancy, maternal low weight gain and placental abruption, impacted on the fetus resulting in an enfeebled anemic newborn.

Low pregnancy weight gain occurred in midpregnancy. In the 10-week period between the twelfth and twenty-second weeks, when the mother should have gained about 8 pounds, she lost a pound. The implication here is plainly that this mother was not well. During the last 20 weeks of the pregnancy, during the time that women put on most of the weight during pregnancy, usually about 16 pounds, this mother gained 2 pounds.

Low weight gain is an ominous sign, indicating a disordered maternal metabolism with consequent poor fetal nutrition, impaired neonatal outcome. The present case is an example of this.

Abruption of the placenta, premature placental detachment, occurred causing vaginal bleeding during the last 2 weeks of the pregnancy. Bleeding became severe; the mother was transfused. A cesarean section was done, terminating the pregnancy at 38 weeks.

Retroplacental hemorrhage was present at delivery, described as "about 40 percent abruption placenta."

With detachment of a part of the placenta, a pocket forms between the placenta and the uterine wall, a pocket filled with blood clot, a retroplacental hematoma. That part of the placenta that is separated, walled off by the clot, is put out of function, leading to placental insufficiency, to interference with fetal oxygenation and nutrition (page 66).

Anemia was present in this newborn, confirmed in the newborn hematology reports: At birth the red blood cell count (RBC) was 3.88 million (normal, 5.14 million). The hemoglobin level was 13.4 grams (normal, 19 grams). The hematocrit level was 40.5 percent (normal, 61 percent).

The anemia present at birth had had its origin during intrauterine life. Prolonged anemia, in the fetus as in the adult human, causes chronic hypoxia. The red cell is the oxygen-carrying vehicle in the blood. The decrease in hematocrit means this fetus existed with less than the average amount of oxygen supply, chronic fetal hypoxia. Intrauterine hypoxia leads to fetal hypoxic visceral damage. The brain is the most sensitive target tissue in the body; with intrauterine hypoxia, the fetus accrues subacute and acute cerebral damage.

The cause of the intrauterine anemia remained open to question, as to whether it was due to fetal gestational deprivation or due to other gestational processes.

Depression of the infant was severe at delivery, with an Apgar score of 2 and 6. This was a weak fetus chronically enfeebled by adversive gestational factors, rendered chronically weakened, anemic, undernourished, unable to tolerate the stress of labor.

Although depressed at first, the infant improved after delivery, breathing on his own, with stable vital signs. Fontanelles were soft, not bulging, indicating there was no acute hypoxic brain swelling. At 5 hours, he was active and breathing well. Vital signs were stable.

This clinical picture, with the newborn infant 5 hours after delivery, active and breathing well, is not the clinical pattern of a newborn infant harboring fresh acute cerebral damage. Infants born with *acute* hypoxic cerebral damage do not improve in the hours after birth; they remain limp and comatose for prolonged periods, with unstable vital function, with respiratory failure, with congestive heart failure, for days. The newborn in this case was not like that after delivery.

The clinical pattern in this case is consistent with the syndromic pattern of latent subacute cerebral damage present at birth, damage incurred a period of time prior to birth, damage related to adversive processes during gestation, damage that is latent, silent at birth.

Seizure activity appeared in the infant during the first day. There is increasing clinical opinion that when seizures appear soon after birth, the process is not attributable to acute intranatal asphyxial brain damage, but rather, the cause must be sought in pathologic processes, brain damage, prior to birth (Chapter 5).

This child developed cerebral palsy. Cerebral palsy is caused by damage to the basal ganglia, located deep in the brain. This deep damage occurs consistently, specifically, only in the immature premature brain, during early fetal life, the consequence of maternal illness, and other complications during pregnancy. Adversive gestational processes exercise their damaging effects through the common denominator of intrauterine hypoxia. When the fetus is damaged during early fetal life, if the fetus survives to term, the infant is born with old subacute brain damage. Deep damage incurred in the premature brain (causing cerebral palsy) at times extends to the cerebral surface, to the cortex, resulting in cortical manifestations of mental retardation and epilepsy. This manifestly occurred in the present case.

The neurologic disabilities became increasingly severe during childhood.

MRI studies at 11 years showed extensive loss of substance of the cerebral walls, the late residual pattern of deep cerebral damage incurred in the premature immature fetus (Figure 494).

Microcephaly of severe degree occurred in this child. Normally the brain enlarges due to elaboration, growth, of the deep strata of the cerebrum. When the deep structures of the cerebrum are blighted during fetal life, growth of the brain is attenuated. With the brain becoming atrophied, shrunken, as in this case, the head remains small, microcephalic.

Figure 494. Cerebral atrophy in a case of severe cerebral palsy, with mental retardation and seizure disorder. MRI of brain at 11 years of age, parasagittal level of the brain. The shrunken cerebrum is separated from the inner surface of the skull, leaving a large space occupied by cerebrospinal fluid. The lateral ventricles are enlarged due to loss of periventricular tissue.

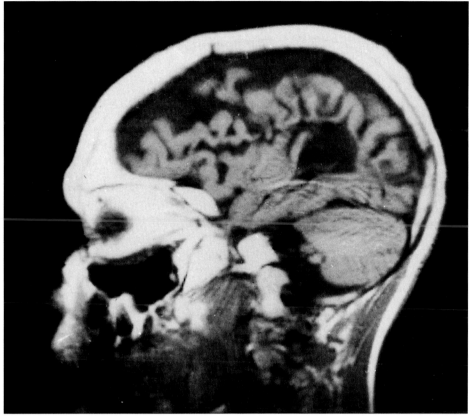

Fig. 494

A Case of   **Twin transfusion syndrome; one twin stillborn; surviving newborn with anemia. Infant later developed hydranencephaly, cerebral palsy, mental retardation, and seizure disorder.**

The present case is concerned with the survivor in a term twin gestation.

Toxemia had complicated the course of the pregnancy. The toxemia, developing in the last weeks of the pregnancy, was mild; there were, in addition to fluid retention, slight proteinuria, slight increase in blood pressure, hyperreflexia, and some apparent visual disturbance, "flashing lights."

Toxemia affects maternal organs, especially the kidneys, liver, brain, and circulatory system. The adverse effects on the fetus are ongoing, beginning with the first signs of the disorder in the mother (page 51).

Any kind of maternal physical or emotional illness directly affects the maternal-placental-fetal complex, compromising the fetus, exercising its effects through the common denominator of intrauterine hypoxia.

Decreased fetal activity was noted by the mother prior to delivery. Death of one of the fetuses was diagnosed. Cesarean section was done.

Twin A, this case, was liveborn. The infant was depressed at birth but responded to resuscitation and improved. Weight was 7 pounds 1 ounce.

Anemia was evident in this infant, described in the delivery room as "pale." The newborn hemoglobin level was 8.9 grams (the average is 18 grams for a term newborn). The infant was immediately transfused.

Twin B was stillborn. This infant, examined at autopsy, was plethoric; congestive heart failure was evident, with cardiac dilatation, with ascites and hydrothorax. Weight was 6 pounds 7 1/2 ounces.

The placenta was monochorionic diamniotic. Pathology examination revealed "vascular crossover apparent" in the placenta.

Taking into account that one twin was anemic and the other twin, stillborn, was plethoric, this case presents characteristics of the twin transfusion syndrome.

In the twin transfusion syndrome, with the circulatory system of the fetuses connected by vascular anastomoses in the placenta, one fetus becomes the donor, sending blood to the other fetus, the recipient. The donor becomes anemic, the recipient becomes plethoric, overloaded with blood and fluid (page 97).

The recipient fetus usually is larger; however in some instances, as in the present case, the fetuses remained about the same size. The pathologic intrauterine processes may lead to death of the anemic donor or to the plethoric recipient, or to death of both fetuses.

The surviving infant in the present case developed cerebral palsy and other cerebral disabilities.

Cerebral palsy is due to damage to the basal ganglia located in the deep portion of the cerebrum. Damage to the deep structures, to the basal ganglia, occurs consistently in the premature (immature) fetus following gestational hypoxia-producing complications. Fetuses that survive to term are born harboring latent subacute lesions in the deep periventricular structures and later develop cerebral palsy.

At the time of the hypoxic process in the premature period, the cerebral damage may extend from the deep structures through the wall of the cerebrum, damaging the cortex, causing (in addition to the cerebral palsy) mental retardation and seizure disorder.

Regarding the cause of the intrauterine hypoxia that led to fetal cerebral damage, while the mother's toxemia compromised fetal well-being, pathologically, most important, is the fact that the surviving newborn had been subjected to chronic anemia, with associated chronic hypoxia, during fetal life.

Chronic anemia, in the fetus as in the adult human, causes chronic hypoxia. The red cell hemoglobin is the oxygen-carrying vehicle of the blood. In the present case, the decrease in hemoglobin to 50 percent of normal means this fetus existed with less than half the average amount of oxygen.

CT scans of the brain taken after the infant developed cerebral palsy and other severe cerebral disabilities, at age 3, showed extreme loss of cerebral substance in a pattern of hydranencephaly (Figure 495).

Hydranencephaly, as in the present case, represents an extreme example of hydrocephalus ex vacuo. The pathogenesis: the enlargement of the ventricles is due to the process of periventricular cerebral hypoxic venous infarction beginning in the premature fetal cerebrum. In the course of time, months, years, after birth, the damaged, necrotic, periventricular strata in the ventricle wall are slowly absorbed, with resulting thinning of the wall from within (page 29).

Figure 495. Hydranencephaly. CT scan of brain at 3 years. In the scan, above and laterally, the cranial vault is translucent, with the structure of the cerebrum effaced, replaced by fluid. In contrast, the lower part of the scan shows the image of the cerebellum and brain stem relatively intact.

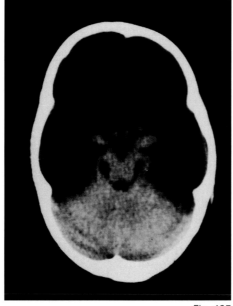

Fig. 495

A Case of **_Cytomegalic viral disease of newborn. Infant
developed cerebral palsy and mental retardation._**

The infant in the present case, in the postnatal clinical course and in the late chronic neurologic pattern, presented substantial manifestations of cytomegaloviral disease. This syndrome disorder, overlooked in the past and now recognized increasingly in neonates, is characterized by postnatal enlargement of the liver and spleen, anemia, hyperbilirubinemia, and neurologically by lethargy and weakness (page 118).

The maternal record in this case revealed no substantial adverse gestational conditions. Delivery occurred at 39 weeks of pregnancy, a spontaneous vaginal birth.

The infant was "very depressed" at birth, and the infant remained lethargic during the postnatal period.

On day 2 jaundice developed, with the bilirubin level rising to 15.2. The liver and spleen were much enlarged. The infant was anemic and leukopenic. Hepatosplenomegaly persisted.

Pathologically there are four common causes of hepatosplenomegaly with jaundice in the newborn: (1) congestive heart failure, (2) isoimmune reaction to Rh incompatibility (erythroblastosis), (3) systemic sepsis associated with acute processes such as pneumonia, urinary tract infection, (4) specific acute neonatal infection, commonly cytomegalovirus disease.

In this case there was no clinical evidence of congestive heart failure or erythroblastosis; there was no septic process diagnosed, such as pneumonia. Elements consistent with cytomegalovirus disease were present clinically and pathologically.

The damage in the brain with cytomegalovirus infection is primarily in periventricular structures (white matter and basal ganglia) and is ongoing during fetal life. In some case, in the newborn, calcifications are evident in x-ray studies of the brain.

Damage to the deep cerebral structures results in manifestations of cerebral palsy, and with extension of the cerebral damage to the cortex, mental retardation and other cortical disabilities result. This was the clinical-pathologic pattern in the present case.

Cytomegalic infection in women is of high incidence (50 to 70 percent have CMV antibodies serologically) but only in a small percent does the maternal infection become transmitted through the placenta and cause fetal-neonatal infection and organic damage during gestation. CMV is asymptomatic during gestation, and the diagnosis is not made prior to delivery. The importance of CMV disease in the newborn was generally overlooked in the past and the diagnosis was missed clinically and pathologically.

CMV is the most frequent perinatal viral disease. It has been estimated to involve 8 per 1,000 births and to be responsible for brain damage in 1 per 1,000 births.

A Case of   *Maternal anemia. Newborn with anemia, with intrauterine growth retardation, developed disseminated intravascular coagulopathy (DIC). Infant later developed cerebral palsy, mental retardation, and seizure disorder.*

The prenatal record indicated two significant details, the mother's anemia and the prelabor decrease of fetal activity.

Anemia in the mother developed in midpregnancy. In the 24-week period between the ninth week and the thirty-third week, the hematocrit dropped from 38.5 percent to 30.5 percent (normal, 35 percent to 47 percent); the hemoglobin level dropped from 12.6 grams to 10.2 grams (normal, 12 to 15 grams).

Although blood levels usually drop somewhat during pregnancy, the reported blood levels in this case were unacceptably low. Maternal anemia is associated with fetal deprivation.

Anemia involves a decrease in the red cells in the blood, a decrease in hemoglobin. Hemoglobin is the oxygen-carrying vehicle in the blood. Accordingly, anemia, as in this case, compromised oxygenation of the mother, with resulting decreased oxygen supply to the placenta and to the fetus.

Fetal activity decreased during the days before labor, indicating that adversive gestational factors, maternal anemia, had impacted on the fetus (page 169).

Nonstress test was nonreactive.

Labor began soon after the nonstress test. The monitor tracing showed late decelerations. Emergency cesarean section was done.

Amniotic fluid was bloody. Retroplacental hemorrhage, a marginal abruption, was found, the cause of the bloody amniotic fluid.

Delivery was at near term, at 37 weeks of gestation.

Depression of the newborn was severe, the infant was almost lifeless. Apgar score was 1 at one minute, 1 at five minutes, 3 at ten minutes.

What was the cause of the neurologic depression of this newborn infant? Was it due to acute fresh brain damage? Or was it due to the fact that this fetus (newborn) was chronically compromised during intrauterine life, with the fetus anemic, enfeebled, unable to tolerate the stress of labor, and with the newborn consequently exhausted, depressed at birth? The infant slowly responded to resuscitation, with improved cardiac function and respiration, improved color, and muscle tone, and was active at 3 hours.

The fontanelles in this baby remained soft, normal, not bulging. This is most important with regard to the presence or absence of acute fresh brain damage. Pathologically, in infants as in adults, acute brain damage causes the brain to "soak up" fluid, causes cerebral edema, causes swelling; this causes the brain to press against the (soft) fontanelles, causing bulging of the fontanelles. Pathologically, the absence of bulging fontanelles, the presence of soft, flat fontanelles, rules out the presence of acute brain damage in this newborn infant.

Intrauterine growth retardation (IUGR) was evident in this newborn infant. This baby was small, at 37 weeks of gestation weighing 2,260 grams (5 pounds), in the tenth percentile for weight. (Average weight at 37 weeks is 2,800 grams, 6 pounds 4 ounces.)

IUGR is associated with inadequate fetal nutrition and inadequate oxygenation, so that the fetus is subject to the accruing of varying severity of silent subacute cerebral damage. Pathologically, this kind of latent subacute damage has been confirmed in the past in autopsy studies, observed in IUGR infants that die during delivery or soon after birth. In infants surviving, the latent cerebral damage ultimately is manifested as cerebral palsy and other cerebral disability. A high incidence of cerebral palsy develops in IUGR infants.

Anemia was apparent early on, with the infant described as pale immediately at birth. Pale means anemia. Anemia was confirmed in the newborn hematology reports.

At birth the red blood cell count (RBC) was 3.82 million (normal, 5.14 million). The hematocrit level was 42.4 percent (normal, 61 percent).

Chronic anemia, in the fetus as in the adult human, causes chronic hypoxia. The red cell hemoglobin is the oxygen-carrying vehicle in the blood. The decrease in hematocrit means this fetus existed with less than the average amount of oxygen supply, chronic fetal hypoxia.

The fact that this was a chronic anemia is indicated by the hematology report of 61 NRBCs, per 100 cells, meaning 61 nucleated red cells per 100 white blood cells. Normally, term newborn infants have an average of 8 nucleated red blood cells per 100 white blood cells. In the present case there were more than seven times the average number of nucleated red blood cells in the blood of this newborn. Nucleated red cells in excessive number in the fetal blood means there has been chronic fetal anemia (page 96).

As in other cases, the cause of the fetal-neonatal anemia is open to question. Significantly, this was a malnourished feeble newborn, reflective of intrauterine deprivation. Anemia present at birth is reflective of intrauterine compromise.

DIC, disseminated intravascular coagulopathy, was diagnosed neonatally, on day 3. DIC is a bleeding disorder that develops in debilitated infants and adults (page 114).

DIC was manifested in the present case as bleeding from the umbilical stump, bloody urine, bloody fluid suctioned from the respiratory tract, and bleeding from needle puncture sites.

DIC is characterized by decreased thrombocytes (platelets) in the blood. In the infant in the present case, the platelet level fell to 20,000 (normally 150,000 to 200,000). The infant was transfused. Bleeding gradually decreased.

Seizure activity in this infant began soon after birth. The occurrence of seizures in the newborn period does not automatically make certain that the underlying cerebral damage was incurred during labor and delivery. There is increasing clinical opinion that when seizures appear soon after birth, the process is not attributable to acute intranatal asphyxial brain damage, but rather, the cause must be sought in pathologic processes, brain damage, prior to birth (Chapter 5).

CT scans of the brain neonatally showed evidence of far-advanced loss of cerebral substance in the newborn infant (Figure 496). This indicates that cerebral damage had originated a long time before birth, during early fetal life.

In summary, this was an enfeebled sick infant who had incurred hypoxic cerebral damage during gestation due to hypoxia-producing effects of maternal anemia and fetal anemia, with adversive effects compounded by postnatal DIC. Hypoxic cerebral damage incurred during early fetal life resulted in the development of cerebral palsy and other cerebral disabilities (Chapter 3).

Figure 496. CT scan of brain showing diffuse low density throughout the cerebral hemispheres, indicating far-advanced loss of substance in the cerebral white matter. Large cavum septi pellucidi, appearing as a midline clear cystic structure; lateral ventricles normal size. Infant of 37 weeks' gestation; CT scan at 18 days of age.

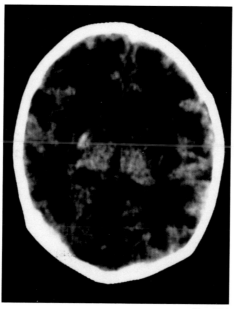

Fig. 496

A Case of **Teenage mother, with prediabetes, excessive pregnancy weight gain. Postmature microcephalic newborn with intrauterine growth retardation, anemia, cardiac malformation. Infant developed cerebral palsy, mental retardation, seizure disorder.**

Teenage pregnancy, as occurred in this case, is a factor adverse to the fetus. The mother had just turned 18 at the beginning of this gestation. This mother was a primipara, also a factor unfavorable to the fetus. There is an increased incidence of fetal and neonatal morbidity and mortality with young primiparous mothers and an increased incidence of cerebral palsy in offspring of young primiparous mothers.

Psychiatric stress was reflected in the circumstances of pregnancy for this unmarried young mother. There is increasing evidence clinically and experimentally that maternal emotional stress, in the same way as physical illness, has adverse effects on the fetus.

Excessive weight gain occurred. This mother indicated her normal weight was 127 pounds. At term, she weighed 177 pounds, a weight gain of 50 pounds. The average optimal weight gain is between 20 and 30 pounds.

Excessive maternal weight gain, of the degree in the present case, is usually of metabolic origin; it reflects endocrine dysfunction, metabolic disorders, such as latent diabetes or thyroid disorder, and exercises an adversive effect on the fetus.

Prediabetes in a latent form was apparent in this mother (page 49). There was a family history of diabetes. The mother gained excessive weight in the pregnancy, common in maternal diabetic conditions.

In people who become diabetic, the bodily dysfunctions have origin many years before the diabetes. Maternal prediabetes (or diabetes) effects an unfavorable uterine environment, exercises a damaging effect on the fetus, extending over the entire length of the gestational period. In these circumstances there is a high incidence of stillbirths.

Malformation of the heart, cardiac hypertrophy, was diagnosed in the newborn infant. This finding is relevant with regard to maternal prediabetes. Cardiac defects are common in offspring of mothers with diabetic conditions (page 48).

In mothers with diabetes, the pathologic mechanism causing stillbirths and malformations, the mechanism causing the injurious effects on the fetus, is not known. Often the newborn infant, born alive, "just doesn't do well." In surviving infants there is a high incidence of cerebral palsy.

Decreased fetal activity was reported by the mother during the last month. Decreased fetal activity reflects fetal compromise, fetal enfeeblement. There is substantial clinical and pathologic evidence that with maternal pregnancy problems exercising adversive effects on the fetus, the compromised fetus, depressed and hypoxic, gradually becomes comatose, paralyzed, manifested as a loss of fetal activity. This may happen before there is a change in fetal heart action. This loss of fetal activity is known as the "fetal alarm signal." The compromised weakened fetus may succumb, or the process may be sublethal with the fetus recovering activity. Fetal kicking may be a better indicator of fetal health than the heartbeat (page 169).

Labor onset did not occur until postterm, at 43 weeks of gestation. After 5 hours of desultory labor, with the fetal monitor tracing showing repeated late deceleration, interpreted to mean fetal distress, cesarean section was done.

Depression of the newborn of moderate degree was evident at birth. The Apgar score was 3 and 6. The infant responded to care in the delivery room, with spontaneous respiration and improved color.

Postmaturity was evidenced by gestational dates, indicating 43 weeks, and by physical findings on examination of the infant. The skin was thick and peeling, evidence of postmaturity. Likewise the footprint showed wide creases, extending to the heel, consistent with postmaturity. The creases on the sole of the foot in the premature appear only on the upper part of the foot and gradually extend downward toward the heel at maturity. In this newborn, as noted, the initial footprint showed creases down into the heel, postmaturity.

IUGR, intrauterine growth retardation, dysmaturity, was apparent in the infant, as well as postmaturity.

The weight-length ratio, known as the Ponderal Index, is a measure of fetal nutrition (page 94). In the present case the PI was 2.06, far below the tenth percentile. As indicated by the low PI, this fetus was chronically deprived, malnourished, dysmature.

Viewed in another way, this newborn weighed 2,820 grams, in the tenth percentile for term, more than a pound underweight. (Average at term is 3,300 grams.) The newborn length was 51.5 centimeters, at the eightieth percentile. This was a long thin newborn, dysmature, IUGR.

Intrauterine growth retardation varies in severity and is due to periods of fetal deprivation resulting from maternal disorders, and other gestational processes that compromise the integrity of the maternal-uterine-placental-fetal complex. Fetal dysmaturity is associated with inadequate fetal nutrition and inadequate oxygenation, so that the fetus is born with varying silent subacute cerebral damage. Pathologically, this kind of latent subacute damage has been confirmed in the past in autopsy studies, observed in dysmature infants that die during delivery or soon after birth. In infants surviving, the latent cerebral damage ultimately is manifested as cerebral palsy and other cerebral disability. A high incidence of cerebral palsy develops in infants with IUGR.

Fetal-neonatal anemia was demonstrated in this newborn. At birth, the hematocrit was 49.9 percent. Normal for newborn is 61 +/- 7.4 percent. The hematocrit measures the quantity of red cells in the blood. In the present case, correspondingly, the hemoglobin level was 15.5 grams (average for newborn is 19 grams).

Chronic anemia, in the fetus as in the adult human, causes chronic hypoxia. The red cell is the oxygen-carrying vehicle in the blood. The decrease in hematocrit means this fetus existed with much less than the average amount of oxygen supply: chronic severe fetal hypoxia.

The fact that this was a longstanding intrauterine anemia is indicated by the hematology report of greatly increased numbers of nucleated red cells (NRBCs), 49.5 per 100 white blood cells, present in the newborn blood count (normal for newborn at term is 8 to 20) (page 96).

One of the important elements in defining the causal mechanism in this case, in defining the pathogenesis of the brain damage, is the fact that this fetus had been subjected to chronic anemia, with associated chronic intrauterine hypoxia.

Microcephaly, an obviously small head, was noted at birth. The head circumference was 31 centimeters, below the tenth percentile. The average circumference at term is 33 to 34 centimeters.

The growth of the head during fetal life reflects the growth, the enlargement, of the brain during fetal life. Growth of the cerebrum is dependent not on an elaboration of surface strata, but on a healthy proliferation of the deep cerebral structures. Damage to deep cerebral structures during early fetal life causes attenuation of growth of the brain, of the head, as was evident at birth in this baby. Delay in head growth continued after birth, a common characteristic in cases of cerebral palsy.

Seizures occurred in this infant soon after birth. The early postnatal occurrence of seizures in the newborn period does not mean that the underlying cerebral damage was incurred during labor and delivery. There is increasing clinical opinion that when seizures appear soon after birth, the process is not attributable to acute intranatal asphyxial brain damage, but rather that the cause must be sought in pathologic processes, brain damage, prior to birth (Chapter 5).

Cerebral palsy developed in this infant. Cerebral palsy is caused by damage to the basal ganglia, located deep in the brain. This deep damage occurs consistently, specifically, only in the immature premature brain, during early fetal life. The deep damage is due to hypoxia-producing gestational processes such as, in this case, maternal disorders and intrauterine fetal anemia.

If the fetus survives, the acute lesions in the cerebrum become subacute, old. With the gestation reaching term, the infant is born harboring latent subacute cerebral damage.

Deep damage incurred in the premature brain (causing cerebral palsy) at times extends to the cerebral surface, to the cortex, later resulting in cortical manifestations of mental retardation and seizure disorder. This is the pattern of pathogenesis manifested in the present case.

A Case of   *Subacute cerebral infarction in newborn infant; macrosomia. Mother with hypotension, syncope; excessive pregnancy weight gain. Infant later developed hemiplegic cerebral palsy.*

The health of this mother during pregnancy was not robust. Although this mother, overall, gained weight excessively, there was a period when, paradoxically, she failed to gain weight appropriately. Apparently she was sick; she failed to come to her regular prenatal visit; she became anemic.

Any kind of maternal illness during pregnancy, physical or emotional illness, directly affects the maternal-placental-fetal complex, compromising the fetus. Pathologically, the causal process exercises its effects through the common denominator of intrauterine hypoxia. Intrauterine hypoxia leads to fetal hypoxia, to cerebral hypoxic damage.

Hypotension, maternal low blood pressure, persisted during this pregnancy, with levels ranging 20 to 30 millimeters below average. With regard to the effect of hypotension on the uterus during pregnancy, just as there was inadequate blood going to the brain and other organs, there would correspondingly be inadequate arterial perfusion to the uterus, to the placenta — fetal hypoxia (page 53).

The mother had a long history of recurrent syncope, fainting spells. Seizures occurred with episodes of syncope, with loss of consciousness. Syncope was related to the mother's chronic low blood pressure, to faulty perfusion of blood to the brain.

Seizures in the mother during pregnancy, associated with apnea and cyanosis, exert stress on the mother, consequently adversive to the fetus.

Excessive weight gain occurred during this pregnancy. The average optimal weight gain is 20 to 25 pounds. This mother's usual weight was 125 pounds. She weighed 169 3/4 pounds at term, an increase of 45 pounds.

Excessive maternal weight gain, of the degree in the present case, is usually of metabolic origin, due to endocrine dysfunctions such as in diabetic conditions.

Was there a factor of latent prediabetes in this case? This mother presented two prime markers of latent diabetes: excessive pregnancy weight gain and a macrosomic baby.

In people who become diabetic, the bodily dysfunctions have origin many years before the diabetes becomes overt. Maternal prediabetes (or diabetes) creates an unfavorable uterine environment, exercises a damaging effect on the fetus, extending over the entire length of the gestational period. In diabetic mothers, the pathologic mechanism causing the macrosomia, the injurious effects on the fetus, is not known. Often the newborn infant, born alive, "just doesn't do well." In surviving infants there is a high incidence of epilepsy and cerebral palsy.

Labor ensued at 41 weeks of pregnancy. Prenatally the fetus was estimated to be large, up to 9 pounds.

After 8 hours of desultory labor, and because of the mother's persisting hypotension, a cesarean section was done.

The newborn infant was in good condition at delivery, with an Apgar of 9 and 9. Initially he was stable and active, recorded as "doing well during the first 24 hours."

Macrosomia was diagnosed at delivery. The newborn weighed 9 pounds 3 ounces (4,134 grams), was oversized, macrosomic, above the ninetieth percentile for weight. Macrosomia of this newborn is attributable to the mother's disordered metabolism, the mother's excessive weight gain. Macrosomic infants are feeble, do not do well. Big does not mean strong, robust. Some are stillborn or die soon after birth. Macrosomia is commonly the first evidence of latent diabetes in the mother. Macrosomic babies, the offspring of mothers with diabetic conditions, have an increased incidence of cerebral palsy.

Seizure activity developed in the infant on day 2, compromising the infant's initial good clinical course. The occurrence of seizures in the newborn period does not automatically make certain that the underlying cerebral damage was incurred during labor and delivery. There is increasing clinical opinion that when seizures appear soon after birth, the process is not attributable to acute intranatal asphyxial brain damage, but rather, the cause must be sought in pathologic processes, brain damage, prior to birth.

CT scans done after the seizure onset on day 2 indicated that there was extensive cerebral damage. The radiologist reported "diminished attenuation is present involving the caudate nucleus on the left and the left parietal lobe. These findings are consistent with infarction" (Figure 497).

When was this infant's brain damage incurred? Was this fresh acute brain damage?

Clinically, the valid assessment of the presence or absence of acute fresh brain damage is determined by the performance of the infant in the hours after delivery. This newborn infant had a good Apgar score and was described as vigorous and active, with good respiratory function, in no distress. On the first day in the nursery he was in an open crib, taking water by mouth, and was bathed and breast-fed. This is not the clinical pattern of a newborn with acute diffuse cerebral damage. Newborn infants who have acute diffuse brain damage are depressed at delivery and stay depressed, comatose, flaccid, with unstable vital signs.

In the present case, considered retrospectively, this was a fetus chronically compromised by adverse maternal gestational processes, a macrosomic feeble newborn who during the first day responded to care and did well, then decompensated after the onset of seizures.

Clinically the pattern in the present case is compatible with the presence of subacute cerebral damage incurred early in fetal life, present at birth.

Pathologically, likewise, the cerebral damage was of subacute nature. The pattern of damage evident in the neonatal CT scan, the degree of disintegration of the damaged tissue, reflects a process of long standing, weeks old, a pattern of subacute damage.

Cerebral palsy developed in this infant. Correlating pathologic and clinical factors — with the cerebral damage more extensive on the left (Figure 498), the cerebral palsy manifestations that developed were more severe on the right side of the body, hemiplegic cerebral palsy.

Figure 497. CT scan of brain on day 2 showing a large subacute cerebral infarction. The left cerebral hemisphere shows an area of decreased density, mainly on the left, involving the deep strata of the frontal and temporal lobes. (The left side of the brain appears on the right in the illustration.) The greatest damage is in the region of the basal ganglia on the left. On the right, in the frontal lobe, the deep white matter appears of decreased density. Ventricles are patent.

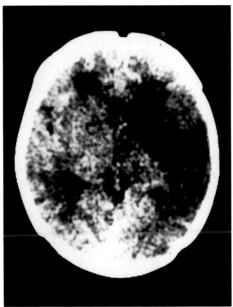

Fig. 497

Figure 498. CT scan of brain at 8 months. Porencephalic cavitation involving the temporoparietal portion of the left cerebrum, extending from the periventricular location, obliterating most of the caudate nucleus and adjoining white matter, leaving a surface layer with cortex in the surrounding insula. In the porencephalic cavity, a V-shaped density, a focus of calcification. The lateral ventricles are enlarged, especially the body of the left lateral ventricle, forming ex vacuo hydrocephalus. Infant with hemiplegic cerebral palsy, with the right extremities mainly affected.

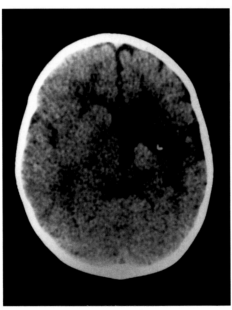

Fig. 498

A Case of **Maternal hypotension, preeclampsia. Newborn with anemia, early-onset seizures, xanthochromic spinal fluid. Infant developed cerebral palsy, mental retardation, seizure disorder, and microcephaly.**

Hypotension, chronic low blood pressure, was noted in this mother's medical records. Through most of this pregnancy the diastolic pressure ranged around 50 to 60 (normal is 80), with the systolic pressure ranging around 100 (normal is 120).

With regard to the effect of hypotension on the uterus during pregnancy, there is inadequate arterial perfusion to the uterus, to the placenta, causing fetal hypoxia. This hypotensive lack of perfusion is increased when the mother is lying down, during the hours of sleep; the condition is well known obstetrically.

Preeclampsia (toxemia) developed during this pregnancy, extending over a period of weeks in midpregnancy, with rapid weight gain (retention of fluid), peripheral edema, severe headache, vision disturbances, and proteinuria. Also, the mother, usually hypotensive, during this time had an elevation of blood pressure.

With toxemia, maternal renal, hepatic, and other metabolic disturbances that occur affect not only the mother but also the fetus. There is a high incidence of fetal and neonatal mortality, from 3 to 10 percent, reported in cases of preeclampsia and eclampsia (page 51).

Birth occurred at term, a spontaneous vaginal delivery.

Depression of severe degree was evident in the infant at birth. The Apgar score was 2 and 5. The infant soon improved and at 1 hour was alert, moving about, with spontaneous respiration.

Anemia was apparent in the newborn infant, noted to be pale at birth. Anemia was confirmed in the newborn hematology reports. The red blood cell count (RBC) was 3.35 million (normal, 5.14 million). The hemoglobin level was 11.1 grams (normal, 19 grams). Hematocrit level was 33.6 percent (normal, 61 percent).

The newborn infant was transfused.

Chronic anemia, in the fetus as in the adult human, causes chronic hypoxia. The red cell is the oxygen-carrying vehicle in the blood. The decrease in hematocrit means this fetus existed with less than the average amount of oxygen supply, chronic fetal hypoxia.

Intrauterine hypoxia leads to fetal hypoxic visceral damage. The brain is the most sensitive target tissue in the body; with intrauterine hypoxia, the fetus accrues acute and subacute cerebral damage.

Regarding the cause of the fetal-neonatal anemia, clinically it was thought this was an example of fetal-maternal transfusion syndrome. The transfer of blood from fetal to maternal circulation occurs regularly, to some degree, in most if not all gestations. The degree, the amount, of transfusion varies, is severe in some instances. The cause, the pathogenesis, of the fetal-maternal transfusion process is thought to be associated with pathologic processes that damage elements of the placenta, as occurs with placental infarction. In the present case there were small infarctions of the placenta. Fetal hemorrhage into the maternal circulation is probably the commonest cause of anemia in the newborn (page 97).

Seizure activity appeared soon after birth, at 14 hours. The question arose as to whether such seizure activity reflected the presence of acute cerebral damage, or whether the seizure activity was due to old subacute damage incurred before birth, due to hypoxia during fetal life prior to term.

The valid assessment of the presence or absence of acute fresh brain damage is determined clinically by the performance of the infant in the hours after delivery. This infant, depressed at birth, soon responded and was awake, alert, moving his extremities, with good suck, grasp, and Moro reflexes. At 2 hours, muscle tone was good; he was crying lustily. This is not the clinical pattern of a newborn with acute diffuse cerebral damage. Newborn infants who have acute diffuse brain damage are depressed at delivery and do not soon improve; they stay depressed, comatose, flaccid, with unstable vital signs.

Did this infant have latent old, subacute cerebral damage, damage not manifested at birth?

A fetus subjected to adverse conditions during intrauterine life often accrues cerebral damage. If the fetus survives to term, the cerebral damage, at first acute, later becomes subacute, old; the infant is born harboring old cerebral damage.

Relevant to the presence of subacute cerebral damage, this newborn was found to have xanthochromic spinal fluid. Xanthochromic spinal fluid was found in the spinal tap done at 15 hours, subsequent to the onset of seizures. The finding of xanthochromic (*xantho-,* yellow; *-chromia,* color) spinal fluid in this case is of major importance in defining the time of incurrence of the cerebral damage. Xanthochromia, yellow coloration of the spinal fluid, is due to the presence of old hemorrhagic damage in the brain.

Regarding the early onset of seizures in this case, with cerebral damage incurred during early intrauterine life, with the damage originating deep in the cerebrum and extending to the cortical surface, with the fetus surviving to term, the lesions in the cortex become subacute, and are capable of causing seizure activity soon after birth (Chapter 5).

This infant developed cerebral palsy. Cerebral palsy is caused by damage to the basal ganglia, located deep in the brain. This deep damage occurs consistently, specifically, only in the immature premature brain, during early fetal life, the consequence of maternal complications and intrauterine fetal pathologic processes. When the fetus is damaged during early fetal life, if the fetus survives to term, the infant is born with old subacute brain damage. Deep damage incurred in the premature brain (causing cerebral palsy) at times extends to the cerebral surface, to the cortex, resulting in cortical manifestations of mental retardation, seizures, and other cortical disabilities.

Microcephaly was evident in early infancy. With deep brain damage occurring during fetal life, with destruction of periventricular tissue, the brain is decreased in size, fails to grow normally, and the head consequently remains relatively small, microcephalic.

A Case of   *Maternal diabetes. Fetal-neonatal anemia.*
              Infant developed cerebral palsy, mental retardation,
              seizure disorder; porencephaly, microcephaly.

Diabetes was diagnosed in the mother during this pregnancy. Characteristic of mothers with diabetic conditions, the mother in the past delivered three oversized, macrosomic, babies, up to 11 pounds in weight. She had a family history of diabetes.

The pathologic processes of diabetes contributed substantially to the fetal compromise, fetal debility, in this case. In people who become diabetic, the bodily dysfunctions have origin many years before the diabetes. Maternal diabetes affects an unfavorable uterine environment, exercises a damaging effect on the fetus, extending over the entire length of the gestational period. Spontaneous abortion is common in diabetic conditions.

In mothers with diabetic processes, the pathologic mechanism causing the injurious effects on the fetus is not well understood. Often infants of mothers with a diabetic condition, even with optimal diabetic control, "just don't do well." In surviving infants there is a high incidence of epilepsy and cerebral palsy.

Characteristic of people who have diabetes, this mother presented two commonly linked medical problems of diabetes — obesity and hypertension — both conditions adverse to fetal well-being.

Hypertension of chronic nature was present in this mother; she was being treated for this during this pregnancy. Pregnancy hypertension jeopardizes the fetus by compromising the uteroplacental blood flow. Compromise of placental blood supply leads to fetal hypoxia (page 52).

Obesity was present in this diabetic mother. At 5 feet 1 inch and weighing 168 pounds, she was described as "appearing obese." Obesity is a hazard to the pregnant mother and her fetus. Obesity is reflective of a disturbed bodily metabolism.

Low pregnancy weight gain occurred. Despite her obesity, she failed to gain weight appropriately in the second trimester, a concern noted in the prenatal clinical record. In a person with diabetes, inappropriate weight gain is an ominous sign. Overall, in the last two trimesters, in a period when she should have gained about 20 pounds, she gained 14 pounds.

Low weight gain is adverse to the fetus and is associated with impaired neonatal outcome.

Labor contractions of mild form were apparent at 38 weeks of the pregnancy. Nonstress tests in the previous two weeks were reactive.

An oxytocin challenge test was done at this time. Late decelerations appeared and were persistent. Delivery by emergency cesarean section was carried out.

Depression of the newborn was present, with the Apgar score being 2 and 6. The infant responded to resuscitation and at ten minutes was given an Apgar score of 10. The infant was of ordinary weight, 7 1/2 pounds. (Although babies of diabetic mothers are overweight, macrosomic, in almost one-third of cases, in the other two-thirds of cases the newborn are average size, as in this infant, or are of low birth weight.)

Anemia was evident at birth. The newborn infant was noted to be pale. Anemia was confirmed in the newborn hematology reports. At birth the red blood cell count (RBC) was 4.1 million (normal, 5.14 million). The hemoglobin level was 15.2 grams (normal, 19 grams). The hematocrit level was 45.7 percent (normal, 61 percent).

The newborn infant was transfused to bring the hematocrit level up.

Chronic anemia, in the fetus as in the adult human, causes chronic hypoxia.

Intrauterine hypoxia leads to fetal hypoxic visceral damage. The brain is the most sensitive target tissue in the body; with intrauterine hypoxia, the fetus accrues subacute and acute cerebral damage.

The cause of the anemia in the present case was thought to be an intrauterine fetal-maternal transfusion process. Regarding the occurrence of the fetal-maternal transfusion syndrome, the transfer of blood from fetal to maternal circulation occurs regularly, to some degree, in most if not all gestations. The degree, the amount of transfusion, varies, but is severe in some instances. The cause, the pathogenesis, of the fetal-maternal transfusion process is thought to be associated with pathologic processes that damage elements of the placenta, as occurs with placental infarction. In the present case there were small infarctions of the placenta. Fetal hemorrhage into the maternal circulation is probably the commonest cause of anemia in the newborn (page 97).

Regarding the newborn depression, considered retrospectively, this was a sick fetus, chronically enfeebled by adverse maternal factors, rendered chronically weakened, anemic, unable to tolerate the stress of labor. Although depressed at first, he continued to improve after delivery, breathing on his own, with stable vital signs. Fontanelles remained soft and flat, indicating there was no acute brain swelling. In the hours after delivery the infant was awake, moving about, responsive.

When was this infant's brain damage incurred? Pathologically, was there *fresh* brain damage present in this newborn at delivery?

Infants born with acute hypoxic cerebral damage do not improve in the hours after birth; they remain limp and comatose for prolonged periods, with unstable vital function, with respiratory failure, with congestive heart failure, with bulging fontanelles.

The newborn in this case was not like that after delivery.

The clinical pattern in this case is consistent with the syndromic pattern of latent subacute cerebral damage present at birth, damage incurred a period of time prior to birth, damage related to adverse pathologic processes during gestation.

Seizure activity developed in the infant soon after birth. The question arose as to whether such seizure activity reflected the presence of acute cerebral damage or whether the seizure activity was due to cerebral damage incurred before birth, due to hypoxic cerebral damage during fetal life prior to term.

The occurrence of seizures in the newborn period does not automatically make certain that the underlying cerebral damage was incurred during labor and delivery. There is increasing clinical opinion that when seizures appear soon after birth, the process is not attributable to acute intranatal asphyxial brain damage, but rather, the cause must be sought in pathologic processes, brain damage, prior to birth.

Cerebral palsy developed in this surviving infant. Cerebral palsy is caused by damage to the basal ganglia, located deep in the brain. This deep damage occurs consistently, specifically, only in the immature premature brain, during early fetal life and is due to hypoxia-producing pathologic intrauterine processes, such as anemia, as occurred in this fetus. When the fetus is damaged during early fetal life, if the fetus survives to term, the infant is born with old subacute brain damage. Deep damage incurred in the premature brain (causing cerebral palsy) at times extends to the cerebral surface, to the cortex, resulting in cortical manifestations of mental retardation and epilepsy.

CT studies of the brain were done over a period of months. In the CT scan done on day 10, the radiologist reported, "There are small areas of increased density adjacent to the mid posterior bodies of the lateral ventricles bilaterally that are believed to represent areas of subependymal hemorrhage. The ventricles are normal in size" (Figure 499). The presence of patent ventricles, together with the absence of bulging fontanelles through the postnatal days, is evidence that no cerebral edema, no swelling of the brain, no acute fresh brain damage was present. Pathologically, acute brain damage, when present, causes the brain to become edematous, swollen. Such cerebral edema, when present, is evidenced in the CT scan by compression of the ventricle spaces and evidenced clinically by bulging fontanelles.

The presence of hemorrhage as noted in the CT scan does not mean that the lesions were fresh, acute. Periventricular lesions originating during early fetal life are hemorrhagic and at times continue to bleed for a prolonged period after birth.

CT scan of the brain done at 2 1/2 months indicated the presence of a porencephalic cavity and hydrocephalus ex vacuo, enlarged cerebral ventricles due to loss of periventricular tissue (Figure 500).

The loss of cerebral periventricular structures, the basal ganglia and deep white matter, correlates with the development of cerebral palsy in this case.

Microcephaly was evident in early infancy. With deep brain damage occurring during fetal life, with destruction of periventricular tissue, the brain is decreased in size, fails to grow normally, leading to decreased head size, microcephaly. As occurred in the present case, microcephaly is common in infants with cerebral palsy.

Figure 499. CT scan of brain at 10 days. Ventricles patent. Dense foci, apparently hemorrhagic lesions, in the periventricular cerebral strata.

Figure 500. CT scan of brain at 2 1/2 months. In the frontal region on the left, near the lateral ventricle, an area of rarefaction, a porencephalic cavity. Ventricles much dilated, hydrocephalus ex vacuo.

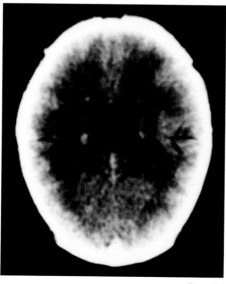

Fig. 499

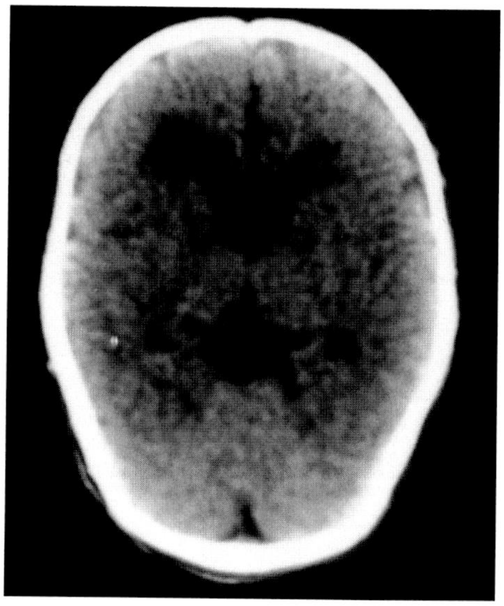

Fig. 500

A Case of **Subdural hemorrhage; macrosomic newborn; DIC. Failed forceps delivery; cesarean section birth. Maternal excessive pregnancy weight gain; latent prediabetes. Infant later developed severe cerebral palsy, mental retardation, and seizure disorder.**

A large supracerebral subdural hemorrhage was discovered in CT scans on day 2 postnatally. The infant, macrosomic, had been delivered by emergency cesarean section following failed forceps effort to deliver the fetus vaginally.

The pregnancy had been complicated by maternal medical problems. The mother had had prolonged nausea and vomiting, extending into midpregnancy. Paradoxically, however, excessive pregnancy weight gain of more than 40 pounds occurred, with the mother weighing 193 pounds at term delivery.

Excessive maternal weight gain, of the degree in the present case, is usually of metabolic origin, due to endocrine dysfunction such as in diabetic conditions.

In this case, the presence of latent prediabetes was evidenced not only by excessive pregnancy weight gain but also, subsequently, by the delivery of a macrosomic baby with multiple malformations — prime markers of maternal diabetic predisposition.

In people who become diabetic, the bodily dysfunctions have origin many years before the diabetes becomes overt, before elevated blood glucose levels and glycosuria appear. Maternal prediabetes (or diabetes) creates an unfavorable uterine environment, exercises a damaging effect on the fetus, extending over the entire length of the gestational period. In these circumstances there is a high incidence of stillbirths.

Decreased fetal activity was noted by the mother in the week prior to delivery. Loss of normal fetal activity reflects fetal compromise, fetal enfeeblement. Pathologic gestational processes have an adversive effect on the fetus, often exercising their effects chronically during intrauterine life, rendering the fetus, as in this case, anemic and weakened. Fetal compromise, enfeeblement, is manifested as loss of normal fetal activity. The compromised weakened fetus may succumb, or the process may be sublethal, with the fetus transiently recovering activity, with depression of the fetus (newborn) reappearing with the stress of labor.

Labor was induced at term; a macrosomic fetus was evident clinically. Following Pitocin induction, the first stage of labor was completed, with the cervix completely dilated. The fetal head descended into the pelvis. At this time fetal distress, with late decelerations, was evidenced.

Forceps were applied but removed during contraction of the uterus. Forceps were reapplied and slipped — a failed forceps delivery. With late decelerations continuing, an emergency cesarean section was done.

Depression of the newborn infant was severe. The infant appeared lifeless, with an initial Apgar score of 0 at 1 minute and 3 at 5 minutes. However, he responded to care; his vital functions improved, with an Apgar rating of 5 at 20 minutes. At 2 hours, the infant had "continued to improve." His fontanelles remained soft and flat through the first day. This is not the clinical pattern of a newborn with acute diffuse cerebral damage. Newborn infants who have acute diffuse brain damage are depressed at delivery and do not soon improve; they stay depressed, with respiratory failure, congestive heart failure, bulging fontanelles. Considered retrospectively, this was a fetus, chronically enfeebled by adversive gestational factors, unable to tolerate the stress of labor. The clinical pattern in the present case, with the infant beginning to improve after delivery, is compatible with the presence of latent subacute cerebral damage at birth, damage accrued during fetal life due to adversive gestational processes (Chapter 2).

Macrosomia was evident at birth. This baby was large, heavy and long. The baby weighed 4,840 grams (10 pounds 12 ounces), over the ninetieth percentile by weight (average newborn term weight, 3,200 grams, 7 pounds to 7 1/2 pounds). The baby was long, 56.75 centimeters (22.3 inches), over the ninetieth percentile. The head also was very large, with a circumference of 35.75 centimeters (average at term, 33.5 centimeters), above the ninetieth percentile for newborn head size.

The excessive size of this newborn, the macrosomia, is attributable to the mother's disordered metabolism, to processes associated with a latent diabetic condition.

Macrosomic babies, as in this case, are feeble, do not do well. Some are stillborn or die soon after birth. The pathologic mechanism causing macrosomia, the injurious effect on the fetus, is not known. Macrosomic infants that survive have an increased incidence of cerebral palsy.

Malformations were noted in this infant, particularly a "vascular ring," a malformation of the aorta, and micrognathia, a small receding lower jaw. Malformations are common in offspring of mothers with diabetic conditions. The malformations had no bearing on the cerebral damage in this case.

The malformations were of induced nature, meaning that some adversive external factor, such as exposure to chemicals, maternal illness, irradiation, occurred during embryonic or early fetal life that affected the development of this embryo (page 141).

In the present case the malformations are attributable to the effects of the mother's prediabetes.

Anemia was evident in this infant. The anemia had origin during fetal life, evidenced by the fact that the infant at delivery was noted to be pale. Anemia was immediately confirmed in the newborn hematology reports. The red blood cell count (RBC) was 3.8 million (normal, 5.14 million). The hemoglobin level was 14.1 grams (normal, 19 grams). The hematocrit level was 43.2 percent (normal, 61 percent).

As to the cause of the fetal-neonatal anemia in this newborn infant, with other causal factors excluded, the anemia was attributable to processes of fetal-maternal transfusion (page 97).

Chronic anemia, in the fetus as in the adult human, causes chronic hypoxia. The red cell is the oxygen-carrying vehicle in the blood. The decrease in hematocrit means this fetus existed with less than the average amount of oxygen supply, chronic fetal hypoxia. Fetal hypoxia leads to the accumulation of fetal hypoxic cerebral damage.

Seizure activity that began soon after delivery interrupted the infant's improvement.

With cerebral damage incurred during the premature period, with the damage originating deep in the cerebrum and extending to the cortical surface, with the fetus surviving to term, the lesions in the cortex become subacute, and are capable of causing seizure activity soon after birth. There is increasing clinical opinion that when seizures appear soon after birth, the process is not attributable to acute intranatal asphyxial brain damage, but rather, the cause must be sought in pathologic processes, brain damage, prior to birth (Chapter 5).

Bleeding, oozing from the umbilical stump and bleeding from the oral cavity and other sites, developed during the first day.

DIC (disseminated intravascular coagulopathy) was diagnosed subsequent to the appearance of the bleeding tendency.

DIC is a syndromic hematologic disorder that occurs in adults and infants, in cases with antecedent ongoing illness, with debilitating conditions, in cases complicated by acute stress (page 114).

Areas of damaged tissue, usually associated with minor hemorrhages, become sites of large hemorrhage when DIC is present.

Caput succedaneum was present at birth in the right temporoparietal region. Caput succedaneum is a localized, round, elevated area of the scalp, created by the firm grasp of the cervical ring against the descending fetal head. It is present regularly with cephalic delivery. Its occurrence is unrelated to forceps application.

Pathologically, the swollen scalp tissue is suffused with edema fluid, often hemorrhagic due to effusion of blood from congested scalp veins. In the presence of the hemorrhagic diathesis, DIC, as occurred in this case, the scalp hemorrhage increased.

Molding of the head in this infant was noted to be of severe degree. The head of the fetus is soft, plastic, and with cephalic presentation, as the fetus descends through the birth canal, the head elongates into a football shape, to more easily get through the pelvis. This is physiologic. Molding is unrelated to forceps delivery.

Following the development of seizures in this infant, CT scans were done on day 2. Subdural hemorrhage was revealed in the initial CT scan (Figure 501). Also, a large caput succedaneum was evident in the CT scan.

The subdural bleeding in the present case was due to two factors: molding of the (very large) head, and the hemorrhagic diathesis (DIC) present.

Pathologically, the initial causal mechanism in subdural hemorrhage is related to the physical effects of parturitional molding. With cephalic presentation, with molding, the dural structures and veins are stretched, at times torn, with bleeding coming from the torn veins.

Subdural hemorrhage over the surface of the cerebrum, as in this case, is due to tearing of the "bridging veins" that extend from the brain surface. These veins pass through the subdural space unsupported, and empty into the dural sinuses. Molding distortion of the head puts a stretch on the bridging veins, resulting in tearing of the veins and subdural bleeding.

In the present case, the presence of an oversized head led to excessive molding, contributing to the occurrence of subdural hemorrhage.

Pathologically, of direct importance is the factor of DIC in the development of the subdural hemorrhage. The subdural hemorrhage accumulated over a period of time after birth. A sonogram done on day 1 at 6 hours showed no intracranial hemorrhage, no subdural hemorrhage. Fontanelles were soft and flat at the time, indicating there was no increased intracranial pressure. The CT scan done on day 2 revealed the development of the subdural hemorrhage (Figure 501). The caput succedaneum, increasing in size on the second day, was also demonstrated on the CT scan.

In the subsequent postnatal period the infant remained in poor condition. Seizure activity continued. There was little spontaneous activity.

CT scans of the brain on day 12 (Figure 502) showed evidence of persisting subdural hemorrhage, now of lesser density, the blood being absorbed. Focal hemorrhage appeared in the substance of the cerebrum, attributable to the bleeding effects of DIC.

CT scans of the brain at 1 month (Figure 503) showed diffuse encephalomalacia, loss of cerebral substance.

The infant remained neurologically obtunded, and presented severe cerebral palsy, mental retardation, and seizure disorder.

MRI study of the brain at 10 months (Figure 504) indicated far-advanced loss of cerebral substance, with resulting ex vacuo hydrocephalus (page 29).

In assessing the cause of the cerebral damage and the cerebral disabilities, it is evident that the impact of adverse processes during gestation resulted in deep cerebral damage with sequelant spastic cerebral palsy (Chapter 3). Superimposed on this is the cerebral damage due to the effects of the subdural hemorrhage and the intracerebral hemorrhages due to DIC.

Figure 501. Subdural hemorrhage. CT scan of the brain on day 2. Density over the left temporo-parietal region representing a subdural collection of blood. On the right, a bulging density external to the calvarium indicating a layer of subcutaneous hemorrhage, a large caput succedaneum. (The right side of the head appears on the left in the illustration.)

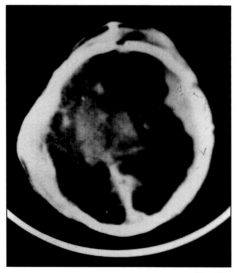

Fig. 501

Figure 502. Chronic subdural hemorrhage; confluent intracerebral hemorrhage. CT scan of the brain on day 12. Deposit of subdural hemorrhage over the left temporoparietal region, evident in Figure 501, now of decreased density, the appearance consistent with a chronic subdural hematoma. The cerebral hemispheres with confluent cloud-like patchy densities, recent areas of intracerebral and subarachnoid hemorrhage. The cerebral lateral ventricles are patent. The caput succedaneum persists.

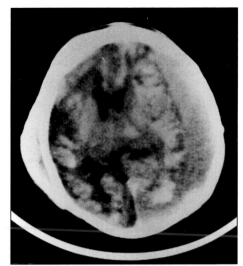

Fig. 502

Figure 503. Cerebrum showing diffuse encephalomalacia, loss of white matter. CT scan of brain at 1 month. Confluent cystic areas of decreased density through the cerebral substance. Lateral ventricles somewhat enlarged.

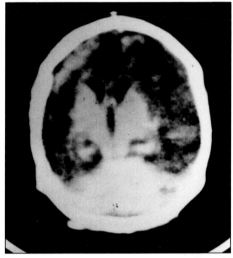

Fig. 503

Figure 504. Hydrocephalus ex vacuo. MRI of the brain at 10 months. Enlargement of the lateral ventricles with corresponding decreased periventricular white matter. Convolutional remnants shrunken and destroyed.

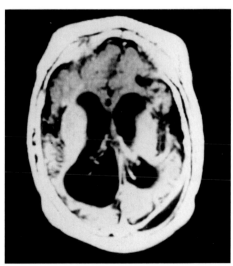

Fig. 504

A Case of **Severe fetal-neonatal anemia; fetal hypoxic cerebral damage; hydrocephalus ex vacuo. Infant developed cerebral palsy, mental retardation, seizure disorder, and microcephaly.**

The mother's health during this pregnancy was not optimal. She was treated for syphilis 3 months prior to this pregnancy. Whether or not the infection was halted by the treatment by the beginning of this pregnancy is open to question. Did the infection affect the gestation? The presence of a syphilitic infection in the mother is harmful to the fetus, especially in the early months of gestation.

An upper respiratory infection, persisting for weeks, occurred at 31 weeks of the pregnancy. That the mother was sick, that this ongoing URI was significant, was evidenced by the fact that she lost weight, lost over 2 pounds in 2 weeks.

Labor developed at 39 weeks. Delivery was vaginal from a breech presentation, with delivery of the aftercoming head assisted with forceps.

Depression of the newborn was severe at delivery, with an Apgar score of 2 and 2.

Pneumothorax was discovered at 1 1/2 hours after birth, and the infant, previously improved, went into a rapid collapse. The pneumothorax was related to positive pressure resuscitation (page 111). After the pneumothorax was evacuated the infant stabilized.

Anemia of severe form was evident at delivery; the newborn infant was noted to be pale. The presence of anemia was confirmed in the hematology reports 11 hours after birth. At birth the red blood cell count (RBC) was 3.3 million (normal, 5.14 million). The hemoglobin level was 10.9 grams (normal, 19 grams). The hematocrit level was 33.7 percent (normal, 61 percent). The newborn infant was transfused to bring the hematocrit level up, with subsequent improvement of the infant.

Chronic anemia, in the fetus as in the adult human, causes chronic hypoxia. With intrauterine hypoxia, the fetus accrues acute and subacute cerebral damage.

As to the cause of the fetal-neonatal anemia, this appeared to be an example of the fetal-maternal transfusion syndrome. The transfer of blood from fetal to maternal circulation occurs regularly to some degree in most if not all gestations; the amount of transfusion varies but is severe in some instances (page 97).

This newborn infant's clinical course was compromised — not by manifestations of acute brain damage — but by ongoing debilitation caused by (fetal) neonatal anemia and by the pneumothorax respiratory complication. Although depressed at birth, he responded to resuscitation and, although severely anemic, and despite the pneumothorax, was maintained oxygenated, pink, and at 5 hours was noted to be active, with spontaneous respiration, with no acute neurologic problem.

As soon as the pneumothorax problem was relieved, the baby was noted to be vigorous. Fontanelles were soft. And, following the blood transfusion for the infant's anemia, he became active with good spontaneous respiration at 17 hours.

The neonatal CT scan in this case provides additional evidence that acute cerebral damage was not present. When there is acute fresh cerebral damage, in the fetus as in the adult — acute damage due to hypoxia, stroke, infection, or any other pathologic process — the brain, in the hours and days after the damage is incurred, becomes edematous, swollen, and stays that way for many days. As a consequence of the edema, the cerebral ventricles become compressed, obliterated. In the present case, the CT scan taken neonatally showed patent ventricles — evidence that no process of acute fresh cerebral damage was present.

Seizure activity began in this infant during the first day after birth.

With cerebral damage incurred during the early premature period, with the damage originating deep in the cerebrum and extending to the cortical surface, and with the fetus surviving to term, the lesions in the cortex become subacute, and are capable of causing seizure activity soon after birth (Chapter 5).

This child developed cerebral palsy. Cerebral palsy is a "dyskinesia," a defect in motor function caused by damage to a certain part of the brain, the basal ganglia, located deep in the brain. This deep damage occurs consistently, specifically, only in the immature premature brain, during early fetal life. Pathologic hypoxia-producing processes such as intrauterine fetal anemia, as occurred in this case, cause hypoxic damage to the fetus, hypoxic cerebral damage. When the fetus is damaged during early fetal life, if the fetus survives to term, the infant is born with old subacute brain damage. Deep damage incurred in the premature brain causing cerebral palsy at times extends to the cerebral surface, to the cortex, resulting in cortical manifestations of mental retardation and epilepsy, as appeared in the present case.

Microcephaly was evident in this infant in the months after birth. The child's head failed to enlarge, measuring 48.5 centimeters at age 6, below the second percentile. As to the cause of the microcephaly, the brain enlarges due mainly to elaboration, growth, of the deep strata of the cerebrum. When the deep periventricular layers of the cerebrum are damaged during fetal life, the development, growth, of the brain eventually is attenuated, with the head consequently appearing microcephalic.

Hydrocephalus was demonstrated in CT scans of the brain at age 7 years (Figure 505). Loss of periventricular tissue due to hypoxic damage in fetal life caused enlargement of the ventricles, ex vacuo hydrocephalus (page 29).

Figure 505. Hydrocephalus ex vacuo. CT scan of brain at 7 years. Loss of periventricular white matter of severe degree with consequent enlargement of the lateral ventricles. Convolutions shrunken, atrophied, due to loss of convolutional white matter. **(a).** Lower level of cerebrum and **(b).** upper level of cerebrum, showing enlarged ventricles.

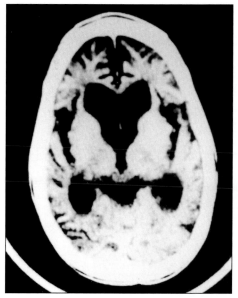 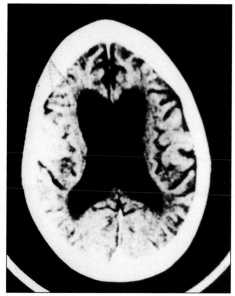

Fig. 505(a)   *(b)*

A Case of   *A macrosomic anemic newborn; xanthochromic spinal fluid. Maternal excessive pregnancy weight gain, latent prediabetes. Infant developed cerebral palsy, seizure disorder, and mental retardation.*

Excessive weight gain occurred during this pregnancy. The mother, although gaining weight excessively, was sick during this pregnancy; she had recurrent fever; she became anemic.

Any kind of maternal illness during pregnancy, physical or emotional illness, directly affects the maternal-placental-fetal complex, compromising the fetus. Pathologically, the causal process exercises its effects through the common denominator of intrauterine hypoxia.

The severity of the maternal illness does not necessarily correspond to the degree of fetal damage. A mild maternal illness may prove disastrous for the fetus; at other times the fetus seems to escape manifest damage.

Regarding the mother's excessive weight gain, her pregravid weight was 136 pounds. She weighed 181 pounds at term, an increase of 45 pounds.

Excessive maternal weight gain, of the degree in the present case, is usually of metabolic origin, due to endocrine dysfunctions such as in diabetic conditions.

Is there a factor of latent prediabetes in this case? This mother presents three prime markers of latent diabetes: a family history of diabetes, excessive pregnancy weight gain, and a macrosomic baby.

In people who become diabetic, the bodily dysfunctions have origin many years before the diabetes becomes overt. Maternal prediabetes (or diabetes) creates an unfavorable uterine environment, exercises a damaging effect on the fetus, extending over the entire length of the gestational period. In these circumstances there is a high incidence of stillbirths. Spontaneous abortion is common in diabetic conditions.

In mothers with diabetic processes, the pathologic mechanism causing the macrosomia and other injurious effects on the fetus is not known.

Labor was induced with Pitocin at 41 weeks. Delivery was augmented with low forceps.

Depression of severe degree was present at birth, with an Apgar score of 1 and 2.

Macrosomia was evident at birth. This baby was large, heavy and long. The baby weighed 4,120 grams (9 pounds 2 ounces), in the ninetieth percentile by weight (average newborn term weight, 3,200 grams, 7 to 7 1/2 pounds). The baby was long, 55 centimeters (21 3/4 inches), at the ninetieth percentile.

With reasonable medical probability, the macrosomia of this baby was related to this mother's disordered metabolism of latent prediabetes.

Macrosomic babies, as in this case, are feeble. Big does not mean strong, robust. Some are stillborn or die soon after birth. Macrosomic babies born alive just don't do well. In surviving infants there is a high incidence of cerebral palsy and seizure disorders (page 49).

Anemia, present in this newborn, manifestly had origin during intrauterine life. At birth the red blood cell count (RBC) was 3.30 million (normal, 5.14 million). The hematocrit was 34.8 percent (average for newborn is 61 percent). The hematocrit measures the quantity of red cells in the blood. In the present case, correspondingly, the hemoglobin level was decreased, 11.5 grams (average for newborn is 19 grams).

Clinically, even prior to the hematology studies, the newborn infant was described as "pale." Pale means anemia. The presence of the anemia in this newborn was very soon recognized, with a transfusion ordered at 9 1/2 hours after birth.

Chronic anemia, in the fetus as in the adult human, causes chronic hypoxia. The red cell is the oxygen-carrying vehicle in the blood. The decrease in hematocrit means this fetus existed with less than the average amount of oxygen supply, chronic severe fetal hypoxia.

Chronic intrauterine hypoxia leads to fetal hypoxic visceral damage. The brain is the most sensitive target tissue in the body; with chronic intrauterine hypoxia, the fetus accrues acute and subacute cerebral damage.

The cause of the anemia present at birth appeared to be a process of fetal-maternal transfusion (page 97).

Although this infant was depressed at delivery, she responded to care, with an Apgar score of 6 at 15 minutes. Respirations were spontaneous. She was moving all her extremities. Fontanelles were flat.

Seizure activity, with onset soon after birth interrupted the infant's clinical improvement.

The question arises as to whether such early seizure activity reflects the presence of acute cerebral damage, or whether the seizure activity was due to cerebral damage incurred before birth, due to hypoxic cerebral damage during fetal life prior to term.

It is well known that epilepsy commonly occurs after brain damage involving the cerebral cortex. Pathologically, the brain lesion forms a seizure-generating (epileptogenic) focus in the cortex. The epileptogenic lesion can be incurred in the fetal brain antenatally, weeks or months before birth. In the premature fetus, brain damage beginning deep in the cerebrum (causing cerebral palsy) may extend to the cortex, causing early-onset seizures.

Xanthochromic spinal fluid was present in the spinal puncture done after the development of seizures. The spinal fluid drawn at 9 1/2 hours after birth was amber, xanthochromic. The finding of xanthochromic (xantho-, yellow; -chromia, color) spinal fluid in this case is of major importance in defining the time of incurrence of the cerebral damage. Xanthochromia, yellow coloration of the spinal fluid, is due to the presence of old hemorrhagic damage in the brain. With hemorrhage in the brain, with blood escaping into the ventricles, into the spinal fluid, red cells becomes lysed, broken down; the hemoglobin from the red cells first gives the spinal fluid a pink color. The hemoglobin gradually degenerates to a yellow pigment and gives the spinal fluid a yellow color — xanthochromia.

This change in color takes many days, and continues to be present for weeks and months when there is an old hemorrhagic lesion in the brain.

Xanthochromia does not develop in a few hours, or even a day or two. The finding of xanthochromia is firm evidence that the brain damage in this fetus, this infant, occurred a long time before labor and delivery (page 173).

In summary, this case illustrates essential processes in the pathogenesis of cerebral palsy:

— This infant developed cerebral palsy. Cerebral palsy is a dyskinesia, a defect in motor function caused by damage to a certain part of the brain, the basal ganglia, located deep in the brain. This deep damage occurs consistently, specifically, only in the immature premature brain, during early fetal life.

— Gestational complications, maternal disorders, pathologic fetal processes, as occurred in this case, cause hypoxic damage to the fetus, cause cerebral damage.

— When the fetus is damaged during early fetal life, if the fetus survives to term the infant is born with old subacute hypoxic brain damage.

— Deep damage incurred in the premature brain (causing cerebral palsy) at times extends to the cerebral surface, to the cortex, resulting in cortical manifestations of mental retardation and epilepsy.

This is the clinical pathologic sequence that occurred in this case.

A Case of

Teenage pregnancy; maternal psychiatric stress, hypotension, chlamydia infection. Fetal-neonatal anemia. Infant developed hydrocephaly; porencephaly; cerebral palsy, mental retardation, and seizure disorder.

This teenage mother confronted substantial medical and emotional pregnancy problems.

The mother was 16 years old at the beginning of this pregnancy, a primipara. There is an increased incidence of fetal and neonatal morbidity and mortality with teenage mothers, especially in primiparous teenage mothers.

Psychiatric stress was present in the circumstances of this pregnancy, an unmarried teenage schoolgirl. Psychologic stress is known to impact unfavorably on gestation, on the fetus. A number of clinical studies on humans and experimental studies in rhesus monkeys confirm the fact that maternal anxiety affects the fetus (page 53).

Hypotension, symptom-producing low blood pressure, was ongoing in the mother during this pregnancy, She had a diastolic blood pressure ranging around 50 to 60 (normal is 80) and at times as low as 40. Clinically she had symptoms of faintness and dizziness related to low blood pressure.

Translating this to the effect on the uterus, just as there was inadequate blood going to the brain, there would correspondingly be inadequate arterial perfusion to the uterus, to the placenta, with resulting fetal hypoxia.

This hypotensive lack of perfusion is increased when the mother is lying down, during the hours of sleep; the condition is well known obstetrically.

Chlamydia infection was diagnosed in this mother. Chlamydia infection, due to the organism *C. trachomatis,* causes enlargement of lymph nodes in the inguinal area and other regions. This mother became ill during the first trimester, was found to have regional lymphadenopathy. Diagnosis of chlamydia infection was made.

It has been pointed out that chlamydia is common among unmarried women pregnant for the first time. Chlamydia infection is known to be injurious to the fetus. Stillbirth and neonatal death occur ten times more often among chlamydia-infected women than among uninfected controls.

Labor developed at 41 weeks of gestation. This was a vertex presentation with spontaneous vaginal delivery. Depression of the infant at birth required resuscitation with positive-pressure oxygen. Apgar score was 1 and 6. The enfeebled infant responded to care and gradually improved, was awake, looking around, crying, during the hours after delivery. Fontanelles were flat.

Anemia was evident; the infant was pale. Anemia was confirmed in the hematology studies. The red cell count (RBC) was 3.71 million (normal at term, 5.14 million). Hemoglobin was 13.4 grams (normal, 19 grams). Hematocrit was 40.9 percent (normal, 61 percent). The infant received two transfusions.

What caused anemia to develop in this fetus? With other anemia-causing processes excluded on clinical bases, it was apparent that the anemia in this case was an example of the fetal-maternal transfusion syndrome.

The anemia, originating during fetal life, was one of the most important elements in defining the cause of the brain damage in this case. The newborn infant had been subjected to chronic anemia, with associated prolonged hypoxia, during fetal life. The brain is the most hypoxia-sensitive target in the body; with chronic intrauterine hypoxia, the fetus accrues subacute cerebral damage.

Taking into consideration clinical and pathologic factors in this case, it is evident that subacute cerebral damage, incurred during fetal life, was present in this infant at birth, that cerebral damage of acute form was not present.

Infants that are born with acute cerebral damage are comatose at birth and remain comatose for prolonged periods, days, with depression of vital function. This was not the pattern in the present case. The infant in this case was alert and crying in the hours after delivery.

Infants born harboring subacute cerebral damage commonly are depressed at delivery but soon respond and are improved in the hours after birth. This pattern appeared in the present case.

Seizure activity was observed late on the first day. Seizures are due to damage to the cerebral cortex (epileptogenic focus). Cerebral damage incurred with hypoxia during fetal life at times extends to the cortical surface. With the fetus surviving to term, the lesions in the cortex become subacute, capable of causing seizure activity soon after birth (Chapter 5).

The CT scan taken neonatally, after the onset of seizures, indicated the absence of cerebral swelling, evidenced by patent lateral ventricles (Figure 506). The cerebral frontal and posterior regions, showed decreased density indicative of far advanced subacute damage.

The cerebral damage evident in Figure 506, damage to the deep cerebral structures incurred during fetal life, resulted clinically in the development of cerebral palsy. Cerebral palsy is known to be due to deep cerebral (basal ganglia) damage incurred at a time during premature, immature, fetal life. At times the deep cerebral damage extends outward to the cerebral cortex, resulting in mental retardation and seizure disorder, as occurred in this case.

Follow-up CT studies done at 1 year (Figure 507) and at 5 years (Figure 508) showed encephaloclastic porencephaly, the consequence pathologically of deep cerebral damage incurred during fetal life. The cerebral damage became subacute; the devitalized tissue became contracted, scarred, leading to ventricular enlargement and porencephalic cavitations.

Figure 506. Subacute cerebral damage present in neonate. CT scan of brain on day 3. Ventricles are patent, indicating absence of acute cerebral swelling. Scattered mottled dense areas in the cerebral walls are attributable to old infarctional damage. Increased translucency frontally and posteriorly indicate loss of cerebral substance, old subacute cerebral damage.

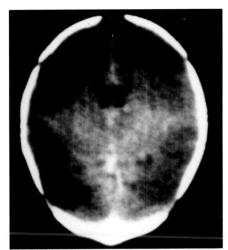

Fig. 506

Figure 507. Hydrocephaly; porencephaly. CT scan of brain at 1 year. Ventricles enlarged due to destruction of surrounding deep cerebral structures, ex vacuo hydrocephalus. Cerebral walls of decreased density, with remnant strands of tissue forming confluent porencephalic cysts.

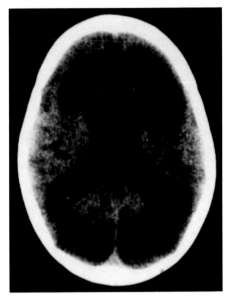

Fig. 507

Figure 508. Hydrocephaly and porencephaly, far advanced. CT scan of brain at 5 years.

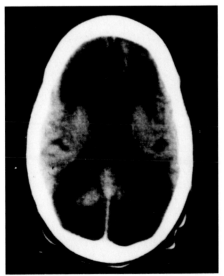

Fig. 508

A Case of **Maternal diabetes, hypothyroidism, low pregnancy weight gain. Newborn macrosomic, hypoglycemic. Infant developed cerebral palsy, mental retardation, and epilepsy.**

Diabetes was present in the mother; she was insulin-dependent (Type I). Diabetes exercises diffuse adversive effects on the fetus. Newborn infants often are defective in structure and function. Control of diabetes during pregnancy is difficult and mothers often are out of diabetic control, especially during the stress of illness. This mother was sick, hospitalized twice during this pregnancy, with the diabetes out of control. With maternal diabetes, even with optimal diabetic control, at times the newborn infant simply does not do well, does not thrive. The underlying cause of the failure to thrive is not well understood. There is an increased incidence of fetal and neonatal deaths associated with maternal diabetes. In infants that survive, there is an increased incidence of cerebral palsy and other developmental disabilities.

Hypothyroidism, diagnosed in the mother at the age of 8 years, required ongoing daily thyroid-supplement medication. The thyroid exercises a major role in maintaining a normal gestation. The hazards to the fetus of maternal hypothyroidism or hyperthyroidism are well known. Although the mother appeared to be in thyroid balance, on thyroid medication, at the onset of pregnancy, the dilemma was — whether she should be given more thyroid medication (and risk creating hyperthyroidism), or whether she should be left alone regarding the thyroid dosage. As the gestation progressed, she showed no specific manifestations of hypothyroidism. Her blood pressure and other vital signs recorded during pregnancy were normal (blood pressure and heart rate are usually affected with thyroid-level imbalance).

Low pregnancy weight gain occurred, with the record noting that the mother "had very poor weight gain in this pregnancy." She had episodic weight loss, reflecting periods of acute illness.

Maternal weight gain during the last months of pregnancy should average 1/2 to 3/4 pound per week. In the present case, in the last 19 weeks of pregnancy she gained 8 pounds; she should have gained twice as much weight in this period, the last half of this pregnancy.

Low maternal weight gain compromises fetal well-being and is associated with impaired neonatal outcome.

Labor began spontaneously at 36 weeks of pregnancy. After 2 hours of desultory labor, with the monitor indicating fetal distress, a cesarean section was done.

Macrosomia was evident at delivery. This baby was oversized, weighing 7 pounds 4 ounces, in the ninetieth percentile for 36 weeks' gestation. She was long, 48.7 centimeters, in the seventy-fifth percentile.

Macrosomic babies are feeble. Big does not mean strong, robust. Some are stillborn or die soon after birth. Macrosomic babies are commonly the offspring of mothers with diabetes. There is an increased incidence of cerebral palsy in these infants. This clinical pattern evolved in the present case.

Hypoglycemia, a blood sugar of 9, was reported soon after birth. Did hypoglycemia in this baby cause acute brain damage?

The nurse's notes for this period record that the newborn was "active" with color of skin pink, with fontanelles normal, with Moro and grasp reflexes normal, and with a normal cry. This description is plainly incongruous with a diagnosis of acute cerebral damage. Infants with acute cerebral damage are comatose, not active and crying; are cyanotic, not pink; are limp without reflexes. They do not cry. They have bulging fontanelles. This newborn infant simply did not fit this picture of acute cerebral damage.

Regarding the hypoglycemia in this infant, relatively low blood sugar levels are very common in clinically well newborn infants. Transient hypoglycemia, in adults as in infants, does not cause brain damage (page 171).

What caused the cerebral damage, the cerebral disabilities, later manifested by the infant in this case? As noted, the good neurologic condition in the postdelivery period rules out the presence of acute brain damage in this newborn infant (Chapter 2).

The clinical-pathologic pattern in this case is consistent with the syndrome of latent subacute cerebral damage present at birth, damage incurred during fetal life.

This infant developed cerebral palsy. Cerebral palsy is due to damage in the basal ganglia located in the deep portion of the cerebrum, damage that occurs in the premature fetus due to hypoxia-producing complications prenatally.

CT scans at age 8 years revealed diffuse loss of cerebral white matter with consequent dilatation of the cerebral ventricles (Figure 509). The cerebral palsy that developed in the infant is related to the loss of substance in the deep cerebral strata, to damage to the white matter and basal ganglia. The deep cerebral damage extended through the wall of the cerebrum damaging the cortex, later causing mental deficiency and seizure disorders. This manifestly occurred in the present case.

Figure 509. CT scans at 8 years of age. **(a).** Loss of cerebral white matter indicated by the decreased density most pronounced in the frontal regions adjoining the lateral ventricles. **(b).** Hydrocephalus ex vacuo, ventricle enlargement due to loss of periventricular white matter.

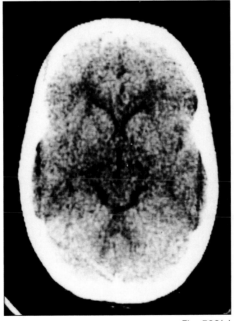
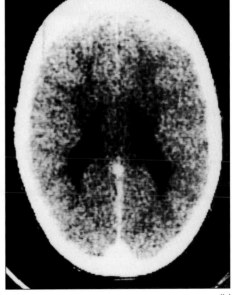

Fig. 509(a)   (b)

A Case of   *Basal ganglia cavitations; infant with cerebral palsy.*
              At birth, macrosomia, xanthochromic spinal fluid.
              Maternal latent prediabetes. Infant also developed
              mental retardation and seizure disorder.

Latent prediabetes was suspected in this mother prenatally because of her delivery previously of a macrosomic baby and because of the presence in this gestation of a large fetus, evident clinically, and because of the mother's excessive pregnancy weight gain, common in diabetic mothers.

Excessive weight gain, over 41 pounds, occurred during this pregnancy (average is 20 to 25 pounds). Excessive maternal weight gain, of the degree in this case, is usually of metabolic origin, due to endocrine dysfunctions as in diabetic conditions. In people who develop diabetes, the bodily metabolic dysfunctions have origin many years before the diabetes becomes clinically overt—the period of latent prediabetes.

Labor began at 42 weeks of pregnancy; a vertex presentation. Labor was desultory, and after 8 hours, with failure of the fetus to descend, a cesarean section was done.

Macrosomia, an oversized baby, was evident at delivery. The infant was large, heavy and long. The infant weighed 11 pounds 6 ounces (5,160 grams), far above the ninetieth percentile for weight. The infant's length was 22 1/8 inches, far above the ninetieth percentile.

Macrosomia in the offspring often is the first sign of a diabetic condition in the mother. Latent diabetes, like overt diabetes, is adversive to the fetus. The macrosomic infants, big but not robust, do not do well at birth. The infants do not thrive. There is a high incidence of fetal-neonatal morbidity and mortality and an increased incidence of cerebral palsy and other developmental disabilities in infants surviving.

Severe depression was present in the infant at birth, with an Apgar score of 2 and 4.

Was this depression due to acute cerebral damage?

The valid assessment of the presence of hypoxic cerebral damage present at birth is determined by the performance of the infant in the period after delivery (page 164). Infants born with fresh acute hypoxic cerebral damage have a consistent clinical pattern: prolonged coma, flaccidity, cyanosis, with evidence of cerebral swelling, with bulging fontanelles. The infant in the present case did not have this pattern. She responded well to the attention given in the delivery room and was soon responsive, with good vital function. Fontanelles were soft, indicating there was no acute brain swelling.

What caused the cerebral damage, the cerebral palsy, later manifested in this infant?

Although there was no sign of acute brain damage in the baby, what is significant, relevant, is the fact that the mother had pregnancy medical problems. Any maternal problem during pregnancy, acute or chronic, directly affects the maternal-placental-fetal complex, compromising the fetus. Pathologically, the causal process exercises its effects through the common denominator of intrauterine hypoxia.

A fetus subjected to hypoxia-producing conditions during intrauterine life accrues hypoxic cerebral damage. If the fetus survives, the acute lesions become subacute, undergo "healing" with scarring, with consequent latent subacute lesions present at birth. The clinical picture in this case reflects this pattern, a macrosomic debilitated fetus and newborn with accrued old subacute brain damage (page 24). In such circumstances, the fetus, compromised during intrauterine life, reacts poorly to the stress of labor. As in this case, infants are depressed at delivery but, characteristically, they soon recover from the stress of labor.

Seizure activity developing during the first day interrupted the postdelivery improvement of this infant. The infant had been observed to be in stable condition neurologically in the nursery, with good grasp, good suck, showing a "remarkable recovery" after being depressed at delivery. However, during the morning after delivery she showed subtle signs of seizure activity, with arching of the back and apneic episodes. There is substantial clinical and pathologic basis for concluding that the seizures were not due to acute cerebral damage, that the seizures were a manifestation of subacute cerebral cortical damage present at birth.

Xanthochromic spinal fluid found in this newborn infant confirmed the presence of old subacute cerebral damage; the spinal tap was done after the onset of seizures. Xanthochromia, yellow discoloration of the spinal fluid, is due to the presence of old hemorrhagic damage to the brain (page 173).

With hemorrhage in the brain, with blood escaping into the ventricles, into the spinal fluid, red cells become lysed, broken down; the hemoglobin from the red cells first gives the spinal fluid a pink color. The hemoglobin gradually degenerates to a yellow pigment and gives the spinal fluid a yellow color—xanthochromia.

This change in color takes many days, and continues to be present for weeks and months when there is an old hemorrhagic lesion in the brain.

Ultrasound studies done on day 3 showed evidence of old hemorrhagic damage in the cerebrum. Correlated with the ultrasound findings, CT scans of the brain at 8 months showed evidence of old infarction in the basal ganglia (putamen) in the cerebrum bilaterally—offering a classic example of the pathogenesis of cerebral palsy (Figure 510).

Figure 510. Basal ganglia damage (arrows) with focal cavitations, residues of old focal infarcts. Decreased cerebral white matter, ex vacuo hydrocephalus; convolutional atrophy. CT scan of brain at 8 months. Infant with cerebral palsy, seizure disorder, and mental retardation.

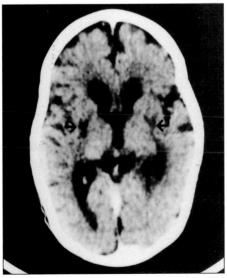

Fig. 510

A Case of **Teenage pregnancy; poor reproductive record; maternal obesity; chlamydia infection. Infant developed hydrocephalus, cerebral palsy, mental retardation, and seizure disorder.**

This mother had medical and emotional problems, problems that affect the fetus. This was a teenage mother, obese, with excessive weight gain, an apparent metabolic dysfunction, not favorable for the well-being of the fetus. She had a poor reproductive history, with two miscarriages prior to the pregnancy in this case. She'd had a recent chlamydia infection.

Any kind of maternal illness during pregnancy, physical or emotional illness, directly affects the maternal-placental-fetal complex, compromising the fetus. Pathologically, the causal process exercises its effects through the common denominator of intrauterine hypoxia.

The reproductive history accumulated by this teenage girl was punctuated by two miscarriages, at 17 and 18 years, the last miscarriage occurring a few months before the conception in the present case. Teenage pregnancy is a factor in itself unfavorable to the mother and the fetus. There is an increased incidence of fetal and neonatal morbidity and mortality with young teenage mothers.

Psychological stress was present in the circumstances of this pregnancy. This unmarried teenage noncompliant mother was living with a foster family. Psychological stress is known to impact unfavorably on gestation, on the fetus (page 53).

Obesity with excessive pregnancy weight gain occurred. Obesity is a hazard to the pregnant mother and her fetus. This mother's pregravid weight was 150 pounds (average appropriate weight for her height, 5 feet 3 3/4 inches is 126 pounds). She gained excessively, put on 50 pounds (appropriate pregnancy weight gain is 25 pounds), reaching 200 pounds at term. The mother was reported to have eaten excessively, ravenously, disregarding orders prescribed about a salt-free diet and limited sweets. Although the obesity in this case is in part psychologically driven, it is also attributable to metabolic factors, to endocrine dysfunction. At times obesity is due to thyroid disease, hypothyroidism. The other common metabolic relationship is with diabetes.

Chlamydia infection was present in this mother. A chlamydia culture was positive a few months before conceiving with the pregnancy in this case. Chlamydia infection is caused by the organism *C. trachomatis*; infection with chlamydia is persistent, becomes chronic.

Chlamydia infection is known to be injurious to the fetus. Clinical studies have shown that chlamydia infection is common among unmarried pregnant women and that stillbirth and neonatal death occurred ten times more often among chlamydia-infected women than among uninfected controls. This clinical pattern fits the present case, a teenage mother with two previous spontaneous abortions (page 123).

Labor was spontaneous at term; this was a cephalic presentation, a spontaneous vaginal delivery.

Severe depression of the infant was present, with an Apgar score of 2 and 2. The infant was pale.

Anemia was diagnosed soon after delivery. The hematocrit was 42 percent (average for newborn is 61 percent). The hematocrit measures the quantity of red cells in the blood. In the present case, correspondingly, the hemoglobin level was decreased, 14.1 grams (average for newborn is 19 grams).

Chronic anemia, in the fetus as in the adult human, causes chronic hypoxia. The red cell is the oxygen carrying vehicle in the blood. The decrease in hematocrit means this fetus existed with less than the average amount of oxygen supply, chronic severe fetal hypoxia.

Chronic intrauterine hypoxia leads to fetal hypoxic visceral damage. The brain is the most sensitive target tissue in the body; with chronic intrauterine hypoxia, the fetus accrues subacute and acute cerebral damage.

The cause of the anemia was apparently due to an intrauterine fetal-maternal transfusion process (page 97).

When was the brain damage later manifested by the infant incurred? Was there fresh brain damage present at birth? There are substantial clinical and pathologic bases indicating that acute fetal brain damage was not incurred during labor, evidence that latent cerebral damage was present in the newborn, damage incurred weeks, months, long before birth, during fetal life.

Tangential to the above question is the other important question—What was the cause of the neurologic depression of this newborn infant? This fetus was chronically compromised during intrauterine life, anemic, enfeebled, unable to tolerate the stress of labor. The newborn, consequently exhausted, was depressed at birth. Although this infant was depressed at delivery, she responded to care and, in the following hour, vital functions improved, with spontaneous respirations beginning. Her color soon was pink; during the second hour her reflexes were intact, fontanelles were soft, and she was moving all her extremities. At 2 hours she was able to take a small feeding by mouth. At 5 hours she was pink, crying, and improved enough to be out to the mother, and was held by the mother and father. During the first night she was awake, with good loud cry, eyes open and following movements with her eyes; fontanelles remained soft. The morning of the first day she was again out to her mother and she was given a bath the first morning, at 17 hours.

Plainly this newborn infant did not act like she had acute diffuse brain damage. Newborn infants that do have acute brain damage show it. They do not soon improve; they stay comatose, depressed, flaccid, with cerebral edema, with bulging, tense fontanelles, with unstable vital signs, for prolonged periods, requiring ICN care, remaining in the hospital for weeks. The infant in this present case was not like that.

Relevantly, of importance clinically, CT scans of the brain on day 3 showed patent cerebral ventricles, evidencing absence of cerebral edema.

Seizure activity developed after the first day. There is increasing clinical evidence that when seizures appear soon after birth, the process is not attributable to acute intranatal asphyxial brain damage, but rather, the cause must be sought in pathologic processes, brain damage, prior to birth (Chapter 5).

CT scans of the brain at 5 months showed decreased cerebral white matter with resulting ventricular enlargement, ex vacuo hydrocephalus. The periventricular white matter in the wall of the cerebrum showed poorly demarcated areas of translucency, apparently cystic foci. This pattern of cerebral damage, with loss of periventricular white matter, is characteristic of cerebral palsy (Figure 511).

The present case is consistent with the syndrome of subacute cerebral damage present at birth, damage incurred a long time before birth, damage capable of triggering early neonatal onset of seizures, damage manifest months, years, later as cerebral palsy, mental retardation, and other cerebral disability.

Figure 511. CT scans of brain at 5 months. **(a).** Ventricular enlargement, ex vacuo hydrocephalus, due to loss of deep cerebral white matter. **(b).** Focal areas of translucency in the cerebral wall, cystic cavitations.

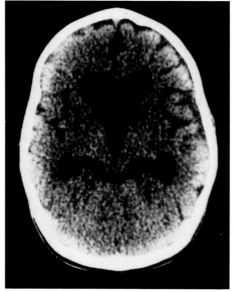 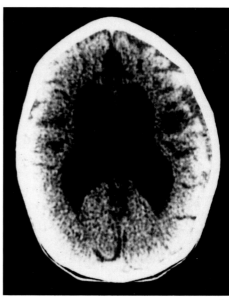

Fig. 511(a)   (b)

A Case of   *Twin gestation. Mother with anemia, obesity, latent prediabetes; complicated delivery; compound presentation of one twin. This infant later developed cerebral palsy, microcephaly; basal ganglia damage.*

This was not a robust pregnancy. The mother was noncompliant; there was no medical record of the first half of the pregnancy, no early prenatal care. Twin gestation was discovered late in the pregnancy.

The mother was apparently sick for a time at 29 weeks of pregnancy. She reported having diarrhea. She failed to gain weight appropriately at this time, in fact, she lost weight.

Any kind of maternal illness during pregnancy, physical or emotional illness, directly affects the maternal-placental-fetal complex, compromising the fetus. Pathologically, the causal process exercises its effects through the common denominator of intrauterine hypoxia.

The severity of the maternal illness does not necessarily correspond to the degree of fetal damage. A mild maternal illness may prove disastrous for the fetus; at other times the fetus seems to escape manifest damage.

Pregnancy obesity was present in this mother. She gained 43 pounds, excessive even for twin gestation, weighing 188 pounds at delivery. Pregnancy obesity is adversive to the well-being of the fetus; it is reflective of an underlying metabolic dysfunction in the mother and predisposes to diabetes.

Latent prediabetes was apparent in this mother. In addition to pregnancy obesity, she had a history of familial diabetes. She was a multipara with a reproductive record of three previous macrosomic babies, with weights up to 10 pounds. Birth of a macrosomic baby often is the first indicator of a diabetic condition in the mother.

Anemia was evident in the mother at midpregnancy, with her hematocrit down to 29 percent. Hematocrit of less than 37 percent in pregnant women is a significant abnormality. Maternal anemia is associated with fetal deprivation, fetal hypoxia (page 45).

Anemia involves a decrease in the red cells in the blood, a decrease in hemoglobin. Hemoglobin is the oxygen-carrying vehicle in the blood. Accordingly, anemia, as in this case, compromises oxygenation of the mother, with resulting decreased oxygen supply to the placenta and to the fetus. While this kind of pregnancy complication may be tolerated by the fetus in many cases, in other instances such oxygen deprivation may lead to intrauterine fetal death or may be sublethal and cause fetal damage, lasting cerebral damage.

Labor was induced at 40 1/2 weeks of the pregnancy. The first fetus, with a vertex presentation, was delivered vaginally, with low forceps. This newborn infant had a good Apgar score (no follow-up information available).

The second fetus descended with a compound presentation with an arm prolapsed alongside the head. The infant was delivered by cesarean section.

Although the mother had delivered macrosomic babies previously, the two babies in this pregnancy were only moderately oversized. Applying the standard reference table for newborn weights (for twins), the first twin, at 6 pounds 7 ounces (2,920 grams), was in the eightieth percentile and the second twin, this case, weighed 7 pounds 3 1/2 ounces (3,360 grams), above the ninetieth percentile.

Depression of severe degree was present in the second twin at birth. Apgar score was 3 and 3. Although depressed at first, she responded to care given and at 20 minutes she had spontaneous respiration and a good cry; her color was pink. At 30 minutes she was actively moving extremities, was grimacing, had a suck reflex. The fontanelles remained soft and flat, indicating there was no acute hypoxic brain swelling. This was confirmed subsequently by ultrasound and CT scans that proved normal. During the first day she remained active, stable, tolerated her feeds well, was out to her mother several times.

This is not the clinical picture of a newborn infant harboring fresh acute cerebral damage incurred intranatally. Infants born with acute hypoxic cerebral damage do not soon improve; they remain limp and comatose for prolonged periods, with unstable vital function, with respiratory failure, with congestive heart failure, for days.

The newborn in this case was not like that after delivery.

The clinical pattern in this case is consistent with the syndromic pattern of latent subacute cerebral damage present at birth, damage incurred a period of time prior to birth, damage related to adversive pathologic processes during gestation.

Seizure activity that began soon after birth interrupted the infant's improvement.

It is well known that epilepsy commonly occurs after brain damage involving the cerebral cortex. Pathologically, the brain lesion forms a seizure-generating (epileptogenic) focus in the cortex. The epileptogenic damage can be incurred in the fetal brain, antenatally, weeks or months before birth. With the fetus surviving to term, the damage in the cortex becomes subacute, capable of causing seizure activity soon after birth.

CT scan and ultrasound studies of the brain in the immediate postnatal days were reported to be normal. This is of major importance in ruling out the presence of acute cerebral edema and other acute pathologic changes. Pertinently, however, these studies of the brain do not rule out the presence of subacute, old, pathologic changes, latent processes often not visualized by CT scan and ultrasound (page 31).

Although the neonatal CT scans did not demonstrate evidence of cerebral damage, the follow-up CT studies at 5 years showed focal cavitations in the basal ganglia. The CT scans showed decreased cerebral white matter, correlating clinically with the development of microcephaly.

Microcephaly was evident in early infancy.

Enlargement of the brain is normally due to growth, thickening, of the deep cerebral layers, the periventricular strata. With deep brain damage occurring during early fetal life, with destruction of periventricular white matter, the brain ultimately fails to grow normally, leading to microcephaly.

This child developed cerebral palsy. Cerebral palsy is caused by damage to the basal ganglia, located deep in the brain (Figure 512).

This deep damage originates consistently, specifically, only in the immature premature brain, during early fetal life. Complications at term (mature) delivery do not cause deep cerebral damage, do not cause cerebral palsy. Maternal illnesses, complications during pregnancy, cause damage to the fetus, cause hypoxic cerebral damage. When the fetus is damaged during early fetal life, if the fetus survives to term, the infant is born with old subacute brain damage. Deep damage incurred in the premature brain (causing cerebral palsy) at times extends to the cerebral surface, to the cortex, resulting in cortical manifestations of mental retardation and epilepsy. This is the clinical-pathologic sequence that evolved in the present case.

Figure 512. Basal ganglia damage in a case of cerebral palsy. Focal area of decreased density bilaterally in the putamen (more prominent on the right side of the illustration). CT scan of brain at 5 years.

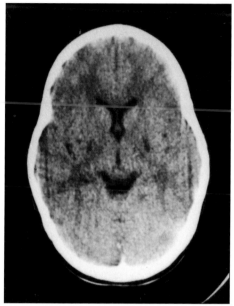

Fig. 512

A Case of   *Subacute cerebral infarction in a postmature dysmature neonate. Infant developed porencephaly, spastic cerebral palsy, and mental retardation.*

Pretoxemia signs appeared in the mother during the last trimester, with a period of sudden weight increase of 10 pounds and the development of peripheral edema. Overall, the mother was described as being "sick through most of the pregnancy."

Labor onset developed at 43 weeks of the pregnancy, with a vertex presentation. After 8 hours of desultory labor, with signs of fetal distress appearing on the monitor tracing, a cesarean section was done.

The newborn infant was depressed at birth with an Apgar score of 3 and 7. She gradually improved during the first day, with stable vital function; she was active, with a good cry. Lungs were clear.

Postmaturity as well as dysmaturity were evident at birth (page 93). The pregnancy by dates, 43 weeks, had been confirmed in prenatal ultrasound studies. At birth there was physical evidence that this fetus (infant) had reached maturity in utero and then remained in utero, acquiring bodily maturation equivalent to an infant 3 weeks old. The pattern of the footprint, the complexity and size of the skin creases, was plainly beyond that as seen in the sole print at 40 weeks.

Another valid measure of maturity-postmaturity is foot length of the newborn. The average foot length at 40 weeks is 7.3 centimeters. The right foot (print) was 8.3 centimeters.

Desquamation of the skin was present; the clinical record of the newborn points out "extensive peeling of the skin," a well-known pathognomic sign of postmaturity.

Postmature infants are at times also dysmature.

Dysmature infants are recognized by their long lean wizened appearance; they show decreased subcutaneous tissue. The newborn infant in this case was long (21 1/2 inches; 53.7 centimeters), above the ninetieth percentile for length. With regard to her weight (7 pounds 6 ounces; 3,345 grams), she was somewhat less than average for 43 weeks. The malnourished appearance of this newborn was noted in the clinical record, "decreased subcutaneous tissue."

Dysmaturity means chronic fetal deprivation, not only of nutriment but also of oxygen, chronic intrauterine hypoxia. Surviving dysmature infants have an increased incidence of cerebral palsy.

The cause of the dysmaturity in most cases is unclear. At times it is related to maternal illness during pregnancy.

Neurologically the infant in the postnatal days was noted to be increasingly lethargic, with a degree of generalized hypotonia.

Seizures of transient nature occurred beginning late on the first day. An EEG on day 9 was abnormal.

CT scan of the brain on day 10 (Figure 513) revealed evidence of far-advanced cerebral damage, an area of subacute infarction (page 33). In the CT scans, the cerebral ventricles are patent, indicating an absence of acute cerebral edema; this is evidence that the large area of cerebral damage was subacute, old, incurred long before birth.

Follow-up CT scans of the brain at 2 1/2 months (Figure 514) showed decreased density over most of the left cerebrum (right side of the illustration), forming a porencephalic cyst (page 28). The cerebral white matter was much decreased.

Microcephaly resulted from the severe cerebral damage, the failure in growth of the cerebrum.

This infant survived with severe developmental delays, with severe mental retardation, and spastic cerebral palsy; spasticity was more severe on the right, reflecting the far-advanced porencephaloclastic cerebral destruction of the left side of the cerebrum.

Cerebral palsy is due to damage to the basal ganglia (the extrapyramidal system) located in the deep portion of the cerebrum. Damage to the deep structures, to the basal ganglia, occurs consistently in the premature (immature) fetus following gestational hypoxia-producing complications. The cerebral damage in the deep cerebral tissues consists of hemorrhagic infarction. Fetuses that survive to term are born harboring old, subacute lesions in the deep periventricular structures and later develop cerebral palsy. At the time of the hypoxic process in the premature period, the cerebral damage may extend from the deep structures through the wall of the cerebrum, damaging the cortex, and later may cause (in addition to the cerebral palsy) mental deficiency and other developmental disabilities.

Figure 513. Subacute cerebral infarction. Large area of decreased density in the left temporoparietal region (right side of the illustration), with some areas of increased density compatible with hemorrhagic infarction. Ventricles are patent. CT scan of the brain at 10 days.

Figure 514. Porencephalic cyst occupying most of the left cerebrum, the result of the large cerebral infarction noted in Figure 513. The porencephalic cyst communicates with the left lateral ventricle. Cerebrum with overall decreased white matter. CT scan of brain at 2 1/2 months.

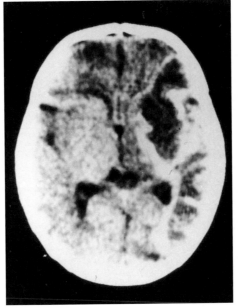

Fig. 513

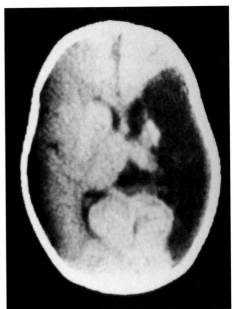

Fig. 514

A Case of   *Maternal morbid obesity; vaginal bleeding. Tight nuchal cord. Infant developed hydranencephaly, with severe cerebral palsy and mental retardation.*

The mother had many medical problems during this pregnancy, processes adverse to the well-being of the fetus: recurrent vaginal bleeding, sore throat, urinary tract infection; she was hospitalized with cholecystitis.

Maternal illness causes fetal deprivation. The damaging effect on the fetus, the common denominator is hypoxia.

Obesity was a problem in this pregnancy. This mother, 5 feet 3 inches tall, weighed 216 pounds at term, was morbidly obese. Obesity, a hazard to the pregnant mother and her fetus, is reflective of a disturbed bodily metabolism. Obesity predisposes to diabetes, common in people who develop diabetes.

Vaginal bleeding, first at 12 weeks of pregnancy, recurred two or more times, with clots up to 3 to 4 inches wide. It was thought that this was prelusive to miscarriage; however, the pregnancy was maintained.

Vaginal bleeding during pregnancy is associated with a high fetal-neonatal mortality and morbidity. Vaginal bleeding during pregnancy is known to lead to a substantial increase in cerebral disabilities in offspring.

Labor developed at term. The fetus presented as a double footling breech. The second stage of labor progressed rapidly. However, during the last 15 minutes the fetal monitor tracing indicated fetal distress.

Severe depression of the newborn was present at delivery, with an Apgar score of 2 and 5.

A nuchal cord, two times tight around the neck, was revealed when the aftercoming head was being delivered (page 83).

With nuchal cord, the fetus may be subjected to hypoxia weeks or months before labor, with resulting total asphyxia and death of the fetus. Or, during the gestation the fetus may be subjected on and off to intermittent hypoxia.

With nuchal cord present during labor, during the descent of the fetus, the loop of cord around the neck tends to become tightened.

The newborn infant responded to resuscitation and at 10 minutes was pink and crying. The record notes there were no apparent clinical problems with the infant in the nursery during the first day.

Thymic atrophy was noted in the x-ray of the thorax. Decreased size of the thymus is a mark of intrauterine fetal deprivation, a consequence of adversive gestational processes (page 94).

The infant survived. The CT studies of the brain in infancy revealed hydranencephaly (Figure 515). Clinically, severe cerebral palsy and mental retardation developed.

When was the manifest brain damage incurred, and to what is the damage attributable?

A fetus subjected to repeated maternal illness, to ongoing adverse conditions during intrauterine life, as in this case, accrues hypoxic cerebral damage. In the premature fetus, prior to 35 weeks' gestation, the damage is located consistently in the deep, periventricular, white matter and adjoining basal ganglia. If the fetus survives and the gestation continues to term, the cerebral lesion becomes subacute. The term fetus is born harboring latent subacute cerebral damage that ultimately leads to cerebral palsy and other cerebral disabilities.

Figure 515. Hydranencephaly; loss of periventricular white matter, of extreme degree, resulting in greatly enlarged ventricles. Frontal region shows confluent large cystic cavitations in the remaining cerebral wall. CT scan of brain at 15 months.

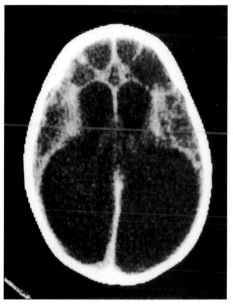

Fig. 515

A Case of   *Teenage pregnancy; near miscarriage; decreased fetal activity. Cranial epidural hematoma present at birth; fetal-neonatal anemia. Infant developed cerebral palsy, mental retardation, and seizure disorder.*

The mother was 16 at the beginning of this gestation. The mother's age, plus being a primipara, are factors unfavorable for the mother and the fetus. There is an increased incidence of fetal and neonatal morbidity and mortality with young primiparous mothers. There is an increased incidence of cerebral palsy in offspring of young primiparous mothers.

Threatened miscarriage occurred. Vaginal bleeding with cramps was present for several days at 27 weeks. Vaginal bleeding with large clots recurred at 34 weeks, with uterine contractions at ten-minute intervals.

Vaginal bleeding is due most often to pathologic processes affecting the placenta, to latent placental abruption or placental infarction, processes that compromise the fetus.

Decreased fetal activity was noted by the mother during the period of the threatened miscarriage. Decreased fetal activity reflects enfeeblement of the fetus. The loss of fetal activity is known as the "fetal alarm signal" (page 169).

Pathologic gestational processes have an adverse effect on the fetus exercising their pathologic effects during intrauterine life, rendering the fetus hypoxic and weakened.

This pregnancy, complicated by premature labor, by threatened miscarriage, was however maintained to term, with the mother receiving prolonged treatment with tocolytic agents and bed rest.

Forceps delivery was decided on in this case. After prolonged labor, with the mother exhausted after pushing for 2 1/2 hours, with the head descended into the pelvis, forceps delivery was undertaken. The procedure proved difficult. After repeated forceps application, the baby was delivered (page 125).

The newborn infant, despite the difficult forceps delivery, was in good clinical condition, with an Apgar score of 7 at one minute and 8 at five minutes.

Anemia was suspected in the infant, pale at birth. The presence of anemia was confirmed in the hematology studies, with the newborn hematocrit reported as low as 25 percent (normal for newborn is 61 ± 7.4 percent).

It is conclusive that this infant, noted to be pale at birth, developed this anemia gradually, chronically, during intrauterine life. Chronic anemia, in the fetus as in the adult human, causes chronic hypoxia. The red cell is the oxygen-carrying vehicle in the blood. The decrease in hematocrit means this fetus existed with much less than the average amount of oxygen supply, chronic severe fetal hypoxia.

The cause of the anemia was not clear, with fetal-maternal transfusion a possibility (page 97).

The condition of the infant at birth, as noted, was good. Although severely anemic, he breathed spontaneously, did not need resuscitation. He was put in the regular nursery. Vital signs were stable. He was bathed and took a feeding the first morning. Examination of the infant at 6 hours indicated the chest was normal, neurological function normal. The infant's well-being during the first day was recorded as normal and the plan was for "routine newborn care."

Plainly, this is not the clinical pattern of a newborn with acute fresh cerebral damage.

Newborn infants who have acute fresh brain damage show it. They are depressed at delivery, do not breathe, have low Apgar scores. After delivery they stay depressed, comatose, flaccid, with unstable vital signs. The newborn infant in the present case was not like that.

The clinical neurologic pattern in the present case — with the infant in good condition during the first day and later developing cerebral palsy — is compatible with the presence of latent subacute cerebral damage, damage that is present at birth but not manifested (page 166).

Seizure activity that developed on the second day compromised the good clinical condition of the baby.

The occurrence of seizures in the newborn period does not automatically make certain that the underlying cerebral damage was incurred during labor and delivery. There is increasing clinical opinion that when seizures appear soon after birth, the process is not attributable to acute intranatal asphyxial brain damage, but rather, the cause must be sought in pathologic processes, brain damage, prior to birth.

A cranial epidural hematoma was evidenced by CT scan of the head on day 2, following the onset of seizures (Figure 516). The radiologist's report stated: "small right-sided epidural hematoma, no evidence of intraparenchymal hemorrhage." The CT scan showed the cerebral ventricles widely patent, evidencing that there was no brain swelling, no cerebral edema, and no acute cerebral damage.

Figure 516a depicts the pathology of an epidural hematoma. Anatomically, from the outside inward, the diagram shows the scalp, the calvarium (skull bone), and the underlying, tightly attached, sheet of dura. With the formation of the epidural hematoma, the dura becomes detached from the calvarium, forming, as in this case, a lentiform clot between the bone and the dura (Figure 516b).

The formation of the epidural hematoma may be related to the difficult forceps delivery. An epidural hematoma in the newborn, as in this case, is attributable to the formation of a so-called "indentation" of the calvarium during delivery of the head.

Indentation of the calvarium appears as a depression in the surface of the infant's head, usually 3 to 4 centimeters wide. Indentations are the result of flicking inward of the flexible resilient plate of bone, like depressing the side of a Ping-Pong ball. Most commonly the deformity is produced as the head is pulled under the promontory of the pelvis during a breech or forceps delivery. The deformity of the skull in most cases corrects itself spontaneously. With indentation, at times tearing of small blood vessels between the dura and the overlying bone occurs, with the formation of a localized epidural hematoma (page 125).

The epidural hemorrhage in the present case was surgically evacuated; the surgeon noted that the hematoma yielded about 20 milliliters of fluid. There was no active bleeding. No subdural bleeding.

Taking into account the CT scan (no cerebral swelling) and the small size of the hematoma, on a pathologic basis, it is conclusive that the hematoma did not cause brain damage.

Cerebral palsy developed in this infant. Cerebral palsy is a "dyskinesia," a defect in motor function caused by damage to the basal ganglia, located deep in the brain. This deep damage occurs consistently, specifically, only in the immature premature brain, during early fetal life. In the present case the brain damage responsible for the cerebral palsy is attributable to gestational hypoxia-producing maternal factors and to the intrauterine anemia of the fetus.

Deep damage incurred in the premature brain (causing cerebral palsy) at times extends to the cerebral surface, to the cortex, resulting in cortical manifestations of mental retardation and epilepsy, as occurred in the present case.

This case demonstrates the late effects pathologically of hypoxic deep cerebral damage seen in cases of cerebral palsy. In infants surviving the damaged deep cerebral structures, necrotic periventricular white matter is gradually absorbed, resulting in ventricular enlargement (Figure 517).

Figure 516(a). Cranial epidural hematoma. Diagram indicating a collection of blood separating the dura from the bone, creating an epidural hematoma.

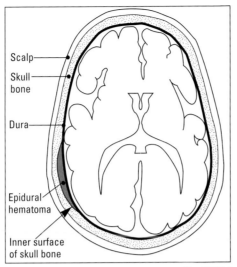

Scalp

Skull bone

Dura

Epidural hematoma

Inner surface of skull bone

Fig. 516(a)

Figure 516(b). Cranial epidural hematoma. In the right parietal region (left side in the illustration), a flat lentiform density under the right parietal bone (indicated by notch in the film), consistent with an epidural collection of blood, an epidural hematoma. The adjacent surface of the cerebrum flattened by the hematoma. Cerebral lateral ventricles patent. CT scan of head on day 2.

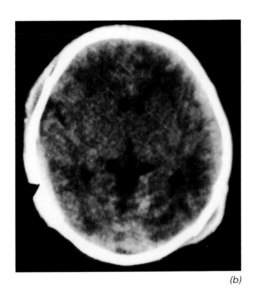

(b)

Figure 517. Ventriculomegaly. Cerebral ventricles enlarged due to shrinkage of damaged periventricular white matter. Late effects of hypoxic deep cerebral damage. CT scan of brain at 2 1/2 months.

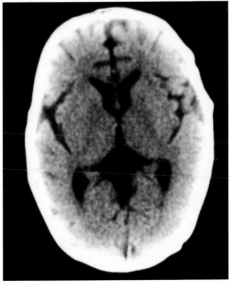

Fig. 517

A Case of **_Twin transfusion syndrome. Anemic newborn twin developed cerebral palsy._**

The twin fetuses were compromised by a complicated pregnancy and delivery and by the development of the twin placental transfusion syndrome.

The mother was a teenage single girl who became pregnant, a primipara who had no prenatal care during the first months of pregnancy. At the time she went to her doctor, at ten weeks, at the first prenatal visit, she was sick with an upper respiratory infection, and was treated with antibiotics.

Emotional stress substantially affects a pregnancy, as in this case — a teenage mother, unmarried, consorting with an abusive man who previously had broken her jaw (he fathered the babies) (page 53).

Essentially, whatever happens to the mother affects the fetus. Maternal pathologic processes exercise an adversive effect on the fetus, causing fetal hypoxia, at times leading to miscarriage — or the fetus, blighted during gestation, surviving to term, is born with old, subacute cerebral damage.

Vaginal bleeding began at 29 weeks of the pregnancy, together with irregular uterine contractions.

The most common cause of vaginal bleeding during midpregnancy is premature partial detachment of the placenta. The placental detachment forms a pocket of blood, a hematoma, behind the placenta. In the present case a partial abruption, a retroplacental hematoma, was present at delivery (pages 44, 68).

Birth of the twins occurred at 31 weeks of gestation.

Twin A, with a vertex presentation, was delivered vaginally with outlet forceps. (Twin A is the infant in the present case.) This infant, although noticeably pale, was in good condition at birth, with an Apgar score of 6 and 7.

Twin B delivery was complicated by a transverse presentation; a cesarean section was done. The infant was depressed at birth, with an Apgar score of 1 and 4, reflecting the stress of the complicated delivery. He responded to care and gradually improved.

Anemia in twin A, evident at birth in the pale infant, was of severe degree, confirmed in the newborn hematology reports. The red blood cell count (RBC) was 2.92 million (normal, 4.2 million). The hematocrit level was 34.2 percent (normal, 46 percent). Hemoglobin was 11.3 grams (normal, 15 grams). (The normal levels quoted here are for infants of 31 weeks' gestational age.)

In twin B, the depressed twin, anemia of a mild degree was present, with an RBC level of 3.57 million, hematocrit of 41.5 percent and hemoglobin of 13.9 grams.

The question arose — In twin A, did the fetal-neonatal anemia cause *acute* brain damage, present at birth, damage that led to cerebral palsy?

The valid assessment of the presence or absence of acute brain damage is based, not on what may or may not have occurred during the events of delivery, but is based on the performance of the newborn. This infant was in stable neurologic condition after delivery, with an Apgar score of 6 and 7, very good for a small preemie, equivalent to a 9 or 10 score in a term baby. He was active, moving all extremities at the time of his initial examination when admitted to the nursery. His Moro reflex was positive, lungs were clear to auscultation. Fontanelles remained soft.

The neurologic picture in this baby, active and alert neonatally, is not the pattern of a newborn with acute fresh cerebral damage (page 166).

The outcome of this gestation, comparing the eventual neurologic development of the twins, was paradoxical. Twin A, in good condition at birth, turned out to have manifest brain damage with sequelant cerebral palsy. Twin B, the depressed newborn, appeared to have escaped brain damage and at the age of 10 years was in grade four in school.

How come?

In retrospect, the main difference in the newborn twins, the process that manifestly had the most impact, was the factor of anemia. Twin A was severely anemic; twin B was not. Anemia in twin A was attributable to twin transfusion syndrome (page 97).

Twin transfusion, transfer of blood fetus-to-fetus, is thought to occur in almost all twin gestations; however, in most instances it is of minor degree. One fetus becomes the donor, the other is the recipient. If the process becomes advanced, the donor fetus gradually becomes anemic, hypoxic.

In summary, the hypoxia-producing anemia that developed in twin A during intrauterine life resulted in an accumulation of hypoxic cerebral damage. As a result, this infant harbored latent old subacute cerebral damage at birth, damage not evident neurologically at birth, damage that later surfaced with manifestations of cerebral palsy and other cerebral disability.

A Case of   *Maternal psychiatric stress. Newborn with severe anemia. Infant later developed microcephaly, cerebral palsy, with mental retardation and seizure disorder.*

Maternal stress, severe and ongoing, was evident in this pregnancy. The mother's history reflected the background of a dysfunctional family. She had had two previous pregnancies, both terminated by abortion. She was unwed, unemployed, indigent, unable to afford prenatal care. Previously, following an abortion, she had attempted suicide by drug overdose.

There is increasing evidence clinically and experimentally that maternal emotional stress, in the same way as physical illness, has adversive effects on the fetus (page 53).

Labor developed spontaneously at term; labor was desultory. Pitocin augmentation was undertaken. Fetal bradycardia developed. Forceps delivery was attempted but was unsuccessful. Cesarean section was done.

Depression of the newborn infant was severe. The infant appeared pale and lifeless, with an Apgar score of 0 and 0. However, she soon responded to resuscitation.

Anemia was evident clinically. The newborn was described in the record as "very pale." Anemia was confirmed in the blood count done within the first hour. The red blood cell count (RBC) was 3.8 million (normal, 5.14 million). The hemoglobin level was 14.4 grams (normal, 19 grams). The hematocrit level was 41 percent (normal, 61 percent).

Transfusions were given beginning at 3 hours of life.

Regarding the cause of the anemia, it became apparent that, with other causes being excluded, this was a case of fetal-maternal transfusion syndrome (page 97).

The presence of fetal-neonatal anemia is an important element in defining the causal mechanism of the brain damage in this case. Anemia, in the fetus as in the adult human, causes chronic hypoxia.

What was the cause of the depression of this newborn infant? Was it due to acute fresh brain damage?

With the adverse effects of the newborn anemia immediately recognized and the infant transfused, within a few hours her vital signs improved, heart action was good, she responded to stimuli. Breath sounds were clear, the infant was crying and moving her extremities. Muscle tone became normal; suck reflex improved.

Ultrasound studies of the infant's brain showed normal structures, no edema, no hemorrhage evident.

Fontanelles were soft and flat at birth and stayed that way. Pathologically, the absence of bulging fontanelles rules out the presence of acute brain damage in this newborn infant.

Newborn infants who have acute diffuse brain damage are depressed at delivery and do not soon improve; they stay depressed for a long time, comatose, flaccid, with unstable vital signs, with bulging fontanelles.

This newborn was not like that.

The clinical pattern in the present case, with the infant improving after delivery, is compatible with the presence of latent subacute cerebral damage at birth.

Infants who are born harboring subacute cerebral damage, characteristically depressed at birth, respond to attention given with improvement in vital function (page 166).

Seizure activity that began soon after birth interrupted the infant's improvement. The occurrence of seizures in the newborn period does not automatically mean that the underlying cerebral damage was incurred during labor and delivery. There is increasing clinical opinion that when seizures appear soon after birth, the process is not attributable to acute intranatal asphyxial brain damage, but rather, the cause must be sought in pathologic processes, brain damage, prior to birth.

This child developed cerebral palsy. Cerebral palsy is a "dyskinesia," a defect in motor function caused by damage to the basal ganglia, located deep in the brain. This deep damage occurs consistently, specifically, only in the immature premature brain, during early fetal life.

Complications during pregnancy, hypoxia-producing pathologic processes such as intrauterine anemia as occurred in this case, cause hypoxic damage to the fetus, cause cerebral damage.

When the fetus is damaged during early fetal life, if the fetus survives to term, the infant is born with old subacute brain damage. Deep damage incurred in the premature brain (causing cerebral palsy) at times extends to the cerebral surface, to the cortex, resulting in cortical manifestations of mental retardation and epilepsy, as occurred in the present case.

MRI scans taken at 4 years showed the residues of early deep cerebral damage, damage to basal ganglia and loss of periventricular white matter leading to enlargement of ventricles (Figure 518). This pattern of cerebral changes is characteristic of cases of cerebral palsy, reflecting damage incurred specifically in the premature immature fetal brain.

Microcephaly developed, with the child's head size smaller than average, in about the tenth percentile.

The brain enlarges due mainly to elaboration, growth, of the deep strata of the cerebrum (not from the cortex). When the deep structures of the cerebrum are blighted during fetal life, the development, growth, of the brain eventually is attenuated; ultimately this becomes manifest as microcephaly during infancy. The compromise of the deep structures of the cerebrum thus leads to microcephaly in cases of cerebral palsy.

Figure 518. Cerebral palsy. Late effects of intrauterine hypoxia due to fetal anemia. MRI of brain at 4 years, frontal section. Decreased periventricular white matter with consequent increased size of ventricles and microcephaly clinically. A cyst-like defect, subependymal, adjoining the right caudate nucleus (left side in the illustration); residual lesion of periventricular infarct incurred during fetal life.

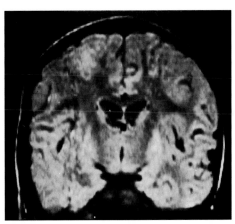

Fig. 518

A Case of   *Cytomegalic viral infection resulting in cerebral palsy.*

During this pregnancy the mother had mononucleosis, thought to be due to cytomegalic viral disease. Her clinical background revealed that prior to this pregnancy she had a variety of sexually transmitted diseases including viral infection that causes venereal warts and chlamydia infection.

Other problems appeared in this pregnancy. This mother had mental health problems. She had a prolonged upper respiratory infection early in pregnancy. Excessive weight gain occurred, reflective of a disorder of metabolism.

The chronic effects of an adverse intrauterine life were evident in this newborn. Although not acutely sick, he obviously was not vigorous, was pale, had feeding problems.

Psychiatric stress during the pregnancy was implicit in this case. This mother previously had been hospitalized with a reactive depression. This was a college student, from an affluent Catholic family, single, pregnant.

There is increasing evidence clinically and experimentally that maternal emotional stress, in the same way as physical illness, has adverse effects on the fetus (page 53).

Excessive weight gain occurred during this pregnancy. The mother's pregravid weight was 160 pounds. This mother weighed 204 pounds at term, a weight gain of 44 pounds. The average optimal pregnancy weight gain is 20 to 25 pounds.

Excessive maternal weight gain, of the degree in the present case, is usually of metabolic origin, due to endocrine dysfunction.

(This mother continued to be obese; and subsequently, in her second pregnancy, she delivered a macrosomic oversized baby of 10 pounds 1 ounce. Macrosomic babies are indicators of disturbed maternal metabolism, prelusive to diabetes.)

The mother developed hypertension.

The clinical factors eventuating in this mother — excessive pregnancy weight gain, increased blood pressure and, later, producing a macrosomic baby — reflect long-existing metabolic imbalance in the mother, present during the first pregnancy, adversive to the fetus.

Cytomegalic viral disease was indicated in this case (page 118). The mother had previously had infectious mononucleosis, an infectious disease commonly due to cytomegalic virus. The infant had a TORCH test (page 117) that was positive for cytomegalic viral infection. The pattern of damage that developed in the cerebrum is characteristic of damage caused by cytomegalic viral infection.

The cytomegalic problem, although not the only problem in this gestation, is with reasonable medical probability the main cause of the cerebral damage.

In addition to the positive TORCH test for CMV and a brain CT scan pattern consistent with CMV, this infant developed microcephaly and deafness, characteristic of a cytomegalic viral infection.

This child developed cerebral palsy. Cerebral palsy is caused by damage to a certain part of the brain, the basal ganglia, located deep in the brain. This deep damage occurs consistently, specifically, only in the immature premature brain, during early fetal life, and in the present case was attributable to cytomegalic viral infection. When the fetus is damaged during early fetal life, if the fetus survives to term, the infant is born with old subacute brain damage. Deep damage incurred in the premature brain (causing cerebral palsy) at times extends to the cerebral surface, to the cortex, resulting in cortical manifestations of mental retardation and epilepsy.

The cerebral palsy that developed in this infant was asymmetrical, with the right limbs more spastic than the left (page 182). This correlates with the pattern of damage evident in the CT scan of the cerebrum with the left cerebral hemisphere more affected than the right. The lateral ventricles in the cerebrum are enlarged, ex vacuo hydrocephalus, more on the left; the ventricular enlargement is the result of antecedent destruction, loss of tissue, in the periventricular strata. This is characteristic of CMV damage in the fetus, the newborn (Figure 519).

Figure 519. Cytomegalic viral disease, cerebral damage; asymmetrical cerebral palsy. Left cerebral hemisphere (on the right in the illustration) smaller than the right hemisphere; left lateral ventricle larger than the right due to greater loss of periventricular white matter. The difference in the size of the cerebral hemispheres correlates with the clinical pattern of asymmetric cerebral palsy, with greater spasticity on the right side of the body. CT of brain at 2½ years of age.

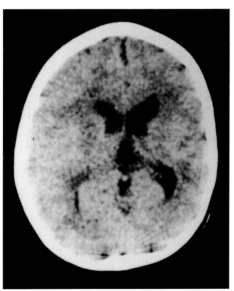

Fig. 519

A Case of **_Polycythemia in a premature newborn. Infant later developed cerebral palsy._**

Polycythemia present in the newborn was the outstanding pathologic factor in this case.

The infant was born prematurely, at 32 weeks of gestation.

Although this pregnancy was characterized as being uncomplicated, this mother did have significant problems during the pregnancy. During the last months of this pregnancy this mother had low weight gain; this was followed by vaginal bleeding at 29 to 30 weeks of the pregnancy.

In this circumstance, in most cases, the bleeding reflects a pathologic process in the placenta. The bleeding represents a late effect, meaning that the underlying pathologic process was ongoing for a time prior to the bleeding onset. All this — the intrauterine pathologic process, the bleeding, the threatened miscarriage, is a major insult to the fetus, predisposing to hypoxia, to hypoxic brain damage.

Manifestly, the fetus survived the intrauterine problem. The fetus got through the stress of labor and vaginal birth; the infant came out in good condition. The Apgar score — 5 to 6 at 5 minutes, with the infant starting to breathe spontaneously — was quite good for a 32-week baby, analogous to a 7 or 8 Apgar for a term infant.

Polycythemia was evident in the newborn hematology examination. Polycythemia literally means excessive number of (red) cells in the blood (page 104).

Hematology studies at 5 hours after birth showed the red cell count (RBC) to be 6.10 million (normal for 32 weeks, 4.2 million); hemoglobin level, 22.5 grams (normal for 32 weeks, 14.7 grams); hematocrit, 65.6 percent (normal for 32 weeks, 46 percent).

Regarding the origin of the polycythemia, red cells are formed in the bone marrow; in polycythemia, excessive red cells are formed in the bone marrow. The excessive red cell formation at times is triggered by the presence of intrauterine hypoxia. During gestation, if the fetus is subjected to hypoxia-producing gestational factors, polycythemia may result. The red cells carry oxygen to the fetus; the increase in red cells in polycythemia is an effort to compensate, to increase oxygenation in the hypoxic fetus.

Polycythemia does not come on suddenly. Plainly, the presence of polycythemia in this newborn is substantial evidence that this fetus was subjected to ongoing chronic hypoxia in the weeks, months, prior to birth.

This infant later developed cerebral palsy. When was this infant's brain damage incurred? Was there *fresh* brain damage present in this newborn at delivery? The valid assessment of the presence or absence of acute fresh brain damage is determined not by the events of labor but by the performance of the infant directly after delivery (page 164).

This infant performed well neurologically. He did not have the clinical pattern of a baby with acute stroke-like damage.

Infants born with acute hypoxic cerebral damage are limp, not moving, are comatose, have bulging fontanelles and have unstable vital function, and they stay that way for prolonged periods.

The newborn in this case was not like that after delivery.

The clinical pattern in this case is consistent with the syndromic pattern of latent subacute cerebral damage present at birth, damage incurred a period of time prior to birth, damage related to adversive pathologic processes to which the fetus was exposed.

Cerebral palsy that developed was due to deep cerebral damage incurred during premature immature fetal life. This deep damage at times extends to the cerebral surface, to the cortex, resulting in cortical manifestations of mental retardation and epilepsy.

In surviving infants, the damaged tissue in the deep cerebral periventricular stratum gradually undergoes scarring and contraction, with resulting increased size of the lateral ventricles. This pathologic condition, with ex vacuo hydrocephalus, is characteristic of late changes in cerebral palsy and was demonstrated in this case in MRI studies of the child at age 10 years (Figure 520).

Figure 520. Cerebral palsy; pattern of changes evident in MRI study of the brain at 10 years of age. **(a).** Scan through anterior level of the cerebrum. Increased periventricular signal indicating scarring of periventricular layer.

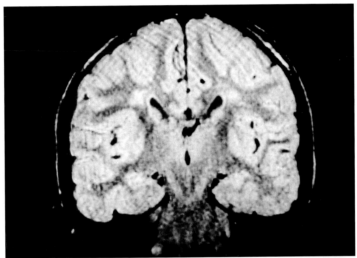

Fig. 520(a)

Figure 520(b). Scan through posterior level of the cerebrum. Decreased cerebral white matter with increase in size of the ventricles.

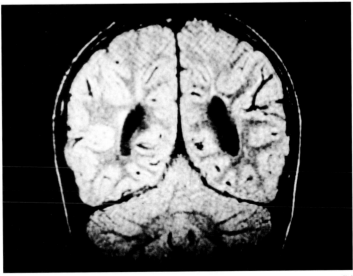

(b)

A Case of   *Nuchal cord; newborn with severe anemia. Infant later developed cerebral palsy, mental retardation, and seizure disorder.*

The mother had a protracted viral-type respiratory infection in the weeks prior to delivery. With viral infection, with fever, the mother's metabolism is elevated, the oxygen requirements of the mother are sharply increased, so that oxygenation of the fetus is depressed.

With gestational problems present during fetal life, the common denominator of these adverse processes is hypoxia — the fetus is subjected to varying degrees of oxygen deprivation that leads to an accruing of subacute cerebral damage in the fetuses surviving to term.

Labor developed prematurely at 36 weeks of the pregnancy. After 10 hours of labor, with failure of the parturition to progress, with the fetus showing evidence of distress on the monitor record, a cesarean section was done.

At delivery a nuchal cord was present. The newborn infant was severely depressed, limp, pale.

Nuchal cord, as present in this case, is an ongoing hazard to the fetus. In some cases, the umbilical cord becomes wound around the neck early on, months before term.

Anemia was recognized at birth, with the infant described as "very pale." Hematology studies revealed an RBC (red cell count) of 3.06 million (normal for 36 weeks is 4.7 million); hemoglobin level was 11.1 grams (normal for 36 weeks, 16 grams); hematocrit was 34.2 percent (normal, 49 percent). The infant received multiple transfusions.

Anemia in this newborn infant had its origin during intrauterine life, fetal-neonatal anemia. Chronic anemia, in the fetus as in the adult human, causes chronic hypoxia. The red cell is the oxygen-carrying vehicle in the blood. The decrease in hematocrit means this fetus existed with less than the average amount of oxygen supply, chronic fetal hypoxia. Intrauterine hypoxia leads to fetal hypoxic visceral damage. The brain is the most sensitive target tissue in the body; with intrauterine hypoxia, the fetus accrues subacute and acute cerebral damage.

The cause of the anemia in the present case was thought to be an intrauterine fetal-maternal transfusion process. Regarding the occurrence of the fetal-maternal transfusion syndrome, the transfer of blood from fetal to maternal circulation occurs regularly, in some degree in most if not all gestations. The degree, the amount of transfusion, varies, at times is severe. The cause, the pathogenesis, of the fetal-maternal transfusion process is thought to be associated with latent pathologic processes in the placenta.

The depression that was present in this newborn, considered retrospectively, is attributable to the fact that this was a sick fetus, chronically enfeebled by adversive maternal factors, compromised by a nuchal cord, rendered chronically weakened, anemic, unable to tolerate the stress of labor. Although depressed at first, he continued to improve after delivery, soon breathing on his own, with stable vital signs. Fontanelles remained soft and flat, indicating there was no acute brain swelling.

Pneumothorax, diagnosed on day one, complicated the postnatal course, rendering the infant hypoxic for hours, until the condition was resolved.

Seizure activity, noted late in the first day, was attributable to cerebral damage during fetal life.

Cerebral palsy developed in this infant. Cerebral palsy is caused by damage to the basal ganglia, located deep in the brain. This deep damage occurs consistently, specifically, only in the immature premature brain, during early fetal life, the consequence of maternal complications and intrauterine fetal pathologic processes. Deep damage incurred in the premature brain (causing cerebral palsy) at times extends to the cerebral surface, to the cortex, resulting in cortical manifestations of mental retardation, seizures, and other cortical disabilities, as in this case.

CT studies of the brain on day 1 and day 11 showed focal high density areas, evidence of hemorrhagic infarction through the left temporal and parietal regions.

CT studies of the brain at 7 months showed porencephalic deep periventricular damage in the temporoparietal region of the cerebrum on the left (Figure 521). This porencephalic damage corresponded to the infarctional damage noted in the neonatal CT scans. Ventricles were enlarged due to loss of deep cerebral white matter.

Microcephaly was evident in early infancy. With deep brain damage incurred in the premature cerebrum, with destruction of periventricular tissue, the brain is decreased in size, fails to grow normally, and the head consequently remains relatively small, microcephalic.

Figure 521. Deep porencephalic damage in the cerebral wall; periventricular area of decreased density in the left temporoparietal region (right side in the illustration). Decreased cerebral white matter with resulting ex vacuo hydrocephalus. CT of brain at 7 months of age.

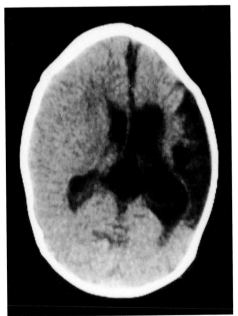

Fig. 521

A Case of   **Malformation of the cerebrum, "schizencephaly."
Infant with profound developmental retardation.**

This infant was born at term. The mother was a primipara; the pregnancy and parturition were said to have been uncomplicated.

Clinical information in the case was sparse. The infant presented equivocal features of Down syndrome. No pathologic neurological findings were recorded. Physically the infant was described as puny. He failed to thrive and died at 5 1/2 months of age.

The brain at autopsy showed a major structural abnormality. A deep cleft extended over the superior and lateral aspects of the cerebrum, along the direction of the precentral sulcus, from the midsagittal plane down to the Sylvian fissure. This pattern of structural abnormality is known as schizencephaly (*schiz-*, split; *-encephaly*, brain) (Figure 522).

Section made through the brain longitudinally, in the parasagittal plane, revealed the clefts extended deeply into the cerebrum. The cleft, viewed in a cut section of the cerebrum, showed irregularly projected ectopic deposits of cortical gray matter extending from the cleft surface into the subjacent white matter (Figure 523).

Pathologically, there is no evidence of a destructive process underlying the cerebral deformity in this case.

This cerebral structural abnormality is considered a true malformation, a localized dysgenesis in the formation of the cerebral wall during early embryonic life (page 150).

Schizencephaly is rare.

Figure 522. Cerebral malformation; schizencephaly. View of the upper aspect of the cerebrum showing a cleft extending transversely across both halves of the cerebrum. Infant with severe developmental retardation. Death at 5 1/2 months.

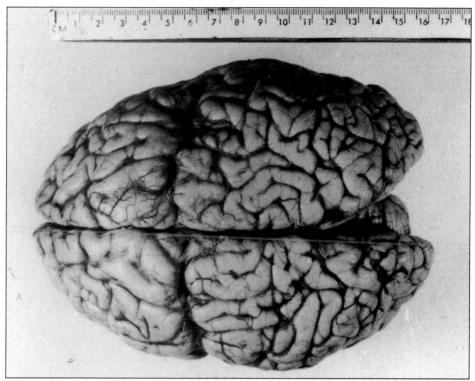

Fig. 522

Figure 523. Schizencephaly. Section of cerebrum through the cleft in Figure 522. Extending around the cleft are irregular ectopic projections of cortical gray tissue into the cerebral white matter.

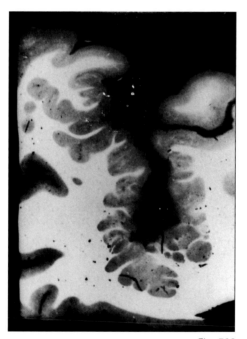

Fig. 523

A Case of **Diffuse chronic hypoxic cerebral damage, present at autopsy, in a one-month-old infant. Mother, teenage, with pregnancy emotional stress, viral infection, excessive weight gain, anemia, and apparent latent diabetes.**

The mother was a young primipara, factors associated with an unfavorable pregnancy outcome. Teenage pregnancy is associated with emotional stress, adversive to the gestation. There is no documented clinical information about this mother's health problems during the first two-thirds of this pregnancy; her first recorded prenatal visit was at approximately 28 weeks of gestation. The mother had evidence of a substantial gestational metabolic problem, with excessive pregnancy weight gain, urinary ketones, and a family history of diabetes. She became marginally anemic. The record indicated that she had a viral upper respiratory infection (URI).

This was a chronically compromised fetus, evident in the manifest decreased fetal activity in the last weeks of gestation (page 169).

Pregnancy was estimated to be 41 weeks. Labor was prolonged, to 28 hours, and with lack of progress, a cesarean section was done.

The newborn infant was depressed, with no spontaneous movements; he remained on a respirator. Fontanelles were soft. CT scans of the brain on day 1 showed open ventricles, no evidence of cerebral swelling; the posterior portion of the left side of the cerebrum showed mottled decreased density (Figure 524).

The infant died at 1 month of age.

Pathologically, there are substantial bases for concluding that the brain damage was incurred a long time before birth, weeks or months prior to labor. The foundation for this conclusion: At autopsy the location of the damage in this brain, the main damage, was in the deep strata of the cerebrum, affecting mainly the white matter, the deep periventricular regions. The cerebral surface was relatively preserved (Figure 525).

On the basis of established information from past clinical and pathology research, it is known that this pattern of cerebral damage, with destruction of the deep cerebral strata, with the surface layer remaining, has its origin specifically in the premature, immature, period of fetal life, related to hypoxic encephaloclastic insult long before term.

Figure 524. CT scan of the cerebrum at 1 day. Ventricles widely patent. Decreased density of the posterior portion of the hemispheres, most pronounced on the left. (Left side of the cerebrum is on the right in the illustration.)

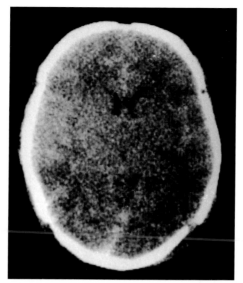

Fig. 524

Figure 525. Hypoxic chronic cerebral damage. Section of the cerebrum, autopsy specimen, shows the two halves of the cerebrum with midline structures of the brain stem. The cerebral hemisphere on the right appears smaller than the left, a distortion due to processing the specimen. The cerebral surfaces show a convolutional pattern that is still recognizable; the deeper strata, the cerebral white matter, are mostly disintegrated, absent, so that the cerebral walls appear as loculated cystic honeycombed structures.

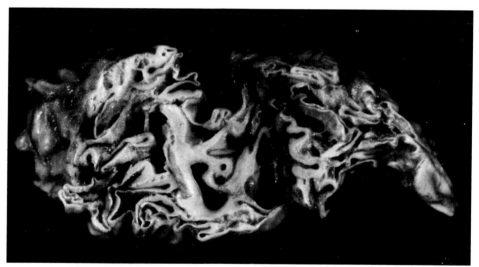

Fig. 525

A Case of   *Premature newborn; bleeding diathesis (DIC);*
              pulmonary hemorrhage; congestive heart failure;
              intracranial hemorrhage.

Premature labor developed spontaneously, with gestation at 30 weeks.

Presentation was vertex. Delivery was vaginal, with low forceps.

The infant was in good condition at birth, with an Apgar score of 8 and 10. Birth weight was 3 pounds 7 1/2 ounces, somewhat more than average for 30 weeks of gestation; physical features of the baby indicated a gestation of 32 weeks or more.

The infant lived 3 days. Respiratory distress developed in the hours after birth and gradually increased, unrelieved by ventilation with oxygen. Cyanosis increased.

A bleeding diathesis was evident on the second day, with oozing around the umbilical catheter and bleeding from needle puncture sites. DIC (disseminated intravascular coagulopathy) was diagnosed (page 114).

Spinal puncture on day 3 yielded xanthochromic fluid, indicating that intracranial bleeding had begun some days before.

Postnatal hypoxic congestive heart failure appeared, marked by peripheral edema and bulging fontanelles, indicative of cerebral edema.

Terminally, on the third day, recurrent episodes of apnea occurred.

At autopsy, the infant was severely cyanotic; the lower extremities were edematous (Figure 526).

The most striking finding at autopsy was the pathologic changes in the lungs. The lungs, externally of an angry bright red color, were firm, rubbery (Figure 527). The lungs were non-air-containing (the lungs sank when suspended in water). Pulmonary hemorrhage was present diffusely, with the tissue suffused with blood grossly and microscopically. The bleeding diathesis, evident prior to death, was the underlying cause of the pulmonary hemorrhage.

Congestive heart failure of severe degree was present. The heart was enlarged, dilated, and together with the large tributary veins in the mediastinum, was distended with blood (Figure 528). Hydrothorax and severe congestion of body viscera were present.

Intracranial hemorrhage was present, evident initially at autopsy by accumulation of subarachnoid blood around the cerebellum and brain stem (Figure 529). Studies of the brain specimen indicated that, with the development of hypoxic congestive heart failure, hemorrhagic infarction of periventricular germinal matrix had occurred (Figure 530). This led to intraventricular and subarachnoid hemorrhage, with the bleeding augmented by the hemorrhagic diathesis present, the DIC.

Figure 526. Severe cyanosis; peripheral edema. Infant of 30 weeks' gestation; lived 3 days.

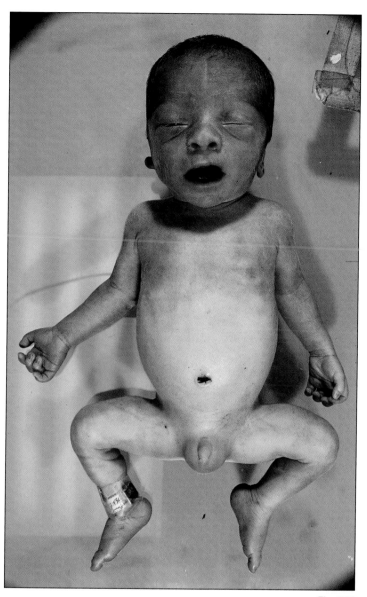

Fig. 526

Figure 527. Pulmonary hemorrhage. At autopsy, lungs reddened and rubbery, suffused with blood grossly and microscopically. Hemorrhagic diathesis developed postnatally. Respiratory failure with increasing hypoxia postnatally.

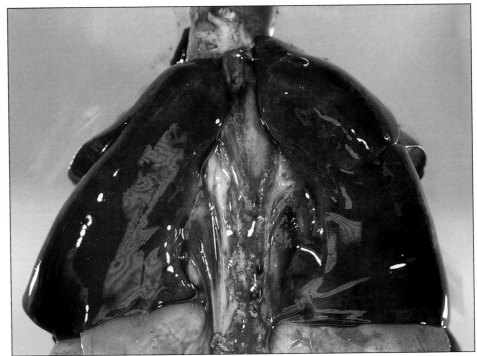

Fig. 527

Figure 528. Congestive heart failure due to hypoxia. Heart and great veins distended with blood. View of thoracic organs at autopsy.

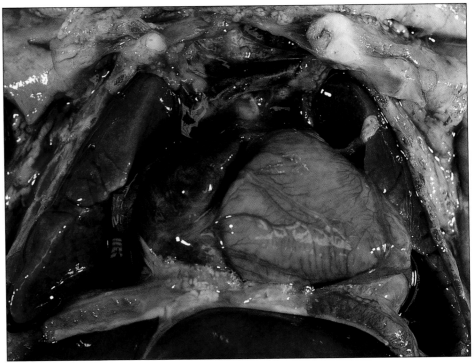

Fig. 528

Figure 529. Subarachnoid hemorrhage around the brain stem and cerebellum.

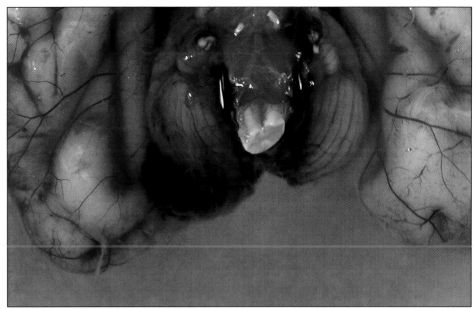

Fig. 529

Figure 530. Periventricular hemorrhagic infarction with intraventricular hemorrhage. Bleeding extending through the ventricles and outward, with resulting subarachnoid hemorrhage (Figure 529).

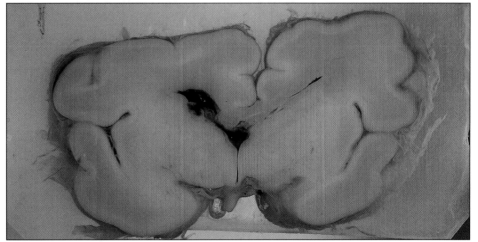

Fig. 530

A Case of

Chronic cerebral damage, frontal lobe and basal ganglia, present at autopsy. Manifestations of mental retardation and cerebral palsy during life.

This child, with severe mental retardation and cerebral palsy, died at age 5 years. At autopsy there was old chronic damage to the frontal lobe and to the basal ganglia.

The mental retardation in this child is related to the severe frontal convolutional scarring (Figures 531 and 532). Cerebral palsy present is related to damage to the deep cerebral structures.

Figure 531. The cerebral hemispheres showing frontal convolutions distorted, irregular, narrow; widened sulci. Posteriorly the convolutions of the cerebrum are relatively preserved.

Figure 532. Section through one side of the cerebrum, frontal region; severe loss of cerebral white matter, shrinking and scarring of convolutions; frontal damage related to severe mental retardation. The lateral ventricle is greatly enlarged, due to loss of cerebral white matter.

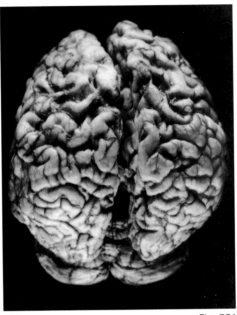

Fig. 531

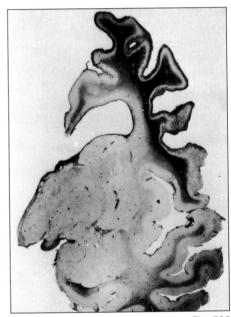

Fig. 532

A Case of   *Down syndrome with the development of Alzheimer's disease manifestations late in life.*

Down syndrome was recognized early in infancy (pages 145, 196). Developmental milestones were delayed. The child never talked plainly. She never went to school. She was institutionalized in a State School at age 2 1/2 years. At 6 1/2 years she was described as impulsive, but was bright and affectionate. Her IQ was estimated to be 32.

During adolescence her affect gradually changed. She had outbursts of temper. She became increasingly hostile, assaultive, and destructive. She had a mania for breaking window glass, broke 35 panes in 3 weeks. The patient was treated with sedation but continued to be disturbed and was transferred to a state mental hospital.

On admission to the hospital she was quiet and cooperative but apparently disoriented. She mumbled and was unresponsive to questions.

She continued to be impulsive in her actions, crying, yelling, and jumping about at times. There was an obvious increasing psychotic element superimposed on the mental deficiency of the Down syndrome.

The deterioration, the changes in behavior and disposition that developed in this woman with age, are common manifestations of Alzheimer's disease.

This woman died at age 52 years. At autopsy the brain showed a typical anatomic pattern of Down syndrome (Figure 96, page 146).

With more and more people with Down syndrome reaching older age, the transition in these cases to a clinical pattern of Alzheimer's disease, as occurred in this case, is increasingly observed (page 146).

A Case of   **A complicated pregnancy, with the offspring developing cerebral palsy, severe mental retardation; ex vacuo hydrocephalus.**

This was a complicated pregnancy with the mother having severe convulsions, eclampsia.

The infant had severe developmental retardation. Physical examination at age 6 years revealed an underdeveloped child, spastic in all extremities. There were periodic irregular convulsive movements; weight was 22 pounds, height 34 3/4 inches. He was poorly developed, poorly nourished and completely helpless. He cried, became excited and held his breath for extended periods. He was unable to perform any useful body movements and required complete custodial and nursing care.

The head was 17 1/2 inches in circumference, microcephalic. The extremities were pipe-stem in character. The upper extremities were maintained in a position of acute flexion at the elbow. The hands were held tightly clenched. The lower extremities were spastic and extended.

The child had frequent episodes of upper respiratory infection, with elevations of temperature up to 106 degrees. The child was in a critical state all of the last year of life. Death occurred at 7 years.

At autopsy, in removing the calvarium, the cerebrum was ruptured and, like a bag filled with water, collapsed onto the base of the skull as the cerebrospinal fluid escaped.

The brain (Figure 533) weighed 310 grams (about one-third of the average weight for the age). The lateral ventricles (Figure 534) were extremely dilated; the cerebral walls were 2 to 3 millimeters thick, with the cerebral white matter reduced to a thin layer. The cerebral hemispheres presented a picture of extreme ex vacuo hydrocephalus (page 29).

Figure 533. Hydrocephalus; microcephalus. Spastic quadriplegia, severe. Seven-year-old boy.

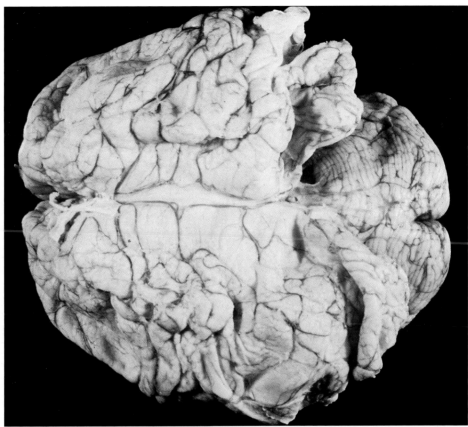

Fig. 533

Figure 534. Hydrocephalus ex vacuo; microcephalus. View of lateral ventricles; extreme thinning of cerebral walls, loss of cerebral white matter.

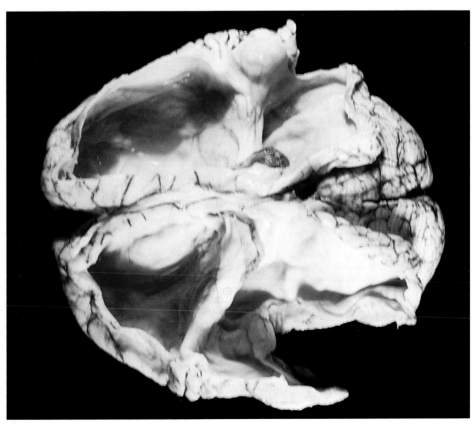

Fig. 534

A Case of   *Lissencephaly; arrest of cerebral and neurologic function.*

This child, born at term, failed to develop mentally and neurologically. There was history of maternal illness during pregnancy.

Retardation of development was evident from birth. The infant was almost completely helpless. Seizures developed at 9 months. The child was unable to walk or talk, was incontinent, had difficulty in chewing and swallowing, and presented complete mental lethargy.

Death occurred at 8 years. Weight was 35 pounds. The head was microcephalic. At autopsy the brain weighed 800 grams (below the second percentile for the age).

The outstanding physical feature of the brain was the smooth surface of the cerebrum. Convolutions were not apparent. On each side a deep fissure appeared, extending from above downward, through the midportion of the cerebrum (Figure 535).

The cerebral cortex, histologically, showed a haphazard scattering of nerve cells, with no organized lamellar pattern.

Lissencephaly represents a form of cerebral dysplasia (page 152).

Figure 535. Lissencephaly, characterized by a generally smooth cerebral surface. A microcephalic 8-year-old with severe lack of mental and neurologic function. **(a).** Side view of the cerebrum.

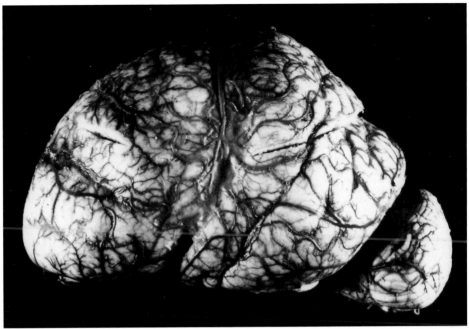

Fig. 535(a)

Figure 535(b). The upper surface of the cerebrum.

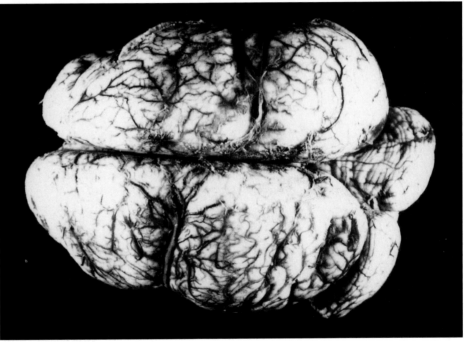

(b)

A Case of *Meningomyelocele (Arnold-Chiari syndrome), cardiac and other malformations. Maternal familial diabetes.*

The mother had a family history of diabetes. The pregnancy was recorded as having been uncomplicated. However, x-ray of the abdomen had revealed a hydrocephalic fetus. The infant, term, was stillborn.

As viewed at autopsy, the head was greatly enlarged. The infant had a "no neck" appearance, the head being attached broadly to the shoulders (Figure 536). As viewed from the side, the back, in the thoracic area, showed a red-brown protrusion. Viewed from the posterior of the body (Figure 537), this protrusion, located in the thoracic area, appeared as a broad midline mass, pathologically a meningomyelocele.

This case is an example of Arnold-Chiari syndrome. The meningomyelocele, containing elements of meninges and cord tissue, anchors the cord in the spinal canal so that as fetal body growth progresses, the medulla and cerebellum are drawn into the spinal canal. As a consequence, circulation of spinal fluid from within the ventricles outward is impeded and results in obstructive hydrocephalus.

In addition to the major nervous system defect in this case, there were other significant structural defects. The diaphragm on the right side was absent, resulting in herniation of the liver and other abdominal organs into the chest. The heart was severely deformed, an example of *cor triloculare*, a malformation with a single atrium.

As previously noted, the mother had a history of familial diabetes. The association between maternal diabetic conditions and the occurrence of malformations of the heart and other viscera is well known. This case is an example of a nervous system abnormality linked to an apparent latent maternal diabetic condition.

Figure 536. Hydrocephalus. Enlarged head, 45 centimeters in circumference (normal, 34 centimeters). "No neck" malformation, the head placed broadly on the shoulders. The side view of the body shows in the midthoracic area a protruding flat red-brown mass, a meningomyelocele (Figure 537).

Figure 537. Meningomyelocele; midportion of the back. In the center, fleshy cystic mass (containing elements of meninges and nervous tissue), a meningomyelocele.

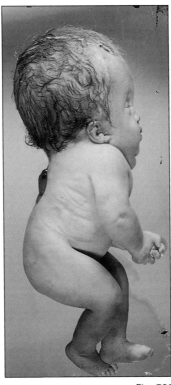

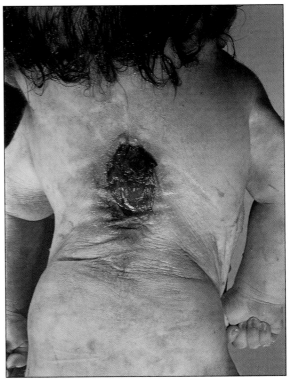

Fig. 536   Fig. 537

A Case of **Down syndrome; cerebral convolutions of abnormal form.**

The parents of this child were in their thirties at the time of the pregnancy. The mother was said to have been under considerable mental stress. This was the third of four children.

The infant showed a typical Down syndrome appearance (page 145). The eyes were slanted. The eyes showed speckling of the irides, Brushfield spots. Characteristic of Down syndrome, the tongue was large, the hands were broad, square, with the fifth fingers incurved.

The infant was institutionalized at an early age. He walked at 2 years. He was never able to talk. His IQ was later estimated to be 8. (The other children in the family showed no mental deficit.) He remained institutionalized and died at age 37 following a respiratory infection.

The brain at autopsy was of abnormal form (Figure 538). The cerebrum was short and had blunted frontal and occipital poles, a pattern common with Down syndrome. The brain weighed 1,300 grams, about average.

The cerebrum, typical of Down syndrome, showed a simplification and distortion of the convolutional pattern, with a lack of tertiary gyri. Convolutions in the frontal region were irregular, some bulging and enlarged, others small and compressed. Histologically, the frontal cortex was distorted, showed a poor lamellar pattern.

Figure 538. Cerebrum in a case of Down syndrome, showing characteristic shortening of the cerebrum and rounded blunting of the frontal pole. The convolutional pattern is simplified and distorted in the frontal region with some convolutions broad and bulging.

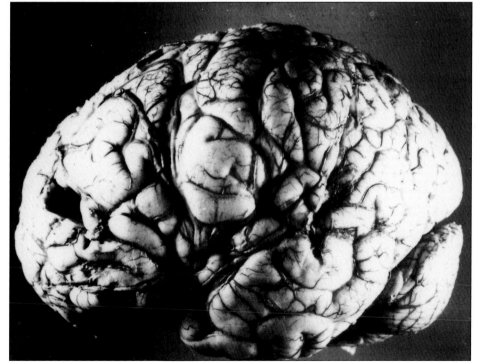

Fig. 538

A Case of **Obstructive hydrocephalus due to aqueductal malformation; atresia of the aqueduct of Sylvius.**

The hydrocephalus in this case had developed during intrauterine life; the newborn infant had a greatly enlarged hydrocephalic head. The infant was institutionalized; she presented severe developmental delays. She walked first at 3 years. She was eventually able to feed herself. She talked very little. Neurologic examination showed hyperactive deep tendon reflexes. Babinskis were negative. Muscle power was generally equal on both sides. The psychological assessment indicated an IQ of 57.

At age 15, her head circumference was 34 inches (85 centimeters) (normal head circumference at 15 years, approximately 22 inches, or 55 centimeters) (Figure 539). She had difficulty balancing her greatly enlarged head. Death occurred at age 15 following a fall, with the development of a traumatic subdural hemorrhage.

At autopsy, the outstanding feature was a massive hydrocephalus. A tan red subdural hemorrhage up to 8 millimeters thick extended over the upper surfaces of the cerebral hemispheres.

In removing the brain, a small laceration of the cerebrum occurred; the ballooned-out cerebral hemispheres collapsed, with the release of tan xanthochromic fluid through the laceration. Transection of the cerebrum revealed greatly dilated lateral ventricles (Figure 540). The wall of the cerebrum varied from 1.8 to 2.2 centimeters.

Anatomic studies of the brain revealed a classic example of aqueductal obstructive hydrocephalus (page 156). Together with the lateral ventricles, the third ventricle was also much dilated. With the third ventricle viewed from within, the opening into the aqueduct was obscured, anatomically closed. At the point normally occupied by the entrance into the aqueduct, the ependymal lining of the third ventricle extended smoothly from side to side with no indication of an entrance into the aqueduct.

Microscopically, study of the mesencephalon showed the proximal portion of the aqueduct, near the third ventricle, obliterated; the distal portion of the aqueduct was patent, intact.

Figure 539. Hydrocephalus; age 15 years. The large head, circumference 34 inches, was a top-heavy burden, difficult to balance.

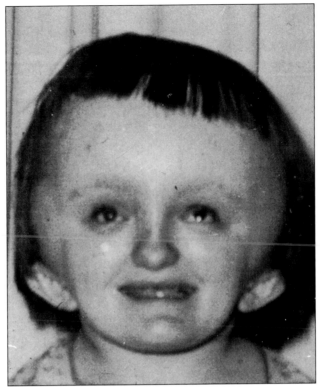

Fig. 539

Figure 540. Hydrocephalus. Greatly dilated lateral ventricles; cerebral walls much reduced in thickness.

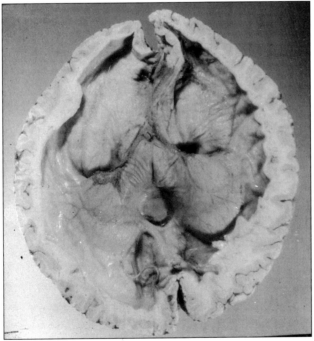

Fig. 540

A Case of **Twin transfusion syndrome. One twin, with encephaloclastic porencephaly, developed cerebral palsy.**

The twin in this case was small and anemic at birth. The other twin was considered normal. This clinical pattern is consistent with the processes of intrauterine placental transfusion syndrome, with the smaller twin, having been the donor fetus, rendered anemic, hypoxic, during intrauterine life (page 97).

The infant developed severe spasticity; he had a seizure disorder and was developmentally retarded. He failed to thrive and died at 11 months.

At autopsy the brain was small, weighed 450 grams; a large amount of fluid escaped from the cerebrum. Section through the cerebrum revealed a large cavitation in the left cerebral wall, approximately 3 centimeters wide, filled with clear fluid and connected to the lateral ventricle (Figure 541). Strands of fibrous tissue traversed the cavity. The wall of the cystic structure was indurated, scarred, and partly calcified.

The cavitation in the cerebral wall is characteristic of encephaloclastic porencephaly (page 28). The cerebral damage is attributable to the processes of intrauterine transfusion syndrome, rendering the smaller fetus hypoxic, with resulting cerebral hypoxic infarctional damage; the devitalized tissue, gradually absorbed postnatally, resulted in the porencephalic cavity.

Figure 541. Encephaloclastic porencephaly. A large cavitation present in the left cerebral wall with strands of tissue traversing the cystic space. Clinical history of twin transfusion syndrome, this twin born undersized and anemic. The cystic lesion is attributable to intrauterine cerebral hypoxic infarctional damage, with the devitalized tissue ultimately absorbed, leaving a cavitation.

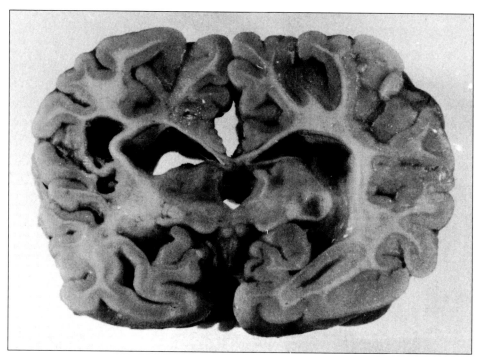

Fig. 541

A Case of *Macrocephaly; mental retardation and psychopathy.*

This was a difficult forceps delivery of a baby with a large head. The infant failed to thrive. At the age of 7 years the child was characterized as feebleminded (page 197). He had an awkward gait. He behaved in a silly manner.

As he became older he was subject to violent temper outbursts. He became assaultive.

He died unexpectedly at age 50; death was due to aspiration of gastric contents.

The brain at autopsy was larger than average size for an adult, weighed 1,560 grams (average adult weight, 1,200 grams). The cerebral convolutions appeared bulky with a paucity of tertiary gyri (Figure 542). Considering the excessive weight of the brain and the simplification of the convolutional pattern, this is an example of cerebral malformation, macrocephaly (page 143).

Figure 542. Macrocephaly. Brain weight, 1,560 grams (average adult weight, 1,200 grams). Cerebral convolutions bulky and simplified with few tertiary sulci. Mental retardation; behavior disorder. Death at 50 years.

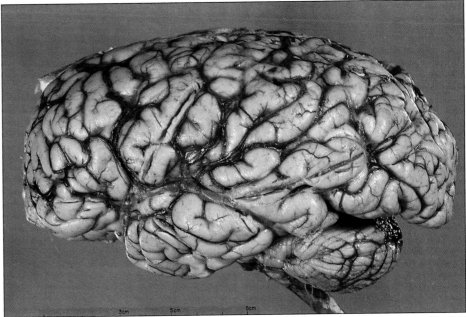

Fig. 542

A Case of   *A child born prematurely after a prolonged labor with subsequent development of cerebral palsy.*

Birth occurred at 32 months of gestation; labor was prolonged, 35 hours, and was difficult.

The premature infant survived but was developmentally severely retarded. He was described as being a low-grade retardate; he was microcephalic. Neurologic examination revealed spasticity of all the extremities with exaggerated deep tendon reflexes. The child developed contractures. The child remained physically enfeebled, malnourished. He developed pneumonia and expired at age 15.

At autopsy, the body was described as that of a puny boy, undersized, with crippled ankylosed joints.

The brain was small, weighed 750 grams (average weight, 1,150 grams). Over the superior surface of the cerebrum externally, over the lateral posterior region of the frontal and parietal lobes bilaterally, convolutions were distorted and shriveled (Figure 543). The surface convolutional distortions proved to be due to a severe loss of supporting convolutional white matter, as evident in Figure 544.

The loss of cerebral white matter — periventricular and convolutional white matter — is characteristic of the pathology of cerebral palsy. The cerebral damage leading to cerebral palsy in this case is attributable to the hypoxia-producing prolonged difficult delivery to which this fetus was exposed.

Figure 543. Microcephalic brain in a case of cerebral palsy and mental retardation (microcephaly is evident in comparing the very small size of the cerebrum with the relatively large size of the cerebellum). The cerebral hemisphere shows a broad area of distorted shrunken convolutions in the posterior frontal and neighboring regions.

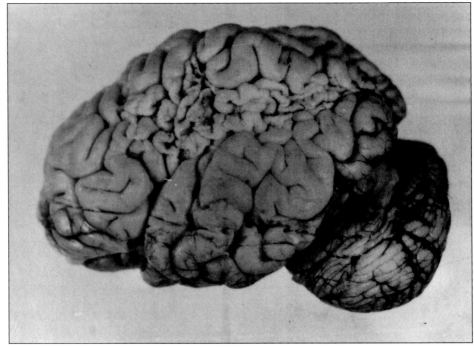

Fig. 543

Figure 544(a). Section through the cerebrum, through the region of distorted convolutions seen in Figure 543. In the regions of the damaged convolutions, although the surface of the convolutions appears relatively intact, the underlying convolutional white matter for the most part is lost. The lateral ventricles are enlarged due to decreased periventricular white matter.

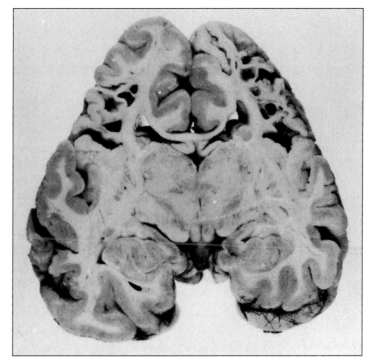

Fig. 544(a)

Figure 544(b). A view of the damaged cerebral wall in higher magnification, corresponding to the damaged cerebral wall seen on the right in Figure 544(a).

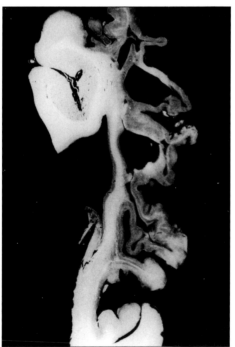

(b)

A Case of   *Maternal toxemia of pregnancy. Premature birth.*
Infant developed cerebral palsy.

The mother had a history of toxemia of pregnancy. Premature labor developed at 31 weeks. The newborn infant weighed 3 pounds 2 ounces. Developmental delays were evident in infancy. Seizure activity began at 2 1/2 months. Microcephaly was evident. Spastic cerebral palsy was evident later in infancy.

The infant developed a severe respiratory infection with fever of 103 degrees, and died at 13 months.

At autopsy, the cerebrum was small, in contrast to the full-size, plump-appearing cerebellum. The brain weighed 268 grams, approximately one-half the average weight for 13 months (Figure 545). It was evident that the low brain weight was due to the very small size of the cerebrum.

Characteristic of the pathologic changes in cases of cerebral palsy, the brain, frontal section (Figure 546), showed loss of periventricular white matter, with consequent ex vacuo hydrocephalus, and diminished appearance of the basal ganglia (page 27).

Figure 545. The brain, lateral view. The illustration shows the brain, approximately its actual size, as it appeared at autopsy. The brain weighed 268 grams. As shown, the smallness of the cerebrum is evident, in contrast to the size of the cerebellum, which is normal. Infant with cerebral palsy, died at 13 months of age.

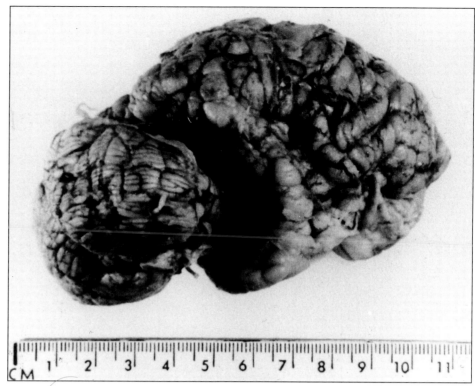

Fig. 545

Figure 546. Section of the brain through the level of the midcerebrum. Extensive loss of periventricular white matter with resulting ex vacuo hydrocephalus; basal ganglia reduced in size.

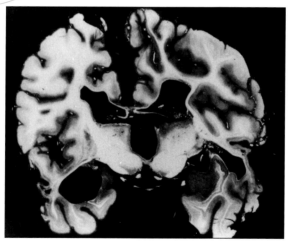

Fig. 546

A Case of **Macrocephaly in a child with mental retardation.**

The history in this case indicated that the pregnancy had been uncomplicated. At delivery it was noted that the infant had a large head. It was thought that this was a case of hydrocephalus in the newborn. Except for the large head, the infant, weighing 8 pounds 7 ounces, did not present any abnormalities. Subsequent radiologic studies indicated that this was not hydrocephalus, that this was a case of macrocephaly (page 143).

Mental development was retarded, with the child limited to the use of only a few words (page 197). The child died at 2 1/2 years of age.

At autopsy the outstanding finding was the large brain, weighing 1,885 grams, approximately 700 grams greater than the average for age 2 1/2 years. The external configuration of the brain was essentially normal (Figure 547). Likewise, the internal structures of the brain showed no apparent abnormalities (Figure 548).

Microscopic study of the brain showed normal arrangement of the cortical layers; no significant abnormalities were evident microscopically in other parts of the brain.

Figure 547. Macrocephaly. Grossly, the brain is oversized, 17 centimeters in AP diameter. The convolutional pattern appears normal.

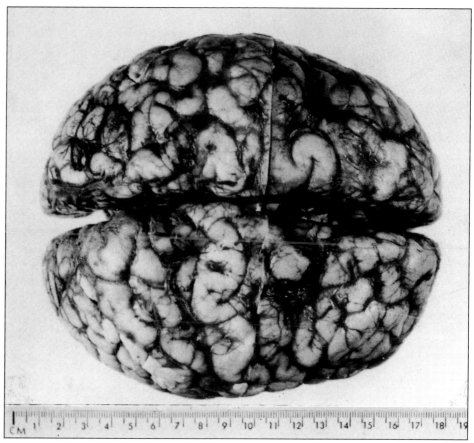

Fig. 547

Figure 548. Section through the brain. No significant structural abnormalities are evident.

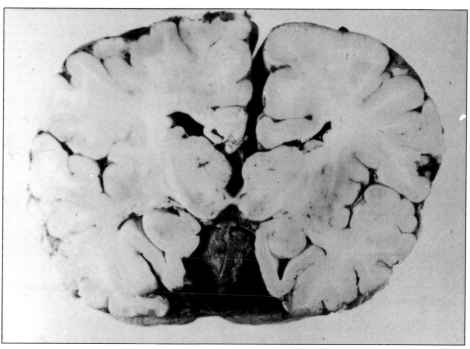

Fig. 548

A Case of **Periventricular and intracranial hemorrhage developing in a dysmature term newborn.**

This term newborn baby was alert and clinically stable during the first 2 days. He suddenly deteriorated neurologically on the third day, with CT scan evidence of periventricular and intraventricular hemorrhage.

In the background of this case, the mother had chronic rheumatic heart disease. She gained weight excessively during this pregnancy. At midpregnancy she was treated for a severe upper respiratory infection, with tonsillitis.

The newborn infant physically showed the effects of adversive gestational conditions, evidence of intrauterine deprivation. This infant was of low birth weight, was long and thin. The Ponderal Index, a measure of fetal nutrition, was 2.08, far below the tenth percentile (page 94).

Despite being underweight, malnourished, the infant's Apgar score was good, 8 at five minutes. In the first 2 days he was active, crying, and nursing well.

What was the etiology of the intracranial hemorrhage, the neurologic collapse, on the third day?

In the first 2 days, this infant plainly did not look like he had fresh acute stroke-like brain damage. Infants with acute cerebral damage show it. They are limp and comatose at delivery and remain that way for prolonged periods.

The baby in the present case was not like that. He had the appearance of a healthy "good baby" until the neurologic collapse on the third day.

The CT scans taken at that time, on day 3, showed evidence of periventricular hemorrhagic infarctional damage and intraventricular hemorrhage (Figure 549). Pertinently, the lateral ventricles were visible, patent.

Clinically, the fontanelles all this time were soft, not bulging. This, together with the CT scan finding of patent ventricles, ruled out the diagnosis of *acute* brain damage. If acute damage were present, the brain would be edematous, swollen, so that the ventricles would be compressed, not patent, and the fontanelles would be bulging (page 167).

The nature of the pathologic process, with acute brain damage ruled out, was consistent with hemorrhage from a previously silent, subacute cerebral lesion. The defining factor here is the periventricular location of the cerebral damage evident in the CT scan. Pathologically, periventricular cerebral damage does not occur in the mature cerebrum; it occurs specifically in the premature cerebrum.

With periventricular damage that originates in the premature cerebrum, if the fetus survives to term, the acute process tends to "quiet down" and the damage pathologically becomes subacute, latent, so that the mature infant is born harboring old subacute periventricular damage without clinical manifestations at first. Subacute lesions have areas of hemorrhagic necrotic tissue. In such circumstances, at times, the latent subacute periventricular lesion, necrotic and hemorrhagic, erupts, causing sudden intracranial hemorrhage, clinically leading to neurologic deterioration, as occurred in this case.

CT scan at 15 months showed loss of periventricular substance with corresponding enlargement of ventricles (Figure 550).

Deep cerebral damage, affecting periventricular white matter and basal ganglia, leads to cerebral palsy and, as occurred in this case, with the damage extending outward through the cerebrum to the cortex, cortical manifestations of seizure disorder and mental retardation may result. Microcephaly developed due to loss of deep cerebral tissue with consequent failure of the cerebrum to grow.

Figure 549. CT scan of brain taken on day 3 following onset of neurologic deterioration, showing evidence of periventricular hemorrhagic infarctional damage with intraventricular hemorrhage. Ventricles are patent indicating absence of cerebral edema.

Figure 550. CT scan of the brain at 1 year 3 months, showing sequelant cerebral changes, with decrease in the periventricular cerebral tissue and consequent ventricular enlargement, ex vacuo hydrocephalus.

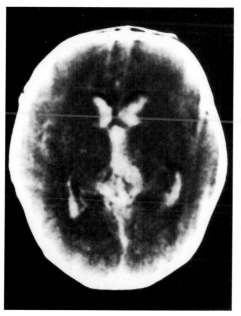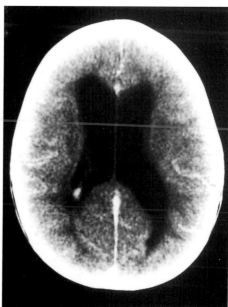

Fig. 549

Fig. 550

A Case of   *Intrauterine growth retardation in a newborn. Mother with pregnancy low weight gain. Child developed cerebral palsy, mental retardation, seizure disorder, and microcephaly.*

This was not a robust pregnancy. This mother failed to gain weight during the first 23 weeks of this pregnancy, a problem reflecting a disturbance in body metabolism, in gestational nutrition. During pregnancy, metabolic disorders exercise unfavorable effects on the fetus as well as the mother.

Adversive conditions during this gestation impacted unfavorably on the fetus, evidenced by this fact that the fetus, the newborn, showed the effects of chronic intrauterine compromise, chronic deprivation, IUGR. This was a chronically sick fetus, a newborn who was described as having a "thin wasted appearance," with dry peeling skin and lacking subcutaneous fat. This is the typical appearance of an IUGR infant, a dysmature infant.

This enfeebled dysmature infant, chronically compromised, depressed during intrauterine life, unable to cope with the stress of labor, was born depressed. This depression is attributable, not to inordinate hypoxia during birth, but was due to the expressed debilitated physical condition of the fetus, the newborn.

Birth occurred at 42 weeks of gestation.

Although the newborn infant was depressed, there was no clinical evidence of *acute* brain damage, based on a consideration of the fontanelles and the CT studies.

The fontanelles in this baby were observed to be soft, normal, not bulging. This is most important, with regard to the presence or absence of acute fresh brain damage. Pathologically, in infants as in adults, acute brain damage causes cerebral edema, swelling; this causes the brain to press against the (soft) fontanelles, causing bulging of the fontanelles. Pathologically, the absence of bulging fontanelles, the presence of soft, normal fontanelles, rules out the presence of acute brain damage in this newborn infant (page 167).

CT studies of the brain on day 4 showed the ventricles were normal; no cerebral edema (Figure 551). If there had been acute cerebral damage, the brain would have become edematous and swollen; this would cause compression, obliteration of the ventricles. The patent ventricles evident in this neonatal CT scan provided conclusive evidence that there was no cerebral edema, no cerebral swelling, no acute fresh cerebral damage.

The CT scan ruled out the presence of *acute* cerebral damage but it did not rule out the presence of old, *subacute*, cerebral damage latently accrued weeks, months before birth.

Cerebral tissue that has severe damage with diffuse loss of nerve cells (evident on microscopic examination) often is not grossly evident, not evident to the naked eye. Accordingly, it cannot be expected that CT scans would validly diagnose the presence or absence of such tissue damage. A CT scan interpretation that indicates no changes are evident in the cerebral structure does not mean there is no damage to the tissue.

Accordingly, in cases in which the brain scans reveal no changes, there may in fact be far-advanced damage, scarring and nerve cell depletion.

In the present case, the CT studies on day 11 showed basal ganglia with focal densities, apparent hemorrhage in areas of subacute infarction (page 185). Ventricles were patent indicating absence of acute brain damage (Figure 552). Presence of focal hemorrhage does not mean acute brain damage; pathologically, old subacute cerebral damage at times becomes hemorrhagic and bleeds.

An MRI taken at 1 1/2 years showed loss of substance in the cerebral white matter with resulting enlargement of the ventricles, ex vacuo hydrocephaly, and evidence of scarring of periventricular tissue (Figure 553).

In overview, this was a case of gestational compromise of a fetus, an infant showing IUGR, born harboring brain damage of subacute nature incurred early during intrauterine life, with the child surviving developing cerebral palsy, mental retardation, and seizure disorder.

Figure 551. CT of the brain taken at 4 days. Ventricles are patent, sharply defined; apparent decreased density in frontal lobes. No evidence of edema or acute cerebral damage.

Figure 552. CT of the brain taken at 11 days. Basal ganglia with focal densities, apparent hemorrhage in the areas of subacute infarction. Ventricles are patent, indicating absence of edema, absence of acute brain damage.

Figure 553. MRI of the brain at 1 1/2 years. Ventricles are much enlarged due to decreased cerebral white matter, ex vacuo hydrocephalus. Periventricular strata of white matter of increased density compatible with scarring, gliosis.

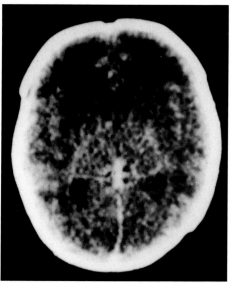

Fig. 551

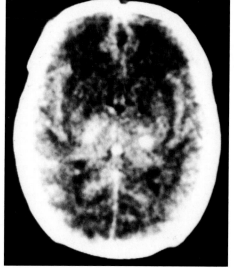

Fig. 552

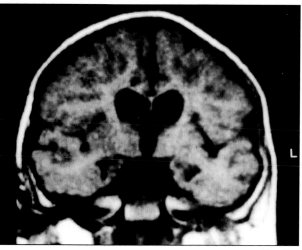

Fig. 553

A Case of   ***Twin transfusion syndrome; one twin stillborn,
one liveborn. Surviving twin with severe anemia
and subacute cerebral damage; subsequent cerebral
palsy, mental retardation, and seizure disorder.***

This case is an example of the placental twin transfusion syndrome exercising severe pathologic effects on the two fetuses, rendering one stillborn and the other, surviving, was enfeebled, anemic, hypoxic, with accrued subacute cerebral damage (page 97).

The surviving fetus proved to be the donor in the placental transfusion process — was rendered chronically anemic, leading to ongoing intrauterine hypoxia.

The placenta was *monochorionic* meaning that the twin fetuses were derived from a single fertilized egg, one placenta serving both twins. With the single placenta having a common vascular network, interchange of blood circulation occurs between the two twins. This sets up the condition for the "twin transfusion syndrome," in which blood flows from one twin to the other twin.

While the donor fetus (the survivor in this case) gradually becomes anemic, the recipient fetus becomes overloaded with blood and goes into congestive heart failure, as occurred in the stillborn fetus in this case.

The surviving fetus, chronically compromised during intrauterine life, enfeebled, severely anemic, although depressed at delivery, soon improved. Following transfusion he was pink and active. The fontanelles remained soft and flat and the neonatal sonogram was normal, showed patent ventricles (Figure 554). In cases that do have acute fresh brain damage, the cerebral tissue "soaks up" fluid, becomes edematous; the brain swells, causing bulging fontanelles and compressed ventricles (page 167). This did not occur in the present case. The findings of normal fontanelles and a normal sonogram, in context with the good postnatal performance of the infant, provided organic evidence that the newborn did not have acute brain damage.

A CT scan of the brain on day 4 showed apparent decreased density in the white matter of the cerebrum (Figure 555). The CT scan showed ventricles were patent, indicating an absence of edema, an absence of acute pathologic process. The changes in the white matter, the apparent depletion of cerebral substance, is attributable to subacute cerebral damage originating during intrauterine life, consequent to the chronic fetal anemia, fetal hypoxia.

A follow-up CT scan study at 11 months showed a progression of the subacute process present neonatally. Pathologically, in the course of time, the devitalized tissue in the periventricular areas of the subacute damage undergoes disintegration and absorption, leading to enlargement of the ventricles, ex vacuo hydrocephalus, as evident in this scan (Figure 556).

The severe loss of deep cerebral tissue led to the development of spastic cerebral palsy; also, there was severe mental retardation and seizure disorder. With the deep strata of the cerebrum damaged, the brain failed to grow, microcephaly.

Figure 554. Sonogram taken at 2 days, shows patent lateral ventricles, indicating absence of cerebral edema. Normal sonogram.

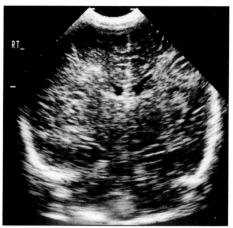

Fig. 554

Figure 555. CT scan of brain at 4 days; cerebral ventricles are patent; no evidence of cerebral edema. Decreased density of white matter.

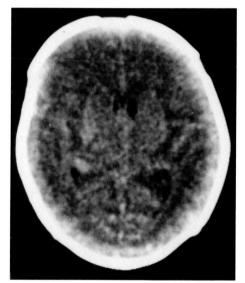

Fig. 555

Figure 556. CT scan of brain at 11 months shows much loss of cerebral white matter, with associated dilatation of the lateral ventricles.

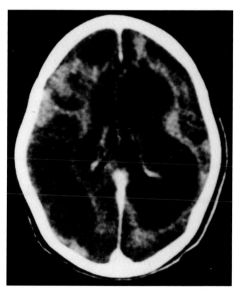

Fig. 556

A Case of   ***Maternal prediabetes, gestational viral infection, vaginal bleeding, placental insufficiency. Macrosomic newborn; porencephaly. Infant survived, developed cerebral palsy, epilepsy, and mild mental retardation.***

This mother had serious intrinsic pregnancy problems, pathologic processes that contributed to cerebral damage during early fetal life. The mother had excessive weight gain, hypertension, manifestations of latent prediabetes, with the delivery of a 9 pound 2 ounce macrosomic infant, characteristic of maternal diabetic condition. She had vaginal bleeding at 10 to 12 weeks of pregnancy, was sick with an upper respiratory infection (URI) at 16 weeks, and lost weight at that time. The placenta was very small, manifestly inadequate to provide sufficient oxygenation for a large fetus.

This mother, with an influenzal respiratory infection with cough at 16 weeks of pregnancy, manifestly was quite sick; she lost 4 pounds during the following 3 weeks. With acute illness, with fever, the metabolic oxygen requirements of the mother are sharply increased, leaving the fetus oxygen-deprived, hypoxic.

This mother had substantial clinical factors associated with latent prediabetes: she had excessive pregnancy weight gain, hypertension, a family history of diabetes, and produced a macrosomic baby (page 48). In people who become diabetic, the bodily dysfunctions have origin many years before the diabetes becomes manifest. Maternal prediabetes (or diabetes) affects an unfavorable uterine environment, exercises a damaging effect on the fetus, extending over the entire length of the gestational period.

The record notes there was prolonged vaginal bleeding during several occasions during this pregnancy. Bleeding during pregnancy is usually due to pathologic processes affecting the placenta, processes that potentially compromise the fetus, causing fetal hypoxia.

There were two abnormalities of the placenta in this case, with regard to the umbilical cord vessels and with regard to the size of the placenta.

The umbilical cord in this case had two vessels. Normally there are three: two arteries and one vein. In the present case there was absence of one of the arteries; this is common in cases of maternal diabetes.

Placental hypoplasia, "microplacenta," was also present. The placenta usually weighs 450 to 475 grams at term. The placenta in the present case weighed 280 grams.

This miniature placenta is an example of placental insufficiency; it could not have adequately oxygenated this big, macrosomic, fetus — thus contributed to chronic intrauterine fetal hypoxia (page 76).

During pregnancy, pathologic processes in the mother, acute and chronic bodily disorders, exercise an adversive effect on the fetus. The common denominator of these adversive processes is hypoxia — the fetus is subjected to varying degrees of oxygen deprivation that leads to an accruing of subacute cerebral damage in the fetuses that survive. Newborn infants, so affected, are born harboring old, subacute cerebral damage.

The occurrence of subacute cerebral damage at birth is well known to pathologists who study neonatal brain damage. It is not well known to clinicians, who tend to attribute cerebral palsy and related cerebral disabilities, automatically, to events that occur during labor and delivery or postnatally.

This child developed dyskinesias of athetoid cerebral palsy.

MRI studies taken at age 15 years (there were no newborn radiologic studies) showed extensive encephaloclastic damage, porencephaly, predominantly in the left cerebrum (Figure 557) (page 28). The right hemisphere appeared essentially unaffected.

Surprisingly, this child, with a severe motor handicap, with an MRI showing massive porencephalic cerebral damage, was described at age 15 years as being quite intelligent, in the seventh grade level in school.

Figure 557. The MRI of the brain at 15 years shows a loss of substance. The left cerebral hemisphere is much reduced in size, with large areas showing loss of substance, a porencephalic cavity, in the frontal region and in the parieto-occipital regions. There is prominent dilatation of the body of the left ventricle, evident in the lower aspect of the left cerebrum. The right hemisphere, much less affected, shows areas with convolutional atrophy in the occipital region.

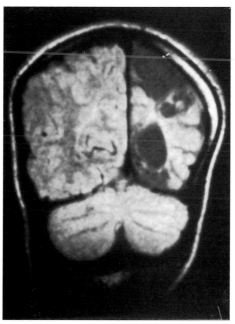

Fig. 557

A Case of **Basal ganglia cavitations in an infant with cerebral palsy.**

The mother had health problems during this pregnancy, problems known to have an adversive hypoxia-producing effect on the fetus. She gave a history of "being sick almost the entire pregnancy, nausea and vomiting." Specifically her pregnancy problem related to obesity, acute illness with gastritis, dehydration, weight loss, and anemia.

This mother was obese, 5 feet 2 inches in height, weighing up to 217 pounds. Marked obesity is a hazard to the pregnant mother and her fetus (page 47).

This mother was acutely ill during pregnancy and was hospitalized for a protracted period with acute gastritis. During this time, although she was obese, she lost weight.

This newborn was depressed at birth but soon improved in the delivery room, with the Apgar score rising to 6 at five minutes, and at 4 hours of age was alert and active, and took a bottle feeding. This is plainly not the picture of a newborn baby with diffuse acute brain damage. Newborn infants with acute hypoxic brain damage are comatose at birth and stay that way for prolonged periods. This newborn was not like that.

There was substantial evidence that brain damage, present at birth in this infant, was of subacute nature pathologically. Evidence of this was afforded in the examination of the spinal fluid. The examination of the cerebrospinal fluid done soon after birth revealed xanthochromic fluid (yellow discoloration). Xanthochromia is due to old decomposed hemoglobin — its presence indicated there was old hemorrhagic cerebral damage in this newborn infant, subacute damage originating long before labor (page 173).

CT scans at 4 months presented structural changes typical of the pathologic pattern that evolves in the brain in cases of cerebral palsy with mental retardation, epilepsy, and microcephaly (Figures 558, 559).

Hypoxic cerebral damage incurred during premature immature fetal life, beginning in the periventricular germinal matrix, at times extends to the neighboring basal ganglia, and to the periventricular cerebral tissue; the damaged periventricular tissue later becomes absorbed, contracted, leaving the ventricles enlarged: ex vacuo hydrocephalus (page 29).

At times, the damaged tissue forms cavitations that are evident grossly and in CT scans, as in the basal ganglia in this case (Figure 558).

The cerebral damage originating in the deep cerebrum at times extends through the cerebral wall to the cerebral surface with resulting surface scarring with convolutional atrophy and cortical destruction (Figure 559). Clinically, the cortical manifestations of seizure disorder and mental retardation are superimposed on the manifest cerebral palsy, as in this case.

This child at 4 years had spastic cerebral palsy, severe mental retardation, epilepsy, and microcephaly.

Figure 558. CT scan of the head taken at 4 months. Cavitations in the basal ganglia (putamen) bilaterally. Loss of periventricular tissue with consequent dilated ventricles. Convolutional shrinking, atrophy (cortical damage), in the frontal lobes.

Figure 559. Scan through the upper level of the cerebrum shows severe convolutional atrophy of the frontal and occipital lobes.

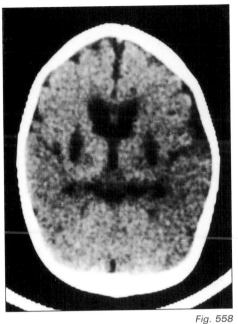

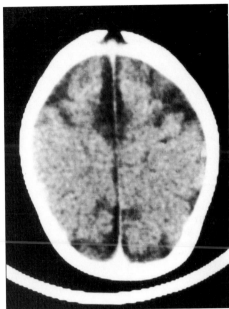

Fig. 558   *Fig. 559*

Index